Micronutrients in Health
and Disease

Micronutrients in Health and Disease

Second Edition

Kedar N. Prasad

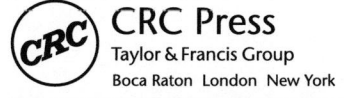

CRC Press
Taylor & Francis Group
Boca Raton London New York

CRC Press is an imprint of the
Taylor & Francis Group, an **informa** business

CRC Press
Taylor & Francis Group
6000 Broken Sound Parkway NW, Suite 300
Boca Raton, FL 33487-2742

First issued in paperback 2021

Printed on acid-free paper

ISBN-13: 978-1-138-50002-0 (hbk)
ISBN-13: 978-1-03-209314-7 (pbk)

Library of Congress Cataloging-in-Publication Data

Names: Prasad, Kedar N., author.
Title: Micronutrients in health and disease / Kedar N. Prasad.
Description: Second edition. | Boca Raton : Taylor & Francis, 2019. |
Includes bibliographical references and index.
Identifiers: LCCN 2018056222| ISBN 9781138500020 (hardback : alk. paper) |
ISBN 9780429243462 (e-ISBN)
Subjects: | MESH: Micronutrients--therapeutic use | Antioxidants--therapeutic
use | Dietary Supplements
Classification: LCC RM258.5 | NLM QU 130.5 | DDC 612.3/9--dc23
LC record available at https://lccn.loc.gov/2018056222

Visit the Taylor & Francis Web site at
http://www.taylorandfrancis.com

and the CRC Press Web site at
http://www.crcpress.com

Contents

Preface

The growing sentiments against the use of micronutrient supplements for improving human health, and disease prevention and treatment outcomes among most academic and practicing physicians, and many health professionals have created confusion and uncertainties in the minds of many consumers and health professionals. These sentiments are primarily based on a few clinical trials in which supplementation with a single dietary antioxidant, mostly vitamin E or beta-carotene, increased the levels of risk factors and/or incidence of the disease in high-risk populations, such as heavy tobacco smokers, patients with coronary artery disease, and cancer survivors. Without critically examining the experimental designs of the trial with respect to the selection of antioxidants, recommendations are being made to not take any micronutrient supplements for health benefits. Such recommendations are alarming from the public health point of view. The adverse health effects of a single antioxidant in high-risk populations were expected, because such populations have high levels of internal oxidative environment in which the individual antioxidants are oxidized and then act as pro-oxidants. A few clinical trials with vitamin E or beta-carotene alone produced no adverse health effects in normal populations that have low levels of internal oxidative environment. I and others have published several reviews in peer-reviewed journals challenging the current trends of using single antioxidants in high-risk populations for preventing the risk of disease or improving the treatment outcomes. These articles failed to have any significant impact on the design of clinical trials, and the inconsistent results on the effect of a single antioxidant continued to be published. The growing anti-micronutrient views promoted by most academic and practicing physicians and science writers of the major news media have alarmed me enough to write the first edition of this book.

In my previous edition of this book, I proposed a unified hypothesis that increased oxidative stress and chronic inflammation are primarily responsible for the initiation and progression of most human chronic diseases as well as accelerated aging. In addition, glutamate release that occurs in certain human chronic diseases such as post-traumatic stress disorder (PTSD), and Huntington's disease, and other anxiety disorders also plays a role in maintenance and progression of the disease. I proposed that multiple micronutrients, including dietary and endogenous antioxidants, might be more useful in prevention and improved management of these diseases than single antioxidants. The central question remains how to optimally and simultaneously reduce these biochemical defects.

In the second edition of this book, additional data are presented in support of my previous hypothesis that increased oxidative stress, chronic inflammation, and glutamate release play an important role in the initiation and progression of human chronic diseases as well as radiation injuries. In order to simultaneously and optimally reduce these biochemical defects, I propose that an elevation of the levels of cytoprotective enzymes, including antioxidant enzymes together with dietary and endogenous antioxidants, may be essential. The levels of antioxidants can easily be increased by an oral supplementation; however, elevating the levels of antioxidant enzymes is complex requiring an elevation of a nuclear transcriptional factor Nrf2. Certain antioxidants and B-vitamins prevent the release and toxicity of glutamate in the laboratory models This edition discusses in detail the regulation of activation of Nrf2 and the release and toxicity of glutamate with respect to each of the relevant disease.

MicroRNAs play an important role in the pathogenesis of chronic diseases. MicroRNAs (miRs) are evolutionarily conserved small non-coding single-stranded RNAs of approximately 22 nucleotides in length, and are present in all living organisms including humans. Each miR binds to its complimentary sequences in the 3′-untranslated region (3′-UTR) of the mRNA, promotes degradation of the mRNA transcript, and prevents translation of the message of protein. In this manner, miRs regulate the translation of proapoptotic or antiapoptotic proteins from their respective mRNAs, depending upon whether they receive damaging or protective signal. The regulation of expression of miRs by oxidative stress, inflammation, and antioxidants has been discussed in each disease.

In this revised edition, I have added 3 additional chapters on Huntington's disease (HD), prion diseases, and Autism spectrum disorder (ASD) because of involvement of increased oxidative stress, inflammation, and excessive release of glutamate in these diseases with diverse inducing agents and disease phenotypes. Except ASD for which current treatments are considered unsatisfactory, HD and prion diseases are progressive, incurable, fatal neurodegenerative disease. A mixture of micronutrients proposed for other diseases may also be useful in the improved management of these neurological diseases.

I have proposed a mixture of micronutrients and phytochemicals that would simultaneously reduce oxidative stress and inflammation by enhancing the levels of antioxidant enzymes through activating the Nrf2 pathway as well as elevating dietary and endogenous antioxidants at the same time. This mixture may also prevent the release and toxicity of glutamate. This micronutrient mixture would be useful in prevention, and in combination with standard care, in improved management of chronic diseases. I have also included current recommendation for diet and lifestyle modifications that would be applicable to all health conditions. I have also proposed experimental designs for primary and secondary prevention, as well as, in combination with standard care, for treatment.

Those who are taking daily multiple micronutrients will be comforted with the information provided in the second edition this book; those who are on the sidelines may decide to take a mixture of micronutrients daily, and some who are currently totally opposed to recommending micronutrient supplements will find this book challenging and may decide to test the proposed idea clinically or may continue to believe that micronutrient supplements may be harmful. In the latter case, they have to provide scientific reasons for their recommendations.

I hope this book will continue to arouse enough passion for and against taking multiple micronutrients that will lead to comprehensive randomized, double blind, and placebo-controlled clinical studies in high-risk and normal populations. Only then can we make a conclusive recommendation about whether a proposed micronutrient mixture is useful for human health, disease prevention, and improved management. In the meanwhile, I recommend that one should continue to take appropriately prepared multiple micronutrients in consultation with his or her physicians and health-care professionals for healthy aging, for reducing the risk of chronic diseases, and for improving current treatment outcomes.

I hope this second edition will continue to serve as a reference book for graduate students in nutrition, instructors teaching courses in nutrition and health, researchers involved in prevention and improved management of diseases using micronutrients, primary care and academic physicians interested in complimentary medicine, and health professionals in complimentary medicine and the nutrition industry.

Kedar N. Prasad

Acknowledgments

This book is dedicated to my family for their encouragement and support.

Author

Kedar N. Prasad obtained a master's degree in Zoology from the University of Bihar, Ranchi, India, and a PhD degree in Radiation Biology from the University of Iowa, Iowa City, in 1963. He received post-doctoral training at the Brookhaven National Laboratory, Long Island. New York, and joined the Department of Radiology at the University of Colorado Health Sciences Center where he became Professor and Director for the Center for Vitamins and Cancer Research. He has published more than 250 articles in peer-reviewed journals and authored and edited 25 books in the area of radiation biology, nutrition and cancer, and nutrition and neurological diseases, particularly Alzheimer's disease and Parkinson's disease. These articles were published in highly prestigious journals such as *Science*, *Nature*, and *Proceedings of the National Academic of Sciences, USA*.

Dr. Prasad has received several honors, which include invitation by the Nobel Prize committee to nominate a candidate for the Nobel Prize in Medicine for 1982. In 2017 he was invited to become a member of the Royal Society of Medicine, London. He was invited for the 1999 Harold Harper Lecture at the meeting of the American College of Advancement in Medicine. He received an award for the best review of 1998–1999 on antioxidant and cancer; and in 1999–2000 on antioxidants and Parkinson's disease by the American College of Nutrition. He was a Fellow of the American College of Nutrition and served as a President of the International Society of Nutrition and Cancer, 1992–2000. Currently, he is Chief Scientific Officer of the Engage Global, Orem, Utah.

1 Basic Facts about Micronutrients

INTRODUCTION

Micronutrients include dietary and endogenous antioxidants, vitamin D3, all B-vitamins, and certain minerals (selenium, zinc, iron, copper and manganese); whereas macronutrients primarily include lipids, carbohydrates, and proteins. Although all micronutrients are essential for growth and development, antioxidants have been subject of extensive laboratory research and clinical studies because of their potential importance in reducing oxidative stress and inflammation that could improve health and reduce the risk of chronic diseases. Before discussing the role of micronutrients in healthy aging, and prevention and improved management of diseases, it is essential to understand certain basic facts about micronutrients.

This chapter describes briefly the evolution of the antioxidant system; provides a historical prospective of some antioxidants, vitamin D3 and B-vitamins; describes the sources, solubility, distribution, storage, absorption, and functions of dietary and endogenous antioxidants; explains antioxidant defense systems and current controversies about antioxidants; and discusses the misuse of antioxidants in clinical studies. In Chapters 4 through 23 of this volume, the detailed role of antioxidants and other micronutrients in health and disease is discussed with respect to aging and specific diseases. Several books have been published on this topic; a few are referenced at the end of this chapter.[1–10]

EVOLUTION OF THE ANTIOXIDANT SYSTEM

Antioxidants are essential for the growth and survival of all organisms that depend on oxygen, including humans. In its early stage, Earth's atmosphere had no oxygen. Anaerobic organisms, which can live without oxygen, thrived in the oceans and rivers. About 2.5 billion years ago, blue-green algae in the ocean acquired the ability to split water (H_2O) into hydrogen (H) and oxygen (O_2). This chemical reaction initiated the release of oxygen into the atmosphere, leading to the extinction of many anaerobic organisms due to the toxicity of oxygen. Those organisms that developed antioxidant defense systems survived—an important biological event that led to the rapid evolution of multicellular organisms that use oxygen for survival. Today, the amount of oxygen in dry air is about 21%, and in water it is about 34%.

HISTORY OF THE DISCOVERY OF MICRONUTRIENTS

Vitamin A: Night blindness, which we now know is caused by vitamin A deficiency, existed for centuries before the discovery of vitamin A. As early as about 1500 BC, the Egyptian knew how to cure this disease. Roman soldiers suffering from night blindness traveled to Egypt, where they would receive liver extract for treatment. It is now well established that liver is a rich source of vitamin A. The treatment of night blindness with liver extract was not performed outside Egypt for centuries; the medical establishment during that period must not have accepted this treatment. It was not until 1912 when Dr. McCollum of the University of Wisconsin discovered vitamin A in butter; and therefore it was initially called a "fat soluble A." The structure of vitamin A was determined in 1930, and this vitamin was synthesized in a laboratory in 1947.

Carotenoids: In 1919 carotenoids pigments were isolated from yellow plants, and in 1930 it was found that some of the ingested carotene was converted to vitamin A. This carotene was referred to as beta-carotene.

Vitamin C: Scurvy is caused by vitamin C deficiency. The symptoms of this disease were known to Egyptians as early as 1,500 BC. In the fifth century BC, Hippocrates described the symptoms of scurvy, which included bleeding gums, hemorrhaging, and death. Native North Americans knew the cure of this disease, but knowledge of the treatment remained limited to this population. During the sea voyages of European explorers between the twelfth and sixteenth centuries, the epidemic of scurvy among sailors forced some to land in Canada where the Native people gave them extract of pine bark and needles (prepared like tea). This treatment completely cured scurvy in these sailors. In 1536 Jacques Cartier, a French explorer, brought this formulation for curing scurvy to France, but the medical establishment rejected it as fraud because it came from Native Americans, who were seen as savages. In 1593, Sir Richard Hawkins recommended that his sailors consume sour oranges and lemons. In 1770, the British Navy began recommending that ships carry sufficient lime juice for all personnel aboard. In 1928, Albert Szent-Gyorgyi, a Hungarian scientist, isolated a substance from the adrenal gland that was called hex-uronic acid. This substance was vitamin C, and in 1932, it was the first vitamin to be synthesized in a laboratory.

Vitamin D: Although rickets, a bone disease, may have existed in human populations for centuries, it was not until 1645, when Dr. Daniel Whistler described the symptoms of rickets, that we now know is due to vitamin D deficiency. In 1922, Sir Edward Mellanby discovered vitamin D while working on a cure for rickets. This vitamin was later found to require sunlight for its formation. The chemical structure of vitamin D was determined by German scientist Dr. Windaus in 1930. Vitamin D3 was chemically characterized in 1936 and was considered a steroid that was effective in the treatment of rickets.

Vitamin E: In 1922, Dr. Herbert Evans from the University of California, Berkeley, observed that rats reared exclusively on whole milk grew normally but were not fertile. The fertility was restored when they were additionally fed wheat germ. However, it took another 14 years (1936) before the active substance responsible for restoring fertility was isolated. Dr. Evans named it *tocopherol*, from the Greek word meaning "to bear offspring" with the ending "ol" signifying its chemical status as an alcohol.

B-Vitamins: All B-vitamins were discovered in the period of 1912–1934. In 1912, the Polish-born biochemist Dr. Casimir Funk isolated the active substance from the rice husks of unpolished rice that prevented the disease beriberi. He named this substance "vitamines" because he thought they were amines, which are derived from ammonia. In 1920, the "e" was dropped when it became known that not all vitamins are amines.

SOURCES AND FORMS OF VITAMINS

Vitamin A and Beta-Carotene: The richest sources of vitamin A are liver (6.5 mg per 100 g liver) from beef, pork, chicken, turkey, and fish; carrot (0.8 mg per 100 g); broccoli leaves (0.8 mg per 100 g); sweet potatoes (0.7 mg per 100 g); kale (0.7 mg per 100 g); butter (0.7 mg per 100 g); spinach (0.5 mg per 100 g); and pumpkin (0.4 mg per 100 g). Other small sources include cantaloupe melon, eggs, apricots, papaya, and mango (40 mg to 170 mg per 100 g). Yellow and red fruits and vegetables are very rich sources of beta-carotene. One molecule of beta carotene is converted to 2 molecules of retinol in the intestinal tract. Vitamin A exists as retinyl palmitate or retinyl acetate, which is coveted into the retinol form in the body. Vitamin A can also exist as a retinoic acid in the cells. It was determined that 1 international unit (IU) equals to 0.3 µg retinol, or 0.6 µg beta-carotene. The activity of vitamin A is also expressed as retinol activity equivalent (RAE). It was determined that 1 µg RAE corresponds with 1µg retinol and 2 µg beta-carotene in oil. Vitamin A and beta-carotene and the synthetic retinoids are also available commercially.

Carotenoids: The richest sources of carotenoids are sweet potatoes, carrots, spinach, mango, cantaloupe, apricot, kale, broccoli, parsley, cilantro, pumpkins, winter squash, and fresh thyme. There are two main forms of carotenoids found in nature: alpha-carotene and beta-carotene. Beta-carotene is the more common form of carotenoids. Other carotenes include lutein, zeaxanthin, and lycopene.

Vitamin C: The richest sources of vitamin C are fruits and vegetables. They include rosehip (2000 mg per 100 g rose hip); red pepper (2000 mg per 100 g red pepper); parsley (2000 mg per 100 g parsley); guava (2000 mg per 100 g guava); kiwi (2000 mg per 100 g kiwi); broccoli (2000 mg per 100 g broccoli); lychee (2000 mg per 100 g lychee); papaya (2000 mg per 100 g papaya); and strawberry (2000 mg per 100 g strawberry). Other sources of vitamin C include orange, lemon, melon, garlic, cauliflower, grapefruit, raspberry, tangerine, passion fruit, spinach, and lime (containing about 30 to 50 mg per 100 g fruits and vegetables). Vitamin C is sold commercially as L-ascorbic acid, calcium ascorbate, sodium ascorbate, or potassium ascorbate.

Vitamin E: The richest sources of vitamin E include wheat germ oil (215 mg per 100 g oil); sunflower oil (56 mg per 100 g oil); olive oil (12 mg per 100 g oil); almond oil (39 mg per 100 g oil); hazelnut oil (26 mg per 100 g oil); walnut oil (20 mg per 100 g oil); and peanut oil (17 mg per 100 g oil). The sources for small amounts of vitamin E (0.1 to 2 mg per 100 g) include kiwi fruit, fish, leafy vegetables, and whole grains. In the United States fortified breakfast cereals are important source of vitamin E. At present, most of the natural form of vitamin E is extracted from vegetable oils, primarily soybean oil.

Vitamin E exists in eight different forms: four tocopherols (alpha-, beta-, gamma-, and delta-tocopherol) and four tocotrienols (alpha-, beta-, gamma- and delta-tocotrienol). Alpha-tocopherol has the most biological activity. Vitamin E can exist in the natural form commonly indicated as *d*, whereas the synthetic form is referred to as *dl*. The stable esterified form of vitamin E is available as alpha-tocopheryl acetate, alpha-tocopheryl succinate, and alpha-tocopheryl nicotinate. The activity of vitamin E is generally expressed in international units (IU). It is determined that 1 IU equals 0.66 mg *d*-alpha-tocopherol, and 1 IU racemic mixture (*dl*-form) equals 0.45 mg *d*-tocopherol.

Glutathione: Glutathione is synthesized from three amino acids, L-cysteine, L-glutamic acid, and glycine, and is present in all cells; however, the liver contains the highest amount, up to 5 mM. Glutathione exists in the cells in reduced or oxidized form. In healthy cells, more than 90% of glutathione is present in the reduced form. The oxidized form of glutathione can be converted to the reduced form by the enzyme glutathione reductase. The reduced form of glutathione acts as an antioxidant.

N-acetylcysteine (NAC): NAC is a synthetic antioxidant made from amino acid L-cysteine that has acetyl group attached. It can directly as a glutathione substitute and indirectly as a precursor of glutathione.

Alpha-lipoic acid: Alpha-lipoic acid, also called thioctic acid, exists in two forms: R-alpha-lipoic acid (natural form) and S-alpha-lipoic acid (synthetic form). It acts as an antioxidant and elevates the levels of glutathione. R-alpha-lipoic acid is found in many vegetables, such as broccoli, yams, potatoes, and brussels sprout. Red meat and organs are rich in alpha-lipoic acid.

Coenzyme Q10: In 1957, Dr. Fredrick Crane isolated coenzyme Q10, and Dr. Wolf, working under Dr. Karl Folkers, determined the structure of coenzyme Q10 in 1958.

L-carnitine: L-carnitine is synthesized from amino acids lysine and methionine and was originally discovered as a growth factor for mealworms. It is primarily synthesized in the liver and kidneys. Vitamin C is necessary for the synthesis of L-carnitine. It exists as L-carnitine, a biologically active form, and as D-carnitine, a biologically inactive form.

B-vitamins: There are 8 different B-vitamins: B1 (thiamine), B2 (riboflavin), B3 (niacin), B5 (pantothenic acid), B6 (pyridoxine), B7 (biotin), B9 (folic acid), and B12 (cyanocobalamine). The major food sources of B-vitamins include meat, eggs, vegetables, and fruits.

Minerals (selenium and zinc): Commonly used selenium is in the form of L-selenomethionine (an organic form) and sodium selenite (an inorganic form). Selenium rich foods include Brazil nuts, lima beans, brown rice, and seeds (sunflower, sesame, and flax). Zinc compounds such as zinc picolinate, zinc gluconate, zinc acetate, and zinc oxide are utilized in the supplement. Rich food sources include oyster, crab, lobster, meat, poultry, legumes, nuts, seeds, and whole grain.

SOLUBILITY OF MICRONUTRIENTS

The lipid-soluble antioxidants include vitamin A, vitamin E, carotenoids, coenzyme Q10, and L-carnitine, and water-soluble antioxidants include vitamin C, glutathione, and alpha-lipoic acid. Vitamin D3 is lipid-soluble. All B-vitamins are soluble in water. Fat-soluble vitamins should be taken with meals, so that they are more readily absorbed. Zinc gluconate is soluble in water, whereas zinc picolinate is only partially soluble in water. Selenium compounds are soluble in water.

DISTRIBUTION OF ANTIOXIDANTS IN THE BODY

Carotenoids: Beta-carotene is one of more than 600 carotenoids found in fruits, vegetables, and plants. It is commercially available in natural or synthetic forms. Natural form of beta-carotene is more effective than the synthetic form. Preparations of natural carotenoids contain primarily beta-carotene; however, the other type of carotenoids is also present. A portion of ingested beta-carotene is converted to retinol (vitamin A) in the intestinal tract before absorption, and the remainder is distributed in the blood and tissues of the body. One molecule of beta-carotene forms two molecules of vitamin A. In humans, the conversion of beta-carotene to vitamin A does not occur if the body has sufficient amounts of vitamin A. Beta-carotene is primarily stored in the eyes and fatty tissues. Other carotenoids such as lycopene accumulate in the prostate more than in other organs, whereas lutein accumulates in the eyes more than in other organs.

Vitamin A: Vitamin A is commercially sold as retinyl palmitate, retinyl acetate, and retinoic acid and its analogues. Retinyl acetate or retinyl palmitate is converted to retinol in the intestine before absorption. Retinol is converted to retinoic acid in the cells. Retinoic acid performs all functions of vitamin A except for maintaining good vision. Retinol is stored in the liver as retinyl palmitate. Vitamin A exists as a protein-bound molecule. The level of retinol can be determined in the plasma.

Vitamin C: Vitamin C is commercially sold as ascorbic acid, sodium ascorbate, magnesium ascorbate, calcium ascorbate, and time-release capsules containing ascorbic acid and vitamin C-ester. Vitamin C is present in all cells. Ascorbic acid is converted to dehydroascorbic acid, which can be reduced to form vitamin C. It is interesting to note that dehydroascorbic acid can cross blood-brain barrier, but vitamin C cannot. All mammals make vitamin C except guinea pigs. An adult goat makes about 13 grams of vitamin C every day. The plasma level of vitamin C may not reflect the tissue levels of vitamin C, but in humans, it is difficult to obtain tissues for determining vitamin C. Vitamin C can recycle oxidized vitamin E to its reduced form, which acts as an antioxidant.

Vitamin E: Among vitamin E isomers, alpha-tocopherol is biologically more active than others. In recent years, the research on tocotrienols has also revealed some important biological functions. Synthetic vitamin E is referred to as the *dl*-form; the natural form is termed as the *d*-form. Vitamin E is commercially sold as *d*- or *dl*-alpha-tocopherol, alpha-tocopheryl acetate (alpha-TA), or alpha-tocopheryl succinate (alpha-TS). The esterified form of vitamin E (alpha-TA and alpha-TS) are more stable than alpha-tocopherol. Alpha-TA has been widely used in the basic research and clinical studies. It has been presumed that alpha-TA or alpha-TS is converted to alpha-tocopherol before absorption. This assumption may be true as long as the stores of alpha-tocopherol in the body are not saturated; however, if the body stores of alpha-tocopherol are saturated, alpha-TS can be absorbed as alpha-TS. Alpha-TS enters the cells more easily than alpha-tocopherol because of its greater solubility. Alpha-TS have some unique functions that cannot be produced by alpha-T. Alpha-TS is now considered the most effective form of vitamin E, but it cannot act as an antioxidant until converted to alpha-T. Alpha-T is located primarily in the membranous structures of the cells. The level of vitamin E can be determined in the plasma.

Glutathione, N-acetylcysteine, and Alpha-lipoic acid: Glutathione is the most important antioxidant within the cells. Glutathione is sold commercially for oral consumption; however, this molecule is degraded totally in the intestine. Therefore, oral administration of glutathione does not increase the cellular level of glutathione. N-acetylcysteine (NAC) increases the cellular levels of glutathione. In the body, N-acetyl is removed from NAC by the enzyme esterase, and then cysteine is used to synthesize glutathione. Alpha-lipoic acid also increases the cellular levels of glutathione by a mechanism that is different than that from NAC and is present in all cells.

Coenzyme Q10: About 95% of energy is generated from the use of coenzyme Q10 by the mitochondria. Therefore, organs such as heart and liver that require high energy have the highest concentrations of coenzyme Q10. Other organelles inside the cells that contain coenzyme Q10 include endoplasmic reticulum, peroxisomes, lysosomes, and Golgi apparatus.

L-carnitine: L-carnitine is made in our body, but it can also be obtained from the diet. The highest concentration of L-carnitine is found in red meat (95 mg per 3.0 oz). In contrast, chicken breast has only 3.9 mg per 3.5 oz. L-carnitine is present in all cells of our bodies.

NADH (reduced form of nicotinamide adenine dinucleotide): Nicotinamide adenine dinucleotide (NAD+) and NADH are present in all cells of our body. NAD+ is an oxidizing agent; therefore, can act as a pro-oxidant, whereas NADH can act as an antioxidant. NAD+ accepts electron from other molecules and is reduced to form NADH. It can recycle oxidized vitamin E to reduce form, which can act as an antioxidant. NADH is essential for mitochondria to generate energy.

Phytochemicals: Phytochemicals, also called polyphenols or phytochemicals, are a group of chemical substances found in plants. They include tannins, lignins, and flavonoids. The largest and best studied polyphenols are flavonoids, which include quercetin, epicatechin, and oligomeric proanthocyanidins. The major sources of flavonoids include all citrus fruits, berries, ginkgo biloba, onions, parsley, tea, red wine, and dark chocolate. More than 5,000 naturally occurring flavonoids have been characterized from various plants. Flavonoids are poorly absorbed by the intestinal tract in humans. All flavonoids possess varying degrees of antioxidants activity.

Melatonin: Melatonin is a naturally occurring hormone produced primarily by the pineal gland in the brain. The retina, the lens, and the gastrointestinal tract also produce it. Melatonin is synthesized from the amino acid tryptophan. Melatonin is also produced by various plants, such as rice. It is readily absorbed from the intestinal tract; however, 50% of melatonin is removed from the plasma in 35 to 50 min. Melatonin has several biological functions, including antioxidant activity, and is necessary for sleep.

STORAGE OF ANTIOXIDANTS

Carotenoids: Most commercially sold carotenoids in solid form can be stored at room temperature away from light for a few years. Beta-carotene in solution, however, degrades within a few days even when stored cold away from light.

Vitamin A: Crystal forms of retinol, retinoic acid, retinyl acetate, and retinal palmitate can be stored at 4°C for several months. A solution of retinoic acid is stable at 4°C, stored away from light, for several weeks.

Vitamin C: Vitamin C should not be stored in solution form because the molecule is easily destroyed within a few days. Crystal or tablet forms of vitamin C can be kept at room temperature, away from light, for a few years.

Vitamin E: Alpha-tocopherol is relatively unstable at room temperature in comparison with alpha-tocopheryl acetate or alpha-tocopheryl succinate. Alpha tocopherol can be stored at 4°C for several weeks, but alpha-tocopheryl acetate or alpha-tocopheryl succinate can be stored at room temperature for a few years. A solution of alpha-tocopheryl succinate is stable for several months at 4°C if kept away from light.

Glutathione, N-acetylcysteine, and Alpha-lipoic acid: Solid forms of glutathione, N-acetylcysteine, and alpha-lipoic acid are stable at room temperature away from light for a few years. The solutions of these antioxidants are stable at 4°C away from the light for several months.

Coenzyme Q10 and NADH: These antioxidants in solid forms are stable at room temperature, away from the light, for a few years. The solutions of these antioxidants are stable at 4°C away from the light for several months.

Phytochemicals: Phytochemicals are very stable at room temperature, stored away from light, for a few years.

Melatonin: The powder form of melatonin is stable at a 4°C for a year or more.

CAN ANTIOXIDANTS BE DESTROYED DURING COOKING?

Carotenoids: Most carotenes, especially lutein and lycopene, are not destroyed during cooking. In fact, their bioavailability improves when they are derived from a cooked or extracted preparation—for example, lycopene from tomato sauce.

Vitamin A: Routine cooking does not destroy vitamin A, but slow heating for a long period of time may reduce its potency. Canning and prolonged cold storage may also diminish the activity of vitamin A. The vitamin A content of fortified milk powder substantially declines after two years.

Vitamin E: Food processing, frying, and freezing destroy vitamin E. The vitamin E content of fortified milk powder is unaffected over a two-year period.

Glutathione, N-acetylcysteine, and Alpha-lipoic acid: They can be partially destroyed during cooking.

Phytochemicals: They are not destroyed during cooking.

Coenzyme Q10 and NADH: They can be partially degraded during cooking.

ABSORPTION OF ANTIOXIDANTS AND ITS SIGNIFICANCE

Antioxidants are absorbed from the intestinal tract and then distributed to various organs of the body. The highest levels of vitamins A, C, and E are present in the liver, and the lowest levels of these antioxidants are present in the brain. Heart and liver have the highest levels of coenzyme Q10. Only about 10% of ingested water-soluble or fat-soluble antioxidants are absorbed from the intestinal tract. It has been argued by some that 90% of antioxidants are therefore wasted. This argument has no scientific merit. During digestion processes, many toxic substances, including mutagens and carcinogens, are formed. Meat eaters formed such toxic substances more than do vegetarians. The consumption of organic food will make no difference in amounts of toxins formed during the digestion of food. A portion of these toxins is absorbed from the gut and could increase the risk of chronic diseases over a long period of time. The presence of excessive amounts of antioxidants markedly reduces the levels of toxins formed during digestion and thereby reduces the risk of these toxins on health and the incidence of chronic diseases. Thus, unabsorbed antioxidants perform very useful function in reducing the levels of mutagens and carcinogens during digestion.

FUNCTIONS OF INDIVIDUAL ANTIOXIDANTS

The functions of antioxidants are varied and complex. Most believe antioxidants have only one function, which is to neutralize free radicals. In view of recent advances in antioxidant research, this belief is incorrect. In addition to neutralizing free radicals, they reduce inflammation, stimulate immune function, act as cofactors for several biological reactions, and regulate expressions of genes involved in proliferation, growth, differentiation, and immune function. Some antioxidant activates a nuclear transcription factor Nrf2, and each alters the expression of different microRNAs.

Vitamin A: In addition to quenching free radicals, vitamin A plays an important role in maintenance of vision; stimulation of immune function; regulation of gene activity in embryonic development and reproduction; bone metabolism, in inhibition of precancer and cancer cell proliferation; and in skin health.

Carotenoids: Beta-carotene is a precursor of vitamin A. Carotenes are also known to protect against ultraviolet light-induced damage. Beta-carotene increases the expression of connexin gene, which codes for gap junction protein, which holds two normal cells together, whereas vitamin A cannot produce such an effect. Beta-carotene is a more effective quencher of free radicals in high atmospheric pressure than vitamin A or vitamin E.

Vitamin D3: Vitamin D3 is essential for bone formation and regulates calcium and phosphorus levels in the blood. Vitamin D3 inhibits parathyroid hormone secretion from the parathyroid glands. It stimulates immune function by promoting phagocytosis and also exhibits antitumor activity.

Vitamin C: Vitamin C acts as an antioxidant and participates as a cofactor of enzymes that are involved in the formation of many vital compounds in the body. Vitamin C helps in the formation of collagen and takes part in the formation of interferon, a naturally occurring antiviral agent. Vitamin C regenerates oxidized vitamin E.

Vitamin E: Vitamin E acts as an antioxidant and regulates gene expression and translocation of certain protein from one compartment to another. It helps maintain good skin texture, reduces scarring, and acts as an anticoagulant. Vitamin E reduces inflammation and stimulates immune function. Its derivative, vitamin E succinate, exhibits a potent anticancer activity.

Alpha-lipoic acid: Alpha-lipoic acid is a more potent antioxidant than vitamin C or vitamin E because it is easily oxidized or reduced. Alpha-lipoic acid is soluble in both water and lipid; therefore, it protects cellular membranes as well as water-soluble compounds. It regenerates tissue levels of vitamin C and vitamin E and markedly elevates glutathione level in the cells. Alpha-lipoic acid acts as a cofactor for multienzyme dehydrogenase complexes.

N-acetylcysteine (NAC): NAC increases the glutathione levels in cells. This function is important because orally administered glutathione is totally degraded in the small intestine. At high doses, N-acetylcysteine binds with metals and removes them from the body.

Glutathione: Glutathione is one of the most important antioxidants that protect cellular components inside the cells. It is needed for detoxification of toxins that are produced as byproducts of normal metabolism or for certain exogenous toxins. Glutathione also acts as a substrate for several enzymes and reduces inflammation.

Coenzyme Q10: This is a weak antioxidant, but it recycles vitamin E. Coenzyme Q10 is essential for energy generation by the mitochondria.

Reduced Nicotinamide adenine dinucleotide (NADH): This also acts as an antioxidant and is essential for generating energy by the mitochondria. NADH has been shown to increase the formation and release of acetylcholine in cholinergic nerve cells responsible for storage of memory.

Phytochemicals: Flavonoids are one of the phytochemicals that have been studied extensively. They exhibit antioxidant activity and reduce inflammation. They also regulate expression of certain genes.

Melatonin: Melatonin is important in regulating circadian rhythms through its receptor. It also acts as an antioxidant and reduces inflammation. Unlike other antioxidants, the oxidation of melatonin is irreversible, and thus, it cannot be regenerated by other antioxidants. It also stimulates immune function. Melatonin prevents the toxicity of beta-amyloid fragments and hyperphosphorylation of tau protein. Beta-amyloid (fragment of amyloid precursor protein) and hyperphosphorylation of tau protein are involved in Alzheimer's disease.

ANTIOXIDANT DEFENSE SYSTEMS

What are antioxidants? Generally speaking, antioxidants are defined as chemical substances that donate an electron to a free radical and convert it into a harmless molecule. The antioxidant defense system in humans can be divided into three groups: antioxidant enzymes, dietary antioxidants, and endogenous antioxidants.

ANTIOXIDANT ENZYMES

Antioxidant enzymes, such as superoxide dismutase (SOD), catalase, and glutathione peroxidase, are made in the body. SOD requires manganese (Mn) or copper (Cu)-zinc SOD for its biological activity. Mn-SOD is present in the mitochondria, whereas Cu-Zn SOD is present in the cytoplasm. They can destroy free radicals and hydrogen peroxide. Catalase requires iron (Fe) for its biological activity; it too destroys hydrogen peroxide in the cell. Selenium itself is not an antioxidant, but glutathione peroxidase, an antioxidant enzyme, requires selenium for its biological activity.

DIETARY ANTIOXIDANTS

Antioxidants are not made in the body and are obtained principally through diet. They include vitamin A, carotenoids, vitamin C, vitamin E, and phytochemicals.

ENDOGENOUS ANTIOXIDANTS

Antioxidant chemicals are primarily made in the body but also consumed through the diet (primarily through meat and eggs) and in the form of supplements. They include glutathione, coenzyme Q10, reduced nicotinamide adenine dinucleotide (NADH), α-lipoic acid, and L-carnitine.

KNOWN FUNCTIONS OF ANTIOXIDANTS

1. They neutralize free radicals by donating electrons to unpaired molecules.
2. They decrease chronic inflammation.
3. They alter gene expression profiles.
4. They activate a nuclear transcriptional factor Nrf2.

5. They alter the expression of microRNAs.
6. They prevent release and toxicity of excessive amounts of glutamate.
7. They act as cofactors for several biological reactions.
8. They induce cell differentiation and apoptosis in cancer cells.
9. They induce cell differentiation in normal cells but not apoptosis.
10. They stimulate immune function.

The functions of antioxidants with respect to aging and each specific disease are discussed in detail in Chapters 4 through 23 of this volume.

CURRENT CONTROVERSIES ABOUT ANTIOXIDANTS

Although antioxidants are essential for human survival and growth, they remain the most misunderstood and misused molecules by most public and health professionals. The reasons for this include inaccurate claims by many in the nutrition industry, inconsistent human data (stemming from epidemiologic studies), and the results of clinical studies in which primarily one dietary or endogenous antioxidant in high-risk populations was administered. Therefore, it is essential to understand antioxidant types, forms, sources, and functions to appreciate how they can potentially be used to improve health and reduce the risk of chronic diseases.

Humans consume some antioxidants such as vitamin A, carotenoids, vitamin C, and vitamin E from their diet, whereas the human body makes some antioxidants such as glutathione, alpha-lipoic acid, coenzyme Q10, and L-carnitine. Despite basic scientific evidence for the role of antioxidants in disease prevention and as an adjunct to standard therapy in the improved management of chronic diseases, the medical establishment has refused to acknowledge their importance. This is not the first time that they have resisted the application of novel agents in the treatment of diseases. As a matter of fact, the history of discovery of antioxidants illustrates some examples of such resistance by the medical establishment. The current controversies regarding the use of micronutrient supplements will be discussed in detail in Chapters 3 through 23.

MISUSE OF ANTIOXIDANTS IN CLINICAL STUDIES

The human body generates different types of inorganic and organic free radicals derived from oxygen and nitrogen in response to the utilization of oxygen. The exposure to various environmental stressors, such as ozone, dust particles, smoke, toxic fumes, toxic chemicals, and ionizing radiation (X-rays or gamma rays) also produces excessive amounts of free radicals. In addition, tobacco smoking, high caloric diet, and obesity can generate excessive amounts of free radicals. Consumption of high levels of trace minerals, such as iron, copper, and manganese in combination with vitamin C generate large amounts of free radicals. Free radical-induced damage is called oxidative damage, which also occurs during the normal aging process and during the initiation and progression of most chronic diseases. If oxidative damage is not repaired, chronic inflammation sets in motion that contributes to aging and ill health.

In order to protect against oxidative stress and chronic inflammation, humans have dietary antioxidants such as vitamins A, C and E, and carotenoids, especially beta-carotene as well as endogenous antioxidants made by the body such as antioxidant enzymes, glutathione, coenzyme Q10, R-alpha-lipoic acid, L-carnitine, and reduced nicotinamide adenine dinucleotide. These antioxidants, together with B-vitamins and certain minerals, are necessary for growth and survival and prevention of chronic diseases.

Extensive studies have suggested that increased oxidative stress and chronic inflammation contribute to the development of most chronic diseases. Therefore, reducing these defects may be useful in reducing the risk of developing such diseases. To address this issue, laboratory experiments on cell culture and animal studies utilized a single antioxidant, which showed that administration of single antioxidants could reduce the risk of developing various diseases. Based on these observations, previous human studies also used single antioxidants in high-risk populations or in patients with early phase of the disease. Unfortunately, the use of single antioxidants in high-risk population or established disease produced inconsistent results varying from transient benefits in early phase of the disease, to no effect, to even harmful effects.

In all human studies with individual antioxidants, the selection of the target population and the statistical analysis have been appropriate, but the selection of single antioxidants, doses, and dose schedule have been without any scientific rationale. This can be demonstrated by a few widely publicized results on antioxidant studies in high-risk populations. In these studies, the synthetic form of beta-carotene was administered orally once a day to male heavy tobacco smokers in order to determine whether beta-carotene would reduce the incidence of lung cancer. The results showed that the incidence of lung cancer in beta-carotene-treated smokers increased by about 17%, prompting the study to be stopped before its completion. Such a treatment has no effect on normal populations. These studies are discussed in the chapter on cancer prevention. Federal agencies then promoted the idea that supplementation with beta-carotene may be harmful to one's health and recommended that consumers not take beta-carotene alone or in a multiple vitamin preparation containing beta-carotene. These erroneous conclusions and recommendations were without any scientific merit.

It had been known before the start of the above human studies that individual antioxidants such as beta-carotene could be oxidized in a high internal oxidative environment to become pro-oxidant. Heavy tobacco smokers have a high internal oxidative environment. Therefore, when beta-carotene is administered to smokers, it is oxidized and acts as a pro-oxidant rather than as an antioxidant. This would then be expected to increase the incidence of cancer in tobacco smokers.

Knowing the above facts about beta-carotene and heavy tobacco smokers, one could have predicted that beta-carotene would increase the risk of lung cancer in smokers. Indeed, the results of the trials confirmed this prediction. In contrast to the adverse effects of beta-carotene in heavy tobacco smokers, the same dose and type of beta-carotene did not increase the risk of cancer among doctors and nurses who were nonsmokers during a five-year follow-up. Again, this result was also expected because populations of nonsmokers do not have a high internal oxidative environment.

The synthetic form of vitamin E has produced inconsistent results in patients with a high risk of cardiovascular disease who have increased an internal oxidative environment. Some studies showed beneficial effects, whereas others showed no effect or even adverse effects in some cases. Harmful effects of vitamin E alone on cardiovascular disease can be attributed to the same biological events as those observed with beta-carotene. At this time, cardiologists do not recommend vitamin E to their patients. There are no human data (intervention studies) to show that the same dose of vitamin E or beta-carotene, when present in an appropriately prepared multiple micronutrients including dietary and endogenous antioxidants, produces adverse health effects among normal or high-risk populations.

The human studies featuring a single antioxidant have also produced inconsistent results in neurological diseases such as Parkinson's disease (PD) and Alzheimer's disease (AD). In both studies, high doses of the synthetic form of vitamin E at a dose of 800 IU per day in PD, and 2,000 IU per day in AD were used. No beneficial effects of vitamin E were observed in PD, but some beneficial effects were observed in early phase AD. These studies were started without careful consideration of the biochemical factors involved in the diseases processes and antioxidant status in the patients. It has been reported that deficiency of the antioxidant glutathione rather than vitamin E is found in both AD and PD patients. In addition, dysfunction of the mitochondria is consistently observed in autopsied samples of brains of patients with PD or AD. Furthermore, evidence of high oxidative damage and chronic inflammation are also found in these brains. Therefore, the idea of supplementation with antioxidants for the prevention and reduction in the rate of progression of disease is very good one. I have proposed simultaneous reduction in the levels of oxidative stress and inflammation may be necessary for the prevention and improved management of PD and AD (to be discussed in detail later in this book). To achieve this goal, it is essential to increase the levels of antioxidant enzymes and dietary and endogenous antioxidants at the same time. The levels of antioxidants can easily be increased by supplementation, but elevating the levels of antioxidant enzymes requires activation of Nrf2, a nuclear transcriptional factor. This proposed strategy would have provided better health outcomes than those obtained by vitamin E alone.

The reasons for producing no effect, transient minimal beneficial effects, or harmful effects by single antioxidants are as follow: (a) the levels of antioxidants in subcellular compartment differ and various antioxidants exhibit different mechanisms of action; therefore, a single antioxidant cannot protect all parts of the cell against different types of free radicals; (b) a single antioxidant in a high internal oxidative environment of high-risk patients with chronic diseases is oxidized and can then itself act as a pro-oxidant rather than as an antioxidant; (c) the body protects against oxidative damage by elevating antioxidant enzymes and dietary and endogenous antioxidants. Antioxidants neutralize free radicals by donating electrons to those with unpaired electron, whereas antioxidant enzymes destroy free radicals by catalysis, converting them to harmless molecules such as water and oxygen; (d) the affinity of various antioxidants with free radicals differs; (e) water-soluble antioxidants such as vitamin C and glutathione protect molecules in the aqueous environment of the cells, whereas lipid-soluble antioxidants such as vitamin A and vitamin E protect molecules in the lipid compartment; (f) vitamin E is more effective in quenching free radicals in a reduced oxygenated cellular environment, whereas vitamin C and alpha-tocopherol are more effective in a higher oxygenated environment of the cells; (g) vitamin C recycles the oxidized form of alpha-tocopherol to the antioxidant form at the lipid/aqueous interface; and (h) antioxidants produce cell protective proteins by altering the expression of different microRNAs (miRs). For example, some antioxidants can activate Nrf2 by upregulating miR-200a that inhibits its target protein Keap1, whereas others activate Nrf2 by downregulating miR-21 that binds with 3′-UTR Nrf2 mRNA.

These studies clearly suggest that use of a single micronutrient in prevention or improved management of human chronic diseases is not expected to yield any beneficial effects. Previous human studies failed to consider the type of antioxidants to be used in the investigation. This was important because in their natural form, certain antioxidants may be more effective than their synthetic counterparts. For example, natural beta-carotene prevented X-ray-induced transformation of normal-like murine fibroblasts in culture, whereas synthetic beta-carotene did not. The natural form of vitamin E (*d*-alpha-tocopherol) accumulated more in various organs than the synthetic form (*dl*-alpha-tocopherol). Furthermore, vitamin E in the form of *d*-alpha-tocopheryl succinate appears to be more effective than other forms of vitamin E.

The doses of antioxidants to be used in human investigation are very important in order to produce optimal health benefits or disease prevention. Low doses (around RDA values) may be useful in reducing some oxidative damage and preventing deficiency; however, they may not be sufficient in reducing oxidative damage and chronic inflammation or in optimizing immune function. The differences in changes in the expression of gene profiles between low and high doses of an antioxidant are very marked. In commercially sold multivitamin preparations, the doses of antioxidants and other micronutrients markedly vary. The selection of appropriated doses of various micronutrients including dietary and endogenous antioxidants that are safe and standardized is essential for health benefits and disease prevention.

The dose schedule of antioxidants to be used in human studies is very critical for achieving the desired health benefits. Most people take once-a-day micronutrient supplement that may not produce optimal health benefits. This is due to the fact that a high degree of fluctuation in the levels of antioxidants in the body may occur because of variation in the plasma half-lives of various micronutrients. In addition, the expression gene profiles of cells markedly changes, depending upon the level of antioxidants in the body; therefore, cells have to readjust their genetic activity all the time, which can stress cells over a long period of time. It is interesting to note that all previous human studies with antioxidants have used the once-a-day schedule in spite of scientific evidence to the contrary.

The published human studies with antioxidants have not taken into consideration the important issues discussed above in the design of experiments; therefore, the results regarding the efficacy of antioxidants have been contradictory.

It is unfortunate that the harmful results obtained with the use of primarily one antioxidant in high-risk populations are often extrapolated to all multiple antioxidant preparations and to all populations. This erroneous extrapolation of data regarding the harmful effects of beta-carotene or vitamin E alone is further propagated by the publication of meta-analysis of published data on the same vitamins with the same conclusion. A meta-analysis publication is often misinterpreted as an original study. In my opinion, a meta-analysis should critically examine an experiment's design instead of just summarizing the results of previous studies. These kinds of experiments and extrapolations have created a wide disconnect between the public and most health professionals—especially physicians—regarding the health benefits of micronutrients. In order to avoid these problems, the subsequent chapters in this book discuss the scientific basis for using multiple micro-nutrients, including dietary and endogenous antioxidants in healthy aging and in reducing the risk of chronic diseases. In addition, the role of these micronutrients in improving the efficacy of standard therapy for various chronic diseases is also discussed.

CONCLUSIONS

Micronutrients include antioxidants, vitamin D3, all B-vitamins, selenium, and other minerals. The sources, stability, forms, subcellular distribution, and function of individual micronutrients were described. Problems associated with the use of single antioxidants in high-risk populations and established disease were discussed. Increased oxidative stress and chronic inflammation are involved in the initiation and progression of aging as well as of chronic diseases. Therefore, reducing these biochemical defects may be useful in prevention, and in combination with standard therapy, in improvement of the management of chronic diseases. It was suggested that elevation of dietary and endogenous antioxidants and antioxidant enzymes might be necessary for an optimal health and disease prevention. High but nontoxic doses of micronutrients including dietary and endogenous antioxidants may be essential for healthy aging and disease prevention. Unfortunately, the clinical studies with antioxidants in populations at high-risk of developing chronic diseases have utilized a single antioxidant that produced inconsistent results. The reasons for this were discussed.

REFERENCES

1. Sen CK, Packer L, Baeuerle PA. *Antioxidants and Redox Regulation of Genes.* New York: Academic Press; 1999.
2. Shils MS, James MO, Ross C. *Modern Nutrition in Health and Disease*, 10th ed. Philadelphia, PA: Lippincott Williams & Wilikins; 2005.
3. Anderson JJB. *Nutrition & Health: An Introduction.* Durham, NC: Carolina Academic Press; 2005.
4. Institute of Medicine. *The Development of DRI's 1994–2004: Lessoned Learned and New Challenges: Workshop.* Wasington, DC: The National Academic Press; 2008.
5. Packer LH, Hiramatsu M, Yoshikawa T. *Antioxidant Food Supplements in Human Health.* New York: Academic Press, Elsevier; 1999.
6. Combs Jr GF. *The Vitamins: Fundamental Aspects in Nutrition & Health*, 2nd Edition. San Diego, CA: Academic Press; 1998.
7. Caballero B, Allen L, Prentice A. *Encyclopedia of Human Nutrition.* Boston, MA: Academic Press, Elsevier; 2005.
8. Cadenas E, Lester P. *Handbook of Antioxidants.* New York: Marcel Dekker, Inc; 1996.
9. Frei B. *Natural Antioxidants in Human Health and Disease.* New York: Academic Press; 1994.
10. Prasad KN. *Neurodegenerative Disease and Micronutrients.* Boca Raton, FL: CRC Press; 2015.

2 Basic Facts about Oxidative Stress, Inflammation, and the Immune System

INTRODUCTION

Increased oxidative stress due to production of excessive amounts of free radicals derived from oxygen and nitrogen plays a central role in the initiation and progression of damage associated with the acute and chronic diseases; therefore, a basic understanding of this process is essential for the development of any preventive or improved treatment strategies. The mechanisms of generating different types of free radicals in the body are very complex; therefore, they are discussed in general terms. The significance of increased oxidative stress in aging, various diseases, and injuries is discussed in Chapters 4 through 23.

Cell injury initiates an important biological event called inflammation, which is considered a protective response following infection with pathogenic organisms or antigens or cellular damage. Inflammation is considered a double-edged sword. It is needed to kill invading pathogenic organisms and for the removal of cellular debris in order to facilitate the recovery process. However, it can also damage normal tissues by releasing a number of toxic chemicals. If cellular damage is not repaired, chronic inflammation sets in motion. The chronic inflammatory responses are more relevant to chronic diseases than the acute inflammatory reactions. Inflammation is a highly complex biological response that is tightly regulated. Therefore, only a brief description of this process in general and simple terms is included in this section. The significance of chronic inflammation in aging and various chronic diseases is discussed in Chapters 4 through 23.

The immune system is an important defense system against invading foreign pathogenic microorganisms and is essential for the healing of injured tissues. Foreign antigens or cell injury evokes an immune response that through complex processes of acute inflammation removes the pathogenic microbes and cellular debris. It is a highly regulated system and is turned off when the invading organisms are killed or injured tissues are healed. Chronic inflammation in response to chronic infection or cellular injury is not turned off; therefore, it is one of the major factors that contribute to chronic diseases through their toxic products. In response of endogenous antigens, the immune cells cannot distinguish between endogenous antigens from foreign antigens, and, consequently, these activated immune cells start damaging the body's own tissues, which produce these antigens causing autoimmune disease. The importance of acute immune response is relevant to HIV infection and cancer prevention and is discussed in Chapters 7 and 14.

This chapter briefly describes the basic concepts of oxidative stress, inflammation, and the immune system in simple and general terms. These issues are huge and complex. This chapter has attempted to describe them in a few pages for basic understanding of the oxidative stress, inflammation, and immune function. For further study of these topics, the references and books that have been used are listed at the end of this chapter.[1–10]

OXIDATIVE STRESS

Increase oxidative stress is caused by excessive production of free radicals derived from oxygen and nitrogen. It is linked with most human chronic diseases such as arthritis, heart disease, Alzheimer's disease, Parkinson's disease, and diabetes.

WHAT ARE FREE RADICALS?

The radicals, also referred to as free radicals, are atoms, molecules, or ions with unpaired electrons. These unpaired electrons are highly reactive and play an important role in several chemical reactions such as combustion, atmospheric chemistry, and polymerization. In living organisms, including humans, they play an important role in several biochemical reactions and gene expressions. In 1900, the first organic free radical, triphenylmethyl radical, was identified by Moses Gomberg of the University of Michigan in the United States. Free radicals can be derived from oxygen or nitrogen and are symbolized by a dot "•".

In the beginning, the earth's atmosphere had no oxygen and anaerobic organisms, which can live without oxygen, thrived. About 2.5 billion years ago, blue-green algae in the ocean acquired the ability to split water (H_2O) into hydrogen (H) and oxygen (O_2). This chemical reaction initiated the release of oxygen into the atmosphere. The increased levels of atmospheric oxygen led to the extinction of many anaerobic organisms from oxygen's toxicity, probably due to the generation of free radicals. This important atmospheric chemical event forced the organisms to acquire antioxidant systems to quench these free radicals. Those who succeeded in developing antioxidant protective systems survived and ultimately led to the evolution of multicellular organisms, including humans, who utilize oxygen for survival, but have a comprehensive antioxidants system to defend against damage produced by free radicals.

TYPES OF FREE RADICALS

There are several different types of free radicals derived from oxygen and nitrogen that are generated in the body. The oxygen-derived free radicals include hydroxyl radical ($OH^\bullet$), peroxyl radical ($ROO^\bullet$), alkoxyl radical ($RO^\bullet$), phenoxyl and semiquinone radicals ($ArO^\bullet$, $HO\text{-}Ar\text{-}O^\bullet$), and superoxide radical ($O_2^{\bullet-}$). The nitrogen-derived free radicals include $NO^\bullet$, $ONOO^-$ (peroxynitrite), and $^\bullet NO_2$.

FORMATION OF FREE RADICALS DERIVED FROM OXYGEN AND NITROGEN

The formation of some of the reactive oxygen species (ROS) is described below.

When molecular oxygen (O_2) acquires an electron, the superoxide anion

$$\left(O_2^{\bullet-}\right) \text{ is formed when } O_2 + e^- = O_2^{\bullet-}$$

Superoxide dismutase (SOD) and H^+ can react with $\left(O_2^{\bullet-}\right)$ to form hydrogen peroxide, H_2O_2:

$$2O_2^{\bullet-} + 2H^+ \text{ plus SOD} \rightarrow H_2O_2 + O_2$$

$$O_2^{\bullet-} + H^+ \rightarrow HO_2^\bullet \text{ (hydroperoxy radical)}$$

$$2H\,O_2^\bullet \rightarrow H_2O_2 + O_2$$

Ferric and ferrous forms of iron can react with superoxide anion and hydrogen peroxide to produce molecular oxygen and hydroxyl radical ($OH^\bullet$), respectively:

$$Fe^{3+} + O_2^\bullet \rightarrow Fe^{2+} + O_2$$

$$Fe^{2+} + H_2O_2 \rightarrow Fe^{3+} + OH^{\bullet} + OH^{-} \text{ (Fenton reaction)}$$

Hydroxyl radical can also be formed from superoxide anion by the Haber-Weiss reaction:

$$O_2^{\bullet-} + H_2O_2 \rightarrow O_2 + OH^{-} + OH^{\bullet}$$

Both the Fenton and Haber-Weiss reactions require a transition metal such as copper or iron. Among ROS, $OH^{\bullet}$ is the most damaging free radical and is very short-lived.

Hydroxyl radical is very reactive with a variety of organic compounds, leading to production of more radical compounds:

$$RH \text{ (organic compound)} + OH^{\bullet} \rightarrow R^{\bullet} \text{ (organic radical)} + H_2O$$

$$R^{\bullet} + O_2 \rightarrow RO_2^{\bullet} \text{ (peroxyl radical)}$$

For example, the DNA radical can be generated by reaction with a hydroxyl radical, and this can lead to strand lesions.

Catalase detoxifies hydrogen peroxide to form water and molecular oxygen:

$$H_2O_2 + \text{catalase} \rightarrow H_2O \text{ and } O_2$$

Reactive nitrogen species (RNS) are represented by nitric oxide ($NO^{\bullet}$). NO is synthesized by the enzyme nitric oxide synthase from L-arginine. $NO^{\bullet}$ can combine with superoxide anion to form peroxynitrite, a powerful oxidant.

$$NO^{\bullet} + O_2^{\bullet-} \rightarrow ONOO^{-} \text{ (peroxynitrite)}$$

When protonated (likely at physiological pH), peroxynitrite spontaneously decomposes to reactive nitric dioxide and hydroxyl radicals:

$$ONOO^{-} + H^{+} \rightarrow {}^{\bullet}NO_2 + OH^{\bullet}$$

Superoxide dismutase (SOD) can also enhance the peroxynitrite-mediated nitration of tyrosine residues on critical proteins, presumably via species similar to the nitronium cation (NO_2^{+}):

$$ONOO^{-} \text{ plus SOD} \rightarrow NO_2^{+} \rightarrow \text{Nitration of tyrosine}$$

There are several oxidizing agents that are formed in the body, in addition to free radicals. They include peroxynitrite, hydrogen peroxide, and lipid peroxide and are very damaging to the cells.

Many other radical species can be formed by biological reactions inside the body. For example, phenolic and other aromatic species can be formed during metabolism of xenobiotic agents. Furthermore, any antioxidant, when oxidized, can act as a free radical.

Oxidative stress occurs when the generation of ROS exceeds the ability of the body's antioxidant defense system to neutralize them. Similarly, nitrosylative stress occurs when the generation of RNS exceeds the ability of the body's antioxidant defense system to neutralize them. Chronic increase in oxidative and nitrosylative stresses has been implicated in the initiation and progression of most human chronic diseases. However, if a short-term increase in oxidative stress, such as seen during viral or bacterial infection, may be important in killing invading organisms, although they can also damage normal tissue. ROS are also used in cell signaling systems that regulate growth, differentiation, and apoptosis. Free radicals can damage DNA (deoxyribonucleic acid), RNA (ribonucleic acid), proteins, carbohydrates, and membranes. The half-lives of various free radicals vary from 10^{-9} seconds to days. This means most are quickly destroyed after causing damage. For example, the half-life of hydroxyl free radicals is 10^{-9} second, whereas that of a superoxide anion is 10^{-5} second, and a lipid peroxyl free radical has a half-life of 7 seconds. The semiquinone free radical half-life is in days, while nitric oxide's is about 1 second, and hydrogen peroxide's is in minutes.

Normally, free radicals are generated in the body during the use of oxygen in the metabolism of certain compounds. Mitochondria—elongated membranous structures present in all cells in varying numbers—use oxygen to produce energy. During this process of generating energy, superoxide anions, hydroxyl radicals, and hydrogen peroxide are produced as byproducts. It is estimated that about 2% of the oxygen consumed by mitochondria remains partially used, and this unused oxygen leaks out of the mitochondria, making about 20 billion molecules of superoxide anions and hydrogen peroxide per cell per day.

During bacterial or viral infection, phagocytic cells are activated and generate high levels of nitric oxide, superoxide anions, and hydrogen peroxide within the infected cells in order to kill infective agents. Excessive production of free radicals by phagocytes can also damage normal cells, and thereby, increase the risk of acute and/or chronic diseases. During the oxidative metabolism of fatty acids and other molecules in the body, free radicals are produced. Certain habits, such as tobacco smoking, and some trace minerals, such as free iron, copper, and manganese, can also increase the rate of production of free radicals in the body. Thus, the human body is exposed daily to different types and varying levels of free radicals.

OXIDATION AND REDUCTION PROCESSES

To understand the role of free radicals and antioxidants in the human body, it is important to grasp the relationship between oxidation and reduction processes, which are constantly taking place in the body. Oxidation is a process in which an atom or molecule gains oxygen, loses hydrogen, or loses an electron. For example, carbon gains oxygen during oxidation and becomes carbon dioxide. A superoxide radical loses an electron during oxidation and becomes oxygen. Thus, an oxidizing agent is a molecule or atom that changes another chemical by adding oxygen to it or by removing electron or hydrogen from it. Examples of oxidizing agents are free radicals, ozone, and ionizing radiation.

Reduction is a process in which an atom or molecule loses oxygen, gains hydrogen, or gains an electron. For example, carbon dioxide loses oxygen and becomes carbon monoxide, carbon gains hydrogen and becomes methane, and oxygen gains an electron and becomes superoxide anion. Thus, a reducing agent is a molecule or atom that changes another chemical by removing oxygen from it or by adding electron or hydrogen to it. All antioxidants can be considered reducing agents. The balanced processes of oxidation and reduction maintain cells in a healthy state. Increased oxidation processes over reduction processes can lead to cellular injury, and eventually chronic diseases or cell death. The role of oxidative stress in various diseases is discussed in Chapters 5 through 23.

WHAT IS INFLAMMATION?

Inflammation in Latin is referred to as *inflammatio*, which means *a setting on fire*. The primary features of inflammation at the affected sites include redness, swelling, warm upon touch, and varying degrees of pain. These characteristics of inflammation were first recognized by a Roman physician, Dr. Cornelius, who lived from about 30 BC to 45 AD. Inflammation is the complex biological response by which the body removes infective agents such as bacteria, viruses, and damaged cells caused by physical agents (such as ionizing radiation or traumatic bodily injuries, or chemical or biological agents). The inflammatory reactions involve the movement of plasma and white blood cells (leukocytes, macrophages, monocytes, lymphocytes, and plasma cells) from the blood to the injured sites. It is a protective response by which the body removes the injurious infective microorganisms as well as initiates the healing process in the damaged tissue. During healing process, the injured tissue is replaced by regeneration of native parenchymal cells by filling the injured site with fibroblastic tissue (scarring), or, most commonly, by a combination of both processes.

TYPES OF INFLAMMATORY REACTIONS

Inflammation is divided into two categories: acute and chronic inflammatory reactions. Acute inflammation occurs following cellular injury or infection with microorganisms. The period of acute inflammation is relatively short, lasting from a few minutes to a few days. The main features of acute inflammations are edema (accumulation of exudation of fluid and plasma in extracellular spaces) and the migration of leukocytes primarily neutrophils to the site of injury. Chronic inflammation also occurs following persistent cellular injury and infection. The period of chronic inflammation is relatively long and can last as long as injury or infection exists. The main features of chronic inflammation are the presence of lymphocytes and macrophages and the proliferation of blood vessels, fibrosis, and tissue necrosis.

Acute inflammation: Acute inflammation causes marked alterations in the blood vessels that allow plasma protein and leukocytes to leave the circulation. Subsequently, the leukocytes migrate to the site of injury by a process called chemotaxis. Leukocytes engulf pathogenic organisms by phagocytosis and kill them by generating burst of ROS and other toxins. They can also engulf cellular debris and foreign antigens by a similar process and then degrade them by lysosomal proteolytic enzymes. On the other hand, leukocytes may release excessive amounts of ROS, pro-inflammatory cytokines, prostaglandins, adhesion molecules, and complement proteins that can damage normal tissues. An acute inflammatory reaction is tightly regulated and turned off soon after the injured sites are healed or invading microbes removed. It is absolutely an important process for removing both pathogens and cellular debris from the damaged site, thus allowing healing to occur.

Acute inflammation is effective only when the injurious stimuli or tissue damage are relatively mild. If the tissue damage is extensive, or the levels of infective organisms are high, acute inflammatory reactions are not tuned off, and consequently, the toxic products of these reactions can enhance the rate of progression of damage that may cause organ failure and eventually even death.

Chronic inflammation: Persistent low-grade cellular injury, exposure to exogenous agents such as particulate silica, or infection can initiate chronic inflammation. In addition, sometimes production of endogenous antigens can evoke a self-perpetuating immune response that causes autoimmune disease such as rheumatoid arthritis and lupus. Chronic inflammation is often associated with most human chronic diseases such as heart disease, Alzheimer's disease, Parkinson's disease, arthritis, diabetes, and HIV/AIDS.

In contrast to acute inflammation, which is characterized by vascular changes, edema, and primarily neutrophilic infiltration, chronic inflammation is characterized by the presence of mononuclear cells, which include macrophages, lymphocytes, and plasma cells, and also tissue damage caused by inflammatory cells. During chronic inflammation, the presence of angiogenesis and fibrosis can be observed at the site of injury.

PRODUCTS OF INFLAMMATORY REACTIONS

During inflammation, several highly reactive agents are released, including cytokines, complement proteins, arachidonic acid (AA) metabolites, and endothelial/leukocyte adhesion molecules. They are briefly described below.

CYTOKINES

Cytokines are proteins released during both acute and chronic inflammation. They are produced by many cell types, primarily by activated lymphocytes and macrophages, but also by many cells such as endothelium, epithelium, and connective tissue cells. Cytokines play an important role in modulating the function of many other cell types. They are multifunctional, and individual cytokines may have both positive and negative regulatory actions. Cytokines mediated their action by binding to specific receptors on target cells. These receptors are regulated by exogenous and endogenous signals.

Cytokines that regulate lymphocyte activation, growth, and differentiation include interleukin-2 (IL-2) and interleukin-4 (IL-4, favors growth), and IL-10, as well as transforming growth factor-beta (TGF-beta). These are negative regulators of immune response. Cytokines involved with natural immunity include inflammatory cytokines, tumor necrosis factor-alpha (TNF-alpha), IL-1Beta, type I interferons (IFN-alpha and IFN-beta), and IL-6. Cytokines that activate inflammatory cells such as macrophages include IFN-gamma, TNF-alpha, TNF-beta, IL-5, IL-10 and IL-12. Cytokines that stimulate hematopoiesis (growth and differentiation of immature leukocytes) include IL-3, IL-7, c-kit ligand, granulocyte-macrophage colony-stimulating factor (G-M-CSF), macrophage colony-stimulating factor (M-CSF), granulocyte CSF, and stem cell factor.

Chemokines are also cytokines that stimulate leukocyte movement and direct them to the site of injury during inflammation. Many classical growth factors may also act as cytokines, and conversely, many cytokines exhibit activities of growth factors.

COMPLEMENT PROTEINS

During inflammation, 20 complement proteins, including their cleavage products, are released into the plasma. When activated, they can cause cell lysis and can exhibit proteolytic activity. They participate in both innate and adaptive immunity for protection against pathogenic organisms. Complement proteins are numbered C1 through C9, each of which has complex mechanisms of action on cells. Some of the complement proteins are also neurotoxic.

ARACHIDONIC ACID (AA) METABOLITES

The AA metabolites include prostaglandins, leukotrienes, and lipoxins: AA is a 20-carbon fatty acid that is derived from the dietary sources or is formed from the essential fatty acid linoleic acid. During inflammation, AA metabolites, also called eicosanoids, are released. These eicosanoids have diverse biological actions, depending upon the cell type. The eicosanoids are synthesized by two major classes of enzymes: Cyclooxygenase (COX) for the synthesis of prostaglandins and thromboxanes and lipoxygenase for the synthesis of leukotrienes and lipoxins. There are two isoforms of cyclooxygenase, COX1 and COX2.

ENDOTHELIAL/LEUKOCYTE ADHESION MOLECULES

The immunoglobulin family molecules include two endothelial adhesion molecules: intracellular adhesion molecule-1 (ICAM-1) and vascular adhesion molecule-1 (VCAM-1). These adhesion molecules bind with leukocyte receptor integrins. They are induced by IL-1 and TNF-alpha. Both ICAM-1 and VCAM-1 are released during inflammatory reactions and have diverse mechanisms of action on cells.

IMMUNE SYSTEM

The immune system plays an important role in defense of the organisms against invading pathogens and is essential for the survival of the organism. Under certain conditions, the immune system can produce toxic chemicals that play an important role in the initiation and progression of chronic diseases, as well as can cause autoimmune diseases.

WHAT IS THE IMMUNE SYSTEM?

The immune system is a highly complex and tightly regulated organ and represents a double-edged sword. On one hand, it defends the body against foreign invading pathogenic microorganisms and antigenic molecules or particles. On the other hand, it has ability to produce toxic chemicals, such as ROS, pro-inflammatory cytokines, complement proteins, adhesion molecules, and prostaglandins that are toxic to tissues and that can increase the risk of chronic diseases such as arthritis, heart disease, Alzheimer's disease, and diabetes. Furthermore, the presence of endogenous antigens can initiate an immune response that damages the body's own tissue, as seen in rheumatoid arthritis. The immune system, once exposed to an antigen and successfully removing it, stores the recognition factor of this antigen in its memory. Thus, during the lifetime of an individual, the immune system stores recognition factors of millions of different antigens and thus protects the body from these antigens all the time. This process of exposure to an antigen and successfully removing it is generally referred to as acquired immunity, which is the basis of vaccination.

The immune system is a network of cells, tissues, and organs that works together in a highly coordinated manner to defend the body against foreign invading organisms or antigenic molecules or particles. The organs of the immune system are located throughout the body. They are lymphoid organs that contain lymphocytes and bone marrow that contain all blood cells, including lymphocytes. Thymus-derived lymphocytes are referred to as T-lymphocytes (T-cells). In blood, T-cell represents about 60%–70% of peripheral lymphocytes. Bone marrow-derived lymphocytes are referred to as B-lymphocytes (B-cells). They constitute about 10%–20% of peripheral lymphocytes in the blood. B-cells mature to plasma cells that secrete specific antibody in response to a particular antigen. Macrophages are derived from monocytes of bone marrow, and are a part of the mononuclear phagocyte system. They exhibit phagocytic activity and play important roles in both the induction and the effector phase of immune responses. A specialized form of cells with numerous fine dendritic cytoplasmic processes, called dendritic cells, do not exhibit phagocytic activity. They play an important role in presenting antigen to T-cells. Natural killer (NK) cells represent about 10%–15% of the peripheral blood lymphocytes and lack T-cell receptors. They can kill tumor cells.

The major components of the immune system are innate immunity and adaptive immunity. The innate immune defenses are non-specific, but it is the dominant system of host defense.[11] The innate immune response is activated when microorganisms are identified by pattern of recognition receptors or when damaged cells send signals to immune system for a defensive response.[12,13] The innate immune responses do not confer long-lasting immunity against pathogenic organisms. The innate immune system responds to infection by inducing inflammation, releasing complement proteins, and recruiting leukocytes. It can also activate the adaptive immunity.

INNATE IMMUNITY

The components of innate include the following inflammation, complement proteins, and leukocytes.

Inflammation: Inflammation is one of the first responses of the immune system to infection with microorganisms. The injured or infected cells release eicosanoids and cytokines as well as growth factors and cytotoxic factors. These cytokines and other chemicals recruit immune cells to the site of infection for the elimination of the invading organisms or promotion of healing of the injured tissue.[14]

Complement proteins: More than 20 complement proteins are released from the activated immune cells in response to infection or injury. These proteins are the major humoral components of the innate immune response.[15] They complement killing of pathogenic microorganisms by the antibodies through complex mechanisms. Complement proteins can also be directly toxic to the organisms or cells.

Leukocytes: Leukocytes are also important components of innate immunity. They include the phagocytes (primarily macrophages and neutrophils), dendritic cells, mast cells, eosinophils, basophils, and natural killer cells. These cells identify and kill microorganisms by phagocytosis. Phagocytosis is an important feature of cellular innate immunity. Neutrophils and macrophages are the most active in phagocytosis following infection with microorganisms. These cells engulf pathogens that are trapped in an intracellular vesicle called phagosomes, which fuse with lysosomes to form phagolysosomes. The pathogens are killed by proteolytic enzymes of the lysosomes aided by bursts of reactive oxygen species released by the phagocytes. Natural killer cells can kill tumor cells or cells infected with viruses.

ADAPTIVE IMMUNITY

The adaptive responses to an antigen are strong and are responsible for storing and recalling immunologic memory for recognizing and eliminating a specific antigen all the time. The lymphocytes (T-cells and B-cells) are responsible for the adaptive immune response. Both T-cells and B-cells carry receptors that recognize specific targets. T-cells can recognize only membrane bound antigens. The cell surface major histocompatibility complex (MHC) molecules binds peptide fragments of foreign proteins for presentation to appropriate antigen-specific T-cells. There are two major subtypes of T-cells: the killer T-cells and the helper T-cells. The killer T-cells can recognize antigens bound to Class I MHC molecules, whereas the helper cells recognize antigens bound to Class II MHC molecules. A minor subtype of T-cells is $\gamma\delta$ T-cells, which recognize intact antigens that are not bound to MHC receptors

In contrast to the T-cells, the surface of a B-cell has antibody molecules for a specific antigen. The antibody molecules recognize whole pathogens and do not need any antigen-presenting mechanism for their action. Each lineage of a B-cell expresses a different antibody. A B-cell first identifies pathogens when an antibody on its surface binds to a specific foreign antigen. This antibody/antigen complex is engulfed by the B-cell where it is converted into peptides by proteolytic enzymes. The B-cells then display on their surface antigenic peptides and Class II MHC molecules that attract matching T-helper cells, which release lymphokines and activate B-cells. The activated B-cells proliferate and differentiate to plasma cells that secrete millions of copies of the antibody that recognize this antigen. These antibodies circulate in the blood and the lymph and bind to pathogens expressing this particular antigen. These antibody/antigen-bound pathogens are destroyed by complement activation or by phagocytes. Antibodies can also neutralize bacterial toxins by directly binding to them and kill bacteria or viruses by interfering with their receptors that are used to infect cells.

CONCLUSIONS

Increased oxidative stress is caused by excessive production of free radicals derived from oxygen and nitrogen. The cell injury initiates an important biological event, called inflammation, which is considered a protective response following infection with pathogenic organisms, antigens, or cellular damage. It is needed to kill invading pathogenic organisms and for the removal of cellular debris in order to facilitate the recovery process. However, it can also damage normal tissues by releasing a number of toxic chemicals. This is a highly complex biological response that is tightly regulated. The immune system plays an important role in defense of the organisms against invading pathogens. Under certain conditions, the immune system can produce toxic chemicals that play an important role in the initiation and progression of chronic diseases as well as can cause autoimmune diseases. Increased oxidative stress and chronic inflammation are associated with the initiation and progression of most chronic human diseases such as cancer, heart disease, arthritis, diabetes, Alzheimer's disease, and Parkinson's disease. Therefore, attenuation of these two biological processes at the same time may reduce the risk of these diseases.

REFERENCES

1. Cotran RSK, Kumar V, Collins T. Disease of immunity. In: *Pathologic Basis of Disease*. New York: W. B. Saunders Company; 1999:188–259.
2. Ryter A. Relationship between ultrastructure and specific functions of macrophages. *Comp Immunol Microbiol Infect Dis*. 1985;8(2):119–133.
3. Langermans JA, Hazenbos WL, van Furth R. Antimicrobial functions of mononuclear phagocytes. *J Immunol Methods*. 1994;174(1–2):185–194.
4. Holtmeier W, Kabelitz D. Gammadelta T cells link innate and adaptive immune responses. *Chem Immunol Allergy*. 2005;86:151–183.
5. Sproul TW, Cheng PC, Dykstra ML, Pierce SK. A role for MHC class II antigen processing in B cell development. *Int Rev Immunol*. 2000;19(2–3):139–155.
6. Kehry MR, Hodgkin PD. B-cell activation by helper T-cell membranes. *Crit Rev Immunol*. 1994;14(3–4):221–238.
7. Asmus K-D., Bonifacio, M. Free radical chemistry. In: Sen CK, Packer L, Hanninen O, eds. *Exercise and Oxygen Toxicity*. New York: Elsevier; 1994:1–47.
8. Vaillancourt F, Fahmi H, Shi Q, Lavigne P, Ranger P, Fernandes JC, Benderdour M. 4-Hydroxynonenal induces apoptosis in human osteoarthritic chondrocytes: The protective role of glutathione-S-transferase. *Arthritis Res Ther*. 2008;10(5):R107.
9. Pryor WA. Oxidants and antioxidants. In: Frei B, ed. *Natural Antioxidants in Human Health and Disease*. New York: Academy press, Inc; 1994:1–24.
10. Kehrer JP, Smith CV. Free radicals in biology: Sources, reactives, and roles in the etiology of human diseases. In: Frei B, ed. *Natural Antioxidants in Human Health and Disease*. New York: Academy Press; 1994:25–62.
11. Litman GW, Cannon JP, Dishaw LJ. Reconstructing immune phylogeny: New perspectives. *Nat Rev Immunol*. 2005;5(11):866–879.
12. Medzhitov R. Recognition of microorganisms and activation of the immune response. *Nature*. 2007;449(7164):819–826.
13. Matzinger P. The danger model: A renewed sense of self. *Science*. 2002;296:301–305.
14. Martin P, Leibovich SJ. Inflammatory cells during wound repair: The good, the bad, and the ugly. *Trends Cell Biol*. 2005;15(11):599–607.
15. Rus H, Cudrici C, Niculescu F. The role of the complement system in innate immunity. *Immunol Res*. 2005;33(2):103–112.

3 Scientific Rationale of Current Trends in Clinical Studies of Micronutrients

INTRODUCTION

Despite extensive basic and clinical research in prevention and progression of chronic diseases such as cancer, heart disease, Alzheimer's disease (AD), and Parkinson's disease (PD) over the past decades, the incidence of these diseases has not significantly changed. As a matter of fact, the incidence of cancer appears to have risen. For example, in 2001, the annual incidence of cancer was 1.1 million new cases; however, in 2017, it was about 1.689 million new cases (CDC 2017). In 2017, the prevalence of cardiovascular disease in the USA was 92.1 million.[1] In 2017, about 5.5 million American suffer from dementia with or without AD. The incidence of AD and other dementia doubles every 5 years beyond the age of 65 years or older, and about 50% of individuals 80 years or older may have dementia with or without AD. Currently, PD affects about 500,000 Americans,[2] and about 50,000 new cases are diagnosed annually.

Despite several randomized, double-blind and placebo-controlled, and non-randomized clinical studies primarily with individual antioxidants in high risk populations, controversy still exists about the usefulness of micronutrient supplements in reducing the risk of chronic diseases. The results of these clinical trials have varied from no effect, beneficial effects, to harmful effects. Repeated reviews and meta-analyses of such clinical studies revealed the same conclusions and recommendations made by the original studies. Fundamental questions arise about whether these clinical trials took into considerations the status of oxidative stress and chronic inflammation that are elevated in high-risk populations, the biology of antioxidants, and the consequences of using a single antioxidant in such populations. After carefully reviewing these studies, I have concluded that the major clinical trials have been performed without the above considerations, and, therefore, the conclusions and recommendations drawn from such clinical studies with respect to the efficacy of antioxidants should be considered inaccurate and misleading.

This chapter discusses the status of oxidative stress and chronic inflammation in high-risk populations, the biology of antioxidants, and the consequences of using a single antioxidant in selected high-risk populations of chronic diseases such as cancer, heart diseases, AD, and PD. This chapter describes an example of a clinical trial (randomized, double-blind, and placebo-controlled) with a single antioxidant for each disease in order to show that these studies were performed without scientific rationale with respect to the use of an antioxidant. The scientific rationale and its supporting evidence for making a shift in the current clinical trial paradigm from one or two micronutrients to multiple micronutrients, together with a high-fiber and low-fat diet to reduce the risk of chronic diseases in high-risk populations are also presented.

LEVELS OF OXIDATIVE STRESS AND CHRONIC INFLAMMATION IN HIGH-RISK POPULATIONS

High levels of oxidative stress and chronic inflammation exist in high-risk populations of cancer, CAD, AD, and PD. However, the sources and mechanisms of inducing increased oxidative stress and chronic inflammations between these high-risk populations may, in part, be different.

HIGH-RISK POPULATIONS OF CANCER

High-risk populations of cancer, which include heavy tobacco smokers and survivors of cancer treatment, have high levels of internal oxidative environment. This is due to the fact that inhalation of smoke generates excessive amounts of free radicals that cause depletion of antioxidants and damage to cells and organs. Long-term survivors of cancer treatment may also have a high internal oxidative environment, because most treatment agents induce increased oxidative stress.[3–5] Markers of pro-inflammatory cytokines such as ineterleukin-6 (IL-6) and tumor necrosis factor-alpha (TNF-alpha) are also elevated in these populations. These high-risk populations are very suitable models to evaluate the efficacy of micronutrients, including antioxidants in reducing the risk of primary cancer (smokers), non-smokers exposed to secondhand smoking, and recurrence of the primary tumor or development of a new cancer (cancer survivors) by well-designed, randomized, double-blind, and placebo-controlled trials.

HIGH-RISK POPULATIONS OF CORONARY ARTERY DISEASE (CAD)

The high-risk populations include individuals with high levels of cholesterol, homocysteine, and C-reactive protein (CRP), and individuals taking a statin with or without any previous cardiac event. The sources of free radicals include cigarette smoking, high homocysteine levels, high glucose levels in diabetes, increase store of free iron, and high-fat and high-caloric diet. In addition to high levels of oxidative stress, high levels of chronic inflammation as evidenced by the presence of increased levels of CRP exist in high-risk populations. These high-risk populations are very suitable models to evaluate the efficacy of micronutrients, including antioxidants in reducing the risk and progression of CAD by well-designed, randomized, double-blind, and placebo-controlled trials.

HIGH-RISK POPULATIONS OF ALZHEIMER'S DISEASE (AD) AND PARKINSON'S DISEASE (PD)

The high-risk populations include individuals over the age of 65 years, individuals with family history, and patients with an early stage disease. The sources of free radicals in the brains of high-risk populations of AD include partially utilized oxygen by the mitochondria, auto-oxidation of acetylcholine, increased production and processing of amyloid precursor proteins (APPs) to beta-amyloid fragments, impaired mitochondrial function, and mutations in APP and presenilins I and II. Reactive microglia releases pro-inflammatory cytokines, which are toxic to cholinergic neurons. The sources of free radicals in the brains of high-risk populations of PD include partially utilized oxygen by the mitochondria, auto-oxidation of dopamine, impaired mitochondrial function, accumulation of free iron in the substantia nigra, overexpression or mutations in alpha-synuclein, and mutations in DJ-1, Parkin, and PINK1 genes, all of which impair mitochondrial function that generate free radicals. Reactive microglia releases pro-inflammatory cytokines, which are toxic to DA neurons. Thus, increased oxidative stress and chronic inflammation exist in both AD and PD. These high-risk populations are very suitable models to evaluate the efficacy of micronutrients including antioxidants in reducing the risk and progression of AD and PD by well-designed, randomized, double-blind, and placebo-controlled trials.

DISTRIBUTIONS AND FUNCTION OF ANTIOXIDANTS

The levels of dietary and endogenous antioxidants markedly vary from one organ to another; they also vary from subcellular compartments to another. Although all antioxidants neutralize free radicals by donating electron to molecules with unpaired electron, they also inhibit the levels of chronic inflammation, markedly alter profiles of several genes, activate a nuclear transcriptional factor Nrf2, and alter expression of microRNAs. It is well established that an individual antioxidant when oxidized acts as a pro-oxidant. Therefore, administration of a single antioxidant in the high-risk populations of cancer, CAD, AD, or PD is expected to increase the risk the chronic diseases after a prolonged consumption because of oxidation of the single antioxidant. Administration of the same single antioxidant with other multiple antioxidants in high-risk populations may produce beneficial effects, because oxidation of a single antioxidant could be counteracted by cooperative reduction by other antioxidants.

The natural forms of vitamin E and beta-carotene are more effective than their synthetic counterparts. For example, natural beta-carotene reduced radiation-induced transformation in mammalian cells in culture, but the synthetic beta-carotene did not.[6] Cells accumulate more of the natural form of vitamin E than the synthetic form.[7] Low doses of vitamin C can stimulate the growth of cancer cells, whereas high doses of the same antioxidant can inhibit the growth of some cancer cells. The results of these studies cannot be extrapolated to humans; however, in high-risk populations of cancer, the possibility of presence of undetectable cancer cells exists. Therefore, administration of low doses of a single antioxidant could enhance the rate of growth of tumor cells, which then become detectable earlier.

It is known that different types of free radicals are produced in the body that has multiple dietary and endogenous antioxidants. Each antioxidant has a different affinity for each of these free radicals, depending upon the cellular environment. Antioxidants are distributed differently in organs and even within the same cells. The gradient of oxygen pressure varies within the cell and tissues. Vitamin E was more effective as a quencher of free radicals in reduced oxygen pressure, whereas beta-carotene and vitamin A are more effective in higher oxygen pressure.[8] Vitamin C is necessary to protect cellular components in aqueous environments, whereas carotenoids and vitamins A and E protect cellular components in nonaqueous environments. Vitamin C also plays an important role in maintaining cellular levels of vitamin E by recycling the vitamin E radical (oxidized) to the reduced (antioxidant) form.[9] Also, the DNA damage produced by oxidized vitamin C can be ameliorated by vitamin E. The form and type of vitamin E used are also important to improve its beneficial effects. It is known that various organs of rats selectively absorb the natural form of vitamin E.[7] It has been established that alpha-tocopheryl-succinate (alpha-TS) is the most effective form of the vitamin E.[10,11] We have reported that oral ingestion of alpha-TS (800 IU/day) for over six months in humans increased plasma levels of not only alpha-tocopherol, but also of alpha-TS, suggesting that alpha alpha-TS can be absorbed from the intestinal tract without hydrolysis to alpha-tocopherol, provided the pool of alpha-tocopherol in the body has become saturated.[11] Selenium is a cofactor of glutathione peroxidase activity, which increases the levels of glutathione. Therefore, selenium supplementation, together with other dietary and endogenous antioxidants, is also essential.

The deficiency of glutathione, an important endogenous antioxidant present in millimolar levels in the cells, is consistently observed in autopsied samples of the brains of both AD and PD patients. Glutathione represents a potent intracellular protective agent against oxidative damage. It catabolizes H_2O_2 and anions and is very effective (in the presence of glutathione peroxidase) in quenching peroxynitrite.[12] Therefore, increasing the intracellular levels of glutathione is essential for the protection of various organelles within the cells. Oral supplementation with glutathione failed to significantly increase plasma levels of glutathione in human subjects,[13] suggesting that this tripeptide is completely hydrolyzed in the gastrointestinal tract. N-acetylcysteine and alpha-lipoic acid enhance the intracellular levels of glutathione by different mechanisms, and therefore, they can also be used in combination with dietary antioxidants. Coenzyme Q10 is needed by the mitochondria to generate energy.

In addition, it also scavenges peroxy radicals faster than alpha-tocopherol,[14] and like vitamin C, can regenerate vitamin E in a redox cycle.[15]

All B-vitamins and vitamin D3 should be combined with multiple antioxidants because at least some studies have reported value of vitamin D3 in cancer risk reduction. B-vitamins are also important for overall health. The importance of B-vitamins and vitamin D3 is discussed in chapters dealing with each chronic disease.

RESULTS OF CLINICAL TRIALS WITH A SINGLE ANTIOXIDANT IN HIGH-RISK POPULATIONS

The issues discussed in the above paragraphs were not considered while designing the clinical trials with antioxidants in high-risk populations of chronic diseases, and this could have contributed to the inconsistent results. Since all clinical studies have been discussed in detail in the chapters of individual diseases, the results of a few clinical trials primarily with one dietary antioxidant in high-risk population of each chronic disease are discussed below. Some of these clinical trials were selected because they are often quoted for not recommending antioxidants in prevention or reducing the rate of progression of chronic diseases.

CANCER

In well-designed clinical studies, an oral administration of synthetic beta-carotene once a day at a dose of 20 mg/day increased the incidence of lung cancer, prostate cancer, and stomach cancer among male heavy tobacco smokers.[16,17] This increase in cancer incidence could have been predicted because beta-carotene in a high internal oxidative environment of heavy smokers would act as a pro-oxidant. In contrast, one would predict that the same dose of beta-carotene would not have a significant effect in normal populations who have a lower internal oxidative environment. Indeed, the same dose of beta-carotene did not affect the incidence of cancer in normal populations who have lower internal oxidative environment than the heavy tobacco smokers.[18] Consumption of vitamin E increased the incidence of secondary cancer after cancer therapy.[19] This observation also could have been predicted for the same reasons as discussed with beta-carotene.

CORONARY ARTERY DISEASE (CAD)

A randomized, double blind, placebo-controlled international trial, Heart Outcomes Prevention Evaluation (HOPE), was conducted from December 21, 1993, to April 15, 1999. One of the objectives of this trial was to evaluate the efficacy of natural vitamin E (400 IU/day) on patients at least 55 years with vascular disease or diabetes; many of them were heavy cigarette smokers in reducing the risk of CAD. The analysis of data published in five separate publications has revealed inconsistent results.

In the analysis published in 2000, the primary endpoints were major cardiac events (myocardial infarction, stroke, and death due to coronary heart disease), and the secondary endpoints were unstable angina, heart failure, revascularization, amputation, or death due to coronary heart disease and complications of diabetes. No significant effect of vitamin E supplementation on primary or secondary endpoints was observed.[20]

In the analysis published in 2001, in a subset of study population, the effect of vitamin E on carotid intimal medial thickness (IMT) as measured by ultrasound was evaluated. The results showed that vitamin E supplementation had no effect on the progression of atherosclerosis.[21]

In the analysis published in 2002, the primary endpoints were same as those in the analysis of 2000, but the secondary endpoints included an additional criterion, nephropathy. The results showed that vitamin E had no effect on either the primary or secondary endpoints.[22]

In the analysis published in 2004, the primary endpoints were the same as those in the analysis of 2000, but the secondary endpoints included an additional criterion, clinical proteinuria (renal insufficiency). The results showed that in people with mild to moderate renal insufficiency, vitamin E had no effect on primary or secondary endpoints.[23]

In the analysis published in 2005, the primary and secondary endpoints were the same as those in the analysis of 2000. The results showed that vitamin E supplementation had no effect on the primary or most secondary endpoints; however, it increased the risk of two secondary endpoints, heart failure by about 13% and hospitalization for heart failure by about 21%.[24]

The analysis of the subpopulation of heavy tobacco smokers revealed that smoking increased the risk of morbidity and mortality among high-risk patients despite the treatment with standard medications known to reduce cardiovascular disease.[25] The is consistent with another independent study (outside HOPE study) in which daily consumption of 800 IU of vitamin E increased the levels of oxidative stress markers in heavy smokers.[26] These studies suggest that smoking plays a dominant role in increasing the morbidity and mortality. If these major cardiac events increased despite gold standard medications that were given to reduce their risk of cardiovascular disease in this population, it is not surprising that administration of vitamin E alone either had no significant effect on all primary endpoints as well as most secondary endpoints or increased the risk of some of the secondary endpoints (heart failure and hospitalization for heart failure) in one study. Individual antioxidant in high-risk populations such as heavy tobacco smokers and type II diabetes may be oxidized because of their high internal oxidative environment and thereby act as a pro-oxidant rather than as an antioxidant.

An analysis of the HOPE study population showed that the levels of markers of inflammation was significantly related to future cardiovascular risk; however, the combination of traditional risk factors and N-terminal pro-brain natriuretic (NTproBNP) provided the best clinical predictive for the secondary prevention population.[27] Thus, the use of single antioxidants in the management of CAD is not recommended.

ALZHEIMER'S DISEASE (AD) AND PARKINSON'S DISEASE (PD)

An analysis of clinical studies revealed that vitamin E may not be useful in the prevention or treatment of AD.[28] Treatment with vitamin E alone produced inconsistent results varying from no effect to some transient beneficial effects. However, a randomized, double-blind, placebo-controlled clinical trial with *dl*-alpha-tocopherol (synthetic form; 2,000 IU/day) in AD patients with moderate to severe impaired cognitive function showed some beneficial effects with respect to rate of deterioration of dementia.[29] The dose of vitamin E used in this trial could produce clotting defects after long-term consumption. This high dose of vitamin E is not recommended for any clinical study or consumption by consumers.

Deprenyl and Tocopherol Antioxidative Therapy of Parkinsonism (DATATOP), a double-blind, placebo-controlled, multicenter clinical trial, was initiated in 1989 in order to evaluate the efficacy of deprenyl (10 mg/day) and dl-tocopherol (2,000 IU/day) individually and in combination in patients with early stage of PD when no therapy was required. The primary outcome was prolongation of the time needed for levodopa therapy. After a follow-up period of 8.2 years, deprenyl significantly delay the time when levodopa therapy was needed, but alpha tocopherol was ineffective.[30,31] The use of single dietary antioxidant vitamin E was a major flaw in this study design in view of the fact that glutathione deficiency in the brain is a consistent finding in most neurodegenerative diseases including PD; therefore, the addition of a glutathione-elevating agent such as alpha-lipoic acid and N-acetylcysteine would have produced at least some transient beneficial effects.. There was another flaw in the DATATOP study design with antioxidant. A multiple vitamin preparation (One A Day™) was allowed for all participants who wished to take it. It was argued that the effect of 30 IU of vitamin E, which was present in the multiple vitamin preparation, would not significantly contribute to the effect of 2,000 IU of vitamin E. This argument may not be valid, since it has been shown that antioxidants, when used individually, had no effect on the growth of mammalian cancer cells in culture, but when they are combined at the same doses produced pronounced effect on the growth inhibition, suggesting antioxidants may interact with each other in a synergistic manner.[32,33] Therefore, the impact of 30 IU of vitamin E in a multiple vitamin preparation would be more pronounced than that produced by 30 IU of vitamin E alone. Hence, the consumption of multiple vitamin preparation with a low dose of vitamin E is likely to create an unacceptable variable while evaluating the efficacy of a high-dose of vitamin E alone in early PD patients. The patients with PD have a high oxidative environment in the brain. It is known that the individual antioxidant, when oxidized, acts as a pro-oxidant. Therefore, the conclusion of the DATATOP study that antioxidants are not useful in reducing the progression of PD is not valid. The extrapolation of data obtained from the use of a single antioxidant to the effects of a multiple antioxidant preparation has no scientific rationale.

WHY THE USE OF A SINGLE ANTIOXIDANT PRODUCED INCONSISTENT RESULTS

Most human epidemiologic studies with the diet showed that certain micronutrients such as antioxidants, and high-fiber and low-fat diet may reduce the risk of chronic diseases such as cancer, heart disease, AD, and PD. However, from these studies it was not clear whether supplementation with antioxidants or low-fat and high-fiber diets can reduce the risk of these diseases. In in vitro and animal models, supplementation with a single antioxidant reduced the levels of oxidative stress and chronic inflammation and inhibited the risk of chemical-induced chronic diseases. This is in contrast to epidemiologic studies in which the diet as a whole, which contain multiple micronutrients including antioxidants, was found to be necessary to reduce the risk of chronic diseases. Most experimental design of clinical trials extrapolated the results of animal studies rather than of epidemiologic studies, and utilized a single antioxidant in order to evaluate its efficacy in reducing the risk or progression of chronic diseases. The results of clinical studies presented above suggested this extrapolation was unfortunate, and future clinical trials should not utilize the results of animal studies in designing clinical trials with antioxidants.

The reasons for individual antioxidants producing no effect, transient beneficial effects, or harmful effect may have been for several reasons: (a) antioxidants show differential subcellular distribution and different mechanisms of action; therefore, a single antioxidant cannot protect all parts of the cell; (b) a single antioxidant in a high internal oxidative environment of patients with neurodegenerative diseases is oxidized and can then itself act as a pro-oxidant rather than as an antioxidant; (c) the body protects against oxidative damage by elevating antioxidant enzymes and dietary and endogenous antioxidants; (d) antioxidants neutralize free radicals by donating electrons to those molecules with unpaired electrons, whereas antioxidant enzymes destroy free radicals by catalysis, converting them to harmless molecules such as water and oxygen. Therefore, both of these events need to be enhanced in concert to achieve substantial therapeutic gain against oxidative damage; (e) the affinity of different antioxidants for free radicals differs, depending upon their lipophilicity; (f) both the aqueous and lipid compartments of the cell need to be protected together. Water-soluble antioxidants such as vitamin C and glutathione protect molecules in the aqueous environment of the cells, whereas lipid soluble antioxidants such as vitamin A and vitamin E protect molecules in the lipid compartment; (g) vitamin E is more effective in quenching free radicals in a reduced oxygenated cellular environment, whereas vitamin C and alpha-tocopherol are more effective in a higher oxygenated environment of the cells[8]; (h) vitamin C is important for recycling the oxidized form of alpha-tocopherol to the antioxidant form at the lipid/aqueous interface[9]; and (i) antioxidants produce cell protective proteins by altering the expression of different microRNAs.[34] For example, some antioxidants can activate Nrf2 by upregulating miR-200a, which inhibits its target protein Keap1, whereas others activate Nrf2 by downregulating miR-21, which binds with 3′-UTR Nrf2 mRNA.[35]

These reasons discussed above suggest that use of a single micronutrient in prevention or improved management of human chronic diseases is not expected to yield any consistent beneficial effects. Nevertheless, most clinical studies continue to utilize a single micronutrient to reduce the risk developing the disease producing inconsistent results. For this reason, a mixture of micronutrients that can simultaneously reduce oxidative stress and inflammation by enhancing the levels of antioxidant enzymes through the activation of Nrf2 pathway together with dietary and endogenous antioxidants for AD and PD has been suggested.[34,36]

Many scientists, researchers, and physicians promote the idea that supplementation with antioxidants can be deleterious to your health and should not be taken by healthy individuals or for reducing the risk of chronic diseases. This idea has no scientific merit.

RESULTS OF CLINICAL STUDIES WITH MULTIPLE DIETARY ANTIOXIDANTS IN CANCER

The administration of multiple dietary antioxidants vitamin A (40,000 IU), vitamin C (2,000 mg), vitamin E (400 IU), zinc (90 mg), and vitamin B6 (100 mg) per day in combination with BCG (Bacilli bilie de Calmette-Guerin) vaccine caused a 50% reduction in the incidence of recurrence of bladder cancer in 5 years, in comparison to control patients who received multiple vitamins containing RDA levels of nutrients and BCG.[37]

Supplementation with antioxidants (vitamin A, 30,000 IU; vitamin C, 1,000 mg; vitamin E, 70 mg) per day reduced the incidence of recurrence of colon polyps from 36% to 6%[38]; however, consumption of synthetic beta-carotene (25 mg), vitamin C (1,000 mg), and vitamin E (400 mg) per day failed to show any beneficial effects on the recurrence of colon polyps.[39] In another study, daily supplementation with vitamin C (4,000 mg) and vitamin E (400 mg) also failed to reduce the risk of colon polyps, but when they were combined with a high fiber diet (more than 12 g/day), there was a significant reduction in the incidence of recurrence of polyps.[40] This study indicated the importance of a high fiber diet in combination with antioxidants in cancer prevention in high- risk populations.

In Linxian General Population Nutrition Interventional Trial, a preparation of multiple dietary antioxidants (beta-carotene, vitamin E, and selenium at doses 2–3 times that of the U.S. RDA) reduced mortality by 10% and cancer incidence by 13%.[41] The beneficial effects of this supplementation on mortality were still evident up to 10 years after the cessation of supplementation and were consistently greater in younger participants.[42]

The combination of vitamins A, C, and E, omega-3 fatty acids, and folic acid significantly reduced recurrence of adenoma in patients after polypectomy.[43] In a randomized placebo-controlled trial involving 80 untreated patients with prostate cancer, daily supplementation with vitamin E, selenium, vitamin C, and coenzyme Q10 did not affect serum levels of prostate specific antigen (PSA).[44] In a randomized, placebo-controlled trial referred to as Selenium and Vitamin E Cancer Prevention Trial (SELECT) involving 35,553 healthy men from 427 participating sites in the United States, Canada, and Puerto Rico with a follow-up period of minimum 7 years and a maximum of 12 years, it was observed that selenium (200 mcg/day) or vitamin E (400 IU/day) alone or in combination did not reduce the risk of prostate cancer.

It is interesting to note that none of the above studies has utilized endogenous antioxidants such as alpha-lipoic acid, N-acetylcysteine, a glutathione-elevating agent, and coenzyme Q10 and L-carnitine. The addition of these antioxidants may have produced consistent beneficial effects in high-risk populations.

From the studies discussed above, it appears that supplementation with one or more dietary antioxidants alone may not be sufficient to produce beneficial and consistent effects on reducing the risk of cancer. Inclusion of endogenous antioxidants may be necessary in any experimental design to test the efficacy of antioxidants in cancer prevention. In recent years, there have been trends to perform meta-analysis of published data in which far-reaching conclusions are made. Since the total number of participating subjects in such analyses becomes huge, numbering hundreds of thousands, the conclusions appear impressive and definitive. However, if the meta-analysis is performed on publications that have flawed experimental designs, the conclusions would be the same that were made in the initial publications. The publications of such meta-analyses are of no scientific value except that they add to the existing misinformation about the value of antioxidants in patients with chronic diseases.

RESULTS OF CLINICAL STUDIES WITH FAT AND FIBER

A review of published data on supplementation with high fiber showed no significant effects on recurrence of adenoma, although most epidemiological studies showed an inverse relationship between consumption of high-fiber diets and cancer incidence. It should be pointed out that a high-fiber diet contains other micronutrients such as multiple antioxidants; thus, the presence of other micronutrients in the diet may have aided to protective effect of a high-fiber diet on cancer incidence. A few clinical studies on supplementation with high fiber alone have produced inconsistent results. These studies are described below.

An intervention study (The Women's health Initiative Dietary Modification Trial) in which postmenopausal women received a low-fat diet (40%) or a high-fat diet (60%) showed that a low-fat diet did not reduce the risk of colorectal cancer during 8.1 years follow-up.[45] I am not sure if a diet in which fat content represents 40% should be considered a low-fat diet. A difference in fat amount of 20% may not be sufficient to exert any protective effect on cancer incidence. I would consider a low-fat diet one that contains no more than 25% of calories from fat. In addition, the protective effect of low fat alone may be minor; therefore, the cancer protective effect of low-fat diet alone cannot be adequately assessed in any intervention trial.

In the Polyp Prevention Trial, dietary intervention with reduced fat and increased consumption of fruits, vegetables, and fibers produced no effect on prostate-specific antigen (PSA) or incidence of prostate cancer in men without prostate cancer.[46] A dietary supplement (13.5 g/day vs. 2 g/day) with wheat-bran fiber did not protect against recurrence of colorectal adenomas.[47] Testing the effect of a high-fiber diet alone in which the difference between control and experimental group is 2 g vs. 13.5 g/day may not yield any significant reduction in cancer incidence, because the effect of additional about 10 g of fiber alone on the risk of cancer may be too small to be detected. Such an interventional trial does not appear to be of any scientific rationale.

In a multi-institutional randomized controlled trial involving 3,088 women previously treated for early stages of breast cancer, supplementation with a diet high in vegetables, fruits, and fiber, and low in fat did not reduce additional breast cancer incidence or mortality during a 7.3 year follow-up period.[4]

The lack of additional micronutrients such as dietary and endogenous antioxidants, B-vitamins, vitamin B3, and calcium may have contributed to the failure of detecting protective effects of a high-fiber and low-fat diet on cancer incidence in the above studies.

No studies have been performed on the role of a high-fiber and low-fat diet in reducing the risk of CAD, AD, or PD. This may be due to the fact that no significant mechanistic studies exist to suggest that they may be important in affecting the incidence or progression of these diseases. However, a low-fat diet could be important for heart, because a high-fat diet can increase levels of cholesterol and triglyceride, a risk factor for CAD. A high-fat diet can also generate increased levels of prostaglandins that contribute to the aggregation of platelets, a risk factor in CAD. Therefore, a high-fiber and low-fat diet is recommended for all chronic diseases discussed in this chapter.

RATIONALE FOR USING A MIXTURE OF MICRONUTRIENTS FOR REDUCING THE RISK AND PROGRESSION OF CHRONIC DISEASES

Increased oxidative stress and chronic inflammation are common effects that initiate and promote most chronic diseases; therefore, attenuation of these abnormalities may reduce the risk and improve management of these diseases. Analysis of studies discussed in above paragraphs suggests that use of a single micronutrient in prevention or improved management of human chronic diseases is not expected to yield any beneficial effects. For this reason, a mixture of micronutrients that can simultaneously reduce oxidative stress and inflammation by enhancing the levels of antioxidant enzymes through the activation of Nrf2 pathway together with dietary and endogenous antioxidants for AD and PD has been suggested.[34,36] Oral supplementation can increase the levels of dietary and endogenous antioxidants; however, elevation of the levels of antioxidant enzymes requires an activation of Nrf2. During acute oxidative stress, ROS is required to activate Nrf2, which then migrate from the cytoplasm to the nucleus where it binds with ARE (antioxidant response element) that allow transcription of genes coding for cytoprotective enzymes, including antioxidant enzymes. During chronic oxidative stress found in chronic diseases, activation of Nrf2 becomes resistant to ROS. However, certain antioxidants and phytochemicals activate Nrf2 without the need for ROS. Activated Nrf2 and certain antioxidants also reduce chronic inflammation.

PROPOSED MIXTURE OF MICRONUTRIENTS FOR REDUCING THE RISK AND PROGRESSION OF CHRONIC DISEASES

A mixture of micronutrients containing vitamin A, mixed carotenoids, vitamin C, α-tocopheryl acetate, α-tocopheryl succinate, vitamin D3, alpha-lipoic acid, N-acetylcysteine, coenzyme Q10, L-carnitine, omega-3 fatty acids, curcumin, resveratrol, all B-vitamins, selenomethionine, and zinc, but without iron, copper, manganese, or heavy metals such as molybdenum and zirconium for healthy aging and for reduction in the functional deficits during aging is proposed. The inclusion of iron, copper, or manganese is not suggested, because these trace minerals, although essential for many biological reactions, combine with vitamin C and generate excessive amounts of free radicals. Furthermore, these minerals are absorbed from the intestine better in the presence of antioxidants than in their absence that could increase body store of free iron, copper, and manganese after long-term consumption. The body has no significant mechanisms of excretion of these trace minerals. Slight increase in the body store of free forms of these trace minerals can increase the risk of most chronic diseases. Heavy metals such as zirconium and molybdenum were not included because the body has no mechanisms of excretion of these heavy metals. Consequently, their levels in the body would increase after long-term consumption. High levels of heavy metals could interfere with the function of organs, including the brain.

It is expected that the proposed micronutrient mixture would increase the levels of antioxidant enzymes by activating the Nrf2 pathway and dietary and endogenous antioxidants that would simultaneously reduce oxidative stress and chronic inflammation.

Most of the clinical studies have utilized a dose schedule of once a day that can create huge fluctuations in the levels of antioxidants in the body. This is because the biological half-lives of micronutrients are highly variable. A 2-fold difference in the levels of certain micronutrients such as alpha-tocopheryl succinate can cause a marked difference in the expression of gene profiles.[48] Therefore, it is recommended that the micronutrient mixture should be taken orally and divided into two doses, half in the morning and the other half in the evening with meals in order to maintain relatively steady levels of micronutrients in the body.

PROPOSED CHANGES IN DIET AND LIFESTYLE FOR REDUCING THE RISK AND PROGRESSION OF CHRONIC DISEASES

Dietary recommendations include daily consuming of a low-fat and high-fiber diet with plenty of fresh fruits and vegetables; avoiding excessive amounts of protein, carbohydrates, or calories; restricting intake of nitrite-rich cured meat or charcoal-broiled or smoked meat or fish; caffeine-containing beverages (cold or hot); and pickled fruits and vegetables.

Lifestyle-related changes include stopping smoking and chewing tobacco; avoiding exposure to secondhand smoke, sun, UV-light for tanning, and hyperbaric therapy for energy; restricting intake of alcohol; reducing stress by vacation, yoga, or meditation; and performing moderate exercise 4–5 times a week.

The efficacy of proposed micronutrient mixtures, together with diet and lifestyle, should be tested by well-designed preclinical and clinical studies. The placebo group in the proposed experimental design should not have any dietary recommendation. Dietary compliances can be monitored by questionnaires, whereas the compliances for the micronutrient group can be monitored by measuring plasma levels of selected micronutrients every six months. The efficacy of proposed micronutrient mixtures in high-risk population of cancer is testable. One may argue that this experimental design is complicated, because at the end of the study we may not know for certain which particular micronutrient was responsible for cancer risk reduction. This argument may not be valid, because the aim of any clinical study is to achieve success in reducing the risk of cancer. For a mechanistic study on micronutrients, animal and cell culture models are most suitable.

Meanwhile, the proposed recommendations may be adopted in consultation with physicians or health professionals. It is expected that these recommendations, if adopted, may reduce the risk of chronic diseases and improve management of these diseases.

CONCLUSIONS

Increased oxidative stress and chronic inflammation are involved in the initiation and progression of most chronic diseases. To address this issue, randomized, double-blind, placebo-controlled, and non-randomized clinical trials primarily with a single dietary antioxidant in high-risk populations, such as cancer, coronary artery disease (CAD), Alzheimer's disease, (AD) and Parkinson's disease (PD) were performed. The results of these trials have varied from no effects, transient beneficial effects, to harmful effects. The scientific reasons for the inconsistent results with single antioxidants were presented and suggested for a shift in the clinical study paradigm from using one dietary antioxidant or endogenous antioxidant alone to multiple micronutrients. In order to simultaneously reduce oxidative stress and chronic inflammation, it is essential to increase the levels of antioxidant enzymes through the activation of Nrf2/ARE pathway, and dietary and endogenous antioxidants. A micronutrient mixture that would achieve the above goal was proposed. Modifications in diet and lifestyle were also suggested. The recommended micronutrient mixture together with changes in diet and lifestyle should be tested in high-risk populations of chronic diseases by well-designed randomized, double-blind, placebo-controlled trials.

REFERENCES

1. Association AH. Heart disease and stroke statistics 2017.
2. NINDS. *Parkinson's Disease: A Research Planning Workshop.* Bethesda, MD: National Instutute of Health; 2008.
3. Rourke MT, Hobbie WL, Schwartz L, Kazak AE. Posttraumatic stress disorder (PTSD) in young adult survivors of childhood cancer. *Pediatr Blood Cancer.* 2007;49(2):177–182.
4. Thomson CA, Stendell-Hollis NR, Rock CL, Cussler EC, Flatt SW, Pierce JP. Plasma and dietary carotenoids are associated with reduced oxidative stress in women previously treated for breast cancer. *Cancer Epidemiol Biomarkers Prev.* 2007;16(10):2008–2015.
5. Zhao W, Diz DI, Robbins ME. Oxidative damage pathways in relation to normal tissue injury. *Br J Radiol.* 2007;80(Spec No 1):S23–S31.
6. Kennedy AR, Krinsky NI. Effects of retinoids, beta-carotene, and canthaxanthin on UV- and X-ray-induced transformation of C3H10T1/2 cells in vitro. *Nutr Cancer.* 1994;22(3):219–232.
7. Ingold KU, Burton GW, Foster DO, Hughes L, Lindsay DA, Webb A. Biokinetics of and discrimination between dietary RRR- and SRR-alpha-tocopherols in the male rat. *Lipids.* 1987;22(3):163–172.

8. Vile GF, Winterbourn CC. Inhibition of adriamycin-promoted microsomal lipid peroxidation by beta-carotene, alpha-tocopherol, and retinol at high and low oxygen partial pressures. *FEBS Letters.* 1988;238(2):353–356.

9. Niki E. Interaction of ascorbate and alpha-tocopherol. *Ann N Y Acad Sci.* 1987;498:186–199.

10. Carini R, Poli G, Dianzani MU, Maddix SP, Slater TF, Cheeseman KH. Comparative evaluation of the antioxidant activity of alpha-tocopherol, alpha-tocopherol polyethylene glycol 1000 succinate and alpha-tocopherol succinate in isolated hepatocytes and liver microsomal suspensions. *Biochem Pharmacol.* 1990;39(10):1597–1601.

11. Prasad KN, Kumar B, Yan XD, Hanson AJ, Cole WC. Alpha-tocopheryl succinate, the most effective form of vitamin E for adjuvant cancer treatment: A review. *J Am Coll Nutr.* 2003;22(2):108–117.

12. Sies H, Sharov VS, Klotz LO, Briviba K. Glutathione peroxidase protects against peroxynitrite-mediated oxidations: A new function for selenoproteins as peroxynitrite reductase. *J Biol Chem.* 1997;272(44):27812–27817.

13. Witschi A, Reddy S, Stofer B, Lauterburg BH. The systemic availability of oral glutathione. *Eur J Clin Pharmacol.* 1992;43(6):667–669.

14. Niki E. Mechanisms and dynamics of antioxidant action of ubiquinol. *Mol Aspects Med.* 1997;18(Suppl):S63–S70.

15. Stoyanovsky DA, Osipov AN, Quinn PJ, Kagan VE. Ubiquinone-dependent recycling of vitamin E radicals by superoxide. *Arch Biochem Biophys.* 1995;323(2):343–351.

16. Albanes D, Heinonen OP, Huttunen JK, et al. Effects of alpha-tocopherol and beta-carotene supplements on cancer incidence in the Alpha-Tocopherol Beta-Carotene Cancer Prevention Study. *Am J Clin Nutr.* 1995;62(6 Suppl):1427S–1430S.

17. Bowen DJ, Thornquist M, Anderson K, et al. Stopping the active intervention: CARET. *Control Clin Trials.* 2003;24(1):39–50.

18. Hennekens CH, Buring JE, Manson JE, et al. Lack of effect of long-term supplementation with beta carotene on the incidence of malignant neoplasms and cardiovascular disease. *N Engl J Med.* 1996;334(18):1145–1149.

19. Bairati I, Meyer F, Gelinas M, et al. Randomized trial of antioxidant vitamins to prevent acute adverse effects of radiation therapy in head and neck cancer patients. *J Clin Oncol.* 2005;23(24):5805–5813.

20. Yusuf S, Dagenais G, Pogue J, Bosch J, Sleight P. Vitamin E supplementation and cardiovascular events in high-risk patients. *N Engl J Med.* 2000;342(3):154–160.

21. Vollset SE, Clarke R, Lewington S, et al. Effects of folic acid supplementation on overall and site-specific cancer incidence during the randomised trials: Meta-analyses of data on 50,000 individuals. *Lancet.* 2013;381(9871):1029–1036.

22. Lonn E, Yusuf S, Hoogwerf B, et al. Effects of vitamin E on cardiovascular and microvascular outcomes in high-risk patients with diabetes: Results of the HOPE study and MICRO-HOPE substudy. *Diabetes Care.* 2002;25(11):1919–1927.

23. Baum MK, Campa A, Lai S, et al. Effect of micronutrient supplementation on disease progression in asymptomatic, antiretroviral-naive, HIV-infected adults in Botswana: A randomized clinical trial. *JAMA.* 2013;310(20):2154–2163.

24. Schneider JM, Fujii ML, Lamp CL, Lonnerdal B, Dewey KG, Zidenberg-Cherr S. Anemia, iron deficiency, and iron deficiency anemia in 12–36-mo-old children from low-income families. *Am J Clin Nutr.* 2005;82(6):1269–1275.

25. Lonn E, Bosch J, Yusuf S, et al. Effects of long-term vitamin E supplementation on cardiovascular events and cancer: A randomized controlled trial. *Jama.* 2005;293(11):1338–1347.

26. Weinberg RB, VanderWerken BS, Anderson RA, Stegner JE, Thomas MJ. Pro-oxidant effect of vitamin E in cigarette smokers consuming a high polyunsaturated fat diet. *Arterioscler Thromb Vasc Biol.* 2001;21(6):1029–1033.

27. Blankenberg S, McQueen MJ, Smieja M, et al. Comparative impact of multiple biomarkers and N-Terminal pro-brain natriuretic peptide in the context of conventional risk factors for the prediction of recurrent cardiovascular events in the Heart Outcomes Prevention Evaluation (HOPE) Study. *Circulation.* 2006;114(3):201–208.

28. Isaac MG, Quinn R, Tabet N. Vitamin E for Alzheimer's disease and mild cognitive impairment. *Cochrane Database Syst Rev.* 2008(3):CD002854.

29. Sano M, Ernesto C, Thomas RG, et al. A controlled trial of selegiline, alpha-tocopherol, or both as treatment for Alzheimer's disease: The Alzheimer's Disease Cooperative Study. *N Engl J Med.* 1997;336(17):1216–1222.

30. Shoulson I. DATATOP: A decade of neuroprotective inquiry—Parkinson Study Group. Deprenyl and Tocopherol Antioxidative Therapy of Parkinsonism. *Ann Neurol.* 1998;44(3 Suppl 1):S160–S166.
31. Group TPS. Effects of tocopherol and deprenyl on the progression of disability in early parkinson's disease. *N Engl J Med.* 1993:176–183.
32. Prasad KN, Hernandez C, Edwards-Prasad J, Nelson J, Borus T, Robinson WA. Modification of the effect of tamoxifen, cis-platin, DTIC, and interferon-alpha 2b on human melanoma cells in culture by a mixture of vitamins. *Nutr Cancer.* 1994;22(3):233–245.
33. Prasad KN, Kumar R. Effect of individual and multiple antioxidant vitamins on growth and morphology of human nontumorigenic and tumorigenic parotid acinar cells in culture. *Nutr Cancer.* 1996;26(1):11–19.
34. Prasad KN. Oxidative stress and pro-inflammatory cytokines may act as one of signals for regulating microRNAs expression in Alzheimer's disease. *Mech Ageing Dev.* 2017;162:63–71.
35. Wu H, Kong L, Tan Y, et al. C66 ameliorates diabetic nephropathy in mice by both upregulating NRF2 function via increase in miR-200a and inhibiting miR-21. *Diabetologia.* 2016;59:1558–1568.
36. Prasad KN. Simultaneous activation of Nrf2 and elevation of antioxidant compounds for reducing oxidative stress and chronic inflammation in human Alzheimer's disease. *Mech Ageing Dev.* 2016;153:41–47.
37. Lamm DL, Riggs DR, Shriver JS, van Gilder PF, Rach JF, DeHaven JI. Megadose vitamins in bladder cancer: A double-blind clinical trial. *J Urol.* 1994;151(1):21–26.
38. Roncucci L, Di Donato P, Carati L, et al. Antioxidant vitamins or lactulose for the prevention of the recurrence of colorectal adenomas: Colorectal Cancer Study Group of the University of Modena and the Health Care District 16. *Dis Colon Rectum.* 1993;36(3):227–234.
39. Greenberg ER, Baron JA, Tosteson TD, et al. A clinical trial of antioxidant vitamins to prevent colorectal adenoma: Polyp Prevention Study Group. *N Engl J Med.* 1994;331(3):141–147.
40. DeCosse JJ, Miller HH, Lesser ML. Effect of wheat fiber and vitamins C and E on rectal polyps in patients with familial adenomatous polyposis. *J Natl Cancer Inst.* 1989;81(17):1290–1297.
41. Blot WJ, Li JY, Taylor PR, et al. Nutrition intervention trials in Linxian, China: Supplementation with specific vitamin/mineral combinations, cancer incidence, and disease-specific mortality in the general population. *J Natl Cancer Inst.* 1993;85(18):1483–1492.
42. Qiao YL, Dawsey SM, Kamangar F, et al. Total and cancer mortality after supplementation with vitamins and minerals: Follow-up of the Linxian General Population Nutrition Intervention Trial. *J Natl Cancer I.* 2009;101(7):507–518.
43. Biasco G, Paganelli GM. European trials on dietary supplementation for cancer prevention. *Ann N Y Acad Sci.* 1999;889:152–156.
44. Hoenjet KM, Dagnelie PC, Delaere KP, Wijckmans NE, Zambon JV, Oosterhof GO. Effect of a nutritional supplement containing vitamin E, selenium, vitamin c and coenzyme Q10 on serum PSA in patients with hormonally untreated carcinoma of the prostate: A randomised, placebo-controlled study. *Eur Urol.* 2005;47(4):433–439; discussion 439–440.
45. Wactawski-Wende J, Kotchen JM, Anderson GL, et al. Calcium plus vitamin D supplementation and the risk of colorectal cancer. *N Engl J Med.* 2006;354(7):684–696.
46. Shike M, Latkany L, Riedel E, et al. Lack of effect of a low-fat, high-fruit, -vegetable, and -fiber diet on serum prostate-specific antigen of men without prostate cancer: Results from a randomized trial. *J Clin Oncol.* 2002;20(17):3592–3598.
47. Alberts DS, Martinez ME, Roe DJ, et al. Lack of effect of a high-fiber cereal supplement on the recurrence of colorectal adenomas. Phoenix Colon Cancer Prevention Physicians' Network. *N Engl J Med.* 2000;342(16):1156–1162.
48. Prasad KN. Alpha-tocopheryl succinate exhibits potent anticancer activity: Its interaction with ionizing radiation and chemotherapy effects. In: Reddy VR, Watson RR, eds. *The Encyclopedia of Vitamin E.* London, UK: CAB International; 2007.

4 Micronutrients in Healthy Aging and Age-Related Decline in Organ Functions

INTRODUCTION

Aging in humans is the result of complex biological processes that are influenced by genetics and environmental-, dietary-, and lifestyle-related factors. Aging in general terms can be defined as a process in which the function of individual organs gradually declines. Most chronic diseases in humans are a reflection of deterioration of the function of individual organs, each of which loses its function at a different rate, depending on genetics and environmental-, dietary-, and lifestyle-related stressors. The higher the levels of one or more of these stressors, the greater would be the rate of loss of organ function. Individual organs may exhibit differential sensitivity to these stressors; therefore, loss of function in the individual organs may appear at a different rate. The loss of function of cholinergic neurons in the brain can lead to Alzheimer's disease (AD), just as the loss of dopaminergic neurons in the brain can lead to Parkinson's disease (PD). In case of familial gene defects, the processes of loss of function in these neurons are accelerated; therefore, these neurological diseases appear at an early age.

The loss of function in one organ may seriously affect other organs, eventually causing death. For example, damage to the vascular system, such as occlusion of major arteries, can cause damage to the heart muscle that can lead to death. Cancer, in which cells gain function, should not be considered part of the normal aging process. Such causes of death should not be taken into consideration while estimating the lifespan of a population.

Aging on the cellular level has been defined on the basis of programmed cell death, which presumes that all cells are genetically programmed to die within a specified time and that no intervention with pharmacological or physiological agents can change this destiny. However, the concept of programmed cell death can be applicable to those dividing cells that are eliminated during embryogenesis, and also those adult precursor cells that divide, differentiate and die within a specified time interval. These precursor cells have a finite lifespan that varies depending upon the organ. I suggest that the concept of programmed cell death should not apply to nondividing cells such as liver cells, muscle cells, and neurons. In these cells, it is the accumulation of the level of epigenetic damage, rather than the genetic damage that determines the rate of cell death. The epigenetic damages can be caused by increased oxidative stress that can cause mitochondrial dysfunction, chronic inflammation, and reduce proteasome activity that progress gradually and eventually lead to cell death. The extent of epigenetic damage is dependent upon the levels of exposure to environmental, dietary, and lifestyle-related stressors.

Aging on the genetic levels is complex. There is no doubt that extensive alterations occur at the transcriptional, post-transcriptional, and pre- and post-translational levels during aging. These changes could be organ-specific and cell-specific. The gene defects causing premature aging have been identified in mice[1] and humans.[2] Mice model of premature aging has been used as an experimental model to study the mechanisms of aging.

Healthy aging is defined as a process during which the rate of loss of organ function is markedly reduced, thereby providing a good quality of life for a long period of time. At present, it is unknown whether the rate of aging can be reduced by pharmacological or physiological intervention.

Despite decades of laboratory research, it has not been possible to develop a rational guideline for healthy aging (reduced rate of loss of function). Among various biochemical and genetic changes that can influence the rate of aging, oxidative stress and pro-inflammatory cytokines released during chronic inflammation appear to be one of the earliest events that play a dominant role in determining the rate of aging. If this is the case, supplementation with nontoxic agents such as antioxidants and phytochemicals that can simultaneously reduce oxidative stress and chronic inflammation would reduce the rate of aging. The linkage between the increased oxidative stress and aging appears to be also applicable to lower organisms such as *Drosophila melanogaster*, nematodes, and birds.

This chapter describes trends of aging in the USA population and presents evidence for the involvement of increased oxidative stress and chronic inflammation in aging. It discusses the role of microRNAs in aging as well as the potential role of activation of Nrf2 (a nuclear transcriptional factor-2) in enhancing the levels of cytoprotective enzymes including antioxidant enzymes and phase-2-detoxifying enzymes. This chapter also proposes that in order to simultaneously reduce oxidative stress and chronic inflammation, it is essential to enhance the levels of cytoprotective enzymes through the activation of Nrf2/ARE pathway and dietary and endogenous antioxidants, and proposes a mixture of micronutrients that together with changes in diet and lifestyle would achieves the above goal.

TRENDS OF AGING POPULATION

It is estimated that the number of people ages 65 years and older would increase from 46 million in 2016 to more than 98 million by 2060. The proportion of this group of population during this period would increase from 15% to 24%. (Fact Sheet: Aging in the United States, The Population Reference Bureau Report, 2016). In 2017, Census Bureau Reports show that the number of people ages 65 years and older grew from 35 million in 2000 to 49.2 million in 2016. The growth proportion of this group of individuals in total population during this period increased from 12.4% to 15.2%. Incidence of age-related chronic diseases such as dementia, diabetes, cancer, heart diseases, and other chronic illnesses are increasing during the last decades. If this trend continues, medical costs of taking care of this population would proportionally increase. Therefore, it is essential to develop novel strategies for healthy aging that would reduce the risk of age-related diseases. In order to develop such strategies, it would be important to identify cellular defects that are associated with aging and age-related chronic diseases.

EVIDENCE FOR INCREASED OXIDATIVE STRESS DURING AGING

Increased production of free radicals causes oxidative damage to cells. This damage is referred to as oxidative stress. If oxidative damage is not repaired, chronic inflammation sets in motion. Among various theories of aging, the free radical theory has strongest support from data obtained from different organisms including flies, birds, mammals, and humans. Direct evidence for the involvement of oxidative stress in aging comes from the studies in which markers of oxidative damage were measured during aging, whereas indirect evidence come from the fact that supplementation with antioxidants or phytochemicals reduce oxidative stress and age-related decline in organ function. Before discussing the evidence for the role of increased oxidative stress in aging, it is important to know about their sources of free radicals and cellular sites where they are produced.

EXTRACELLULAR SOURCES FOR PRODUCTION OF FREE RADICALS

Environmental stressors that can increase oxidative stress in humans include extreme heat and cold, high levels of ozone in air, excessive amounts of dust particles in air, intense sound or vibration, and pathogenic bacteria or viruses. Dietary factors include high-caloric intake, daily consumption of increased amounts of iron, manganese, or copper, and ingestion of xenobiotic substances. Free radicals are produced during normal metabolism of certain compounds. During degradation of fatty acids and oxidative metabolism of ingested xenobiotic substances, free radicals are produced. Some enzymes during their normal degradation of their substrates generate free radicals. Monoamine oxidase, tyrosine hydroxylase, and L-amino acid oxidases produce hydrogen peroxide as a normal by-product of their activity.[3] Other enzymes such as xanthine oxidase and aldehyde oxidase also form superoxide anions during metabolism of their substrates. Auto-oxidation of ascorbate and catecholamines generate free radicals.[4] In addition, calcium-dependent activation of phospholipase A2 releases arachidonic acid, which liberates $O_2^{\bullet-}$ during the synthesis of eicosanoids.[5] Stimulation of glutamate receptor NMDA (n-methyl-D-aspartate) produces excessive amounts of $O_2^{\bullet-}$ and OH$^{\bullet}$.[6] Certain lifestyle-related factors such as cigarette smoking can increase the level of nitric oxide (NO)[7,8] and oxidation of NO produces peroxynitrite, a highly reactive species of radicals. Smoking also depletes antioxidants[9,10] and thereby further increases the oxidative stress in smokers. Free iron and copper can increase oxidative stress by combining with the molecules like vitamin C.[11]

CELLULAR SITES OF PRODUCTION OF FREE RADICALS

Mitochondria are the major site where free radicals derived from oxygen are generated[12–14]; they include superoxide (O_2^-), hydrogen peroxide (H_2O_2), hydroxyl radical (HO$^{\bullet}$), and nitric oxide (NO$^{\bullet}$). The oxidation of NO$^{\bullet}$ forms another type of free radicals called peroxynitrite, which is very damaging to cells, especially nerve cells. Free radicals are also produced in the cytoplasm by oxidases. This theory of free radicals in aging proposes that increased production of free radicals by mitochondria contribute to the cellular damage during advancing age.[15,16] During normal aerobic respiration, the mitochondria of one nerve cell of a rat will process about 10^{12} oxygen molecules and reduce them to water. During this process, superoxide anion ($O_2^{\bullet-}$), hydrogen peroxide (H_2O_2), and hydroxyl (OH$^{\bullet}$) radicals are produced. It has been estimated that about 2% of partially reduced oxygen are leaks out from the mitochondria to generate approximately 20 billion molecules of superoxide anion and hydrogen peroxide per cell.[12,17] The mitochondria are very susceptible to oxidative damage because the mitochondrial DNA (mt DNA) is not protected by histones or DNA-binding proteins. Therefore, it is not surprising that they are easily damaged by free radicals during aging. The damaged mitochondria can produce more free radicals. The role of oxidative stress in aging has been reviewed.[18,19] Based on the published studies, I propose that free radical-induced damage to mitochondria is the first damage that initiate cascade of events such as more production of free radicals, shortening of telomeres, reduced proteasome activity, chronic inflammation, and impaired immune function that are associated with aging. These cellular abnormalities contribute to age-related decline in organ function and chronic diseases.

Phagocytes also produce free radicals that include superoxide, hydrogen peroxide, nitric oxide, and hypochlorous (HOCl).[13,20,21] Hypochlorous is a strong inducer of inflammation and also acts as a strong oxidizing and chlorinating agent and can form nitryl chloride (NO_2Cl) and nitrogen dioxide ($NO_2^{\bullet}$), in the presence of nitrite,[22] all of which are toxic to cells. In addition to phagocytes, activated human polymorphonuclear neutrophils convert nitrite into NO_2Cl and $NO_2^{\bullet}$.[23] Thus, increased production of reactive oxygen species (ROS), reactive nitrogen species (RNS), and chlorinated species that can increase oxidative stress and thereby increase the rate of aging.

In addition to reactive oxygen and nitrogen species, there are other damaging molecules produced by lipid peroxidation. For example, peroxidation of membrane phospholipids acyl chains generates reactive carbonyl species (alpha-, beta-unsaturated aldehydes, di-aldehydes, and keto-aldehydes), which are relatively stable. These carbonyl species can diffuse from one subcellular compartment to another within the same cell or they can escape from the cells and damage targets far away from the site of formation. These carbonyl species react with cellular constituents and form advanced lipoxidation end products (ALEs), and they play an important role in accelerating aging process.[24]

This is supported by the fact that the level of ALEs in several tissues and species increases with age, and dietary restriction that increases the lifespan and decreases the levels of AELs.

The oxidation and nitration of intracellular proteins play an important role in aging because they can induce loss of function.[25] The oxidized proteins can easily form aggregates that also contribute to the loss of cell function. Normally, damaged proteins are removed by the proteasome activity; however, if this pathway is impaired, the damaged proteins will accumulate to cause progressive loss in cell function, and, eventually, cell death. A progressive increase in oxidative stress in the brain is strongly implicated in the gradual decline of cognitive function with aging.

Heavy metals at high concentrations are toxic to humans and animals. Metal homeostasis is regulated by a metal-responsive transcriptional factor (MTF-1). Mutation in the MTF-1 reduced the lifespan of *Drosophila melanogaster*, suggesting that the wild-type MTF-1 is an essential component for maintaining the normal lifespan. The overexpression of MTF-1 in neurons protects against oxidative damage and prolongs the lifespan of Cu/Zn superoxide dismutase-deficient flies.[26]

OXIDATIVE STRESS-INDUCED AGE-RELATED DECLINE IN ORGANELLE FUNCTIONS

MITOCHONDRIAL DYSFUNCTION

Among various organelles in the cells, mitochondria exhibit unique functions. They are present in all cells but most abundantly in nondividing cells such as liver cells, neurons, and muscle cells. The main function of mitochondria is to generate energy. However, they are the major source of free radicals derived from oxygen, and at the same time, they are very vulnerable to free radicals. Damaged mitochondria produce more free radicals, and this creates a vicious cycle of damage by free radicals and production of more free radicals.

Various organs may age at a different rate depending upon the levels of oxidative damage to the mitochondria in the individual cells of that organ. Several studies suggest that damage to the mitochondria may initiate degenerative changes in the cells during aging of at least nondividing organs such as liver, brain, muscle, and bone. Several animal studies have shown that age-associated increase in the generation of free radicals by the mitochondria occurs. For example, the levels of $(O_2^{\cdot-})$ and H_2O_2 increased with aging in the mitochondria isolated from the aged heart of gerbils.[27] The generation of H_2O_2 by mitochondria from older hepatocytes of rats increases by 23%.[28] In houseflies, the rate of the production of H_2O_2 progressively increases with age.[29]

The increased production of free radicals by the mitochondria with age may cause increased rate of mutation in the mitochondrial DNA (mtDNA) and oxidative damage to proteins. Indeed, it has been proposed that mutations in the mitochondria may contribute to accelerated aging.[30] The mtDNA is especially sensitive to oxidative damage, because it is not protected by histones or DNA-binding proteins. It also has either no repair mechanisms, or repair mechanisms are less efficient in comparison to nuclear DNA.[31] The progressive damage to mitochondria may reduce production of energy and, therefore, can cause progressive degenerative changes in the cells during aging, and eventually, loss of function of organs involved. Mitochondrial dysfunction leads to reduced lifespan in yeast.[32] In mammals, aged tissues produce reduced amounts of ATP by oxidative phosphorylation.[33] Indeed, aging of the mammalian brain exhibits a gradual but continuous decrease in production of ATP by reduced oxidative phosphorylation in the mitochondria.[34]

Mitochondrial dysfunction also plays a major role in vascular aging.[35,36] Vascular aging is primarily characterized by an impaired endothelium-dependent vasodilation that is regulated by nitric oxide (NO). The expression of endothelial nitric oxide synthase (eNOS) is markedly upregulated in the endothelial cells with increasing age, resulting in production of excessive amounts of NO. Increased levels of super oxide $(O_2^{\cdot-})$ are also produced. The combination of superoxide and nitric oxide can form peroxynitrite ($ONOO^-$). Peroxynitrite causes oxidative modification of proteins that contribute to vascular aging.

The plasma cysteine/acid soluble thiol ratio, an indicator of redox state, is increased in old age, and this increase may account for the loss of body cell mass that is associated with aging in humans. This is further supported by the fact that supplementation with N-acetylcysteine caused an increase in body cell mass of healthy subjects with high plasma cysteine/thiol ratio.[37,38] Increased oxidative stress and mitochondrial dysfunction are also associated with some age-related neurological diseases such as AD and Parkinson's disease,[39–41] as well as the genetic basis of these neurological diseases. A few reviews have further elucidated the role of mitochondrial dysfunction in aging.[42,43]

IMPAIRMENT OF PROTEASOME AND LYSOSOMAL-MEDIATED PROTEOLYTIC ACTIVITIES

Progressive loss of muscle mass (sarcopenia) during aging occurs in both humans and rodents. There could be several reasons for this. It has been proposed that reduced degradation of oxidized proteins may be one of the factors that contribute to sarcopenia.[44] The cells can respond successfully to oxidative damage of proteins only when the ability of proteasome and lysosome to degrade altered proteins remains intact. Increased oxidative stress can impair proteasome activity as well as lysosomal-mediated proteolytic activity. Indeed, during aging these two biological processes are impaired.[44–47]

OXIDATIVE STRESS-INDUCED CHANGES IN CELL CULTURE MODELS

Treatment of young and older human endothelial cells in culture with H_2O_2 (hydrogen peroxide) showed a progressive increase in TBARS (thiobarbituric acid-reactive substances), a marker of oxidative damage, and decrease in expression of deacetylase Sirtuin 1 (Sirt1) and its target gene forkhead box O3a (Foxo3a) in both cell types, but the extent of these biochemical changes was more in older cells than in young cells. In addition, the levels of beta-galactosidase, a marker of senescence, markedly increased in older cells compared with young cells.[48]

OXIDATIVE STRESS-INDUCED CHANGES IN ANIMAL MODELS

The degeneration of lumbar intervertebral disc is associated with aging. In order to investigate the role of oxidative stress in this disease, youth, adult, and geriatric rats were used. The results showed that the levels of antioxidant enzyme SOD gradually declined with age in both serum and intervertebral disc, whereas the levels of MDA and advanced oxidation of protein products (AOPPs), markers of oxidative damage, increased.[49] Loss of bones was also associated with increased levels of AOPPs and MDA and decreased levels of SOD in older rats.[50] In senescence-accelerated mouse 10 (SAMP10), the levels of SOD decreased and the levels of MDA increased in the brain tissue. These biochemical changes were associated with deceased thickness of cortical regions and the number of Nissl bodies.[51]

OXIDATIVE STRESS-INDUCED SHORTENING OF THE LENGTH OF TELOMERE

Telomeres consist of a repetitive sequences of TTAGGG located at the end of chromosome needed for the replication of DNA. Telomerase reverse transcriptase (TRT) is the catalytic subunit of telomerase enzyme that is responsible for maintaining telomere length by adding telomere repeats TTAGGG at the end. On the other hand, telomeric repeat-binding factor-2 (TRF-2) is needed for the telomere maintenance, cell cycle progression, and protection of the ends to avoid chromosomal fusion.[52,53] One of the widely held hypotheses is that aging of mammalian cells is due to the shortening of telomere length.[54] This is supported by the fact that point mutations within the telomere cause accelerated attrition of telomere length and also lead to premature aging.[55] There is substantial evidence to show that increased oxidative stress and inflammation play a central role in shortening the length of telomeres possibly by decreasing the activity of telomerase and/or TRF-2 level. The data on the role of telomere in human aging come primarily from the normal human fibroblasts or other normal cells in culture. These studies suggest that telomere shortening is associated with aging and that increased oxidative stress accelerates the rate of telomere shortening.[56,57] Increased oxidative stress induced translocation of nuclear telomerase reverse transcriptase (TERT) from the nucleus to the cytoplasm.[58] Treatment with N-acetylcysteine (NAC) reduced the translocation of nuclear TERT from the nucleus to the cytoplasm.[58] The increase in oxidative stress caused pre-mature aging of normal endothelial cells in culture. The role of oxidative stress in telomere shortening is further supported by the fact that dietary antioxidants vitamin C[59] and vitamin E[60] reduced the rate of telomere shortening. The role oxidative stress and inflammation in shortening of telomere length associated with aging and age-related chronic diseases have been recently reviewed.[61]

EVIDENCE FOR CHRONIC INFLAMMATION DURING AGING

If oxidative damage of cells is not repaired, chronic inflammation sets in motion. During chronic inflammation, pro-inflammatory cytokines such as tumor necrosis factor-alpha (TNF-alpha) and interleukin-6 (IL-6) are released. Prostaglandins, adhesion molecules, and complement proteins are also released all of which are toxic to the cells. The increased levels of these products of chronic inflammation can enhance the rate of degenerative changes in the cells and enhance the rate of aging and the risk of age-related chronic diseases. The microglia in the aged brain have increased levels of a pro-inflammatory cytokine TNF-alpha.[62] Treatment with TNF-alpha plus beta-amyloid (Aβ-42), a fragment of amyloid precursor protein (APP), caused more toxicity in the older neurons than in the younger neurons.[62] In addition, it has been suggested that TNF-alpha treatment caused nuclear translocation of nuclear factor kappa-beta (NF-kappa-B) in neurons.[63] This phenomenon together with the lower level of Bcl-2 promoted cell death in older neurons.[63] It has been reported that treatment of neuron obtained from middle-aged rats with TNF-alpha and Aβ-42 increased TNF receptors (TNFR1 and TNFR2); however, similarly treated older neurons do not increase these surface receptors of TNF-alpha.[64] Chronic inflammation also has been linked with several age-related chronic diseases such as Alzheimer's disease, Parkinson's disease, cardiovascular disease, and diabetes type II.[40,65–67] Higher blood levels of pro-inflammatory cytokine IL-6 are associated with increased risk of knee osteoarthritis progression.[68] Higher levels of IL-6 and TNF-alpha in the skeletal muscle impair regenerative capacity of skeletal muscle in the older population.[69]

Increased mitochondrial oxidative stress activates NF-kappa-B in the endothelial cells of blood vessels that enhances the expression of inflammatory genes.[70] Age-related increase in oxidative stress may promote vascular inflammation.[71] Thus, aged blood vessels exhibit increased NF-kappaB activity. This was attributed to increased oxidative stress that occurs during aging.[70]

Higher plasma concentrations of IL-6 and TNF-alpha are associated with lower muscle mass and lower muscle strength in well-functioning older men and women.[72] This suggests that pro-inflammatory cytokines contribute to the loss of muscle mass and muscle strength that are associated with aging. In another study, higher plasma levels of IL-6 and C-reactive proteins increased the risk of loss of muscle strength in older men and women, whereas higher levels of alpha1-antichymotrypsin decreased the risk of muscle strength loss.[73] Higher plasma levels of IL-6 predict onset of disability in older individuals.[74] This may be due to the fact that increased levels of IL-6 contribute to muscle atrophy and may increase the risk of certain chronic diseases.

IMPAIRED IMMUNE FUNCTION IN AGING

Phagocytes are one of the major sources of free radicals and represent one of the functions of immune system. Normally, phagocytes attack and eliminate invading pathogenic organisms by generating excessive amounts of oxidants such as superoxide ($O^{•-}$), nitric oxide ($NO^{•}$), H_2O_2, and HOCl, and engulfing them through phagocytosis. The engulfed microorganisms are killed and eliminated by a combination of oxidants and lysosomal digestive enzymes.[18]

It has been reported that free radicals production is a function of aging. For example, older macrophages produce reduced levels of free radicals,[75–77] suggesting the phagocytic activity of macrophages may be reduced in older individuals. Others have reported that production of ROS appears to increase in older peritoneal macrophages.[78]

In mice, the antitumor activity of macrophages is reduced in older animals.[79,80] Furthermore, macrophages from old mice were less responsive to the activation signals of lipopolysaccharide (LPS) plus interferon-gamma (INF-gamma) for macrophage-mediated tumoricidal activity.[81] It has been shown that natural killer (NK) activity of macrophages decreases as a function of age due to an increase in suppressor function of adherent cells.[82] These studies suggest that the immune functions are impaired in older individuals, possibly because of increased oxidative damage caused by free radicals and pro-inflammatory cytokines. The levels of pro-inflammatory genes such as NFKB1 (nuclear factor NF-kappaB1), TRAF6 (TNF receptor Associated factor 6), TLR4 (Toll like receptor 4), IL1R1 (interleukin 1 receptor type1), TSPO (translocator protein), and GFAP (glial fibrillary acidic protein) were upregulated, whereas the levels of neurotrophic and synaptic integrity genes such as BDNF (brain-derived nerve growth factor), NGF (nerve growth factor), PDGFA (platelet derived growth factor subunit A), Syn (synapsin), and DBN1 (debrin1) were downregulated during aging in humans.[83] High circulating levels of pro-inflammatory markers are associated with multiple adverse health effects and T cells undergo senescence due to activation of NF-KB in older individuals.[84] Increased levels of chronic inflammation contribute to the age-related macular degeneration due to damage to the blood-retina barrier leading to retinal lesions.[85] Inflammation associated transcriptional factors NF-KB, STAT1, and STAT3 were elevated in the renal cortex of older individuals. Stimulation of renal tubular epithelial cells with a pro-inflammatory cytokine IL-6 (an activator of STAT3), Interferon-gamma (a STAT1 activator) or TNF-alpha (an activator of NF-KB) induced alterations in age-associated gene expression.[86] In vivo using the positron emission tomography (PET) radioligand ^{18}F-FEEPPA, a marker of microglia activation, it was demonstrated that the levels of mitochondrial 18k DA Translocator Protein (TSPO) did not change as a function of aging in healthy individuals. This finding may suggest that chronic inflammation as measured by microglia activation may not play any role in healthy aging and that neuroinflammation may be present in neurodegenerative diseases.[87]

CHANGES IN THE ANTIOXIDANT DEFENSE SYSTEMS DURING AGING

Antioxidant defense system constitutes antioxidant enzymes and dietary and endogenous antioxidant compounds. The changes in the levels of individual antioxidant enzymes or individual antioxidant compounds vary from no effect, to decline, or to increase in their levels in aged animals or humans despite the presence of increased oxidative stress and chronic inflammation. In the same experiment, the levels of individual antioxidants and the levels of all antioxidant enzymes are seldom measured. In order to simultaneously reduce oxidative stress and chronic inflammation, it is essential both components of antioxidant defense system should be elevated at the same time. Depending upon the experimental conditions and systems, increase in antioxidant enzymes or individual antioxidant compound in the presence of high oxidative stress and chronic inflammation may reflect a transient adaptive response to the cellular injury.

ANTIOXIDANT ENZYMES

Antioxidant enzymes represented by glutathione peroxidase, catalase, and cytosolic Cu/Zn-SOD and mitochondrial Mn-SOD play an important role in protecting cells against oxidative damage. Glutathione peroxidase is one of the major antioxidant enzymes that neutralize hydrogen peroxide and lipid peroxide and is present in both cytosol and mitochondria. Catalase found in the cytosol and mitochondria also metabolized H_2O_2 into water and oxygen. There are two forms of SOD distributed differently within the cell. Cu/Zn-SOD is present in the cytosol, whereas Mn-SOD is present in the mitochondria. Some of these enzymes respond to increased oxidative stress by elevating their activities. This response is referred to as an adaptive response that is an indicator of the presence of high oxidative stress in the cells. However, the activities of some of these antioxidant enzymes may not change or may even decline as a function of aging.

CHANGES IN ANTIOXIDANT ENZYMES ACTIVITIES IN ANIMALS

The changes in the activities of antioxidant enzymes in animals (primarily rodents) as a function of aging are variable, depending upon the organs. It has been reported that antioxidant enzymes activities gradually increase as a function of aging in the skeletal muscle of rats.[88] The increase in the activity of catalase in the heart, skeletal muscle, brain, and Cu/Zn-SOD in the skeletal muscle was observed in rats.[88,89] The increase in antioxidant enzymes activities is considered as an adaptive response to the increased oxidative stress, because markers of oxidative damage and chronic inflammation are elevated in spite of an increase in activities of antioxidant enzymes. These studies suggest that the increased levels of certain antioxidant enzymes are not sufficient to downregulate the level of oxidative stress and chronic inflammation.

The activity of glutathione peroxidase in the brain and Cu/Zn SOD in the heart showed no significant changes in enzyme activity in rats as a function of aging.[89] However, in other organs such as the liver, brain, and heart, a decrease in catalase activity was reported.[89] Prostaglandin E2 (PGE2) is one of the toxic products released during chronic inflammation. PGA1, which is formed during extraction of PGE2, is stable and used in experimental systems. We have reported that PGA1-induced degeneration of murine differentiated neuroblastoma cells increased the expression of catalase gene, decreased the expression of glutathione peroxidase and Mn-SOD genes without changing the expression of Cu/Zn-SOD as determined by gene array and confirmed by real time PCR.[90] The protein levels of glutathione peroxidase increased, whereas the protein level of Mn-SOD decreased and the levels of catalase and Cu/Zn-SOD did not change as determined by the Western blot.[90]

The activities of antioxidant enzymes as a function of aging varied in different organs. The phenomenon of adaptive response to increased oxidative stress was observed for only certain antioxidant enzymes and in certain organs. The markers of oxidative damage and chronic inflammation were elevated and immune functions were impaired in older animals irrespective of changes in the activities of antioxidant enzymes. Thus, increased activities of certain antioxidant enzymes are not sufficient to downregulate increased oxidative stress and chronic inflammation. Additional studies in which antioxidant enzymes activities, and markers of oxidative damage and chronic inflammation are measured at the same time in the same animals are needed.

CHANGES IN ANTIOXIDANT ENZYMES ACTIVITIES IN HUMANS

There is very limited information on changes in antioxidant enzymes activities as a function of aging in humans. However, based on a few studies, it appears that changes in enzyme activities as a function of aging are in part different from those observed in rodents. One major difference is that an adaptive response of certain antioxidant enzymes to increased oxidative stress that is found in rodents has not been observed in humans thus far. In older humans, the serum concentrations of SOD, glutathione peroxidase, and albumin were lower than those found in younger individuals, but the activity of catalase did not change.[91] The total antioxidant capacity decreased and lipid peroxides level increased in older subjects, as compared to younger ones.[91] In another study, the activities of catalase and SOD in serum did not change as a function of aging; however, the activity of glutathione peroxidase declined in older subjects.[92] Furthermore, age-related increases in lipid peroxidation and protein oxidation were observed.[92] In the human skeletal muscle, total SOD decreased as a function of aging, although Mn-SOD increased in older individuals.[93] The activities of catalase and glutathione peroxidase did not change.[93] These observations are opposite to those observed on the skeletal muscle of rats.[88] Thus, the results on changes in the antioxidant enzymes activities in rodents cannot be extrapolated to humans, in whom no increase in enzyme activity as an adaptive response to increased oxidative stress was observed. This may be due to the fact that the adaptive response of enzymes to increased oxidative stress in humans is very sensitive to damage or that the increased levels of oxidative damage in humans overwhelms the adaptive response of antioxidant enzymes.

In older individual with a disease, the changes in antioxidant enzyme activity were different from those found in older individuals without the disease. It is established that age-related macular degeneration (AMD) is the leading cause of irreversible blindness in developed countries. It appears that increased oxidative stress and decrease in certain antioxidant enzymes play an important role in pathophysiology of AMD. It has been reported that SOD and glutathione peroxidase were lower in both plasma and RBC of patients with maculopathy in comparison to those found in age- and sex-matched control subjects; however, the catalase activity in RBC remained unchanged.[94] The activity of alpha-ketoglutarate dehydrogenase complex, a mitochondrial enzyme, is decreased in the brains of Alzheimer's disease (AD) patients compared with matched control subjects.[95] It is interesting to observe that, in AD patients who carry ApoE4 allele of ApoE gene, the Clinical Dementia Rating (CDR) correlated better with KGDHC activity than with the densities of extracellular neuritic plaques and intracellular neurofibrillary tangles. However, in patients with AD who do not carry ApoE4 allele, the CDR correlated better with the densities of extracellular neuritic plaques and intracellular neurofibrillary tangles. The activity of glutamine synthetase decreased in the autopsied samples of the brain of AD patients,[96] and the levels of glutathione peroxidase in ventricular cerebral spinal fluid (CSF) also decreased in AD patients compared to age-matched control subjects.[97] Substantia nigra samples from autopsied brains of Parkinson disease patients showed reduced levels of antioxidant enzymes.[98,99] These studies suggest that the activities of certain antioxidant enzymes in the brain of patients with neurodegenerative diseases decline more than those found in age-matched control subjects.

CHANGES IN DIETARY AND ENDOGENOUS ANTIOXIDANTS LEVELS

In addition to antioxidant enzymes, dietary (vitamin A, beta-carotene, vitamin C, vitamin E, and selenium) and endogenous (glutathione, coenzyme Q10, L-carnitine, and alpha-lipoic acid) antioxidants play an important role in reducing oxidative stress and chronic inflammation. The organ, cellular, and subcellular distributions of these antioxidants appear to be highly variable for the same antioxidant. The levels of different dietary and endogenous antioxidants also differ in their distributions. Therefore, measurements of the plasma, whole tissue or cell levels may not be true reflection of changes in the levels of antioxidants in the subcellular fractions that may be critical in determining the rate of progression of aging or the risk of age-related chronic diseases. In addition, the levels of different antioxidants distributed in the subcellular fractions of most mammals (primarily rodents) may be different from those found in humans, because most mammals except guinea pigs synthesize their own vitamin C that could affect the level of other antioxidants in the body. Therefore, it is impossible to extrapolate the value of antioxidant level obtained from the animal studies to humans. Most studies in animals or humans have measured antioxidant levels primarily in the plasma. Only the values for a few antioxidants as function of aging are available, primarily in rodents, and these values are highly variables.

VITAMIN C

Vitamin C is a water-soluble antioxidant that has multiple biological functions. One of them includes regeneration of oxidized glutathione and vitamin E to reduced form in order to maintain their antioxidant function. The plasma level of vitamin C declines as a function of age in various species.[35,100–102] This result cannot be extrapolated to humans, since they do not synthesize their own vitamin C; they primarily rely on dietary sources for vitamin C, and consumption of this vitamin from the diet is highly variable among US population. Therefore, changes in the vitamin C levels as a function of aging is meaningless with respect to its role in aging. This is further confounded by the fact that the plasma half-life of vitamin C is rather short (a few hours).

GLUTATHIONE

Glutathione is also a water-soluble antioxidant present in cells in millimolar concentrations. It maintains glutathione peroxidase activity and prevents oxidation of vitamin E and vitamin C along with several other functions. Some studies have shown that glutathione levels increase in the brain of mice as a function of aging,[103,104] but others have reported no significant change in the brain of old rats.[105] Increased glutathione levels have been found in the plasma, heart, and liver.[104,105] Some studies have reported that the level of glutathione in the skeletal muscle increases as a function of aging.[88,104] Other studies have reported no change in the level of glutathione in the liver of rodents.[104,106,107] In contrast, some studies have reported a decline in the glutathione levels in the brain[106,107] and eye lens[102] as a function of aging. These studies suggest that the levels of glutathione in most tissues except the brain of rodents increase or show no significant change as a function of aging. In contrast to the level of glutathione found in whole tissues of rodents, the levels in the subcellular fractions consistently showed decline as a function of aging. For example, the levels of glutathione in the cerebral cortex synaptosomes[108] and mitochondria of the liver, kidney, and brain[109] declined as a function of aging. In a model of prematurely aging mice, the levels of glutathione decreased and the levels of MDA increased compared to normal mice.[110]

Changes in the levels of glutathione as a function of aging are not available in humans; however, in age-related diseases such as Parkinson disease, the autopsied brain tissues consistently showed decline in the levels of glutathione.[111–113] The serum levels of vitamins A, E, and beta-carotene were lower in well-nourished AD patients than in control subjects.[114]

VITAMIN E

Like the levels of water-soluble antioxidants, the lipid-soluble antioxidant vitamin E levels also revealed variable changes in rodents as a function of aging. For example, vitamin E levels increased in the certain regions of brain, lung, liver,[115] aortic wall of the blood vessel,[35] and serum.[116] There were, however, no changes in vitamin E levels in the heart,[117] liver,[100] blood,[118] and membranes.[116] There was a decline in the levels of vitamin E in the plasma[100] and substantia nigra region of the brain[119] as a function of aging. These studies suggest that the levels of vitamin E increased, decreased, or showed no change as a function of aging in most studies in rodents.

In elderly humans, the plasma levels of vitamin E declined by 70% compared with younger subjects, whereas the plasma levels of retinol did not change significantly. However, on the basis of the ratio of lipid-adjusted vitamin E to plasma lipids, only 12% showed decline in vitamin E levels.[120] No data are available on changes in tissue vitamin E levels as a function of aging in humans.

COENZYME Q10

Coenzyme Q10 recycles vitamin C and vitamin E. Tissue levels of coenzyme Q10 decrease with age.[119] Many studies with rodents revealed that the activities of antioxidant enzymes and the levels of certain antioxidants (vitamin E and glutathione) increased as a function of aging, although some studies reported no changes or decline in their levels. How can one explain the existence of increased oxidative stress and increased levels of certain markers of pro-inflammatory cytokines (tumor necrosis factor-alpha and IL-6) in the presence of increased, decreased, or no change in antioxidant enzymes and antioxidants? I propose that increased physiological activity of antioxidant enzymes or single antioxidants levels alone is not sufficient to decrease oxidative stress or chronic inflammation. In order to reduce these two biological processes that play a crucial role in aging and age-related chronic diseases, the pharmacological doses of dietary and endogenous antioxidants are needed. Indeed, supplementation with high doses of one more dietary or endogenous antioxidants decreased oxidative stress and chronic inflammation in rodents.

MicroRNAs IN AGING

MicroRNAs

MicroRNAs (miRs) are evolutionarily conserved small noncoding single-stranded RNAs of approximately 22 nucleotides in length, and are present in all living organisms including humans.[121–124] The biogenesis of miRs is very complex and involves multiple biochemical steps. The majority of miRs are transcribed by RNA polymerase II (Pol II), while some are transcribed by RNA polymerase III (Pol III) from the noncoding region of the DNA to produce primary miRs (pri-miRs). Pri-miRs undergo a nuclear cleavage by ribonuclease III Drosa to generate precursor-miRs (pre-miRs) that migrate to the cytoplasm where they are further cleaved by ribonuclease III Dicer to ultimately form mature single-stranded miRs with the help of another protein argonaute (Ago).[123,125–127] Each microRNA binds to its complementary sequences in the 3′-untranslated region (3′-UTR) of the mRNA, promotes degradation of the mRNA transcript, and prevents translation of the message of protein. In this manner, miRs regulate the translation of proapoptotic or anti-apoptotic proteins from their respective mRNAs, depending upon whether they receive damaging or protective signal.

MicroRNAs in Age-Related Diseases

MicroRNAs are involved in the pathogenesis of age-related neurodegenerative diseases such as Alzheimer's disease (AD)[128] and Parkinson's disease (PD).[67] Reactive oxygen species (ROS) and pro-inflammatory cytokines play a major role in the initiation and progression of these diseases; therefore, they can alter the expression of miRs that activate pro-apoptotic and inflammatory pathways in neurons. It is unknown whether ROS- and pro-inflammatory cytokines-induced upregulation and downregulation of microRNAs could be due to alterations in their transcription, processing by Drosa in the nucleus and Dicer in the cytoplasm or stability.

MicroRNAs and Their Target Proteins in Aged Animals

Since increased oxidative stress and chronic inflammation are also involved in aging, it is possible they can also alter the expression of microRNAs. Indeed, several studies suggest that a large number of microRNAs are differently expressed during cellular aging. The changes in expression of microRNAs with their target proteins during aging are presented in Table 4.1.

There were 18 microRNAs that were upregulated, which decreased genes associated with energy metabolism, cell proliferation, antioxidant defense, and extracellular matrix degradation, and 7 microRNAs that were downregulated, which enhanced genes associated with the inflammatory responses and cell-cycle arrest in the aged rat kidneys.[129] Further analysis revealed that the expression of miR-335 and miR-34a were upregulated that inhibited the levels of SOD2 and thioredoxin reductase 2 (Txnrd2) by binding to the 3′-UTRmRNA of each protein in aging mesangial cells. The expression of miR-34a and miR-93 was upregulated and their respective target proteins Nrf2 (nuclear transcriptional factor 2), SP1 (transcriptional factor specificity protein1), sirt1 (silent mating type information regulator 2 homolog 1), and Mgst1 (microsomal glutathione S-transferase) were decreased[130] in rat liver. Increased expression of miR-34a inhibited all four proteins, whereas increased expression of miR-93 inhibited only Sp1, sirt1, and Mgst1. In the aged human umbilical cord vein endothelial cells and heart and spleen of mice, the expression of miR-34a was upregulated and downregulated its target protein sirt1.[131] The expression of miR-195 was upregulated and the

TABLE 4.1

Alterations in the Expression of MicroRNAs in Aging

Cell Type	Upregulated miRs	Downregulated Target Proteins
Rat mesanglial cells	miR-325, miR-34a	SOD2, thioredoxin reductase 2
Rat liver	miR-34a, miR-93	SP1, Nrf2, Sirt1, Mgst1
HUVEC, heart, spleen	miR-349	Sirt1
Mice skeletal myoblasts	miR-195	Sirt1, TERT
Human keratinocytes	miR-325	LOX, IDH1, Aven
Human PBMC	miR-34a, miR-9	Sirt1
Human PBMC	miR-96, miR-145	IGF-1R
	miR-96, miR-145, miR-9	FOXO1
IMR-90	miR-760, miR-186	CK2-alpha
	miR-337-3p, miR-216b	
MSCs	miR-29c-3p	CNOT6
Rodent muscle	miR-29	p85a, IGF-1, B-myb
Human skin fibroblasts	miR-377, miR-217	DNMT1

SOD2, Mn-dependent mitochondrial superoxide dismutase; SP1, specificity protein1; Nrf2, nuclear transcriptional factor-2; sirt1, silent mating type information regulation 2 homolog 1; MGST1, microsomal glutathione S transferase 1; TERT, telomere reverse transcriptase; PBMC, peripheral blood mononuclear cell; IGF-1R, Insulin growth factor receptor 1; FOXO1, forkhead box protein O1; IMR-90, human lung fibroblast; C2k, alpha subunit of protein kinase ck2; MSCs, mesenchymal stem cells; p85a, a regulator protein of phosphatidylinositol-3-kinase (PI3K); IGF, insulin growth factor; B-myb, avian myeloblastosis viral oncogene B; DNMT1, DNA methyltransferase1.

levels of sirt1 and TERT (telomere reverse transcriptase) were downregulated in the old skeletal myoblasts (SkMs) from mice compared with young SkMs.[132] The expression of miR-30a was upregulated in old human keratinocytes and inhibited its target proteins LOX (encoding lysyl oxidase, a regulator of proliferation/differentiation balance of keratinocytes), IDH1 (encoding isocitrate dehydrogenase, an enzyme for cellular metabolism), and AVEN (encoding a caspase inhibitor).[133] Overexpression of miR-34a and miR-9 reduced its target protein Sirt1 in old human peripheral blood mononuclear cells (PBMC) compared with young cells.[134] In old PBMC, overexpression of miR-96 and miR-145 reduces the levels of their target protein IGF-1R (insulin growth factor receptor 1), whereas overexpression of miR-96, miR-145, and miR-9 reduced the levels of their target protein FOXO1 (forkhead box protein O1).[135] Overexpression of miR-29c-3p reduced its target protein CNOT6 (chemokine receptor 4 (CCR4)-not transcription complex subunit6) in old mesenchymal stem cells (MSCs), suggesting that upregulation of this microRNA promotes senescence in these cells.[136] The expression of miR-29 was higher in aged rodent muscle than in younger muscle. Overexpression of this microRNA downregulated the levels of its target proteins p85a, IGF-1, and B-myb and suppressed the proliferation and increased the levels of cellular arrest proteins.[137] In human skin fibroblasts, overexpression of miR-377 and miR-217 downregulate their target protein DNA methyltransferase1 (DNMT1) that regulates DNA methylation, and induce senescence in young fibroblasts.[138,139]

Most microRNAs discussed above were upregulated in aged cells; however, in the aged mice skeletal muscle, the expression of miR-434-3p was downregulated and the levels of its target protein eukaryotic translation initiation factor 5A1 (elF5A1) were upregulated, and cause apoptosis. On the other hand, overexpression of miR-434-3p inhibited apoptosis by reducing the levels of elF5A1. The expression of miR-92a was elevated in aged vascular endothelial cells. Transfection with an inhibitor of, promoted cell proliferation, decreased caspase-3 activity, levels of ROS, expression of TNF-alpha, IL2, and KEAP1, and enhanced the activity and activation of Nrf2 in these cells.[140]

Serum levels of miR-92a, miR-222, and miR-375 were upregulated, whereas miR-29b, miR-106b, miR-130b, miR-142-5p, and miR-340 were downregulated with aging in humans. It is not certain whether alteration in these microRNAs levels can be used as a predictive value for aging.

OXIDATIVE STRESS AND PRO-INFLAMMATORY CYTOKINE REGULATE EXPRESSION OF MicroRNAs

We have suggested that increased oxidative stress and chronic inflammation are one of the early events in the initiation and promotion of age-related neurodegenerative diseases such as Alzheimer's disease (AD)[66] and Parkinson's disease (PD).[141] We have also shown that oxidative stress and pro-inflammatory cytokines regulate the expression of microRNAs and their associated target proteins that cause neurodegeneration in age-related AD[128] and PD.[67] It is likely that the levels of microRNAs may be altered in cells following exposure to these stressors. Additional direct evidence on the effect of free radicals on the expression of microRNAs is described here.

Treatment of human endothelial cells with H_2O_2 enhanced the expression of miR-192-5p, and its target mRNAs for the cell cycle, DNA repair, and stress response were downregulated, suggesting that increased oxidative stress contributes to senescence and cell death.[142] Treatment with H_2O_2 also increased the p53-dependent apoptotic pathway. In premature fibroblast senescence model, treatment with H_2O_2 increased the expression of miR-24 and miR-424. The levels of p53 were increased in miR-24 overexpressing cells, but decreased in cells overexpressing miR-424.[143] Furthermore, it was demonstrated that overexpression of miR-24 induced senescence by decreasing the levels of its target protein DNA topoisomerase1 (TOP1). This was further confirmed by showing that knocking down TOP1 induced senescence in the fibroblasts. Increased oxidative stress enhanced the expression of miR-153 that reduced the expression of Nrf2 by binding to its 3'-UTR region of Nrf2 mRNA.[144] Mutation in miR-153 restored the oxidative stress-induced reduction in Nrf2 activity.

ANTIOXIDANTS REGULATE EXPRESSION OF MicroRNAs

Previous reviews proposed that antioxidants regulate expression of microRNAs that allow translation of only protective proteins in varieties of cell type and health conditions such as Alzheimer's disease (AD)[66] and Parkinson's disease (PD).[141] Since antioxidants protect against age-related decline in organ functions, it is possible that they may also alter the expression of microRNAs in order to provide protection during aging. No direct studies have been performed to evaluate the role of antioxidants in altering microRNAs expressions during aging.

EFFECTS OF INDIVIDUAL ANTIOXIDANTS ON AGE-RELATED FUNCTIONAL DEFICITS

VITAMIN E

Supplementation with vitamin E restores mitochondrial dysfunction in the aged brain and liver.[33] In healthy elderly humans, supplementation with vitamin E and fish oil was more effective in reducing the levels of pro-inflammatory cytokines (IL-6 and tumor necrosis factor-alpha) than fish oil alone.[145] Age-dependent loss of T helper1 (Th1) cytokines especially interferon-gamma (INF-gamma) that plays an important role in defending against influenza infection occurs.[146] In addition, the production prostaglandin E2 (PGE2) that suppresses Th1 cytokines increases with age in mice. Vitamin E supplementation reduced influenza titer in old mice. This antiviral effect of vitamin E is mediated through reduced production of PGE2 and enhanced production of Th1 cytokines.[146] Other antioxidants such as glutathione, melatonin, or strawberry extract, which reduced oxidative stress, did not affect the level of influenza titer.[147]

Vitamin E supplementation increased the activity of SOD in old trainee rats; however, exercise alone failed to increase SOD activity and reduced oxidative damage in these older animals.[148] It has been shown that vitamin E supplementation plus exercise improved age-related deficit in antioxidant enzymes in the cerebral cortex and hippocampus regions of rat brain.[149] Age-related increase in lipid peroxidation and protein oxidation was reduced in the brain of older rats by vitamin E supplementation.[150] Reduced level of SOD was found in cerebral cortex of old rats, whereas it was highest in the hippocampus region of the brain; however, vitamin E supplementation increased it.[150] Vitamin E, in combination with fish oil, reduced pro-inflammatory cytokines more than fish oil alone in healthy elderly subjects.[145] In contrast, the immune-enhancing effect of vitamin E alone was reduced in healthy elderly men and women when fish oil was taken concomitantly. This may be due to the fact that plasma levels of vitamin E increased by smaller amounts in the presence of fish oil.[151] From this one study, it appears that supplementation with fish oil interferes with the absorption of vitamin E. Additional studies are needed to substantiate this observation.

COENZYME Q10

Supplementation with coenzyme Q10 prolonged lifespan of animals fed on polyunsaturated fatty acids-6-enriched diet. It decreased oxidative stress and cardiovascular risk and reduced inflammation during aging.[152,153] Combination of vitamin E and coenzyme Q10 improved age-related learning deficits in mice, but the individual agent failed to do so.[154] Administration of coenzyme Q10 increased the levels of vitamin E in the mitochondria that was related to regenerating effect of coenzyme Q10.[155] In mice and rats, ingestion of coenzyme Q10 elevated coenzyme Q9, the predominant homologue in mitochondria. It has been reported that the rate of mitochondrial superoxide anion radical generation is directly proportion to mitochondrial coenzyme Q9 and inversely related to coenzyme Q10.[156]

CAROTENOIDS AND ZINC

Intake of dietary lutein and zeaxanthin or zinc reduced the risk of age-related macular degeneration (AMD); however, higher consumption of beta-carotene was associated with increased risk of AMD.[157] Another study showed no effect of vitamin E or beta-carotene supplementation on the risk of AMD.[158]

MELATONIN

Supplementation with melatonin for 30 days reversed age-related retention deficits in mice.[159] Melatonin regulates circadian rhythms through the hypothalamic suprachiasmatic nucleus (SCN). Age-related loss of sensitivity to melatonin occurs in the SCN of mice.[160]

FLAVONOIDS

Quercetin is a bioflavonoid that exhibits a strong antioxidant property. Supplementation with quercetin for 30 days reversed age-related retention deficits in mice.[161] Others have reported that supplementation with flavonoids (apigenin-7-glucoside and quercetin) reversed age-related and lipopolysaccharide-induced retention deficits in mice.[162]

GLUTATHIONE AND N-ACETYLCYSTEINE (NAC)

In a model of prematurely aging mice, treatment with NAC plus thioproline increased chemotaxis, phagocytosis, and IL-beta release, and decreased superoxide levels and TNF-alpha production.[163] This suggests that antioxidant supplementation can protect against early decline in immune function in prematurely aging mice. These antioxidants also reversed age-related behavioral dysfunction in prematurely aging mice.[164]

ALPHA-LIPOIC ACID

A combination of alpha lipoic acid and acetyl-L-carnitine reduced mitochondrial decay and oxidative damage in rat brain during aging.[165] These results support many other studies discussed previously that oxidative damage of mitochondria plays a central role in increasing the risk of age-related chronic diseases and organ functional deficits. Alpha-lipoic acid and acetyl-L-carnitine are substrates for mitochondrial enzyme carnitine acetyltransferase (CAT). In the brains of older rats, the activity of CAT and its binding affinity with substrates declined compared to younger rats.[166] Feeding old rats with high doses of acetyl-L-carnitine and alpha-lipoic acid can ameliorate oxidative damage, carnitine acetyltransferase activity and its binding affinity with substrates, and mitochondrial dysfunction.[166]

MULTIPLE DIETARY ANTIOXIDANTS

The effects of supplementation with antioxidants (vitamin C, 500 mg; vitamin E, 400 IU; and beta-carotene, 15 mg); zinc, 80 mg as zinc oxide and copper, 2 mg as cupric oxide; or antioxidant plus zinc on age-related macular degeneration (AMD) were investigated.[167] The results showed that antioxidants or zinc reduced the risk of developing advanced AMD in higher risk groups; however, the combination was more effective than the individual agents. Diet supplementation with antioxidants protected against early decline in immune function and behavior in prematurely aging mice.[110] It has been shown that the macrophages of prematurely aging mice exhibit depressed chemotaxis and phagocytosis activity. However, supplementation with dietary antioxidants (vitamin C, vitamin E, beta-carotene, zinc, and selenium) decreased the levels of pro-inflammatory cytokines and improved natural killing cell activity, lymphocyte chemotaxis activity, and proliferation response of lymphocytes to concanavalin A,[168] as well as decreased oxidative stress.[169] Dietary antioxidant supplementation protected immune function against oxidative damage and improved lifespan.[170] Psychomotor performance is decreased with aging, and this could be related to increased oxidative damage and increased levels of pro-inflammatory cytokine IL-6. Supplementation with dietary antioxidants improved psychomotor performance in old mice, and decreased the levels of oxidative damage and IL-6.[171]

The studies primarily in cell culture and animal models discussed above suggest that single antioxidants can reduce certain age-related functional deficits. No such studies have been performed during aging in humans. However, the use of single antioxidants in humans with high risk of developing chronic diseases has produced inconsistent results varying from transient beneficial effects to no effect.

STUDIES WITH INDIVIDUAL ANTIOXIDANTS ON AGE-RELATED NEURODEGENERATIVE DISEASES IN HUMANS

Treatment with individual antioxidants such as vitamin E[172,173] and curcumin[174] did not improve cognitive function, whereas alpha-lipoic acid,[175] vitamin E,[176] and omega-3-fatty acids[177,178] produced transient and limited improvements in cognitive function only in early phases of Alzheimer's disease (AD). In the case of Parkinson's disease, high doses of coenzyme Q10 produced transient improvements in some symptoms.[179] The reasons for individual antioxidants producing no effect or transient beneficial effects may have been for several reasons: (a) antioxidants show differential subcellular distribution and different mechanisms of action; therefore, a single antioxidant cannot protect all parts of the cell; (b) a single antioxidant in a high internal oxidative environment of patients with neurodegenerative diseases is oxidized and can then itself act as a pro-oxidant rather than as an antioxidant; (c) the body protects against oxidative damage by elevating antioxidant enzymes and dietary and endogenous antioxidants; (d) antioxidants neutralize free radicals by donating electrons to those molecules with unpaired electron, whereas antioxidant enzymes destroy free radicals by catalysis, converting them to harmless molecules such as water and oxygen. Therefore, both of these events need to be enhanced in concert to achieve substantial therapeutic gain against oxidative damage; (e) the affinity of different antioxidants for free radicals differs, depending upon their lipophilicity; (f) both the aqueous and lipid compartments of the cell need to be protected together. Water-soluble antioxidants such as vitamin C and glutathione protect molecules in the aqueous environment of the cells, whereas lipid soluble antioxidants such as vitamin A and vitamin E protect molecules in the lipid compartment; (g) vitamin E is more effective in quenching free radicals in a reduced oxygenated cellular environment, whereas vitamin C and alpha-tocopherol are more effective in a higher oxygenated environment of the cells[180]; (h) vitamin C is important for recycling the oxidized form of alpha-tocopherol to the antioxidant form at the lipid/aqueous interface[181]; (i) antioxidants produce cell protective proteins by altering the expression of different microRNAs.[128] For example, some antioxidants can activate Nrf2 by upregulating miR-200a that inhibits its target protein Keap1, whereas others activate Nrf2 by downregulating miR-21 that binds with 3'-UTR Nrf2 mRNA.[182]

These studies suggest that use of a single micronutrient in prevention or improved management of human neurodegenerative diseases is not expected to yield any beneficial effects. For this reason, a mixture of micronutrients that can simultaneously reduce oxidative stress and inflammation by enhancing the levels of antioxidant enzymes through the activation of Nrf2 pathway together with dietary and endogenous antioxidants for AD and PD has been suggested.[66,128] The same suggestion is proposed for maintaining healthy aging and improving age-related functional deficits. Oral supplementation can increase the levels of dietary and endogenous antioxidants; however, elevation of the levels of antioxidant enzymes requires an activation of Nrf2. Therefore it is essential to understand the regulation of activation of Nrf2.

REGULATION OF ACTIVATION OF Nrf2

Reactive Oxygen Species (ROS) Activates Nrf2

Normally, during acute oxidative stress, ROS is needed to activate Nrf2 which then dissociates itself from Keap1-Cul-Rbx1 complex and translocates in the nucleus where it heterodimerizes with a small Maf protein, and binds with the ARE (antioxidant response element) leading to increased expression of target genes coding for several cytoprotective enzymes including antioxidant enzymes.[183–185] In this manner, activation of Nrf2 increases the levels of cytoprotective enzymes including antioxidant enzymes and phase-2-detoxifying enzymes.[186,187]

Binding of Nrf2 with ARE in the Nucleus

Activation of Nrf2 alone may not be sufficient to increase the levels of antioxidant enzymes. Activated Nrf2 must bind with antioxidant response element (ARE) in the nucleus for increasing the expression of its target genes. This binding ability of Nrf2 with ARE was impaired in aged rats, and this defect was restored by supplementation with alpha-lipoic acid.[188]

Existence of ROS-Resistant Nrf2

Activation of Nrf2 by ROS becomes impaired in aged cells. This is evidenced by the fact that increased oxidative stress occurs in these cells despite the presence of Nrf2. In aging mice model (SAMP8), lower levels of nuclear Nrf2 were associated with increased oxidative stress. Phosphorylation of GSK-3 beta (glycogen synthase kinase 3-beta and protein kinase B (Akt), a serine/threonine-specific protein kinase, that is involved in translocation of Nrf2 from the cytoplasm is lowered in SAMP8 mice compared with normal mice (SAMR1). The decrease in translocation of Nrf2 may account for the decreased levels of nuclear Nrf2 in SAMP8 mice.[189] Nrf2 signaling pathway is impaired in old retinal pigment epithelial cells compared with younger cells.[190]

ANTIOXIDANTS AND PHYTOCHEMICALS ACTIVATE ROS-RESISTANT Nrf2

Activation of Nrf2 becomes unresponsive to ROS in aged cells. Some dietary antioxidants and phytochemicals can activate Nrf2 without requiring ROS. These include vitamin C,[191,192] vitamin E,[193] endogenous antioxidants such as alpha-lipoic acid[188] and coenzyme Q10,[194] synthetic antioxidant N-acetylcysteine (NAC),[195] omega-3-fatty acids,[196,197] and phytochemicals such as curcumin[198] and resveratrol.[199,200]

L-CARNITINE ACTIVATES Nrf2 BY A ROS-DEPENDENT MECHANISM

Treatment with L-carnitine activates Nrf2 by a ROS-dependent mechanism,[201] probably by generating transient ROS.

ACTIVATION OF Nrf2 BY MicroRNAs

The complex of Keap1-Nrf2 in the cytoplasm prevents activation of Nrf2. Overexpression of miR-200a reduced Keap-1 levels allowing Nrf2 to migrate to the nucleus where it binds to the ARE that enhanced the transcription of target cytoprotective genes including antioxidant enzymes.[202] Some antioxidants can activate Nrf2 by downregulating miR-21 that binds with 3'-UTR Nrf2 mRNA.[182]

SUPPRESSION OF CHRONIC INFLAMMATION

The activation of Nrf2 also suppresses chronic inflammation.[186,187] Some antioxidant compounds also reduce markers of chronic inflammation.[203–208]

PROPOSED MIXTURE OF MICRONUTRIENTS FOR HEALTHY AGING AND FOR REDUCING AGE-RELATED FUNCTIONAL DEFICITS

Based on the studies discussed above, a mixture of micronutrients containing vitamin A, mixed carotenoids, vitamin C, α-tocopheryl acetate, α-tocopheryl succinate, vitamin D3, alpha-lipoic acid, N-acetylcysteine, coenzyme Q10, L-carnitine, omega-3-fatty acids, curcumin, resveratrol, all B-vitamins, selenomethionine, and zinc, but without iron, copper, manganese, or heavy metals such as molybdenum and zirconium for healthy aging and for reduction in functional deficits in aging is proposed. The inclusion of iron, copper, or manganese is not suggested, because these trace minerals, although essential for many biological reactions, combine with vitamin C to generate excessive amounts of free radicals. Furthermore, these minerals are absorbed from the intestine better in the presence of antioxidants than in their absence that could increase body store of free iron, copper, and manganese after a long-term consumption. The body has no significant mechanisms of excretion of these trace minerals. Slight increase in the body store of free forms of these trace minerals can increase the risk of most chronic diseases. Heavy metals such as zirconium and molybdenum were not included because the body has no mechanisms of excretion of these heavy metals. Consequently, their levels in the body would increase after long-term consumption. High levels of heavy metals could interfere with the function of organs including the brain.

It is expected that the proposed micronutrient mixture would increase the levels of antioxidant enzymes by activating the Nrf2 pathway, and dietary and endogenous antioxidants that may simultaneously reduce oxidative stress and chronic inflammation.

The recommended micronutrient mixture should be taken orally and divided into two doses, half in the morning and the other half in the evening with meal. This is because the biological half-lives of micronutrients are highly variable which can create high levels of fluctuations in the tissue levels of micronutrients. A 2-fold difference in the levels of certain micronutrients such as alpha-tocopherol succinate causes a marked difference in the expression of gene profiles.[209] In order to maintain relatively steady levels of micronutrients in the body, the proposed dose-schedule is necessary.

PROPOSED CHANGES IN DIET AND LIFESTYLE FOR HEALTHY AGING AND FOR REDUCING AGE-RELATED FUNCTIONAL DEFICITS

Dietary recommendations include daily consuming of low-fat and high-fiber diet with plenty of fresh fruits and vegetables, avoiding excessive amounts of protein, carbohydrate, or calories, restricting intake of nitrite-rich cured meat, charcoal-broiled or smoked meat or fish, caffeine-containing beverages (cold or hot), and pickled fruits and vegetables.

Lifestyle-related changes include stopping smoking and chewing tobacco, avoiding exposure to secondhand smoke, sun, UV-light for tanning, and hyperbaric therapy for energy, restricting intake of alcohol, reducing stress by vacation, yoga, or meditation, and performing moderate exercise 4–5 times a week.

The efficacy of proposed micronutrient mixture together with diet and lifestyle should be tested by well-designed preclinical and clinical studies. In the meanwhile, the proposed recommendations may be adopted by the individuals in consultation with their physicians or health professionals for healthy aging. It is expected that these recommendations, if adopted, may help in maintaining healthy aging and in reducing age-related organ functional deficits.

CONCLUSIONS

Increased oxidation caused by generation of excessive amounts of free radicals and pro-inflammatory cytokines produced during chronic inflammation contribute to the age-related decline in organ function and chronic diseases. Mitochondria are not only the first target to be damaged by free radicals, but they are also the most sensitive targets to oxidative stress. Damaged mitochondria produce more free radicals that initiate cascade of events that reduce proteasome activity, length of telomere, immune function, and increase lysosomal proteolytic activity.

Changes in the antioxidant enzymes during aging have been investigated more in rodents than in humans, and they are highly variable. In rodents, an increase, no change, or a decline in antioxidant enzymes activities in the presence of elevated levels of markers of oxidative damage and inflammation have been observed; however, in humans, the activities of antioxidant enzyme consistently showed either decrease or no change as a function of aging. An increase in the activities of certain antioxidant enzymes in the presence of elevated levels of markers of oxidative stress and inflammation suggests that they were not sufficient to downregulate oxidative stress and chronic inflammation. An adaptive response of certain antioxidant enzymes to increased oxidative stress that is found in rodents, but is not observed in humans.

Very limited data exist with respect to changes in the levels of dietary and endogenous antioxidants as a function of aging in rodents or in humans. In rodents, plasma vitamin C and tissue coenzyme levels declined, but plasma glutathione and vitamin E levels were elevated as function of aging. In contrast, the plasma level of vitamin E decreased, and retinol did not change in elderly humans.

MicroRNAs that regulate the translation of mRNAs into their respective proteins are altered in aged cells and in animal models of aging. Since increased oxidative stress and chronic inflammation are involved in aging, it is not surprising that their expressions are altered.

We have proposed that in order to simultaneously reduced oxidative stress and chronic inflammation, it is necessary to elevate the levels of cytoprotective enzymes including antioxidant enzymes and phase-2-detoxyfying enzyme through activation of the Nrf2/ARE pathway as well as dietary and endogenous antioxidants. Activation of Nrf2 becomes resistant during chronic oxidative stress; however, certain antioxidants and phytochemicals activate Nrf2 without ROS. This chapter proposes a mixture of micronutrients that would achieve the above goal, and recommends changes in diet and lifestyle for healthy aging and for reduction in age-related functional deficits. Preclinical and clinical studies to test the efficacy of proposed micronutrient mixture together with modifications in diet and lifestyle should be performed.

REFERENCES

1. de Boer J, Andressoo JO, de Wit J, et al. Premature aging in mice deficient in DNA repair and transcription. *Science.* 2002;296(5571):1276–1279.
2. Coppede F. Premature aging syndrome. *Adv Exp Med Biol.* 2012;724:317–331.
3. Coyle JT, Puttfarcken P. Oxidative stress, glutamate, and neurodegenerative disorders. *Science.* 1993;262(5134):689–695.
4. Graham DG. Oxidative pathways for catecholamines in the genesis of neuromelanin and cytotoxic quinones. *Mol Pharmacol.* 1978;14(4):633–643.
5. Chan PH, Fishman RA. Transient formation of superoxide radicals in polyunsaturated fatty acid-induced brain swelling. *J Neurochem.* 1980;35(4):1004–1007.
6. Lafon-Cazal M, Pietri S, Culcasi M, Bockaert J. NMDA-dependent superoxide production and neurotoxicity. *Nature.* 1993;364(6437):535–537.
7. Kiyosawa H, Suko M, Okudaira H, et al. Cigarette smoking induces formation of 8-hydroxydeoxyguanosine, one of the oxidative DNA damages in human peripheral leukocytes. *Free Radic Res Commun.* 1990;11(1–3):23–27.
8. Reznick AZ, Cross CE, Hu ML, et al. Modification of plasma proteins by cigarette smoke as measured by protein carbonyl formation. *Biochem J.* 1992;286 (Pt 2):607–611.
9. Duthie GG, Arthur JR, James WP. Effects of smoking and vitamin E on blood antioxidant status. *Am J Clin Nutr.* 1991;53(4 Suppl):1061S–1063S.
10. Schectman G, Byrd JC, Hoffmann R. Ascorbic acid requirements for smokers: Analysis of a population survey. *Am J Clin Nutr.* 1991;53(6):1466–1470.
11. Winterbourn CC. Toxicity of iron and hydrogen peroxide: The Fenton reaction. *Toxicol Lett.* 1995;82–83:969–974.
12. Boveris A, Chance B. The mitochondrial generation of hydrogen peroxide. General properties and effect of hyperbaric oxygen. *Biochem J.* 1973;134(3):707–716.
13. Chance B, Sies H, Boveris A. Hydroperoxide metabolism in mammalian organs. *Physiol Rev.* 1979;59(3):527–605.
14. Giulivi C, Poderoso JJ, Boveris A. Production of nitric oxide by mitochondria. *J Biol Chem.* 1998;273(18):11038–11043.
15. Harman D. Aging and disease: Extending functional lifespan. *Ann N Y Acad Sci.* 1996;786:321–336.
16. Harman D. Aging: Phenomena and theories. *Ann N Y Acad Sci.* 1998;854:1–7.
17. Ames BN, Shigenaga MK, Hagen TM. Oxidants, antioxidants, and the degenerative diseases of aging. *Proc Natl Acad Sci USA.* 1993;90(17):7915–7922.
18. Pollack ML, Leeuwenburgh C. Molecular mechanisms of oxidative stress in aging: Free radicals, aging, antioxidants and disease. In: Sen CKP, Packer L. Hanninen O, ed. *Handbook of Oxidants and Antioxidants in Exercise.* New York: Elesvier Science B.V.; 1999:881–923.
19. Droge W. Oxidative stress and aging. *Adv Exp Med Biol.* 2003;543:191–200.
20. Hurst JK, Barrette WC, Jr. Leukocytic oxygen activation and microbicidal oxidative toxins. *Crit Rev Biochem Mol Biol.* 1989;24(4):271–328.
21. Klebanoff SJ. Oxygen metabolism and the toxic properties of phagocytes. *Ann Intern Med.* 1980;93(3):480–489.
22. Eiserich JP, Cross CE, Jones AD, Halliwell B, van der Vliet A. Formation of nitrating and chlorinating species by reaction of nitrite with hypochlorous acid. A novel mechanism for nitric oxide-mediated protein modification. *J Biol Chem.* 1996;271(32):19199–19208.

23. Eiserich JP, Hristova M, Cross CE, et al. Formation of nitric oxide-derived inflammatory oxidants by myeloperoxidase in neutrophils. *Nature.* 1998;391(6665):393–397.
24. Pamplona R. Membrane phospholipids, lipoxidative damage and molecular integrity: A causal role in aging and longevity. *Biochim Biophys Acta.* 2008;1777(10):1249–1262.
25. Squier TC. Oxidative stress and protein aggregation during biological aging. *Exp Gerontol.* 2001;36(9):1539–1550.
26. Bahadorani S, Mukai S, Egli D, Hilliker AJ. Overexpression of metal-responsive transcription factor (MTF-1) in *Drosophila melanogaster* ameliorates life-span reductions associated with oxidative stress and metal toxicity. *Neurobiol Aging.* 2008;31(7):1215–1226.
27. Sohal RS, Agarwal S, Sohal BH. Oxidative stress and aging in the Mongolian gerbil (Meriones unguiculatus). *Mech Ageing Dev.* 1995;81(1):15–25.
28. Hagen TM, Yowe DL, Bartholomew JC, et al. Mitochondrial decay in hepatocytes from old rats: Membrane potential declines, heterogeneity and oxidants increase. *Proc Natl Acad Sci USA.* 1997;94(7):3064–3069.
29. Sohal RS. Hydrogen peroxide production by mitochondria may be a biomarker of aging. *Mech Ageing Dev.* 1991;60(2):189–198.
30. Miquel J. An update on the oxygen stress-mitochondrial mutation theory of aging: Genetic and evolutionary implications. *Exp Gerontol.* 1998;33(1–2):113–126.
31. Yakes FM, Van Houten B. Mitochondrial DNA damage is more extensive and persists longer than nuclear DNA damage in human cells following oxidative stress. *Proc Natl Acad Sci USA.* 1997;94(2):514–519.
32. Aerts AM, Zabrocki P, Govaert G, et al. Mitochondrial dysfunction leads to reduced chronological lifespan and increased apoptosis in yeast. *FEBS Lett.* 2008;583(1):113–117.
33. Navarro A, Boveris A. The mitochondrial energy transduction system and the aging process. *Am J Physiol Cell Physiol.* 2007;292(2):C670–C686.
34. Boveris A, Navarro A. Brain mitochondrial dysfunction in aging. *IUBMB Life.* 2008;60(5):308–314.
35. van der Loo B, Koppensteiner R, Luscher TF. How do blood vessels age? Mechanisms and clinical implications. *Vasa.* 2004;33(1):3–11.
36. van der Loo B, Schildknecht S, Zee R, Bachschmid MM. Signaling processes in endothelial aging in relation to chronic oxidative stress and their potential therapeutic implications. *Exp Physiol.* 2008;94(3):305–310.
37. Hack V, Breitkreutz R, Kinscherf R, et al. The redox state as a correlate of senescence and wasting and as a target for therapeutic intervention. *Blood.* 1998;92(1):59–67.
38. Droge W. Aging-related changes in the thiol/disulfide redox state: Implications for the use of thiol antioxidants. *Exp Gerontol.* 2002;37(12):1333–1345.
39. Pope S, Land JM, Heales SJ. Oxidative stress and mitochondrial dysfunction in neurodegeneration; cardiolipin a critical target? *Biochim Biophys Acta.* 2008;1777(7–8):794–799.
40. Prasad KN, Cole WC, Prasad KC. Risk factors for Alzheimer's disease: Role of multiple antioxidants, non-steroidal antiinflammatory and cholinergic agents alone or in combination in prevention and treatment. *J Am Coll Nutr.* 2002;21(6):506–522.
41. Prasad KN, Cole WC, Kumar B. Multiple antioxidants in the prevention and treatment of Parkinson's disease. *J Am Coll Nutr.* 1999;18(5):413–423.
42. Kong Y, Trabucco SE, Zhang H. Oxidative stress, mitochondrial dysfunction and the mitochondria theory of aging. *Interdiscip Top Gerontol.* 2014;39:86–107.
43. Cedikova M, Pitule P, Kripnerova M, Markova M, Kuncova J. Multiple roles of mitochondria in aging processes. *Physiol Res.* 2016;65(Suppl. 5):S519–S531.
44. Combaret L, Dardevet D, Bechet D, Taillandier D, Mosoni L, Attaix D. Skeletal muscle proteolysis in aging. *Curr Opin Clin Nutr Metab Care.* 2009;12(1):37–41.
45. Shringarpure R, Davies KJ. Protein turnover by the proteasome in aging and disease. *Free Radic Biol Med.* 2002;32(11):1084–1089.
46. Dirks AJ, Hofer T, Marzetti E, Pahor M, Leeuwenburgh C. Mitochondrial DNA mutations, energy metabolism and apoptosis in aging muscle. *Ageing Res Rev.* 2006;5(2):179–195.
47. Davies KJ, Shringarpure R. Preferential degradation of oxidized proteins by the 20S proteasome may be inhibited in aging and in inflammatory neuromuscular diseases. *Neurology.* 2006;66(2 Suppl 1):S93–S96.
48. Conti V, Corbi G, Simeon V, et al. Aging-related changes in oxidative stress response of human endothelial cells. *Aging Clin Exp Res.* 2015;27(4):547–553.
49. Hou G, Lu H, Chen M, Yao H, Zhao H. Oxidative stress participates in age-related changes in rat lumbar intervertebral discs. *Arch Gerontol Geriatr.* 2014;59(3):665–669.

50. Zhang YB, Zhong ZM, Hou G, Jiang H, Chen JT. Involvement of oxidative stress in age-related bone loss. *J Surg Res.* 2011;169(1):e37–e42.
51. Wang J, Lei H, Hou J, Liu J. Involvement of oxidative stress in SAMP10 mice with age-related neurodegeneration. *Neurol Sci.* 2015;36(5):743–750.
52. Hanaoka S, Nagadoi A, Nishimura Y. Comparison between TRF2 and TRF1 of their telomeric DNA-bound structures and DNA-binding activities. *Protein Sci.* 2005;14(1):119–130.
53. Kim H, Lee, O-H, Xin H, et al. TRF2 functions as a protein hub and regulates telomere maintenance by recognizing specific peptide motifs. *Nat Struct Mol Biol.* 2009;16:372–379.
54. Mikhelson VM, Gamaley IA. Telomere shortening is a sole mechanism of aging in mammals. *Curr Aging Sci.* 2012;5(3):203–208.
55. Fyhrquist F, Saijonmaa O. Telomere length and cardiovascular aging. *Ann Med.* 2012;44(Suppl 1):S138–S142.
56. Kawanishi S, Oikawa S. Mechanism of telomere shortening by oxidative stress. *Ann N Y Acad Sci.* 2004;1019:278–284.
57. Kurz DJ, Decary S, Hong Y, Trivier E, Akhmedov A, Erusalimsky JD. Chronic oxidative stress compromises telomere integrity and accelerates the onset of senescence in human endothelial cells. *J Cell Sci.* 2004;117(Pt 11):2417–2426.
58. Haendeler J, Hoffmann J, Diehl JF, et al. Antioxidants inhibit nuclear export of telomerase reverse transcriptase and delay replicative senescence of endothelial cells. *Circ Res.* 2004;94(6):768–775.
59. Furumoto K, Inoue E, Nagao N, Hiyama E, Miwa N. Age-dependent telomere shortening is slowed down by enrichment of intracellular vitamin C via suppression of oxidative stress. *Life Sci.* 1998;63(11):935–948.
60. Tanaka Y, Moritoh Y, Miwa N. Age-dependent telomere-shortening is repressed by phosphorylated alpha-tocopherol together with cellular longevity and intracellular oxidative-stress reduction in human brain microvascular endotheliocytes. *J Cell Biochem.* 2007;102(3):689–703.
61. Prasad KN, Wu M, Bondy SC. Telomere shortening during aging: Attenuation by antioxidants and anti-inflammatory agents. *Mech Ageing Dev.* 2017;164:61–66.
62. Viel JJ, McManus DQ, Smith SS, Brewer GJ. Age- and concentration-dependent neuroprotection and toxicity by TNF in cortical neurons from beta-amyloid. *J Neurosci Res.* 2001;64(5):454–465.
63. Patel JR, Brewer GJ. Age-related differences in NFkappaB translocation and Bcl-2/Bax ratio caused by TNFalpha and Abeta42 promote survival in middle-age neurons and death in old neurons. *Exp Neurol.* 2008;213(1):93–100.
64. Patel JR, Brewer GJ. Age-related changes to tumor necrosis factor receptors affect neuron survival in the presence of beta-amyloid. *J Neurosci Res.* 2008;86(10):2303–2313.
65. You T, Nicklas BJ. Chronic inflammation: Role of adipose tissue and modulation by weight loss. *Curr Diabetes Rev.* 2006;2(1):29–37.
66. Prasad KN. Simultaneous activation of Nrf2 and elevation of antioxidant compounds for reducing oxidative stress and chronic inflammation in human Alzheimer's disease. *Mech Ageing Dev.* 2016;153:41–47.
67. Prasad KN. Oxidative stress, pro-inflammatory cytokines, and antioxidants regulate expression levels of microRNAs in Parkinson's disease. *Curr Aging Sci.* 2017;10(3):177–184.
68. Greene MA, Loeser RF. Aging-related inflammation in osteoarthritis. *Osteoarthr Cartil.* 2015;23(11):1966–1971.
69. Merritt EK, Stec MJ, Thalacker-Mercer A, et al. Heightened muscle inflammation susceptibility may impair regenerative capacity in aging humans. *J Appl Physiol.* 2013;115(6):937–948.
70. Ungvari Z, Orosz Z, Labinskyy N, et al. Increased mitochondrial H_2O_2 production promotes endothelial NF-kappaB activation in aged rat arteries. *Am J Physiol Heart Circ Physiol.* 2007;293(1):H37–H47.
71. Csiszar A, Wang M, Lakatta EG, Ungvari Z. Inflammation and endothelial dysfunction during aging: Role of NF-kappaB. *J Appl Physiol.* 2008;105(4):1333–1341.
72. Visser M, Pahor M, Taaffe DR, et al. Relationship of interleukin-6 and tumor necrosis factor-alpha with muscle mass and muscle strength in elderly men and women: The Health ABC Study. *J Gerontol A Biol Sci Med Sci.* 2002;57(5):M326–M332.
73. Schaap LA, Pluijm SM, Deeg DJ, Visser M. Inflammatory markers and loss of muscle mass (sarcopenia) and strength. *Am J Med.* 2006;119(6):526, e529–e517.
74. Ferrucci L, Harris TB, Guralnik JM, et al. Serum IL-6 level and the development of disability in older persons. *J Am Geriatr Soc.* 1999;47(6):639–646.
75. Alvarez E, Machado A, Sobrino F, Santa Maria C. Nitric oxide and superoxide anion production decrease with age in resident and activated rat peritoneal macrophages. *Cell Immunol.* 1996;169(1):152–155.

76. Alvarez E, Santa Maria C. Influence of the age and sex on respiratory burst of human monocytes. *Mech Ageing Dev.* 1996;90(2):157–161.

77. Santa Maria C, Ayala A, Revilla E. Changes in superoxide dismutase activity in liver and lung of old rats. *Free Radic Res.* 1996;25(5):401–405.

78. Lavie L, Weinreb O. Age- and strain-related changes in tissue transglutaminase activity in murine macrophages: The effects of inflammation and induction by retinol. *Mech Ageing Dev.* 1996;90(2):129–143.

79. Khare V, Sodhi A, Singh SM. Age-dependent alterations in the tumoricidal functions of tumor-associated macrophages. *Tumour Biol.* 1999;20(1):30–43.

80. Wallace PK, Eisenstein TK, Meissler JJ, Jr., Morahan PS. Decreases in macrophage mediated antitumor activity with aging. *Mech Ageing Dev.* 1995;77(3):169–184.

81. Khare V, Sodhi A, Singh SM. Effect of aging on the tumoricidal functions of murine peritoneal macrophages. *Nat Immun.* 1996;15(6):285–294.

82. Irimajiri N, Bloom ET, Makinodan T. Suppression of murine natural killer cell activity by adherent cells from aging mice. *Mech Ageing Dev.* 1985;31(2):155–162.

83. Primiani CT, Ryan VH, Rao JS, et al. Coordinated gene expression of neuroinflammatory and cell signaling markers in dorsolateral prefrontal cortex during human brain development and aging. *PLoS One.* 2014;9(10):e110972.

84. Bektas A, Schurman SH, Sen R, Ferrucci L. Human T cell immunosenescence and inflammation in aging. *J Leukoc Biol.* 2017;102(4):977–988.

85. Chen M, Xu H. Parainflammation, chronic inflammation, and age-related macular degeneration. *J Leukoc Biol.* 2015;98(5):713–725.

86. O'Brown ZK, Van Nostrand EL, Higgins JP, Kim SK. The inflammatory transcription factors NFkappaB, STAT1 and STAT3 Drive Age-Associated Transcriptional Changes in the Human Kidney. *PLoS Genet.* 2015;11(12):e1005734.

87. Suridjan I, Rusjan PM, Voineskos AN, et al. Neuroinflammation in healthy aging: A PET study using a novel Translocator Protein 18kDa (TSPO) radioligand, [(18)F]-FEPPA. *Neuroimage.* 2014;84:868–875.

88. Leeuwenburgh C, Fiebig R, Chandwaney R, Ji LL. Aging and exercise training in skeletal muscle: Responses of glutathione and antioxidant enzyme systems. *Am J Physiol.* 1994;267(2 Pt 2):R439–R445.

89. Yu B, ed. *Free Radicals in Aging.* Boca Raton, FL: CRC Press; 1993.

90. Yan XD, Kumar B, Nahreini P, Hanson AJ, Prasad JE, Prasad KN. Prostaglandin-induced neurodegeneration is associated with increased levels of oxidative markers and reduced by a mixture of antioxidants. *J Neurosci Res.* 2005;81(1):85–90.

91. Tokunaga K, Kanno K, Ochi M, et al. Lipid peroxide and antioxidants in the elderly. *Rinsho Byori.* 1998;46(8):783–789.

92. Kasapoglu M, Ozben T. Alterations of antioxidant enzymes and oxidative stress markers in aging. *Exp Gerontol.* 2001;36(2):209–220.

93. Pansarasa O, Bertorelli L, Vecchiet J, Felzani G, Marzatico F. Age-dependent changes of antioxidant activities and markers of free radical damage in human skeletal muscle. *Free Radic Biol Med.* 1999;27(5–6):617–622.

94. Evereklioglu C, Er H, Doganay S, et al. Nitric oxide and lipid peroxidation are increased and associated with decreased antioxidant enzyme activities in patients with age-related macular degeneration. *Doc Ophthalmol.* 2003;106(2):129–136.

95. Gibson GE, Haroutunian V, Zhang H, et al. Mitochondrial damage in Alzheimer's disease varies with apolipoprotein E genotype. *Ann Neurol.* 2000;48(3):297–303.

96. Koppal T, Drake J, Yatin S, et al. Peroxynitrite-induced alterations in synaptosomal membrane proteins: Insight into oxidative stress in Alzheimer's disease. *J Neurochem.* 1999;72(1):310–317.

97. Lovell MA, Xie C, Markesbery WR. Decreased glutathione transferase activity in brain and ventricular fluid in Alzheimer's disease. *Neurology.* 1998;51(6):1562–1566.

98. Ambani LM, Van Woert MH, Murphy S. Brain peroxidase and catalase in Parkinson disease. *Arch Neurol.* 1975;32(2):114–118.

99. Kish SJ, Morito C, Hornykiewicz O. Glutathione peroxidase activity in Parkinson's disease brain. *Neurosci Lett.* 1985;58(3):343–346.

100. De AK, Darad R. Age-associated changes in antioxidants and antioxidative enzymes in rats. *Mech Ageing Dev.* 1991;59(1–2):123–128.

101. Panda AK, Ruth RP, Padhi SN. Effect of age and sex on the ascorbic acid content of kidney, skeletal muscle and pancreas of common Indian toad, Bufo melanostictus. *Exp Gerontol.* 1984;19(2):95–100.

102. Rikans LE, Moore DR. Effect of aging on aqueous-phase antioxidants in tissues of male Fischer rats. *Biochim Biophys Acta.* 1988;966(3):269–275.

103. Hussain S, Slikker W, Jr., Ali SF. Age-related changes in antioxidant enzymes, superoxide dismutase, catalase, glutathione peroxidase and glutathione in different regions of mouse brain. *Int J Dev Neurosci.* 1995;13(8):811–817.

104. Ohkuwa T, Sato Y, Naoi M. Glutathione status and reactive oxygen generation in tissues of young and old exercised rats. *Acta Physiol Scand.* 1997;159(3):237–244.

105. Barja de Quiroga G, Perez-Campo R, Lopez Torres M. Anti-oxidant defences and peroxidation in liver and brain of aged rats. *Biochem J.* 1990;272(1):247–250.

106. Farooqui MY, Day WW, Zamorano DM. Glutathione and lipid peroxidation in the aging rat. *Comp Biochem Physiol B.* 1987;88(1):177–180.

107. Ravindranath V, Shivakumar BR, Anandatheerthavarada HK. Low glutathione levels in brain regions of aged rats. *Neurosci Lett.* 1989;101(2):187–190.

108. Favilli F, Iantomasi T, Marraccini P, et al. Relationship between age and GSH metabolism in synaptosomes of rat cerebral cortex. *Neurobiol Aging.* 1994;15(4):429–433.

109. de la Asuncion JG, Millan A, Pla R, et al. Mitochondrial glutathione oxidation correlates with age-associated oxidative damage to mitochondrial DNA. *Faseb J.* 1996;10(2):333–338.

110. Viveros MP, Arranz L, Hernanz A, Miquel J, De la Fuente M. A model of premature aging in mice based on altered stress-related behavioral response and immunosenescence. *Neuroimmunomodulation.* 2007;14(3–4):157–162.

111. Perry TL, Godin DV, Hansen S. Parkinson's disease: A disorder due to nigral glutathione deficiency? *Neurosci Lett.* 1982;33(3):305–310.

112. Riederer P, Sofic E, Rausch WD, et al. Transition metals, ferritin, glutathione, and ascorbic acid in parkinsonian brains. *J Neurochem.* 1989;52(2):515–520.

113. Sofic E, Lange KW, Jellinger K, Riederer P. Reduced and oxidized glutathione in the substantia nigra of patients with Parkinson's disease. *Neurosci Lett.* 1992;142(2):128–130.

114. Zaman Z, Roche S, Fielden P, Frost PG, Niriella DC, Cayley AC. Plasma concentrations of vitamins A and E and carotenoids in Alzheimer's disease. *Age Ageing.* 1992;21(2):91–94.

115. Matsuo M, Gomi F, Dooley MM. Age-related alterations in antioxidant capacity and lipid peroxidation in brain, liver, and lung homogenates of normal and vitamin E-deficient rats. *Mech Ageing Dev.* 1992;64(3):273–292.

116. Laganiere S, Yu BP. Effect of chronic food restriction in aging rats. I. Liver subcellular membranes. *Mech Ageing Dev.* 1989;48(3):207–219.

117. Vatassery GT, Angerhofer CK, Knox CA. Effect of age on vitamin E concentrations in various regions of the brain and a few selected peripheral tissues of the rat, and on the uptake of radioactive vitamin E by various regions of rat brain. *J Neurochem.* 1984;43(2):409–412.

118. Sawada M, Carlson JC. Changes in superoxide radical and lipid peroxide formation in the brain, heart and liver during the lifetime of the rat. *Mech Ageing Dev.* 1987;41(1–2):125–137.

119. Albano CB, Muralikrishnan D, Ebadi M. Distribution of coenzyme Q homologues in brain. *Neurochem Res.* 2002;27(5):359–368.

120. Panemangalore M, Lee CJ. Evaluation of the indices of retinol and alpha-tocopherol status in free-living elderly. *J Gerontol.* 1992;47(3):B98–B104.

121. Lee RC, Feinbaum RL, Ambros V. The C. elegans heterochronic gene lin-4 encodes small RNAs with antisense complementarity to lin-14. *Cell.* 1993;75(5):843–854.

122. Wightman B, Ha I, Ruvkun G. Posttranscriptional regulation of the heterochronic gene lin-14 by lin-4 mediates temporal pattern formation in C. elegans. *Cell.* 1993;75(5):855–862.

123. Macfarlane LA, Murphy PR. MicroRNA: Biogenesis, function and role in cancer. *Curr Genomics.* 2010;11(7):537–561.

124. Londin E, Loher P, Telonis AG, et al. Analysis of 13 cell types reveals evidence for the expression of numerous novel primate- and tissue-specific microRNAs. *Proc Natl Acad Sci USA.* 2015;112(10):E1106–E1115.

125. Denli AM, Tops BB, Plasterk RH, Ketting RF, Hannon GJ. Processing of primary microRNAs by the Microprocessor complex. *Nature.* 2004;432(7014):231–235.

126. Lee Y, Ahn C, Han J, et al. The nuclear RNase III Drosha initiates microRNA processing. *Nature.* 2003;425(6956):415–419.

127. Hutvagner G, McLachlan J, Pasquinelli AE, Balint E, Tuschl T, Zamore PD. A cellular function for the RNA-interference enzyme Dicer in the maturation of the let-7 small temporal RNA. *Science.* 2001;293(5531):834–838.

128. Prasad KN. Oxidative stress and pro-inflammatory cytokines may act as one of signals for regulating microRNAs expression in Alzheimer's disease. *Mech Ageing Dev.* 2017;162:63–71.

129. Bai XY, Ma Y, Ding R, Fu B, Shi S, Chen XM. miR-335 and miR-34a promote renal senescence by suppressing mitochondrial antioxidative enzymes. *J Am Soc Nephrol.* 2011;22(7):1252–1261.

130. Li N, Muthusamy S, Liang R, Sarojini H, Wang E. Increased expression of miR-34a and miR-93 in rat liver during aging, and their impact on the expression of Mgst1 and Sirt1. *Mech Ageing Dev.* 2011;132(3):75–85.

131. Ito T, Yagi S, Yamakuchi M. MicroRNA-34a regulation of endothelial senescence. *Biochem Biophys Res Commun.* 2010;398(4):735–740.

132. Kondo H, Kim HW, Wang L, et al. Blockade of senescence-associated microRNA-195 in aged skeletal muscle cells facilitates reprogramming to produce induced pluripotent stem cells. *Aging Cell.* 2016;15(1):56–66.

133. Muther C, Jobeili L, Garion M, et al. An expression screen for aged-dependent microRNAs identifies miR-30a as a key regulator of aging features in human epidermis. *Aging (Albany NY).* 2017;9(11):2376–2396.

134. Owczarz M, Budzinska M, Domaszewska-Szostek A, et al. miR-34a and miR-9 are overexpressed and SIRT genes are downregulated in peripheral blood mononuclear cells of aging humans. *Exp Biol Med (Maywood).* 2017;242(14):1453–1461.

135. Budzinska M, Owczarz M, Pawlik-Pachucka E, Roszkowska-Gancarz M, Slusarczyk P, Puzianowska-Kuznicka M. miR-96, miR-145 and miR-9 expression increases, and IGF-1R and FOXO1 expression decreases in peripheral blood mononuclear cells of aging humans. *BMC Geriatr.* 2016;16(1):200.

136. Shang J, Yao Y, Fan X, et al. miR-29c-3p promotes senescence of human mesenchymal stem cells by targeting CNOT6 through p53-p21 and p16-pRB pathways. *Biochim Biophys Acta.* 2016;1863(4):520–532.

137. Hu Z, Klein JD, Mitch WE, Zhang L, Martinez I, Wang XH. MicroRNA-29 induces cellular senescence in aging muscle through multiple signaling pathways. *Aging (Albany NY).* 2014;6(3):160–175.

138. Xie HF, Liu YZ, Du R, et al. miR-377 induces senescence in human skin fibroblasts by targeting DNA methyltransferase 1. *Cell Death Dis.* 2017;8(3):e2663.

139. Wang B, Du R, Xiao X, et al. Microrna-217 modulates human skin fibroblast senescence by directly targeting DNA methyltransferase 1. *Oncotarget.* 2017;8(20):33475–33486.

140. Liu H, Wu HY, Wang WY, Zhao ZL, Liu XY, Wang LY. Regulation of miR-92a on vascular endothelial aging via mediating Nrf2-KEAP1-ARE signal pathway. *Eur Rev Med Pharmacol Sci.* 2017;21(11):2734–2742.

141. Prasad KN. Simultaneous activation of Nrf2 and elevation of dietary and endogenous antioxidants for prevention and improved managment of Parkinson's disease. In: Bondy SCC A., ed. *Inflammation, Aging and Oxidative Stress.* New York: Springer; 2016:277–301.

142. Fuschi P, Carrara M, Voellenkle C, et al. Central role of the p53 pathway in the noncoding-RNA response to oxidative stress. *Aging (Albany NY).* 2017;9(12):2559.

143. Bu H, Baraldo G, Lepperdinger G, Jansen-Durr P. Mir-24 activity propagates stress-induced senescence by down regulating DNA topoisomerase 1. *Exp Gerontol.* 2016;75:48–52.

144. Narasimhan M, Riar AK, Rathinam ML, Vedpathak D, Henderson G, Mahimainathan L. Hydrogen peroxide responsive miR153 targets Nrf2/ARE cytoprotection in paraquat induced dopaminergic neurotoxicity. *Toxicol Lett.* 2014;228(3):179–191.

145. Wu D, Han SN, Meydani M, Meydani SN. Effect of concomitant consumption of fish oil and vitamin E on production of inflammatory cytokines in healthy elderly humans. *Ann N Y Acad Sci.* 2004;1031:422–424.

146. Han SN, Wu D, Ha WK, et al. Vitamin E supplementation increases T helper 1 cytokine production in old mice infected with influenza virus. *Immunology.* 2000;100(4):487–493.

147. Han SN, Meydani M, Wu D, et al. Effect of long-term dietary antioxidant supplementation on influenza virus infection. *J Gerontol A Biol Sci Med Sci.* 2000;55(10):B496–B503.

148. Asha Devi S, Prathima S, Subramanyam MV. Dietary vitamin E and physical exercise: II. Antioxidant status and lipofuscin-like substances in aging rat heart. *Exp Gerontol.* 2003;38(3):291–297.

149. Devi SA, Kiran TR. Regional responses in antioxidant system to exercise training and dietary vitamin E in aging rat brain. *Neurobiol Aging.* 2004;25(4):501–508.

150. Jolitha AB, Subramanyam MV, Asha Devi S. Modification by vitamin E and exercise of oxidative stress in regions of aging rat brain: Studies on superoxide dismutase isoenzymes and protein oxidation status. *Exp Gerontol.* 2006;41(8):753–763.

151. Wu D, Han SN, Meydani M, Meydani SN. Effect of concomitant consumption of fish oil and vitamin E on T cell mediated function in the elderly: A randomized double-blind trial. *J Am Coll Nutr.* 2006;25(4):300–306.

152. Santos-Gonzalez M, Gomez Diaz C, Navas P, Villalba JM. Modifications of plasma proteome in long-lived rats fed on a coenzyme Q10-supplemented diet. *Exp Gerontol.* 2007;42(8):798–806.

153. Quiles JL, Ochoa JJ, Huertas JR, Mataix J. Coenzyme Q supplementation protects from age-related DNA double-strand breaks and increases lifespan in rats fed on a PUFA-rich diet. *Exp Gerontol.* 2004;39(2):189–194.

154. McDonald SR, Sohal RS, Forster MJ. Concurrent administration of coenzyme Q10 and alpha-tocopherol improves learning in aged mice. *Free Radic Biol Med.* 2005;38(6):729–736.

155. Lass A, Sohal RS. Effect of coenzyme Q(10) and alpha-tocopherol content of mitochondria on the production of superoxide anion radicals. *Faseb J.* 2000;14(1):87–94.

156. Sohal RS, Forster MJ. Coenzyme Q, oxidative stress and aging. *Mitochondrion.* 2007;7(Suppl):S103–S111.

157. Tan JS, Wang JJ, Flood V, Rochtchina E, Smith W, Mitchell P. Dietary antioxidants and the long-term incidence of age-related macular degeneration: The Blue Mountains Eye Study. *Ophthalmology.* 2008;115(2):334–341.

158. Evans JR, Henshaw K. Antioxidant vitamin and mineral supplements for preventing age-related macular degeneration. *Cochrane Database Syst Rev.* 2008(1):CD000253.

159. Raghavendra V, Kulkarni SK. Possible antioxidant mechanism in melatonin reversal of aging and chronic ethanol-induced amnesia in plus-maze and passive avoidance memory tasks. *Free Radic Biol Med.* 2001;30(6):595–602.

160. von Gall C, Weaver DR. Loss of responsiveness to melatonin in the aging mouse suprachiasmatic nucleus. *Neurobiol Aging.* 2008;29(3):464–470.

161. Singh A, Naidu PS, Kulkarni SK. Reversal of aging and chronic ethanol-induced cognitive dysfunction by quercetin a bioflavonoid. *Free Radic Res.* 2003;37(11):1245–1252.

162. Patil CS, Singh VP, Satyanarayan PS, Jain NK, Singh A, Kulkarni SK. Protective effect of flavonoids against aging- and lipopolysaccharide-induced cognitive impairment in mice. *Pharmacology.* 2003;69(2):59–67.

163. Guayerbas N, Puerto M, Alvarez P, de la Fuente M. Improvement of the macrophage functions in prematurely ageing mice by a diet supplemented with thiolic antioxidants. *Cell Mol Biol (Noisy-le-grand).* 2004;50:OL677–681.

164. Guayerbas N, Puerto M, Hernanz A, Miquel J, De la Fuente M. Thiolic antioxidant supplementation of the diet reverses age-related behavioural dysfunction in prematurely ageing mice. *Pharmacol Biochem Behav.* 2005;80(1):45–51.

165. Long J, Gao F, Tong L, Cotman CW, Ames BN, Liu J. Mitochondrial decay in the brains of old rats: Ameliorating effect of alpha-lipoic acid and acetyl-L-carnitine. *Neurochem Res.* 2008;34(4):755–763.

166. Liu J, Killilea DW, Ames BN. Age-associated mitochondrial oxidative decay: Improvement of carnitine acetyltransferase substrate-binding affinity and activity in brain by feeding old rats acetyl-L-carnitine and/or R-alpha-lipoic acid. *Proc Natl Acad Sci USA.* 2002;99(4):1876–1881.

167. Group A-REDS. A randomized, placebo-contolled, clinical trial of high-dose supplementation with vitamins C and E, beta-carotene, and zinc for age-related macular degeneration and vision loss: AREDS report no. 8. *Arch Opthamol.* 2001;119:1417–1436.

168. Alvarado C, Alvarez P, Jimenez L, De la Fuente M. Improvement of leukocyte functions in young prematurely aging mice after a 5-week ingestion of a diet supplemented with biscuits enriched in antioxidants. *Antioxid Redox Signal.* 2005;7(9–10):1203–1210.

169. Alvarado C, Alvarez P, Puerto M, Gausseres N, Jimenez L, De la Fuente M. Dietary supplementation with antioxidants improves functions and decreases oxidative stress of leukocytes from prematurely aging mice. *Nutrition.* 2006;22(7–8):767–777.

170. De la Fuente M. Effects of antioxidants on immune system ageing. *Eur J Clin Nutr.* 2002;56(Suppl 3):S5–S8.

171. Richwine AF, Godbout JP, Berg BM, et al. Improved psychomotor performance in aged mice fed diet high in antioxidants is associated with reduced ex vivo brain interleukin-6 production. *Brain Behav Immun.* 2005;19(6):512–520.

172. Isaac MG, Quinn R, Tabet N. Vitamin E for Alzheimer's disease and mild cognitive impairment. *Cochrane Database Syst Rev.* 2008(3):CD002854.

173. Farina N, Isaac MG, Clark AR, Rusted J, Tabet N. Vitamin E for Alzheimer's dementia and mild cognitive impairment. *Cochrane Database Syst Rev.* 2012;11:CD002854.

174. Hamaguchi T, Ono K, Yamada M. REVIEW: Curcumin and Alzheimer's disease. *CNS Neurosci Ther.* 2010;16(5):285–297.

175. Hager K, Kenklies M, McAfoose J, Engel J, Munch G. Alpha-lipoic acid as a new treatment option for Alzheimer's disease—A 48 months follow-up analysis. *J Neural Transm Suppl.* 2007(72):189–193.

176. Dysken MW, Sano M, Asthana S, et al. Effect of vitamin E and memantine on functional decline in Alzheimer disease: The TEAM-AD VA cooperative randomized trial. *JAMA*. 2014;311(1):33–44.

177. Fiala M, Terrando N, Dalli J. Specialized pro-resolving mediators from omega-3 fatty acids improve amyloid-beta phagocytosis and regulate inflammation in patients with minor cognitive impairment. *J Alzheimers Dis*. 2015;48(2):293–301.

178. Chiu CC, Su KP, Cheng TC, et al. The effects of omega-3 fatty acids monotherapy in Alzheimer's disease and mild cognitive impairment: A preliminary randomized double-blind placebo-controlled study. *Prog Neuropsychopharmacol Biol Psychiatry*. 2008;32(6):1538–1544.

179. Shults CW, Oakes D, Kieburtz K, et al. Effects of coenzyme Q10 in early Parkinson disease: Evidence of slowing of the functional decline. *Arch Neurol*. 2002;59(10):1541–1550.

180. Vile GF, Winterbourn CC. Inhibition of adriamycin-promoted microsomal lipid peroxidation by beta-carotene, alpha-tocopherol and retinol at high and low oxygen partial pressures. *FEBS Letters*. 1988;238(2):353–356.

181. Niki E. Interaction of ascorbate and alpha-tocopherol. *Ann N Y Acad Sci*. 1987;498:186–199.

182. Wu H, Kong L, Tan Y, et al. C66 ameliorates diabetic nephropathy in mice by both upregulating NRF2 function via increase in miR-200a and inhibiting miR-21. *Diabetologia*. 2016;59:1558–1568.

183. Itoh K, Chiba T, Takahashi S, et al. An Nrf2/small Maf heterodimer mediates the induction of phase II detoxifying enzyme genes through antioxidant response elements. *Biochem Biophys Res Commun*. 1997;236(2):313–322.

184. Williamson TP, Johnson DA, Johnson JA. Activation of the Nrf2-ARE pathway by siRNA knockdown of Keap1 reduces oxidative stress and provides partial protection from MPTP-mediated neurotoxicity. *Neurotoxicology*. 2012;33(3):272–279.

185. Jaramillo MC, Zhang DD. The emerging role of the Nrf2-Keap1 signaling pathway in cancer. *Genes Dev*. 2013;27(20):2179–2191.

186. Li W, Khor TO, Xu C, et al. Activation of Nrf2-antioxidant signaling attenuates NFkappaB-inflammatory response and elicits apoptosis. *Biochem Pharmacol*. 2008;76(11):1485–1489.

187. Kim J, Cha YN, Surh YJ. A protective role of nuclear factor-erythroid 2-related factor-2 (Nrf2) in inflammatory disorders. *Mutat Res*. 2010;690(1–2):12–23.

188. Suh JH, Shenvi SV, Dixon BM, et al. Decline in transcriptional activity of Nrf2 causes age-related loss of glutathione synthesis, which is reversible with lipoic acid. *Proc Nantl Acad Sci USA*. 2004;101(10):3381–3386.

189. Tomobe K, Shinozuka T, Kuroiwa M, Nomura Y. Age-related changes of Nrf2 and phosphorylated GSK-3beta in a mouse model of accelerated aging (SAMP8). *Arch Gerontol Geriat*. 2012;54(2):e1–e7.

190. Sachdeva MM, Cano M, Handa JT. Nrf2 signaling is impaired in the aging RPE given an oxidative insult. *Exp Eye Res*. 2014;119:111–114.

191. Mostafavi-Pour Z, Ramezani F, Keshavarzi F, Samadi N. The role of quercetin and vitamin C in Nrf2-dependent oxidative stress production in breast cancer cells. *Oncol Lett*. 2017;13(3):1965–1973.

192. Katsuyama Y, Tsuboi T, Taira N, Yoshioka M, Masaki H. 3-O-Laurylglyceryl ascorbate activates the intracellular antioxidant system through the contribution of PPAR-gamma and Nrf2. *J Dermatol Sci*. 2016;82(3):189–196.

193. Xi YD, Yu HL, Ding J, et al. Flavonoids protect cerebrovascular endothelial cells through Nrf2 and PI3K from beta-amyloid peptide-induced oxidative damage. *Curr Neurovasc Res*. 2012;9(1):32–41.

194. Choi HK, Pokharel YR, Lim SC, et al. Inhibition of liver fibrosis by solubilized coenzyme Q10: Role of Nrf2 activation in inhibiting transforming growth factor-beta1 expression. *Toxicol Appl Pharm*. 2009;240(3):377–384.

195. Ji L, Liu R, Zhang XD, et al. N-acetylcysteine attenuates phosgene-induced acute lung injury via up-regulation of Nrf2 expression. *Inhal Toxicol*. 2010;22(7):535–542.

196. Gao L, Wang J, Sekhar KR, et al. Novel n-3 fatty acid oxidation products activate Nrf2 by destabilizing the association between Keap1 and Cullin3. *J Biol Chem*. 2007;282(4):2529–2537.

197. Saw CL, Yang AY, Guo Y, Kong AN. Astaxanthin and omega-3 fatty acids individually and in combination protect against oxidative stress via the Nrf2-ARE pathway. *Food Chem Toxicol*. 2013;62:869–875.

198. Trujillo J, Chirino YI, Molina-Jijon E, Anderica-Romero AC, Tapia E, Pedraza-Chaverri J. Renoprotective effect of the antioxidant curcumin: Recent findings. *Redox Biol*. 2013;1(1):448–456.

199. Steele ML, Fuller S, Patel M, Kersaitis C, Ooi L, Munch G. Effect of Nrf2 activators on release of glutathione, cysteinylglycine, and homocysteine by human U373 astroglial cells. *Redox Biol*. 2013;1(1):441–445.

200. Kode A, Rajendrasozhan S, Caito S, Yang SR, Megson IL, Rahman I. Resveratrol induces glutathione synthesis by activation of Nrf2 and protects against cigarette smoke-mediated oxidative stress in human lung epithelial cells. *Am J Physiol. Lung Cell Mol Physiol.* 2008;294(3):L478–L488.
201. Zambrano S, Blanca AJ, Ruiz-Armenta MV, et al. The renoprotective effect of L-carnitine in hypertensive rats is mediated by modulation of oxidative stress-related gene expression. *Eur J Nutr.* 2013;52(6):1649–1659.
202. Eades G, Yang M, Yao Y, Zhang Y, Zhou Q. miR-200a regulates Nrf2 activation by targeting Keap1 mRNA in breast cancer cells. *J Biol Chem.* 2011;286(47):40725–40733.
203. Abate A, Yang G, Dennery PA, Oberle S, Schroder H. Synergistic inhibition of cyclooxygenase-2 expression by vitamin E and aspirin. *Free Radic Biol Med.* 2000;29(11):1135–1142.
204. Fu Y, Zheng S, Lin J, Ryerse J, Chen A. Curcumin protects the rat liver from CCl4-caused injury and fibrogenesis by attenuating oxidative stress and suppressing inflammation. *Mol Pharmacol.* 2008;73(2):399–409.
205. Lee HS, Jung KK, Cho JY, et al. Neuroprotective effect of curcumin is mainly mediated by blockade of microglial cell activation. *Pharmazie.* 2007;62(12):937–942.
206. Rahman S, Bhatia K, Khan AQ, et al. Topically applied vitamin E prevents massive cutaneous inflammatory and oxidative stress responses induced by double application of 12-O-tetradecanoylphorbol-13-acetate (TPA) in mice. *Chem Biol Interact.* 2008;172(3):195–205.
207. Suzuki YJ, Aggarwal BB, Packer L. Alpha-lipoic acid is a potent inhibitor of NF-kappa B activation in human T cells. *Biochem Biophys Res Commun.* 1992;189(3):1709–1715.
208. Zhu J, Yong W, Wu X, et al. Anti-inflammatory effect of resveratrol on TNF-alpha-induced MCP-1 expression in adipocytes. *Biochem Biophys Res Commun.* 2008;369(2):471–477.
209. Prasad KN. Alpha-tocopheryl succinate exhibits potent anticancer activity: Its interaction with ionizing radiation and chemotherapy effects. In: Reddy VR, Watson RR, ed. *The Encyclopedia of Vitamin E.* London, UK: CAB International; 2007.

5 Role of Micronutrients in Prevention of Coronary Artery Disease and Improvement of the Standard Therapy

INTRODUCTION

In the Unites States, cardiovascular diseases remain the leading cause of death and accounts for about 801,000 deaths—that means 1 in every 3 deaths. It is estimated that about 2,200 American die of this disease each day, an average of 1 death every 40 seconds.[1] Despite current dietary and lifestyle recommendations, methods of early detection, advanced surgical intervention, wide use of cholesterol-lowering and antiplatelet aggregation drugs, coronary artery disease (CAD) remains the number-one cause of death in the USA. The exact reasons for the failure of the current approaches to affect overall mortality from heart disease are unknown. However, it is possible that the major risk factors that initiate and promote CAD are not being optimally reduced at the same time.

In order to devise an effective prevention and improved management of CAD, it is essential to identify extracellular and intracellular risk factors that initiate and promote this disease. Extracellular risk factors include tobacco smoking, obesity, lack of physical activity, poor nutrition, diabetes, and aging. Implementation of recommended dietary and lifestyle can reduce some extracellular risk factors except aging. However, human behaviors are difficult to change; therefore, these recommendations have not had significant impact on reducing extracellular risk factors. Intracellular risk factors include increased oxidative stress, chronic inflammation, high levels of homocysteine and cholesterols, particularly LDL-cholesterol, triglycerides, platelet aggregation, and heritable gene defects. Although cholesterol-lowering and antiplatelet aggregation drugs have been useful in reducing the risk of heart attack, the other cellular risk factors are not optimally and simultaneously attenuated. The evidence for intracellular risk factors is discussed in detail later in this chapter.

One of the nontoxic micronutrients that could simultaneously reduce oxidative stress, chronic inflammation, and homocysteine levels has not been utilized on the basis of scientific rationale. This is evidenced by the fact that use of a single antioxidant or B-vitamins alone in high-risk population of CAD has produced inconsistent results, varying from no effect to some transient effects on certain clinical outcomes. These results were in contrast to animal studies in which a single antioxidant produced consistent benefits on cardiac health.

This chapter briefly describes incidence, prevalence, cost, and evidence for increased oxidative stress, chronic inflammation, and homocysteine levels in the initiation and progression of CAD. It describes involvement of microRNAs that regulate the translation of proteins from their respective mRNAs transcripts in the pathogenesis of CAD. It also presents results of epidemiologic and intervention studies on the effects of primarily individual micronutrients in management of CAD, and discusses potential reasons for obtaining inconsistent results varying from no effect to transient benefits on some risk factors. A single micronutrient cannot simultaneously reduce oxidative stress and inflammation that are required for optimal benefit in the prevention and, in combination with standard therapy, improved management of CAD. In order to accomplish the above goal, it is essential to increase the levels of cytoprotective enzymes including antioxidant enzymes through activation of the Nrf2/ARE pathway and dietary and endogenous antioxidants. This chapter suggests a mixture of micronutrients that would reduce oxidative stress, chronic inflammation, and homocysteine levels at the same time and thereby would help in the prevention and improved management of CAD.

PREVALENCE, INCIDENCE, AND COST

About 92.1 million are living with cardiovascular disease. Annual incidence of heart disease is about 790,000 cases; 114,000 die of this disease. The incidence of heart attack estimated to be 580,000 new cases and 210,000 recurrent cases each year.[1] The direct and indirect cost is estimated to be $316 billion. The incidence of diagnosed heart attack and fatal coronary heart disease is age and gender dependent.[2]

Age (years)	Number per 1000/year	
	Men	Women
45–54	75	35
55–64	125	60
65–74	125	70
75–84	120	84
85+	80	110

It is interesting to note that incidences of heart disease continue to increase in women as a function of age; however, in men, it decreases after the age of 75 years.

EVIDENCE FOR INCREASED OXIDATIVE STRESS IN CAD

The direct evidence for increase in oxidative stress comes from elevated levels of markers of oxidative stress in the blood, and the indirect evidence is supported by the experiments in which antioxidant protect against heart disease by reducing oxidative damage. Numerous articles and reviews have been published on this issue. Only a few of them are presented here.

The levels of malondialdehyde (MDA), a marker of oxidative stress, and DNA strand breaks, and indicator of decreased efficiency of DNA repair were elevated, whereas the levels of ascorbic acid and glutathione were reduced in patients with CAD compared with control subjects.[3] In Thai patients with stable CAD, the levels of MDA were higher, but the plasma total protein thiols levels were lower than in control subjects.[4] Patients with CAD and psoriasis had similar higher levels of MDA, IL-6, carotid-femoral pulse wave velocity (PWVc) and central augmentation index (CAI) carotid intima media thickness (IMT), and lower levels of flow-mediated dilation (FMD) of the brachial artery, left ventricular global longitudinal strain (GLS), coronary flow reserve (CFR), and GLS rate (GLSR) compared with controls.[5] In erythrocytes from CAD patients, the levels of lipid peroxidation and total cholesterol were elevated, whereas the levels of membrane fluidity, and activities of catalase and SOD were decreased compared with control subjects.[6] The elevated serum levels of gamma-glutamyl transferase (GGT), a product of increased cellular oxidative stress, which is associated with poor prognosis of CAD, were also enhanced in CAD patients who have undergone coronary angiography.[7,8] In Pakistani patients with early CAD, serum levels of GGT were enhanced. This marker of oxidative stress positively correlated with blood pressure, cholesterol, blood glucose, and smoking and negatively correlated with antioxidants levels.[9]

In patients with microvascular angina and with CAD, the plasma and RBC levels showed increased amounts of inhibitors of nitric oxide (NO) synthesis and reduced expression of NO synthase. These patients showed enhanced oxidative stress.[10] Levels of 8-isoprostane, a marker of oxidative stress in the plasma, were associated with the severity of CAD.[11] Among elderly patients with CAD, women had higher levels of serum hydroperoxides than men.[12] The levels of MDA, nitrite/nitrate, and DNA damage in CAD patients were higher than those found in control subjects, suggesting involvement of increased oxidative and nitrosylative stresses in pathophysiology of this disease.[13] The serum levels of 8-hydroxy-2′-deoxyguanosine (8-OHdG) were higher in CAD patients than in normal subjects.[14] This marker of oxidative stress was associated with the severity of CAD.

CONSEQUENCES OF INCREASED OXIDATIVE STRESS

LDL-cholesterol is commonly referred to as "bad cholesterol" because it is easily oxidized by free radicals. Oxidized LDL-cholesterol may be one of the early events that initiate plaque formation by increasing the formation of foam cells; enhancing platelet adhesion and aggregation; triggering thrombosis; and impairing elasticity of the coronary arteries.[15,16] Oxidized LDL-cholesterol can also increase vascular smooth muscle cell proliferation by activating c-myc oncogene, and its binding partner MAX, the carboxyl-terminal domain-binding factors activator protein-2 (AP-2), and elongation 2-factor (E2F) in human coronary artery smooth muscle cells.[17] Oxidized LDL-cholesterol is engulfed by the macrophages to form foam cells, and C-reactive protein increases the uptake of oxidized LDL-cholesterol by the macrophages and thereby increased the number of foam cells.[18] Both foam cells and increased proliferation of vascular smooth muscle cells contribute to the formation of plaque in the coronary arteries. Once the plaque is formed, it serves as a continuous stimulus for increased inflammatory reactions that release reactive oxygen species (ROS) and pro-inflammatory cytokines. Using cultured monocyte/mononuclear cells obtained from CAD patients and normal persons, it was demonstrated that long-term exposure to oxidized LDL-cholesterol enhanced cytoplasmic IkappaB phosphorylation and NF-kappaB translocation, and increased endothelial adhesiveness of monocyte/mononuclear. Oxidized LDL-cholesterol also significantly enhanced TNF-alpha-stimulated ROS production and endothelial adhesiveness of monocyte/mononuclear cells. This increase in oxidative stress contributes to atherogenesis.[19] Thus, the lowering the level of LDL-cholesterol and preventing its oxidation should reduce the risk of developing plaques.

Endothelial cells of the vascular wall are damaged by the free radicals, secretary products of inflammatory reactions (ROS, pro-inflammatory cytokines, adhesion molecules, complement proteins and prostaglandin E_2), and homocysteine. It is now recognized that endothelial cell dysfunction may also be one of the early events in the development of CAD.[20,21] Damage to endothelial cells may impair the nitric oxide synthase (NOS) pathway, which in turn may reduce endothelium-dependent coronary artery dilation. Thus, deficiency in the production of NO may interfere with the function of the vessel wall. The levels of inducible NOS (iNOS) mRNA in vascular smooth muscle cells of a healthy arterial wall is low, but the levels of iNOS mRNA and protein in macrophages, and smooth muscle cells are high in CAD.[22] This suggests that high levels of iNOS may release excessive amounts of NO that could be oxidized to form peroxynitrite, which can induce arterial dysfunction. Thus, the role of NO in maintaining normal vascular function depends upon maintaining the proper levels of NO. Both deficiency and excess production of NO can impair vasomotion and enhance endothelial dysfunction. Therefore, protecting the endothelial cells from damage produced by free radicals should be considered useful in reducing the risk and progression of CAD.

EVIDENCE FOR INCREASED CHRONIC INFLAMMATION IN CAD

Oxidative damage, if not repaired, chronic inflammation sets in motion. Chronic infection also induced prolonged inflammation. During this biological event, ROS, pro-inflammatory cytokines, complement proteins, and adhesion molecules are released all of which are toxic to cells. High blood levels of C-reactive proteins, a marker of chronic inflammation, were present in CAD patients.[18] Increased levels of plasma CRP were independently associated with coronary atherosclerosis burden.[23] Elevated plasma concentrations were more frequently observed in patients who had undergone coronary artery bypass grafting surgery who died than those who survived.[24] Increased plasma levels of CRP, neoptrin, matrix metalloproteinase-9, soluble intercellular adhesion molecule-1, and previous history of unstable angina were associated with rapid progression of CAD.[25] Increased plasma levels of CRP are considered an independent risk factor for CAD and independently predicts enhanced platelet aggregation in stable CAD patients.[26]

Increased concentrations of the pro-inflammatory cytokines IL-17, IL-6, IL-8, and heat-sensitive CRP, and decreased levels of IL-10 were found in the plasma of patients with unstable angina and acute myocardial infarction.[27] The levels of IL-6, IL-8, IL-10, and TNF-alpha were higher in patients with myocardial infarction and unstable angina than in patients with stable angina or control subjects.[28] Plasma concentrations of IL-9 were elevated in asymptomatic and symptomatic patients with coronary and carotid atherosclerosis compared with healthy controls. IL-9 enhanced the release of IL-17 in the peripheral blood mononuclear cells from patients with coronary and carotid atherosclerosis compared with control subjects.[29] Markers of inflammation are associated with CAD. Enhanced amounts of CRP, fibrinogen, IL-6, stoma-derived factor-1, CXC motif ligand 16, macrophage migration inhibitory factor, RANTES (Regulated on Activation, Normal T cell Expressed and Secreted), calprotectin, and copeptin were associated with increased risk of cardiovascular events in CAD patients.[26]

EVIDENCE FOR INCREASED LEVELS OF HOMOCYSTEINE IN CAD

Increased levels of plasma homocysteine are considered a risk factor for CAD.[30] High homocysteine levels in the plasma were associated with age, male gender, hypertension, renal failure, family history of CAD, previous cardiovascular event, previous myocardial infarction, ejection fraction, higher baseline creatinine, treatment with nitrate, calcium antagonists, diuretics, Ace inhibitors, clopidogrel, hemoglobin, white blood cells count, total cholesterol, and low-density lipoproteins (LDL). The plasma levels of homocysteine were correlated with the extent of CAD.[31] Higher levels of plasma homocysteine and CRP, and older age, and reduced creatine-clearance were indicative for CAD. Furthermore, the levels of homocysteine were correlated with neopterin levels, and CRP and accumulation of this compound was associated with impaired renal and heart function.[32] High plasma homocysteine levels contribute to the low-dose aspirin resistance in CAD patients, and to platelet aggregation.[33] Elevated plasma homocysteine levels were independent predictor of suboptimal response to antiplatelet therapy by acetylsalicylic acid.[34] Higher levels of homocysteine were associated with lower number of circulating endothelial progenitor cells and their impaired migratory capacity and ability to adhere to fibronectin, and CAD.[35] Enhanced plasma levels of homocysteine but not cysteine were inversely related to ApoA-1 and HDL-cholesterol and directly related to risk of CAD. Furthermore, combination of increased plasma levels of homocysteine and cysteine was associated with decreased levels of ApoA-1 and HDL-cholesterol, and with increased risk of CAD.[36] High plasma levels of homocysteine were associated with left ventricular dysfunction and congestive heart failure.[37] These studies suggest that increased plasma levels of homocysteine play an important role in the pathogenesis of CAD.

MicroRNAs IN CAD

Increased oxidative stress and chronic inflammation play a central role in the pathogenesis of CAD. Previous reviews have revealed that oxidative damage and pro-inflammatory cytokines alter the expression of microRNAs in some neurodegenerative diseases such as Alzheimer's disease (AD)[38] and Parkinson's disease (PD).[39] Therefore, it is likely that they also play an important role in the development of CAD. Indeed, altered levels of microRNAs were found in the plasma and serum of CAD patients that have been suggested to be of diagnostic value, and in the cells that may lead to cardiac dysfunction.

MicroRNAs

MicroRNAs (miRs) are evolutionarily conserved small noncoding single-stranded RNAs of approximately 22 nucleotides in length, and are present in all living organisms including humans.[40–43] The biogenesis of miRs is very complex and involves multiple biochemical steps. The majority of miRs are transcribed by RNA polymerase II (Pol II), while some are transcribed by RNA polymerase III (Pol III) from the non-coding region of the DNA to produce primary miRs (pri-miRs). Pri-miRs undergo a nuclear cleavage by ribonuclease III Drosa to generate precursor-miRs (pre-miRs) that migrate to the cytoplasm where they are further cleaved by ribonuclease III Dicer to ultimately form mature single-stranded miRs with the help of another protein argonaute (Ago).[42,44–46] Each microRNA binds to its complementary sequences in the 3′-untranslated region (3′-UTR) of the mRNA, promotes degradation of the mRNA transcript, and prevents translation of the message of protein. In this manner, miRs regulate the translation of proapoptotic or antiapoptotic proteins from their respective mRNAs, depending upon whether they receive damaging or protective signal. Damaging signals may include oxidative damage and pro-inflammatory cytokines and protective signals may include antioxidants and phytochemicals.

Circulating MicroRNAs in CAD

Table 5.1 summarizes changes in the expression of circulating microRNAs in patients with CAD. Plasma levels of three microRNAs (miR-19b-3p, miR-134-5p, and miR-186-5p) were enhanced in early stage of acute myocardial infarction (AMI).[47] The expression of miR-145 and miR-126-5p in the plasma was lower in patients with severe CAD compared with control subjects.[48,49] Plasma levels of miR-941were elevated in patients with non-ST elevation acute coronary syndrome (ACS)

TABLE 5.1

Plasma Levels of MicroRNAs in Coronary Artery Disease (CAD)

CAD Status	Upregulation	Downregulation
AMI	miR-19b-3p, miR-134-5p, miR-186-5p	None[47]
CAD severity	None	miR-145[48]
CAD severity	None	miR-126-5p[49]
NSTE-ACS STEMI	miR-941	None[50]
CAD stable STEMI	miR-15a-5p, miR-16-5p, miR-93-5p miR-499a-5p	miR-146a-5p[51]
CAD stable	None	miR-126, miR-17, miR-92a, miR-155[52]
CAD stable	miR-126, miR-199a	None[53]
CVS death	miR-132, miR-140-3p, miR-210	None[54]
CAD atypical	miR-487a, miR-502, miR-208 miR-215	miR-29b[55]
CAD early	None	miR-196-5p, miR-3163-3p miR-145-3p, miR-190a-5p[56]
CCC	miR-155[57]	miR-146a[58]
CAD death	miR-197, miR-223	None[59]
CAD	miR-18a, miR-17, miR-92a, miR-106b	None[60]

Note: NSTE-ACS, non-SF elevation acute coronary syndrome; STEMI, St segment elevation myocardial infarction; CVS, cardiovascular disease; CCC, coronary collateral circulation.

(NSTE-ACS) and ST-segment elevation myocardial infarction (STEMI) compared with non-CAD subjects.[50] Elevated plasma levels of miR-15a-5p, miR-16-5p, and miR-93-5p were found in stable CAD patients, whereas miR-146a-5p level was decreased compared with control subjects. Furthermore, the expression of miR-499a-5p was elevated in patients with STEMI.[51] Plasma levels of miR-126, miR-17, miR-92a, and miR-155 were reduced in patients with stable CAD compared with control subjects.[52] Enhanced expression of miR-126 and miR-199a in circulating microvesicles was associated with a lower risk of major adverse cardiovascular event rate.[53] Elevated plasma levels of miR-132, miR-143-3p, and miR-210 were predictor of cardiovascular death in patients with acute coronary syndrome.[54] Increased serum expression of miR-487a, miR-502, miR-208, and miR-215, and decreased expression of miR-29b were associated with atypical CAD.[55] Decreased expression of miR-196-5p, miR-3163-3p, miR-145-3p, and miR-190a-5p was found in the serum of patients with early-onset of CAD.[56] Increased plasma expression of miR-155 and decreased levels of its target protein VCAM-1 in CAD patients with poor coronary collateral circulation (CCC),[57] while reduced expression of miR-146a was associated with poor CCC.[58] Elevated serum levels of miR-197 and miR-223 were predictor of future CAD death.[59] Increased plasma levels of miR-17, miR-18a, miR-92a, and miR-106b were associated with CAD. Furthermore, the expression of miR-17 was positively correlated with total cholesterol, LDL-cholesterol, and apolipoprotein B, the expression of miR-92a was positively correlated with HDL-cholesterol but negatively correlated with apo-lipoprotein A, and the expression of miR-106b was positively correlated with apolipoprotein A and HDL-cholesterol.[60] These studies discussed above suggest that certain circulating microRNAs could be used as a predictor of CAD.

Cellular MicroRNAs in CAD

Table 5.2 summarizes changes in the expression of cellular microRNAs in CAD patients. Reduced expression of miR-31 leads in to the elevation of the levels of its target proteins FAT atypical cadherin 4 and thromboxane A2 receptor in the endothelial progenitor cells (EPCs) from patients with CAD.[61] Overexpression of miR-31 in CAD EPCs restored their ability to participate in angiogenesis

TABLE 5.2

Cellular Levels of MicroRNAs in Coronary Artery Disease (CAD)

Upregulation	Downregulation	Target proteins
	miR-31	Atypical cadherin 4
		Thromboxane A2 receptors
	miR-720	Vasoinhibition 1[61]
miR-410-3p, miR-497-5p, miR-2355-5p		VEGFR2[65]
miR-21		FOXP3, TGF1β, Smad7[66]
	miR-181a	TLR/NFkB[67]
miR-206		PIK3C-α[62]
miR-23a		EGFR[63]
miR-214		VEGF[64]

Note: VEGFR2, Vascular endothelial growth factor receptor 2; FOXP3, forkhead boxP3; TGF1β,transforming growth factor 1β; TLR/NFkB, toll-like receptor/ nuclear factor-kappaB; PIK3G2-α, phosphatidylinositol 4,5-bisphosphate 3-kinase catalytic subunitA isoform.

and vasculogenesis in both in vitro and in vivo. Furthermore, lower expression of miR-720 leads to increased levels of its target protein vasohibin-1 in the EPCs from patients with CAD. Thus, downregulation of miR-31 and miR-720 contribute to the pathogenesis of CAD. The expression of miR-206 was elevated and its target protein phosphatidylinositol 4,5-bisphosphate 3-kinase catalytic subunitA isoform (PIK3G2-α) in EPCs from CAD patients. Deletion of miR-206 restored angiogenesis and vasculogenesis functions of EPCs.[62] Elevated expression of miR-23a downregulated its target protein epidermal growth factor receptor (EGFR) in EPCs from CAD patients. Knockingdown of miR-23a restored functions of EPCs and enhanced blood flow recovery in ischemic limbs of mice.[63] The expression of miR-214 was enhanced and its target protein vascular endothelial growth factor (VEGF) was reduced in EPCs from patients with CAD. Deletion of miR-214 restored normal function of EPCs.[64]

The expression of miR-410-3p, miR-497-5p, and miR-2355-5p was elevated in EPCs from CAD patients and their target protein vascular endothelial growth factor receptor-2 (VEGFR2) was reduced. Knockingdown these microRNAs restored the levels of VEGFR2 and increased angiogenic activities of CAD endothelial colony-forming cells (ECFCs) in vitro, and facilitated blood flow recovery in ischemic limbs in mice model. Since similar levels of these microns were also found in plasma of CAD patients, they may be useful biomarkers for CAD.[65]

The expression of miR-21 was upregulated in peripheral blood mononuclear cells (PBMCs) from patients with CHD (acute myocardial infarction, unstable angina, stable angina). This microRNA showed a progressive enhancement from stable angina to unstable angina to AMI. The upregulation of miR-21 led to reduced levels of its target proteins forkhead box p3 (Foxp3), transforming growth factor beta-1 (TGF-b1) and Smad7, and decreased number of PBMCs.[66]

The expression of miR-181a was downregulated and its target proteins Toll-like receptor/nuclear factor-kappaB (TLR/NFkB) levels were enhanced in monocyte from CAD patients. An association of changes with CAD remained intact even after adjustment for CAD traditional risk factors such as obesity and the metabolic syndrome.[67]

The studies discussed above suggest that upregulation and downregulation of microRNAs are involved in the pathogenesis of CAD. In addition, the results show that one microRNA can prevent the translation of multiple mRNAs transcripts into proteins, and multiple microRNAs can prevent the translation of mRNA transcript of one protein.

OXIDATIVE STRESS AND PRO-INFLAMMATORY CYTOKINE REGULATE EXPRESSION OF MicroRNAs

We have also shown that oxidative stress and pro-inflammatory cytokines regulate the expression of microRNAs and their associated target proteins that cause neurodegeneration in Alzheimer's disease[38] and Parkinson's disease.[39] It is likely that the levels of microRNAs may be altered in CAD. Additional direct evidence on the effect of free radicals on the expression of microRNAs is described here.

Treatment of human endothelial cells with H_2O_2 enhanced the expression of miR-192-5p, and its target mRNAs for the cell cycle, DNA repair, and stress response were downregulated, suggesting that increased oxidative stress contributes to senescence and cell death.[68] Treatment with H_2O_2 also increased the p53-dependent apoptotic pathway. In premature fibroblast senescence model, treatment with H_2O_2 increased the expression of miR-24 and miR-424. The levels of p53 were increased in miR-24 overexpressing cells, but decreased in cells overexpressing miR-424.[69] Furthermore, it was demonstrated that overexpression of miR-24 induced senescence by decreasing the levels of its target protein DNA topoisomerase1 (TOP1). This was further confirmed by showing that knocking down TOP1 induced senescence in the fibroblasts. Increased oxidative stress enhanced the expression of miR-153 that reduced the expression of Nrf2 by binding to its 3'-UTR region of Nrf2 mRNA.[70] Mutation in miR-153 restored the oxidative stress-induced reduction in Nrf2 activity.

Antioxidants Regulate Expression of MicroRNAs

Previous reviews proposed that antioxidants regulate expression of microRNAs that allow translation of only protective proteins in varieties of cell type and health conditions such as Alzheimer's disease (AD)[71] and Parkinson's disease (PD).[72] Since antioxidants protect against some components of CAD, it is possible that they may also alter the expression of microRNAs in order to provide protection against the development of CAD.

ROLE OF ANTIOXIDANTS IN CAD

Since increased oxidative stress and chronic inflammation are early events that initiate and promote damage leading to CAD, and since antioxidants can neutralize free radicals and reduce inflammation, they should be considered one of the rational strategies for the prevention of CAD. Indeed, the US Prevention Service Task Force recommends multiple vitamin supplements to reduce the risk of cancer and CAD.[73,74] However, these recommendations do not provide guidelines with respect to type of micronutrients that should be included and excluded. The doses and dose schedule were also not described in the above recommendation.

Animal Studies after Treatment with Antioxidants

Animal studies consistently showed that individual antioxidants such as vitamin E alone reduced the incidence and/or rate of progression of CAD.[75–77] In rats, supplementation with vitamin C and vitamin E reduced hyperhomocysteinemia-induced increase in myocardial oxidative stress and myocardial fibrosis.[78] The beneficial effects of one or two dietary antioxidants on cardiac events in animals have not been consistently observed in patients with CAD. This suggests that the data obtained on animal models should not be extrapolated to humans because the absorption, distribution, and metabolism of antioxidants is different in each. Furthermore, rodents, except guinea pigs, make their own vitamin C, while humans do not.

Epidemiologic Studies with Antioxidants

Despite numerous confounding factors associated with the epidemiologic investigations, 6 out of 8 studies with vitamin E alone showed an inverse relationship between vitamin E intake and the risk of CAD. The remaining two studies showed no beneficial effects. In a WHO/MONICA study (an International Collaborative World Health Organization Monitoring of Trends and Determinants in Cardiovascular Disease), there was a high inverse association between age-specific mortality from ischemic heart disease and lipid-standardized vitamin E levels.[79] In a Polish study, plasma levels of vitamin E were significantly lower in patients with stable and unstable angina compared to healthy control persons.[80] In a UK study, an inverse association between plasma vitamin E levels and the risk of angina was reported.[81]

In a Harvard study of 39,910 male health professionals, a 36% lower relative risk of CAD was demonstrated among those consuming 60 IU of vitamin E per day, compared to those who consume less than 7.5 IU of vitamin E per day.[82] Men who took at least 100 IU of vitamin E per day for at least 2 years had a 37% lower risk of CAD than those who did not take vitamin E. Another Harvard study of 87, 245 healthy nurses with a follow-up period of 8 years revealed that women in the top fifth of vitamin E intake had a 34% lower relative risk of major cardiac events compared to those in the lowest fifth.[83] The relative risk of CAD was 48% lower in women taking vitamin E supplements of more than 100 mg/day for at least 2 years. Vitamin E obtained only from the diet provided no such protection.

In another US study of 11,000 people of age 67 or over with a follow-up period of 6 years found that vitamin E supplementation was associated with a 47% reduction in mortality from CAD.[84] Further reduction was observed in people who were taking vitamin E supplements together with vitamin C.

In contrast to the above 6 investigations, 2 studies failed to observe any association between serum selenium, vitamin A, or vitamin E and the risk of death from CAD.[85,86] None of the epidemiologic studies have examined the role of endogenous antioxidants such as glutathione, alpha-lipoic acid, L-carnitine, or coenzyme Q10 in reducing the risk of CAD.

It has been reported that the serum levels of neopterin, a marker of inflammation, were elevated in patients with CAD compared to controls.[87] The average serum levels of vitamin C, gamma-tocopherol, lycopene, lutein, zeaxanthin, alpha-carotene, and beta-carotene (BC) were lower in patients with CAD compared to controls. These results suggest that the serum level of neopterin was inversely related to the serum levels of antioxidants in patients with CAD, and that increased inflammation plays an important role in the etiology of CAD.

INTERVENTION HUMAN STUDIES AFTER TREATMENT WITH ANTIOXIDANTS

Based on the consistency of data on the beneficial effects of vitamin E alone, vitamin C alone, or both in combination on CAD obtained from animal and epidemiologic studies, it was tempting to think that similar beneficial effects of these dietary antioxidants could be observed when used individually or in combination in human populations at high risk of developing CAD. However, in view of the fact that the high-risk populations, such as heavy tobacco smokers and patients with type II diabetes, have a high internal oxidative environment, and that administration of vitamin E or vitamin C alone can result in oxidation of these antioxidants, such a temptation should have been resisted. Nevertheless, a few clinical studies with vitamin E alone were initiated in patients with CAD, and as expected, they all produced inconsistent results varying from no effect, to beneficial effects, to harmful effects. Other reasons were that the form, type, number, dose and dose-schedule of antioxidants, study end points, observation periods, and patient populations differ from one study to another (Tables 5.3 through 5.5). When endogenous antioxidants were used individually, similar inconsistent results were obtained. When dietary antioxidants were used in combination with cholesterol-lowering drugs, similar inconsistent results were also noted (Tables 5.6 and 5.7).

TABLE 5.3
Summary of Intervention Trials with Vitamin E Alone in High-Risk CAD Patients Showing Beneficial Effects

Name of Study	No. of Patients	Type of Antioxidant	Criteria of Study	Follow-up Period	Results
CHAOS	2,002[a]	Vitamin E (d-α) 400 or 800 IU	Death, non-fatal M.I.	510 d	Reduced[92]
	42[b]	Vitamin E(α-TA) 544 IU	FMD	4 months	Improved[90]
	100[c] Vitamin E 1200 IU	Stenosis	4 months	Reduced[88]	
	75[d] Vitamin E 1200 IU	C-reactive protein	5 months	Reduced[89]	
	33[e]	Vit. E (d-αT) 800 IU	LDL oxidation	12 weeks	Reduced[91]

Note: CHAOS, Cambridge Heart Antioxidant Study; M.I., myocardial infarction; FMD, endothelial-dependent flow-mediated dilation.

All vitamins were given once a day until specified otherwise. The number in superscript indicates reference number.

[a] Proven atherosclerosis disease.

[b] Hypercholesterolemia, smokers and smokers with hypercholesterolemia.

[c] Angioplasty.

[d] Type II diabetes.

[e] Patients undergoing peritoneal dialysis (N = 17) or hemodialysis (N = 16).

TABLE 5.4

Summary of Intervention Trials with Vitamin E in Combination with Vitamin C in High-Risk CAD Patients Showing Beneficial Effects

No. of Patients	Type of Antioxidant	Criteria of Study	Follow-up Period	Results
19[a]	Vitamin E-400 IU Vitamin C-500 mg	Coronary atherosclerosis	1 year	Reduced[94]
520[b]	Vitamin E, slow release	Atherosclerosis	6 years	Reduced[96]
20[c]	Vitamin E 800 IU Vitamin C-1g	FMD	6 hours	Increased[95]
182[b]	Multivitamins	Homocysteine	6 months	Reduced[93]

Note: FMD, Endothelial-dependent flow-mediated dilation; LDL-C, LDL-cholesterol.

All vitamins were given once a day until specified otherwise. The number in superscript indicates reference number.

[a] Cardiac transplant.

[b] Hypercholesterolemia.

[c] Normal individuals consuming high-fat meal.

TABLE 5.5

Dietary Antioxidants Producing No Effects or Adverse Effects in High-Risk CAD Patients

Study	Treatment	End Points	Results
ATBC trial	High serum alpha-T	Mortality	Decreased[98]
	DL-alpha-T (50 mg/day)	CAD risk	No effect[99]
	DL-alpha-T (50 mg/day)	Cerebral infarction	Decreased[100,101]
	DL-alpha-T (50 mg/day)	Fatal HS	Increased[100]
ATBC trial	Synthetic BC (50 mg/day)	CAD risk	Increased[99]
	Synthetic BC (50 mg/day)	Intracerebral hemorrhage	Increased[100]
	Synthetic BC (50 mg/day)		No effect[101]
HOPE trial	Natural alpha-T 400 IU/day	Major cardiac events (myocardial infarction, Stroke and death)	No affect[102–106]
		Secondary cardiac events (Unstable angina, Renal insufficiency, nephropathy)	No effects[102–106]
		Risk for heart failure, Hospitalization for heart failure	Increased[106]
Wave trial	Vitamin E 400 IU + Vitamin C 500 mg	MLD	No effect[110] Decreased[a110]
	" " "	FMD	No effect[111]
	" " "	MLD	Increased[b112]

Note: ATBC, Alpha-Tocopherol, Beta-Carotene Cancer Prevention; HOPE, Heart Outcomes Prevention Evaluation; WAVE, Women's Angiographic Vitamin and Estrogen; Alpha-T, alpha-tocopherol; Fatal HS, fatal hemorrhagic strokes; CAD, coronary artery disease; MLD, median luminal diameter; FMD, flow-mediated dilation.

All vitamins were given once a day until specified otherwise. The number in superscript indicates reference number.

[a] Potential harm (decrease in MLD) was suggested only when patients who died or had myocardial infarction during the trial period was included in the analysis.

[b] Patients with haptoglobin allele showing beneficial effect.

TABLE 5.6

Beneficial or No Effects of Antioxidants in Combination with Cholesterol-Lowering Drugs in High-Risk CAD Patients

Name of Study	No. of Patients	Type of Antioxidant + Cholesterol-Lowering Drugs	Criteria of Study	Follow-up Period	Results
	7[a]	Simvastatin + Vit. E-300 IU	FMD NMD	8 weeks	Improved[122]
	126[b]	Standard therapy + Co-enzyme Q10 33.3 mg (thrice/day)	Cardiac muscle function, cardiomyopathy	6 years	Improved[123,124]
CLAS	156[c]	Colestipol + niacin Vit. E-100 IU or more	Progressive atherosclerosis	2 years	Reduced[125]
HPS	20,500[a]	Simvastatin + Vit. E-650 mg Vit. C-250 mg	Cardiac events	5.5 years no better than than drug alone[126]	
		Beta-carotene-20 mg			

Note: HPS, Heart Protection Study; CLAS, Cholesterol-Lowering Atherosclerosis Study; FMD, endothelium-dependent flow-mediated dilation; NMD, endothelium-independent nitroglycerine-mediated dilation.

All vitamins were given once a day until specified otherwise. The number in superscript indicates reference number.

[a] Hypercholesterolemia.

[b] Idiopathic dilated cardiomyopathy.

[c] Coronary bypass surgery.

TABLE 5.7

Summary of Intervention Trials with One or More Dietary Antioxidants in Combination with Cholesterol-Lowering Drugs in High-Risk Patients Showing No Effects or Adverse Effects

Name of Study	No. of Patients	Antioxidants + Cholesterol-Lowering Drugs	Criteria of Study	Follow-up Period	Results
HATS	160[a]	Simvastatin + niacin+ Vitamin E 800 IU Vitamin C-1g β-carotene—25 mg, Selenium-100 mcg (N = 46)	Stenosis	3 year	Reduced drug[127] Effectiveness, more effective than control
HATS	153[b]	Same	HDL	1 year	Reduce drug[128] Effectiveness
HATS		Same	Markers of cholesterol synthesis and absorption		No effect[129]

Note: HATS, HDL-Atherosclerosis Treatment Study; HDL, high density lipoprotein cholesterol; N, sample size for the group.

All vitamins were given once a day until specified otherwise. The number in superscript indicates reference number.

[a] Women with diabetics.

[b] Coronary disease with low HDL-cholesterol.

The published intervention trials utilizing antioxidants with or without cholesterol-lowering drugs can be divided into five groups:

1. Dietary antioxidants producing beneficial effects;
2. Dietary antioxidants producing no effect or adverse effects;
3. Endogenous antioxidants producing no effects or beneficial effects;
4. Dietary antioxidants in combination with cholesterol-lowering drugs producing beneficial effects; and
5. Dietary antioxidants in combination with cholesterol-lowering drugs producing no effects or adverse effects.

VITAMIN E ALONE PRODUCING BENEFICIAL EFFECTS

Table 5.3 summarizes the effect of vitamin E alone on various cardiac risk factors.[88–92] It can be noted that the dose of vitamin E varied from 400 IU to 1200 IU and the number and type of patients, criteria of study, and follow-up period also varied. It is well established that when vitamin E is oxidized, it acts as a pro-oxidant. Since the observation period was short, the adverse effects of oxidized vitamin E were not apparent. Table 5.4 primarily shows the effect of vitamin E in combination with vitamin C on the risk factors for CAD.[93–96] The variables described in the Table 5.3 can also be seen in the Table 5.4. These studies showed that the beneficial effects of two dietary antioxidants on CAD risk factors could be observed. Even though these studies produced some short-term beneficial effects, I do not recommend the use of one or two dietary antioxidants for the prevention or improved treatment of CAD, because they do not take into account other cardiac risk factors and do not utilize other antioxidants.

VITAMIN C ALONE PRODUCING BENEFICIAL EFFECTS

During a 10-year follow-up, 4,647 major cardiac events occur in 293,172 subjects who were free of CAD at baseline. The results showed that the supplemental vitamin C at high doses reduced major cardiac events.[97]

DIETARY ANTIOXIDANTS PRODUCING NO EFFECTS OR ADVERSE EFFECTS

A prospective cohort study of 29,092 Finnish male smokers aged 50–69 years who participated in the Alpha-Tocopherol, Beta-Carotene Cancer Prevention (ATBC) study was carried out to determine the risk of cardiac events. Fasting baseline of serum alpha-tocopherol concentration was determined. Only about 10% of participants reported the use of vitamin E supplement. The analysis of data presented in 4 separate publications has produced inconsistent results (Table 5.5). The results showed that higher serum concentrations of alpha-tocopherol were associated with lower total and cause-specific (cancer and cardiovascular disease) mortality in male heavy smokers.[98]

In the ATBC study, the effect of daily oral supplementation once-a-day dose of synthetic (dl) alpha-tocopherol 50 mg or synthetic beta-carotene 20 mg on CAD was investigated 6 years after the completion of the trial period of 5–8 years. At the beginning of posttrial follow-up, 23,144 men were at risk for a first major cardiac event, and 1255 men with pretrial history of myocardial infarction (MI) were at risk for major cardiac events. The results showed that alpha-tocopherol supplementation did not significantly affect the outcomes in either patient population compared to placebo control subjects. However, BC supplementation increased the risk of major cardiac events by about 14%, nonfatal myocardial infarction by about 16%, and fatal coronary heart disease by about 11%. However, no such effects were observed in the population that had a history of pretrial MI.[99] In the same study population, vitamin E prevented cerebral infarction, but increased the risk of fatal hemorrhagic strokes; BC increased the risk of Intracerebral hemorrhage.[100] In the same study population, another investigation showed that alpha-tocopherol increased the risk of cerebral infarction, while BC had no effect.[101] The reasons for this discrepancy in the analysis of the same population are unknown. During a 10-year follow-up, 4,647 major cardiac events occur in 293,172 subjects who were free of CAD at the baseline. The results showed that supplementation with vitamin E alone did not reduce the major cardiac events.[97]

A randomized, double blind, placebo-controlled international trail, Heart Outcomes Prevention Evaluation (HOPE), was conducted from December 21, 1993, to April 15, 1999. One of the objectives of this trial was to evaluate the efficacy of natural vitamin E (400 IU/day) in reducing the risk of CAD for patients at least 55 years of age with vascular disease or diabetes, many of who were heavy cigarette smokers. The analysis of data from this study presented in five separate publications has produced inconsistent results (Table 5.5).

In the analysis published in 2000, the primary end points were major cardiac events (MI, stroke, and death due to coronary heart disease), and the secondary end points were unstable angina, heart failure, revascularization, amputation, death due to coronary heart disease, and complications of diabetes. No significant effect of vitamin E supplementation on the primary or the secondary end points was observed.[102]

In the analysis published in 2001, the effect of vitamin E on carotid intimae medial thickness (IMT) as measured by ultrasound was evaluated in a subset of study population. The results showed that vitamin E supplementation had no effect on the progression of atherosclerosis.[103] In the analysis published in 2002, the primary end points were the same as those in the analysis of 2000, but the secondary end points included an additional criterion, nephropathy. The results showed that vitamin E had no effect on either the primary or the secondary end points.[104]

In the analysis published in 2004, the primary end points were the same as those in the analysis of 2000, but the secondary end points included an additional criterion, clinical proteinuria (renal insufficiency). The results showed that in people with mild to moderate renal insufficiency, vitamin E had no effect on the primary or the secondary end points.[105]

In the analysis published in 2005, the primary and secondary end points were the same as those in the analysis of 2000. The results showed that vitamin E supplementation had no effect on the primary or most secondary end points; however, it increased the risk of two secondary end points: heart failure by about 13%, and hospitalization for heart failure by about 21%.[106] The analysis of subpopulation of heavy tobacco smokers revealed that smoking increased the risk of morbidity and mortality among the high-risk patients, despite the treatment with gold standard medications known to reduce cardiovascular disease.[107] This is consistent with another independent study outside of the HOPE study, in which daily consumption of 800 IU of vitamin E increased the levels of oxidative stress markers in heavy smokers.[108] These studies suggest that smoking plays a dominant role in increasing morbidity and mortality. If these major cardiac events increased despite gold standard medications that were given to reduce the risk of cardiovascular disease in this population, it is not surprising that administration of vitamin E alone either had no significant effect on any primary end points or most secondary end points, or increased the risk of two of the secondary end points (heart failure and hospitalization for heart failure) in one study. Individual antioxidant in high-risk populations, such as tobacco smokers and type II diabetes, may be oxidized because of high internal oxidative environment and, thereby, act as a pro-oxidant rather than as an antioxidant.

A recent analysis of HOPE study population showed that the levels of markers of inflammation was significantly related to future cardiovascular risk; however, the combination of traditional risk factors and the levels of N-terminal pro-brain natriuretic peptide (NT proBNP) were the best clinical predictive for future cardiac events.[109]

The Women's Angiographic Vitamin and Estrogen (WAVE) trial was conducted on postmenopausal women suffering from progressive CAD with at least one 15%–75% coronary stenosis at baseline coronary angiography. The trial was conducted from July 1997 to January 2002. Antioxidants (vitamin E 400 IU plus vitamin C 500 mg twice daily) were administered orally. The primary end point was annualized mean changes in minimum luminal diameter (MLD). The results showed that in postmenopausal women with progressive coronary disease, antioxidant supplements provided no cardiovascular benefits in these patients (Table 5.5). The potential for harm was suggested only when patients who died or had MIs during the trial period were included in the data analysis.[110] In the analysis published in 2005, antioxidant treatment did not improve flow-mediated dilation (FMD).[111] The analysis of subgroup of patients with haptoglobin (hp) alleles showed a significant beneficial changes in MLD with antioxidant therapy compared with placebo in patients with Hp 1-allele homozygote (Hp-1-1). This effect was more pronounced in women with diabetes.[112] Again, because of inconsistencies of the results with one or two dietary antioxidants, I do not recommend the use of such antioxidants in the prevention or improved treatment of CAD.

Administration of vitamin E (400 IU) plus vitamin C (1000 mg) for 8 weeks improved arterial stiffness and endothelial-dependent vasodilation in patients with essential hypertension.[113] The combination of vitamin E and vitamin C reduced 30-day cardiac mortality in diabetic patients with AMI by about 14%, but this beneficial effect was not observed in patients with AMI who did not have diabetes.[114] Another study revealed that dietary intake of vitamins C and E, and supplemental intake of vitamin E had an inverse association with CAD risk.[115] In contrast, administration of vitamin E (800 IU) plus vitamin C (1000 mg) for six months did not improve coronary and brachial endothelial vasomotor function.[116] A combination of 400 IU of vitamin E, 500 mg vitamin C, and 12 mg beta-carotene or 800 IU vitamin E, 1000 mg vitamin C, and 24 mg BC did not significantly affect brachial reactivity.[117] These studies suggested that supplementation with dietary antioxidants alone may not be sufficient to reduce the risk of CAD. Addition of endogenous antioxidants and other micronutrients may be necessary.

In a recent analysis of published data on the use of diet, and dietary or supplemental dietary antioxidants,[118] it has been suggested that a strong inverse relationship between intake of vegetables, nuts, and Mediterranean diet patterns with CAD exists. A moderate inverse relationship exists between intake of fish, marine omega-3-fatty acids, folate, whole grain, dietary vitamin E, C, and BC, alcohol, and fruits and fiber with CAD. However, insufficient evidence exists regarding the value of supplemental vitamin E, vitamin C, saturated and polyunsaturated fatty acids, total fats, alpha-linolenic acid (ALA), meat, eggs, and milk in reducing the risk of CAD when used individually. These studies revealed that diet modifications together with other micronutrients might be important in reducing the risk of CAD.

ENDOGENOUS ANTIOXIDANTS PRODUCING NO EFFECTS OR BENEFICIAL EFFECTS

Like dietary antioxidants, endogenous antioxidants such as glutathione-elevating agent N-acetylcysteine (NAC) and alpha-lipoic acid produced inconsistent results when used individually. In a study with 100 patients, prophylactic use of NAC in patients undergoing coronary artery bypass grafting did not improve clinical outcomes or biochemical markers.[119] However, in another study involving 40 patients, prophylactic administration of NAC attenuated myocardial oxidative stress in the heart of patients undergoing cardiopulmonary bypass.[120] In a short-term (8 weeks) study involving 36 patients, an oral administration of NAC and alpha-lipoic acid increased brachial artery diameter and reduced arterial tone as well as decreased systolic blood pressure in patients with CAD.[121] Based on these results, I do not recommend the use of one or two endogenous antioxidants in any prevention or treatment strategy for CAD.

DIETARY AND ENDOGENOUS ANTIOXIDANTS WITH CHOLESTEROL-LOWERING DRUGS

A summary of three interventional trials in high-risk patients with vitamin E or coenzyme Q10 alone or in combination with cholesterol-lowering drugs is described in Table 5.6. The number, type, dose and dose schedules of antioxidants, patient population, observation period and criteria of study were different. It has been reported[122] that vitamin E supplementation (300 IU/day), together with simvastatin for an 8-week period, improved endothelial-dependent flow-mediated dilation (FMD) as well as endothelial-dependent nitroglycerine-mediated dilation (NMD) in the brachial artery of patients with hypercholesterolemia more than that produced by simvastatin alone. Similarly, coenzyme Q10 in combination with standard therapy improved the function of damaged cardiac muscle associated with congestive heart failure[123] and idiopathic dilated cardiomyopathy.[124] One study using 156 men with previous coronary bypass surgery who were receiving a cholesterol-lowering drug combination (colestipol-niacin) alone or in combination with vitamin E 100 IU/day showed that the vitamin E-treated group revealed less progression of the narrowing of their coronary arteries compared to cholesterol-lowering drugs alone during a 4-year trial period.[125] In The Heart Protection Study[126] involving 20,500 patients at high risk, supplementation with antioxidants (vitamin E 650 mg, vitamin C 250 mg, and α-carotene 20 mg) together with simvastatin for a period of 5.5 years did not interfere with the efficacy of cholesterol-lowering drugs.

MULTIPLE DIETARY ANTIOXIDANTS WITH CHOLESTEROL-LOWERING DRUGS

In the HDL Atherosclerosis Treatment Study (HATS), the effects of the dietary antioxidants in combination with cholesterol-lowering drugs on stenosis and HDL-cholesterol were evaluated in CAD patients with low HDL.[127,128] Dietary antioxidants vitamin C (1000 mg/day), vitamin E as D-α-tocopherol (800 IU/day), natural BC (25 mg/day, and selenium (100 µg/day) were given together with simvastatin-niacin in a subset of patients with low levels of HDL-cholesterol (Table 5.7). The results revealed that simvastatin-niacin-induced elevation of HDL-cholesterol was reduced by antioxidant supplements. The same group of investigators using the same formulation reported that a mixture of dietary antioxidants reduced the degree of proximal artery stenosis compared to placebo controls; however, in combination with simvastatin-niacin antioxidant supplementation was less effective than the simvastatin-niacin treatment alone in reducing the degree of stenosis. Because of the small sample size (40 patients per group) and unusually large variations in the results (200%–700% variation around the mean value),[127] no conclusion regarding the value of antioxidants in combination with standard therapy in the management of stenosis can be drawn. This was further confirmed by the analysis of plasma levels of markers of cholesterol synthesis and absorption in the same study population. In this study, simvastatin-niacin treatment reduced plasma levels of desmosterol and lathosterol (markers of cholesterol synthesis) by 46% and 36%, respectively, whereas simvastatin-niacin plus antioxidant reduced each of them by 37% and 31%, respectively, suggesting no significant difference between two groups. Similarly, simvastatin-niacin treatment increased plasma levels of campesterol and beta-sitosterol (markers of cholesterol absorption) by 70% and 59%, respectively; whereas, simvastatin-niacin plus antioxidant increased each of them by 54% and 46%, respectively, suggesting no significant difference between two groups.[129] Nevertheless, the authors concluded that mean changes in percent stenosis was positively associated with a percent change in the lathosterol level and negatively associated with a percent change in the β-sitosterol level. This conclusion does not appear to be consistent with their data on the markers of cholesterol synthesis and absorption. Thus, the conclusion that antioxidant supplementation can increase the level of stenosis in the group of CAD patients with low HDL receiving simvastatin-niacin therapy, may not be valid. These intervention studies with one or multiple dietary antioxidants in combination with cholesterol-lowering drugs, produced inconsistent results because other cardiac risk factors were not addressed, and appropriate preparation of antioxidants were not used in these studies.

RESVERATROL AND OMEGA-3 FATTY ACIDS

RESVERATROL

Several epidemiological and experimental studies have shown that mild to moderate drinking of wine particularly red wine reduced the risks for cardiovascular, cerebrovascular, and peripheral vascular diseases.[130–133] The cardioprotective effects of wine were primarily due to the presence of antioxidants, primarily resveratrol (trans-3,5,4'-trihydroxystilbene) found in grape skin, and proanthocyanidins found in grape seed. The white wine also appears to provide cardioprotection in animal models that was primarily due to the presence of antioxidants, especially tyrosol and hydroxytyrosol.[134] These antioxidants increased the activities of mitochondrial complex (I-IV). Resveratrol reduced infarct size and prevented cardiac mitochondrial swelling in rats during reperfusion injury.[135] It also protected against H_2O_2-induced apoptosis in cardiomyocytes.[136] This effect of resveratrol on apoptosis is mediated through activation of AMP-activated kinase in cardiomyocytes[137] Administration of resveratrol significantly reduced the MI-induced ventricular tachycardia and ventricular fibrillation. The infract size and mortality were reduced in resveratrol-treated rats.[138] It has been demonstrated that lower doses of resveratrol provided cardioprotection on the criteria of improved post-ischemic ventricular recovery, reduction of myocardial infarct size, and cardiomyocyte apoptosis by upregulating antiapoptotic and redox proteins Akt and Bcl-2 in ischemic/ reperfusion rats. However, higher doses of resveratrol produced adverse effects on the heart by down-regulating redox proteins and upregulating proapoptotic proteins.[139] The biphasic effects of resveratrol, depending upon the dose, should be carefully considered while considering the doses to be used in any clinical studies.

The identified mechanisms of cardioprotection by components of red or white wine include antioxidant, anti-inflammatory, and antifibrotic. Oxidized LDL-reduced antiplatelet activity of endothelial cells, and nitric oxide synthase protein in endothelial cells, but pre-treatment of these cells with resveratrol attenuated the above effects of oxidized HDL.[140] Resveratrol and quercetin inhibited the expression of C-reactive protein (CRP) induced by IL-1 beta +IL-6) by activating phosphorylation of p38 and p44/42 MAP kinases.[141] Resveratrol treatment inhibited ICAM-1 gene expression induced by cytokines (TNF-alpha and IL-6) by reducing STAT3 phosphorylation.[142]

Treatment with resveratrol inhibited collagen-and epinephrine-induced aggregation of platelets obtained from patients who exhibited aspirin-resistance.[143] In an ischemic/reperfusion rats with hypercholesterolemia, it was observed that treatment with resveratrol, statin or resveratrol plus statin improved left ventricular function recovery better, and infract size smaller compared to control animals. The lipid levels were decreased in all treatment groups compared to controls, but more so in statin- and statin-plus-treated groups than in the resveratrol-treated group. The reduction in apoptosis was more in the group treated with statin plus resveratrol than in other treated groups.[144] In a rat myocardial MI model, it was demonstrated that resveratrol treatment upregulated the protein expression profiles of vascular endothelial growth factor (VEGF) and its tyrosine kinase receptor, FIK-1, after inducing MI. Pretreatment with resveratrol also increased iNOS and eNOS together with increased anti-apoptotic and pro-angiogenic factors NF-kappaB and specificity (SP)-1. Resveratrol treatment also improved left ventricular function and increased capillary density 3 weeks after MI.[145]

OMEGA-3 FATTY ACIDS

Omega-3 fatty acids are essential fatty acids consisting of alpha-linolenic acid (ALA), eicosapentaenoic acid (EPA), and docosahexaenoic acid (DHA). These fatty acids are not synthesized in the body but are obtained from the diet. EPA and DHA are formed from ALA in the body. Several reviews on the efficacy of omega-3 fatty acids have revealed that supplementation with omega-3 from the fish or in the capsules reduced the risk of cardiac events in patients with CAD.[146–151] It has been reported that certain CAD patients with angina and some individuals with a history of ventricular arrhythmia may not derive any benefit from omega-3 fatty acids supplementation.[152] Atrial fibrillation is a common complication after coronary artery bypass grafting operation. A review of studies suggests that omega-3 fatty acids supplementation is associated with a lower incidence of atrial fibrillation in patients who underwent cardiac surgery. It also reduced the incidence of sudden death in survivors of MI.[153] Oral administration of omega-3 fatty acids significantly reduced the rate of postoperative atrial fibrillation. Preoperative intravenous infusion of omega-3 fatty acids also reduced the incidence of atrial fibrillation after cardiac surgery and shortened a stay in the intensive care unit and in the hospital.[154,155] An analysis of published studies on the effects of omega-3 fatty acids on the incidence of recurrent ventricular arrhythmia in patients with implantable cardioverter defibrillator (ICD) showed that these fatty acids did not provide any protection in these patients.[156] Prescription omega-3 fatty acids, in combination with statin, improved lipid profiles better than statin alone.[157] An analog of omega-3 fatty acids, omega-3 ethyl esters, in combination with simvastatin, improved lipid profiles better than simvastatin alone.[158] Administration of omega-3 fatty acid and not statin (rosuvastatin) significantly reduced death and admission to hospital for cardiovascular reasons.[159] Chronic kidney disease is associated with increased risk of CAD. In a randomized, double-blind, placebo-controlled trials involving 85 non-diabetic patients with chronic kidney disease, it was observed that omega-3 fatty acid supplementation reduced blood pressure, heart rate, and triglycerides.[160] A review of literatures has confirmed that supplementation with omega-3 fatty acids significantly improved arterial hypertension.[161] Omega-3 fatty acids also exhibit a wide-range of biological activity, including regulation of both vasomotor tone and renal sodium excretion. They also reduce angiotensin-converting enzyme (ACE) activity, angiotensin II formation, tumor growth factor-beta (TGF-beta) expression, as well as enhance production of endothelial nitric oxide and activate the parasympathetic nervous system.

Based on cellular and animal models, the mechanisms of action of omega-3 fatty acids involve reduction of inflammation and platelet aggregation and improvement of endothelial dysfunction.[162] The western diet contains a high ratio of omega-6/omega-3 that has been implicated to be associated with increased incidence of chronic diseases, including CAD. Omega-3 fatty acids reduced the levels of interleukin-1beta (IL-1beta), TNF-alpha, and interleukin-6 (IL-6).[163] The studies discussed above are convincing to suggest that supplementation of omega-3 fatty acids could be of value when combine with other micronutrients for the prevention and improved treatment of CAD.

INTERVENTION STUDIES WITH B-VITAMINS TO LOWER HOMOCYSTEINE LEVELS

All patients included in four studies (Table 5.8) were at high risk for MI, stroke, and death from CAD. It is interesting to note that high-dose folic acid plus vitamin B6 and vitamin B12 increased the risk of recurrence of myocardial infarction, stroke, and death from CAD in one study[164] but had no significant effect in the other three studies.[165–167] The exact reasons for this discrepancy are

TABLE 5.8
Effect of B-Vitamins on Cardiac Events Showing No Effects or Adverse Effects

Patients Type	Vitamin Treatment	End Points	Results
3749 patients with M.I.	Folic acid (0.8 mg) Vitamin B-6 (40 mg) Vitamin B12 (0.4 mg)	MI, stroke, death	Increase
5522 patients with vascular disease or diabetes	Folic acid (2.5 mg) Vitamin B-6 (50 mg) Vitamin B12 (1 mg)	MI, stroke, death	No effect
Same patients	Same B-vitamins	Thrombosis	No effect
3680 with nondisabling cerebral infarction	Multiple vitamins with high dose or low	MI, Stroke, dose B-vitamins	No effect death

Note: MI—Myocardial infarction.

unknown; however, the patient population and criteria of end points in these studies were different. In the first study,[164] the patients who had MI within one week were randomized; whereas, in other studies,[165–167] patients with vascular disease and diabetes were randomized for the study. The latter patient population was considered at the lower risk for CAD compared to those in the first study. These studies concluded that high-dose B-vitamins should not be recommended to these patients in order to reduce the risk of cardiac events. These well-designed studies were performed in order to reduce the risk of major cardiac events; however, they did not take into account of the oxidative stress through which homocysteine mediated its action on endothelial cells of the vessel walls. Therefore, a modest reduction in homocysteine level is not expected to have any significant effect on any of the major cardiac events. Other risk factors, such as increased oxidative stress generated by mechanisms other than homocysteine, chronic inflammation, and oxidation of LDL-cholesterol were not affected by supplementation with B-vitamins alone. Therefore, consumption of B-vitamins alone is not expected to produce any beneficial effects on the cardiac events in high-risk populations.

POTENTIAL REASONS FOR THE FAILURE OF INDIVIDUAL MICRONUTRIENTS IN PRODUCING SUSTAINED AND CONSISTENT BENEFITS IN CAD

The reasons for individual antioxidants producing no effects on the primary end points, transient benefits on some markers of CAD, and harmful effects on some secondary end points may have been for several reasons: (a) antioxidants show differential subcellular distribution and different mechanisms of action; therefore, a single antioxidant cannot protect all parts of the cell; (b) a single antioxidant in a high internal oxidative environment of patients with neurodegenerative diseases is oxidized and can then itself act as a pro-oxidant rather than as an antioxidant; (c) the body protects against oxidative damage by elevating antioxidant enzymes and dietary and endogenous antioxidants; (d) antioxidants neutralize free radicals by donating electrons to those molecules with unpaired electron, whereas antioxidant enzymes destroy free radicals by catalysis, converting them to harmless molecules such as water and oxygen. Therefore, both of these events need to be enhanced in concert to achieve substantial therapeutic gain against oxidative damage; (e) the affinity of different antioxidants for free radicals differs, depending upon their lipophilicity; (f) both the aqueous and lipid compartments of the cell need to be protected together. Water-soluble antioxidants such as vitamin C and glutathione protect molecules in the aqueous environment of the cells, whereas lipid soluble antioxidants such as vitamin A and vitamin E protect molecules in the lipid compartment; (g) vitamin E is more effective in quenching free radicals in a reduced oxygenated cellular environment, whereas vitamin C and alpha-tocopherol are more effective in a higher oxygenated environment of the cells[168]; (h) vitamin C is important for recycling the oxidized form of alpha-tocopherol to the antioxidant form at the lipid/aqueous interface[169]; (i) antioxidants produce cell protective proteins by altering the expression of different microRNAs.[38] For example, some antioxidants can activate Nrf2 by upregulating miR-200a that inhibits its target protein Keap1, whereas others activate Nrf2 by downregulating miR-21 that binds with 3′-UTR Nrf2 mRNA.[170]

These studies suggest that use of a single micronutrient in prevention or improved management of human CAD is not expected to yield any beneficial effects. For this reason, a mixture of micronutrients that can simultaneously reduce oxidative stress and inflammation by enhancing the levels of antioxidant enzymes through the activation of Nrf2 pathway together with dietary and endogenous antioxidants for AD and PD has been suggested.[38,71] The same suggestion is proposed for prevention and improved management of CAD. Oral supplementation can increase the levels of dietary and endogenous antioxidants; however, elevation of the levels of antioxidant enzymes requires an activation of Nrf2. Therefore, it is essential to understand the regulation of activation of Nrf2.

REGULATION OF ACTIVATION OF Nrf2

REACTIVE OXYGEN SPECIES (ROS) ACTIVATES Nrf2

Normally, during acute oxidative stress, ROS is needed to activate Nrf2, which then dissociates itself from Keap1-CuI-Rbx1 complex and translocates in the nucleus where it heterodimerizes with a small Maf protein and binds with the ARE (antioxidant response element), leading to increased expression of target genes coding for several cytoprotective enzymes including antioxidant enzymes.[171–173] In this manner, activation of Nrf2 increases the levels of cytoprotective enzymes, including antioxidant enzymes and phase-2-detoxifying enzymes.[174,175]

BINDING OF Nrf2 WITH ARE IN THE NUCLEUS

Activation of Nrf2 alone may not be sufficient to increase the levels of antioxidant enzymes. Activated Nrf2 must bind with antioxidant response element (ARE) in the nucleus for increasing the expression of its target genes. This binding ability of Nrf2 with ARE was impaired in aged rats and this defect was restored by supplementation with alpha-lipoic acid.[176]

EXISTENCE OF ROS-RESISTANT Nrf2 IN CAD

There are limited investigations on activation of Nrf2 in CAD. The fact that increased oxidative stress and chronic inflammation are present in patients with CAD suggests that activation of Nrf2 in impaired. The expression of Nrf2/ARE in peripheral blood mononuclear cells (PBMCs) and the levels of plasma levels of glutathione were lower in patients with CAD than in control subjects.[177] Activation of Nrf2 reduced infarct size and cardiac hypertrophy in mouse models of heart failure.[178] Furthermore, activation of the Nrf2/ARE pathway may also be necessary in ischemic preconditioning in which the heart suffers one or more episodes of nonlethal myocardial ischemic/reperfusion (I/R) before the sustained occlusion of coronary artery. Methanol extract of Chinese herbal mixture activated Nrf2, which translocated from the cytoplasm to the nucleus where it binds with ARE to increase the transcription of genes coding for cytoprotective enzymes including antioxidant enzymes and phase-2-detoxifying enzyme in cardiomyocytes (H9c2).[179] Resveratrol increased the expression of Nrf2 in a dose-dependent manner in cultured coronary arterial endothelial cells. This effect of resveratrol was attenuated by downregulation Nrf2 or overexpression of Keap-1.[180] Furthermore, in high-fat diet (HFD) Nrf2 (+/+) mice, resveratrol treatment reduced oxidative stress, improved acetylcholine-induced vasodilation, and diminished apoptosis in branches of the femoral artery; however, this protective effect of resveratrol was reduced in HFD Nrf2 (−/−) mice.

ANTIOXIDANTS AND PHYTOCHEMICALS ACTIVATE ROS-RESISTANT Nrf2

Activation of Nrf2 becomes impaired to ROS. Some dietary antioxidants and phytochemicals can activate Nrf2 without requiring ROS. These include vitamin C,[181,182] vitamin E,[183] endogenous antioxidants such as alpha-lipoic acid,[176] and coenzyme Q10,[184] synthetic antioxidant N-acetylcysteine (NAC),[185] omega-3-fatty acids,[186,187] and phytochemicals such as curcumin[188] and resveratrol.[189,190]

L-CARNITINE ACTIVATES Nrf2 BY A ROS-DEPENDENT MECHANISM

Treatment with L-carnitine activates Nrf2 by a ROS-dependent mechanism,[191] probably by generating transient ROS during chronic oxidative stress.

Activation of Nrf2 by MicroRNAs

The complex of Keap1-Nrf2 in the cytoplasm prevents activation of Nrf2. Overexpression of miR-200a reduced Keap-1 levels allow Nrf2 to migrate to the nucleus where it binds to the ARE that enhanced the transcription of target cytoprotective genes including antioxidant enzymes.[192] Some antioxidants can activate Nrf2 by downregulating miR-21 that binds with 3′-UTR Nrf2 mRNA.[170]

SUPPRESSION OF CHRONIC INFLAMMATION

The activation of Nrf2 also suppresses chronic inflammation.[174,175] Some antioxidant compounds also reduce markers of chronic inflammation.[193–198]

PROPOSED MIXTURE OF MICRONUTRIENTS FOR PREVENTION AND IMPROVED MANAGEMENT OF CAD

Based on the studies discussed above, a mixture of micronutrients containing vitamin A, mixed carotenoids, vitamin C, α-tocopheryl acetate, α-tocopheryl succinate, vitamin D3, alpha-lipoic acid, N-acetylcysteine, coenzyme Q10, L-carnitine, omega-3-fatty acids, curcumin, resveratrol, all B-vitamins, selenomethionine, and zinc, but without iron, copper, manganese, or heavy metals such as molybdenum and zirconium for prevention and improved management of CAD is proposed. The inclusion of iron, copper, or manganese is not suggested because these trace minerals, although essential for many biological reactions, combine with vitamin C and generate excessive amounts of free radicals. Furthermore, these minerals are absorbed from the intestine better in the presence of antioxidants than in their absence that could increase body store of free iron, copper, and manganese after long-term consumption. The body has no significant mechanisms of excretion of these trace minerals. Slight increase in the body store of free forms of these trace minerals can increase the risk of most chronic diseases. Heavy metals such as zirconium and molybdenum were not included because the body has no mechanisms of excretion of these heavy metals. Consequently, their levels in the body would increase after long-term consumption. High levels of these heavy metals could be toxic.

It is expected that the proposed micronutrient mixture would increase the levels of antioxidant enzymes by activating the Nrf2/ARE pathway and dietary and endogenous antioxidants that would simultaneously reduce oxidative stress and chronic inflammation.

The recommended micronutrient mixture should be taken orally and divided into two doses, half in the morning and the other half in the evening with meal. This is because the biological half-lives of micronutrients are highly variable which can create high levels of fluctuations in the tissue levels of micronutrients. A 2-fold difference in the levels of certain micronutrients such as alpha-tocopheryl succinate causes a marked difference in the expression of gene profiles.[199] In order to maintain relatively steady levels of micronutrients in the body, the proposed dose-schedule is necessary.

PROPOSED CHANGES IN DIET AND LIFESTYLE FOR PREVENTION AND IMPROVED MANAGEMENT OF CAD

Dietary recommendations include daily consuming of a low-fat and high-fiber diet with plenty of fresh fruits and vegetables, increasing the intake of nuts, avoiding excessive amounts calories, and minimizing sugar consumption.

Lifestyle-related changes include stopping smoking and chewing tobacco, avoiding exposure to secondhand smoke, maintaining normal weight for your age and height, restricting intake of alcohol, reducing stress by vacation, yoga, or meditation, and performing moderate to vigorous exercise 4–5 times per week.

The efficacy of proposed micronutrient mixture together with diet and lifestyle should be tested by well-designed preclinical and clinical studies. In the meanwhile, the proposed recommendations may be adopted by the individuals in consultation with their physicians or health professionals for reducing the risk and improved management of CAD.

PREVENTION AND IMPROVED MANAGEMENT OF CAD

PRIMARY PREVENTION

Primary prevention includes individuals who have not developed any risk biomarkers associated with CAD. Despite rationale diet modifications and lifestyle changes for primary prevention, the incidence of CAD has not significantly changed. The proposed mixture of micronutrients together with modifications in diet and lifestyle may reduce the development of cardiac risk factors by reducing oxidative stress and chronic inflammation.

SECONDARY PREVENTION

Secondary prevention includes individuals who have one or more cardiac risk factors but has not suffered a heart attack. Current strategies include antiplatelet drugs including low-dose aspirin and cholesterol-lowering drugs such as statins, together with modifications in diet and lifestyle. This strategy has been useful in secondary prevention. However, some individuals resistant to low-dose aspirin and high doses of statins can experience damage to the muscle and reduce energy levels. Coenzyme Q10, which is used by the mitochondria to generate energy, is in the same pathway as cholesterol; therefore, statin treatment could lower the levels of coenzyme Q10.

Low-dose aspirin (acetylsalicylic acid) has been shown to reduce major cardiac or cerebral events by 25%.[200] It does so by irreversibly inhibiting cyclooxygenase-1 enzyme activity, thus preventing the production of thromboxane-A2, which is responsible for aggregation of platelet.[201] However, it has been reported that about 5%–12% of patients with CAD develop resistance to aspirin,[202,203] and about 24% of patients taking aspirin become semiresponders.[204] Another study estimated that 8%–45% of patients taking aspirin develop aspirin resistance.[201] This has required physicians to increase aspirin doses. However, the aspirin resistance continued to be present in some cases, in spite of increased aspirin doses. Aspirin resistance may increase the risk of major cardiac events.[205] The exact mechanisms of aspirin resistance remain to be elucidated. The proposed mechanisms include genetic polymorphism, alternate pathway of platelet activation, insensitivity of cyclooxygenase-1 enzyme, and drug interactions.[206] In addition, it has been reported that endothelial dysfunction is one of the mechanisms of aspirin resistance, and increased oxidative stress plays no significant role in this process.[206] It has been reported that the risk of major cardiac events may increase by about 3-fold in aspirin resistant patients.[203] Therefore, resolving the issue of aspirin resistance has become a new challenge for researchers in cardiology.

The propose mixture of micronutrients may increase the effectiveness of aspirin. This is due to the fact that vitamin E in the micronutrient mixture in combination with aspirin is more effective in inhibiting cyclooxygenase-1-enzyme activity than the individual agent.[193]

The proposed micronutrient mixture in combination with aspirin and cholesterol-lowering drugs may enhance their effectiveness in secondary prevention. This is due to the fact that the levels of oxidative stress and chronic inflammation would be simultaneously and optimally would be reduced by the above strategy in patients with CAD.

IMPROVED MANAGEMENT OF CAD

The individuals who have had one or more heart attacks, undergone surgical intervention such as angioplasty procedure, ablation therapy to treat atrial fibrillation, or bypass surgery are on standard drug therapy. It is expected that addition of proposed micronutrient mixtures may allow faster recovery and may enhance the effectiveness of standard therapy.

CONCLUSIONS

Despite current prevention recommendation and improved treatment outcomes due to advances in surgical technique, early detection equipment, and discovery of cholesterol-lowering drugs, coronary artery disease (CAD) remains the number-one cause of death in the USA. The risk factors for CAD include increased oxidative stress, chronic inflammation, and homocysteine. Altered expression of microRNAs in plasma or serum has been suggested to be of diagnostic value, while changes in the expression of microRNAs in the cells contribute to the pathogenesis of CAD. In order to reduce oxidative stress and chronic inflammation, use of single micronutrients has produced inconsistent results varying from no effect, to harmful effects. To reduce optimally and simultaneously, it is essential to increase the levels of cytoprotective enzymes including antioxidant enzymes, and dietary and endogenous antioxidants. Oral supplementation can increase the levels of antioxidants, but increasing the levels of antioxidant enzymes requires activation of Nrf2/ARE pathway that becomes impaired to ROS stimulation in CAD. Certain antioxidants and phytochemicals activate Nrf2 without ROS stimulation. A mixture of micronutrients that would activate Nrf2/ARE pathway, enhance the levels of dietary and endogenous antioxidants, and reduce homocysteine level is proposed. This micronutrient mixture together with modifications in the diet and lifestyle is expected to reduce all major risk factors in healthy individuals (primary prevention), enhance the effectiveness of aspirin and cholesterol-lowering drugs (secondary prevention), and improve the efficacy of standard therapy (improved management). The efficacy of proposed recommendations can be tested by well-designed clinical trials. In the meanwhile, individuals interested in reducing the risk or improved treatment of CAD may like to adopt these recommendations in consultation with their doctors.

REFERENCES

1. Association AH. Heart Disease and Stroke Statistics at-a-Glance, pp1–2, 2017.
2. Mozaffarian D, Benjamin EJ, Go AS, et al. Heart disease and stroke statistics—2015 update: A report from the American Heart Association. *Circulation*. 2015;131(4):e29–e322.
3. Simon AS, Chithra V, Vijayan A, Dinesh RD, Vijayakumar T. Altered DNA repair, oxidative stress and antioxidant status in coronary artery disease. *J Biosci*. 2013;38(2):385–389.
4. Tosukhowong P, Sangwatanaroj S, Jatuporn S, et al. The correlation between markers of oxidative stress and risk factors of coronary artery disease in Thai patients. *Clin Hemorheol Microcirc*. 2003;29(3–4):321–329.
5. Ikonomidis I, Makavos G, Papadavid E, et al. Similarities in coronary function and myocardial deformation between psoriasis and coronary artery disease: The role of oxidative stress and inflammation. *Can J Cardiol*. 2015;31(3):287–295.
6. Pytel E, Olszewska-Banaszczyk M, Koter-Michalak M, Broncel M. Increased oxidative stress and decreased membrane fluidity in erythrocytes of CAD patients. *Biochem Cell Biol*. 2013;91(5):315–318.
7. Mao Y, Qi X, Xu W, et al. Serum gamma-glutamyl transferase: A novel biomarker for coronary artery disease. *Med Sci Monit*. 2014;20:706–710.
8. Celik O, Cakmak HA, Satilmis S, et al. The relationship between gamma-glutamyl transferase levels and coronary plaque burdens and plaque structures in young adults with coronary atherosclerosis. *Clin Cardiol*. 2014;37(9):552–557.
9. Shabbir S, Khan DA, Khan FA, Elahi MM, Matata BM. Serum gamma glutamyl transferase: A novel biomarker for screening of premature coronary artery disease. *Cardiovasc Revasc Med*. 2011;12(6):367–374.

10. Porro B, Eligini S, Veglia F, et al. Nitric oxide synthetic pathway in patients with microvascular angina and its relations with oxidative stress. *Oxid Med Cell Longev.* 2014;2014:726539.

11. Vassalle C, Botto N, Andreassi MG, Berti S, Biagini A. Evidence for enhanced 8-isoprostane plasma levels, as index of oxidative stress in vivo, in patients with coronary artery disease. *Coron Artery Dis.* 2003;14(3):213–218.

12. Vassalle C, Maffei S, Boni C, Zucchelli GC. Gender-related differences in oxidative stress levels among elderly patients with coronary artery disease. *Fertil Steril.* 2008;89(3):608–613.

13. Rajesh KG, Surekha RH, Mrudula SK, Prasad Y, Sanjib KS, Prathiba N. Oxidative and nitrosative stress in association with DNA damage in coronary heart disease. *Singapore Med J.* 2011;52(4):283–288.

14. Xiang F, Shuanglun X, Jingfeng W, et al. Association of serum 8-hydroxy-2'-deoxyguanosine levels with the presence and severity of coronary artery disease. *Coron Artery Dis.* 2011;22(4):223–227.

15. Holvoet P, Collen D. Oxidized lipoproteins in atherosclerosis and thrombosis. *FASEB J.* 1994;8(15):1279–1284.

16. Reaven PD, Khouw A, Beltz WF, Parthasarathy S, Witztum JL. Effect of dietary antioxidant combinations in humans. Protection of LDL by vitamin E but not by beta-carotene. *Arterioscler Thromb.* 1993;13(4):590–600.

17. de Nigris F, Youssef T, Ciafre S, et al. Evidence for oxidative activation of c-Myc-dependent nuclear signaling in human coronary smooth muscle cells and in early lesions of Watanabe heritable hyperlipidemic rabbits: Protective effects of vitamin E. *Circulation.* 2000;102(17):2111–2117.

18. Becker AE, de Boer OJ, van Der Wal AC. The role of inflammation and infection in coronary artery disease. *Annu Rev Med.* 2001;52:289–297.

19. Belli A, Sen J, Petzold A, et al. Extracellular N-acetylaspartate depletion in traumatic brain injury. *J Neurochem.* 2006;96(3):861–869.

20. Anderson TJ, Gerhard MD, Meredith IT, et al. Systemic nature of endothelial dysfunction in atherosclerosis. *Am J Cardiol.* 1995;75(6):71B–74B.

21. Drexler H. Nitric oxide and coronary endothelial dysfunction in humans. *Cardiovasc Res.* 1999;43(3):572–579.

22. Luoma JS, Yla-Herttuala S. Expression of inducible nitric oxide synthase in macrophages and smooth muscle cells in various types of human atherosclerotic lesions. *Virchows Arch.* 1999;434(6):561–568.

23. Quaglia LA, Freitas W, Soares AA, et al. C-reactive protein is independently associated with coronary atherosclerosis burden among octogenarians. *Aging Clin Exp Res.* 2014;26(1):19–23.

24. De Lorenzo A, Pittella F, Rocha A. Increased preoperative C-reactive protein levels are associated with inhospital death after coronary artery bypass surgery. *Inflammation.* 2012;35(3):1179–1183.

25. Zouridakis E, Avanzas P, Arroyo-Espliguero R, Fredericks S, Kaski JC. Markers of inflammation and rapid coronary artery disease progression in patients with stable angina pectoris. *Circulation.* 2004;110(13):1747–1753.

26. Larsen SB, Grove EL, Wurtz M, Neergaard-Petersen S, Hvas AM, Kristensen SD. The influence of low-grade inflammation on platelets in patients with stable coronary artery disease. *Thromb Haemost.* 2015;114(3):519–529.

27. Hashmi S, Zeng QT. Role of interleukin-17 and interleukin-17-induced cytokines interleukin-6 and interleukin-8 in unstable coronary artery disease. *Coron Artery Dis.* 2006;17(8):699–706.

28. Rajappa M, Sen SK, Sharma A. Role of pro-/anti-inflammatory cytokines and their correlation with established risk factors in South Indians with coronary artery disease. *Angiology.* 2009;60(4):419–426.

29. Gregersen I, Skjelland M, Holm S, et al. Increased systemic and local interleukin 9 levels in patients with carotid and coronary atherosclerosis. *PLoS One.* 2013;8(8):e72769.

30. Verhoef P, Kok FJ, Kruyssen DA, et al. Plasma total homocysteine, B vitamins, and risk of coronary atherosclerosis. *Arterioscler Thromb Vasc Biol.* 1997;17(5):989–995.

31. Schaffer A, Verdoia M, Cassetti E, et al. Relationship between homocysteine and coronary artery disease. Results from a large prospective cohort study. *Thromb Res.* 2014;134(2):288–293.

32. Schroecksnadel K, Grammer TB, Boehm BO, Marz W, Fuchs D. Total homocysteine in patients with angiographic coronary artery disease correlates with inflammation markers. *Thromb Haemost.* 2010;103(5):926–935.

33. Karolczak K, Kamysz W, Karafova A, Drzewoski J, Watala C. Homocysteine is a novel risk factor for suboptimal response of blood platelets to acetylsalicylic acid in coronary artery disease: A randomized multicenter study. *Pharmacol Res.* 2013;74:7–22.

34. Verdoia M, Schaffer A, Pergolini P, et al. Homocysteine levels influence platelet reactivity in coronary artery disease patients treated with acetylsalicylic acid. *J Cardiovasc Pharmacol.* 2015;66(1):35–40.

35. Huang C, Zhang L, Wang Z, Pan H, Zhu J. Endothelial progenitor cells are associated with plasma homocysteine in coronary artery disease. *Acta Cardiol*. 2011;66(6):773–777.

36. Xiao Y, Zhang Y, Lv X, et al. Relationship between lipid profiles and plasma total homocysteine, cysteine, and the risk of coronary artery disease in coronary angiographic subjects. *Lipids Health Dis*. 2011;10:137.

37. May HT, Alharethi R, Anderson JL, et al. Homocysteine levels are associated with increased risk of congestive heart failure in patients with and without coronary artery disease. *Cardiology*. 2007;107(3):178–184.

38. Prasad KN. Oxidative stress and pro-inflammatory cytokines may act as one of signals for regulating microRNAs expression in Alzheimer's disease. *Mech Ageing Dev*. 2017;162:63–71.

39. Prasad KN. Oxidative stress, pro-inflammatory cytokines, and antioxidants regulate expression levels of microRNAs in Parkinson's disease. *Curr Aging Sci*. 2017;10(3):177–184.

40. Lee RC, Feinbaum RL, Ambros V. The C. elegans heterochronic gene lin-4 encodes small RNAs with antisense complementarity to lin-14. *Cell*. 1993;75(5):843–854.

41. Wightman B, Ha I, Ruvkun G. Posttranscriptional regulation of the heterochronic gene lin-14 by lin-4 mediates temporal pattern formation in C. elegans. *Cell*. 1993;75(5):855–862.

42. Macfarlane LA, Murphy PR. MicroRNA: Biogenesis, function, and role in cancer. *Curr Genomics*. 2010;11(7):537–561.

43. Londin E, Loher P, Telonis AG, et al. Analysis of 13 cell types reveals evidence for the expression of numerous novel primate- and tissue-specific microRNAs. *Proc Natl Acad Sci USA*. 2015;112(10):E1106–E1115.

44. Denli AM, Tops BB, Plasterk RH, Ketting RF, Hannon GJ. Processing of primary microRNAs by the microprocessor complex. *Nature*. 2004;432(7014):231–235.

45. Lee Y, Ahn C, Han J, et al. The nuclear RNase III Drosha initiates microRNA processing. *Nature*. 2003;425(6956):415–419.

46. Hutvagner G, McLachlan J, Pasquinelli AE, Balint E, Tuschl T, Zamore PD. A cellular function for the RNA-interference enzyme Dicer in the maturation of the let-7 small temporal RNA. *Science*. 2001;293(5531):834–838.

47. Wang KJ, Zhao X, Liu YZ, et al. Circulating miR-19b-3p, miR-134-5p and miR-186-5p are promising novel biomarkers for early diagnosis of acute myocardial infarction. *Cell Physiol Biochem*. 2016;38(3):1015–1029.

48. Gao H, Guddeti RR, Matsuzawa Y, et al. Plasma levels of microRNA-145 are associated with severity of coronary artery disease. *PLoS One*. 2015;10(5):e0123477.

49. Li HY, Zhao X, Liu YZ, et al. Plasma microRNA-126-5p is associated with the complexity and severity of coronary artery disease in patients with stable angina pectoris. *Cell Physiol Biochem*. 2016;39(3):837–846.

50. Bai R, Yang Q, Xi R, Li L, Shi D, Chen K. miR-941 as a promising biomarker for acute coronary syndrome. *BMC Cardiovasc Disord*. 2017;17(1):227.

51. JF OS, Neylon A, McGorrian C, Blake GJ. miRNA-93-5p and other miRNAs as predictors of coronary artery disease and STEMI. *Int J Cardiol*. 2016;224:310–316.

52. Fichtlscherer S, De Rosa S, Fox H, et al. Circulating microRNAs in patients with coronary artery disease. *Circ Res*. 2010;107(5):677–684.

53. Jansen F, Yang X, Proebsting S, et al. MicroRNA expression in circulating microvesicles predicts cardiovascular events in patients with coronary artery disease. *J Am Heart Assoc*. 2014;3(6):e001249.

54. Karakas M, Schulte C, Appelbaum S, et al. Circulating microRNAs strongly predict cardiovascular death in patients with coronary artery disease-results from the large AtheroGene study. *Eur Heart J*. 2017;38(7):516–523.

55. Wang J, Pei Y, Zhong Y, Jiang S, Shao J, Gong J. Altered serum microRNAs as novel diagnostic biomarkers for atypical coronary artery disease. *PLoS One*. 2014;9(9):e107012.

56. Du Y, Yang SH, Li S, et al. Circulating microRNAs as novel diagnostic biomarkers for very early-onset (</=40 years) coronary artery disease. *Biomed Environ Sci*. 2016;29(8):545–554.

57. Wang J, Yan Y, Song D, Liu L, Liu B. The association of plasma miR-155 and VCAM-1 levels with coronary collateral circulation. *Biomark Med*. 2017;11(2):125–131.

58. Wang J, Yan Y, Song D, Liu B. Reduced plasma miR-146a is a predictor of poor coronary collateral circulation in patients with coronary artery disease. *Biomed Res Int*. 2016;2016:4285942.

59. Schulte C, Molz S, Appelbaum S, et al. miRNA-197 and miRNA-223 predict cardiovascular death in a cohort of patients with symptomatic coronary artery disease. *PLoS One*. 2015;10(12):e0145930.

60. Liu F, Li R, Zhang Y, Qiu J, Ling W. Association of plasma miR-17-92 with dyslipidemia in patients with coronary artery disease. *Medicine* (*Baltimore*). 2014;93(23):e98.

61. Bai H, Liu R, Chen HL, et al. Enhanced antioxidant effect of caffeic acid phenethyl ester and Trolox in combination against radiation induced-oxidative stress. *Chem Biol Interact.* 2014;207:7–15.

62. Tang Y, Zhang Y, Chen Y, Xiang Y, Xie Y. Role of the microRNA, miR-206, and its target PIK3C2alpha in endothelial progenitor cell function—Potential link with coronary artery disease. *FEBS J.* 2015;282(19):3758–3772.

63. Wang S, He W, Wang C. miR-23a Regulates the vasculogenesis of coronary artery disease by targeting epidermal growth factor receptor. *Cardiovasc Ther.* 2016;34(4):199–208.

64. Jin Y, Yang CJ, Xu X, Cao JN, Feng QT, Yang J. miR-214 regulates the pathogenesis of patients with coronary artery disease by targeting VEGF. *Mol Cell Biochem.* 2015;402(1–2):111–122.

65. Su SH, Wu CH, Chiu YL, et al. Dysregulation of vascular endothelial growth factor receptor-2 by multiple miRNAs in endothelial colony-forming cells of coronary artery disease. *J Vasc Res.* 2017;54(1):22–32.

66. Li S, Fan Q, He S, Tang T, Liao Y, Xie J. MicroRNA-21 negatively regulates Treg cells through a TGF-beta1/Smad-independent pathway in patients with coronary heart disease. *Cell Physiol Biochem.* 2015;37(3):866–878.

67. Hulsmans M, Sinnaeve P, Van der Schueren B, Mathieu C, Janssens S, Holvoet P. Decreased miR-181a expression in monocytes of obese patients is associated with the occurrence of metabolic syndrome and coronary artery disease. *J Clin Endocrinol Metab.* 2012;97(7):E1213–E1218.

68. Fuschi P, Carrara M, Voellenkle C, et al. Central role of the p53 pathway in the noncoding-RNA response to oxidative stress. *Aging (Albany NY).* 2017;9(12):2559.

69. Bu H, Baraldo G, Lepperdinger G, Jansen-Durr P. miR-24 activity propagates stress-induced senescence by down regulating DNA topoisomerase 1. *Exp Gerontol.* 2016;75:48–52.

70. Narasimhan M, Riar AK, Rathinam ML, Vedpathak D, Henderson G, Mahimainathan L. Hydrogen peroxide responsive miR153 targets Nrf2/ARE cytoprotection in paraquat induced dopaminergic neurotoxicity. *Toxicol Lett.* 2014;228(3):179–191.

71. Prasad KN. Simultaneous activation of Nrf2 and elevation of antioxidant compounds for reducing oxidative stress and chronic inflammation in human Alzheimer's disease. *Mech Ageing Dev.* 2016;153:41–47.

72. Prasad KN. Simultaneous activation of Nrf2 and elevation of dietary and endogenous antioxidants for prevention and improved managment of Parkinson's disease. In: Bondy SCC A, ed. *Inflammation, Aging and Oxidative Stress.* New York: Springer; 2016:277–301.

73. Al Moutaery K, Al Deeb S, Ahmad Khan H, Tariq M. Caffeine impairs short-term neurological outcome after concussive head injury in rats. *Neurosurgery.* 2003;53(3):704–711; discussion 711–702.

74. Riley SJ, Stouffer GA. Cardiology grand rounds from the University of North Carolina at Chapel Hill. The antioxidant vitamins and coronary heart disease: Part 1. Basic science background and clinical observational studies. *Am J Med Sci.* 2002;324(6):314–320.

75. Smith TL, Kummerow FA. Effect of dietary vitamin E on plasma lipids and atherogenesis in restricted ovulator chickens. *Atherosclerosis.* 1989;75(2–3):105–109.

76. Verlangieri AJ, Bush MJ. Effects of d-alpha-tocopherol supplementation on experimentally induced primate atherosclerosis. *J Am Coll Nutr.* 1992;11(2):131–138.

77. Wojcicki J, Rozewicka L, Barcew-Wiszniewska B, et al. Effect of selenium and vitamin E on the development of experimental atherosclerosis in rabbits. *Atherosclerosis.* 1991;87(1):9–16.

78. Armstrong GT, Liu Q, Yasui Y, et al. Late mortality among 5-year survivors of childhood cancer: A summary from the Childhood Cancer Survivor Study. *J Clin Oncol.* 2009;27(14):2328–2338.

79. Gey KF, Puska P. Plasma vitamins E and A inversely correlated to mortality from ischemic heart disease in cross-cultural epidemiology. *Ann N Y Acad Sci.* 1989;570:268–282.

80. Sklodowska RW, Gromadzinska W, Miroslaw J, Malczyk W, Goch JH. Selenium and vitamin econcentrations in plasma and erythrocytes of angina pectoris patients. *Trace Elem Med.* 1991;8:113–117.

81. Riemersma RA, Wood DA, Macintyre CC, Elton RA, Gey KF, Oliver MF. Risk of angina pectoris and plasma concentrations of vitamins A, C, and E and carotene. *Lancet.* 1991;337(8732):1–5.

82. Rimm EB, Stampfer MJ, Ascherio A, Giovannucci E, Colditz GA, Willett WC. Vitamin E consumption and the risk of coronary heart disease in men. *N Engl J Med.* 1993;328(20):1450–1456.

83. Stampfer MJ, Hennekens CH, Manson JE, Colditz GA, Rosner B, Willett WC. Vitamin E consumption and the risk of coronary disease in women. *N Engl J Med.* 1993;328(20):1444–1449.

84. Losonczy KG, Harris TB, Havlik RJ. Vitamin E and vitamin C supplement use and risk of all-cause and coronary heart disease mortality in older persons: The established populations for epidemiologic studies of the Elderly. *Am J Clin Nutr.* 1996;64(2):190–196.

85. Kok FJ, de Bruijn AM, Vermeeren R, et al. Serum selenium, vitamin antioxidants, and cardiovascular mortality: A 9-year follow-up study in the Netherlands. *Am J Clin Nutr.* 1987;45(2):462–468.

86. Salonen JT, Salonen R, Penttila I, et al. Serum fatty acids, apolipoproteins, selenium and vitamin anti-oxidants and the risk of death from coronary artery disease. *Am J Cardiol.* 1985;56(4):226–231.

87. Goodson AG, Cotter MA, Cassidy P, et al. Use of oral N-acetylcysteine for protection of melanocytic nevi against UV-induced oxidative stress: Towards a novel paradigm for melanoma chemoprevention. *Clin Cancer Res.* 2009;15(23):7434–7440.

88. DeMaio SJ, King 3rd SB, Lembo NJ, et al. Vitamin E supplementation, plasma lipids and inci-dence of restenosis after percutaneous transluminal coronary angioplasty (PTCA). *J Am Coll Nutr.* 1992;11(1):68–73.

89. Devaraj S, Jialal I. Alpha tocopherol supplementation decreases serum C-reactive protein and mono-cyte interleukin-6 levels in normal volunteers and type 2 diabetic patients. *Free Radic Biol Med.* 2000;29(8):790–792.

90. Heitzer T, Yla Herttuala S, Wild E, Luoma J, Drexler H. Effect of vitamin E on endothelial vaso-dilator function in patients with hypercholesterolemia, chronic smoking or both. *J Am Coll Cardiol.* 1999;33(2):499–505.

91. Islam KN, O'Byrne D, Devaraj S, Palmer B, Grundy SM, Jialal I. Alpha-tocopherol supplementation decreases the oxidative susceptibility of LDL in renal failure patients on dialysis therapy. *Atherosclerosis.* 2000;150(1):217–224.

92. Stephens NG, Parsons A, Schofield PM, Kelly F, Cheeseman K, Mitchinson MJ. Randomised controlled trial of vitamin E in patients with coronary disease: Cambridge Heart Antioxidant Study (CHAOS). *Lancet.* 1996;347(9004):781–786.

93. Earnest CP, Wood KA, Church TS. Complex multivitamin supplementation improves homocysteine and resistance to LDL-C oxidation. *J Am Coll Nutr.* 2003;22(5):400–407.

94. Fang JC, Kinlay S, Beltrame J, et al. Effect of vitamins C and E on progression of transplant-associated arteriosclerosis: A randomised trial. *Lancet.* 2002;359(9312):1108–1113.

95. Plotnick GD, Corretti MC, Vogel RA. Effect of antioxidant vitamins on the transient impairment of endothelium-dependent brachial artery vasoactivity following a single high-fat meal. *JAMA.* 1997;278(20):1682–1686.

96. Salonen JT. Clinical trials testing cardiovascular benefits of antioxidant supplementation. *Free Radic Res.* 2002;36(12):1299–1306.

97. Knekt P, Ritz J, Pereira MA, et al. Antioxidant vitamins and coronary heart disease risk: A pooled analysis of 9 cohorts. *Am J Clin Nutr.* 2004;80(6):1508–1520.

98. Wright ME, Lawson KA, Weinstein SJ, et al. Higher baseline serum concentrations of vitamin E are associated with lower total and cause-specific mortality in the Alpha-Tocopherol, Beta-Carotene Cancer Prevention Study. *Am J Clin Nutr.* 2006;84(5):1200–1207.

99. Tornwall ME, Virtamo J, Korhonen PA, et al. Effect of alpha-tocopherol and beta-carotene supplemen-tation on coronary heart disease during the 6-year post-trial follow-up in the ATBC study. *Eur Heart J.* 2004;25(13):1171–1178.

100. Leppala JM, Virtamo J, Fogelholm R, et al. Controlled trial of alpha-tocopherol and beta-carotene supplements on stroke incidence and mortality in male smokers. *Arterioscler Thromb Vasc Biol.* 2000;20(1):230–235.

101. Tornwall ME, Virtamo J, Korhonen PA, Virtanen MJ, Albanes D, Huttunen JK. Postintervention effect of alpha tocopherol and beta carotene on different strokes: A 6-year follow-up of the Alpha Tocopherol, Beta Carotene Cancer Prevention Study. *Stroke.* 2004;35(8):1908–1913.

102. Heart Outcomes Prevention Evaluation Study I, Yusuf S, Dagenais G, Pogue J, Bosch J, Sleight P. Vitamin E supplementation and cardiovascular events in high-risk patients. *N Engl J Med.* 2000;342(3):154–160.

103. Lonn E, Yusuf S, Dzavik V, et al. Effects of ramipril and vitamin E on atherosclerosis: The study to evaluate carotid ultrasound changes in patients treated with ramipril and vitamin E (SECURE). *Circulation.* 2001;103(7):919–925.

104. Lonn E, Yusuf S, Hoogwerf B, et al. Effects of vitamin E on cardiovascular and microvascular out-comes in high-risk patients with diabetes: Results of the HOPE study and MICRO-HOPE substudy. *Diabetes Care.* 2002;25(11):1919–1927.

105. Mann JF, Lonn EM, Yi Q, et al. Effects of vitamin E on cardiovascular outcomes in people with mild-to-moderate renal insufficiency: Results of the HOPE study. *Kidney Int.* 2004;65(4):1375–1380.

106. Lonn E, Bosch J, Yusuf S, et al. Effects of long-term vitamin E supplementation on cardiovascular events and cancer: A randomized controlled trial. *Jama.* 2005;293(11):1338–1347.

107. Dagenais GR, Yi Q, Lonn E, et al. Impact of cigarette smoking in high-risk patients participating in a clinical trial. A substudy from the Heart Outcomes Prevention Evaluation (HOPE) trial. *Eur J Cardiovasc Prev Rehabil.* 2005;12(1):75–81.

108. Weinberg RB, VanderWerken BS, Anderson RA, Stegner JE, Thomas MJ. Pro-oxidant effect of vitamin E in cigarette smokers consuming a high polyunsaturated fat diet. *Arterioscler Thromb Vasc Biol.* 2001;21(6):1029–1033.

109. Blankenberg S, McQueen MJ, Smieja M, et al. Comparative impact of multiple biomarkers and N-Terminal pro-brain natriuretic peptide in the context of conventional risk factors for the prediction of recurrent cardiovascular events in the Heart Outcomes Prevention Evaluation (HOPE) Study. *Circulation.* 2006;114(3):201–208.

110. Waters DD, Alderman EL, Hsia J, et al. Effects of hormone replacement therapy and antioxidant vitamin supplements on coronary atherosclerosis in postmenopausal women: A randomized controlled trial. *JAMA.* 2002;288(19):2432–2440.

111. Kelemen M, Vaidya D, Waters DD, et al. Hormone therapy and antioxidant vitamins do not improve endothelial vasodilator function in postmenopausal women with established coronary artery disease: A substudy of the Women's Angiographic Vitamin and Estrogen (WAVE) trial. *Atherosclerosis.* 2005;179(1):193–200.

112. Levy AP, Friedenberg P, Lotan R, et al. The effect of vitamin therapy on the progression of coronary artery atherosclerosis varies by haptoglobin type in postmenopausal women. *Diabetes Care.* 2004;27(4):925–930.

113. Plantinga Y, Ghiadoni L, Magagna A, et al. Supplementation with vitamins C and E improves arterial stiffness and endothelial function in essential hypertensive patients. *Am J Hypertens.* 2007;20(4):392–397.

114. Jaxa-Chamiec T, Bednarz B, Herbaczynska-Cedro K, Maciejewski P, Ceremuzynski L, Group MT. Effects of vitamins C and E on the outcome after acute myocardial infarction in diabetics: A retrospective, hypothesis-generating analysis from the MIVIT study. *Cardiology.* 2009;112(3):219–223.

115. Ye Z, Song H. Antioxidant vitamins intake and the risk of coronary heart disease: Meta-analysis of cohort studies. *Eur J Cardiovasc Prev Rehabil.* 2008;15(1):26–34.

116. Kinlay S, Behrendt D, Fang JC, et al. Long-term effect of combined vitamins E and C on coronary and peripheral endothelial function. *J Am Coll Cardiol.* 2004;43(4):629–634.

117. McKechnie R, Rubenfire M, Mosca L. Antioxidant nutrient supplementation and brachial reactivity in patients with coronary artery disease. *J Lab Clin Med.* 2002;139(3):133–139.

118. Mente A, de Koning L, Shannon HS, Anand SS. A systematic review of the evidence supporting a causal link between dietary factors and coronary heart disease. *Arch Intern Med.* 2009;169(7):659–669.

119. El-Hamamsy I, Stevens LM, Carrier M, et al. Effect of intravenous N-acetylcysteine on outcomes after coronary artery bypass surgery: A randomized, double-blind, placebo-controlled clinical trial. *J Thorac Cardiovasc Surg.* 2007;133(1):7–12.

120. Tossios P, Bloch W, Huebner A, et al. N-acetylcysteine prevents reactive oxygen species-mediated myocardial stress in patients undergoing cardiac surgery: Results of a randomized, double-blind, placebo-controlled clinical trial. *J Thorac Cardiovasc Surg.* 2003;126(5):1513–1520.

121. McMackin CJ, Widlansky ME, Hamburg NM, et al. Effect of combined treatment with alpha-Lipoic acid and acetyl-L-carnitine on vascular function and blood pressure in patients with coronary artery disease. *J Clin Hypertens (Greenwich).* 2007;9(4):249–255.

122. Neunteufl T, Kostner K, Katzenschlager R, Zehetgruber M, Maurer G, Weidinger F. Additional benefit of vitamin E supplementation to simvastatin therapy on vasoreactivity of the brachial artery of hypercholesterolemic men. *J Am Coll Cardiol.* 1998;32(3):711–716.

123. Judy WV, Folker K, Hall JH. Improved long-term survival in coenzyme Q10 treated congestive heart failure patients compared to conventionally treated patients. In: Folkers K, Littarru, GP, Yamagami, T, eds. *Biomedical and Clinical Aspects of Coenzyme Q10.* Amsterdam, the Netherlands: Elsevier; 1991; 4:291–298.

124. Langsjoen PH, Langsjoen PH, Folkers K. Long-term efficacy and safety of coenzyme Q10 therapy for idiopathic dilated cardiomyopathy. *Am J Cardiol.* 1990;65(7):521–523.

125. Hodis HN, Mack WJ, LaBree L, et al. Serial coronary angiographic evidence that antioxidant vitamin intake reduces progression of coronary artery atherosclerosis. *JAMA.* 1995;273(23):1849–1854.

126. Perry RT, Collins JS, Wiener H, Acton R, Go RC. The role of TNF and its receptors in Alzheimer's disease. *Neurobiol Aging.* 2001;22(6):873–883.

127. Albanes D, Till C, Klein EA, et al. Plasma tocopherols and risk of prostate cancer in the Selenium and Vitamin E Cancer Prevention Trial (SELECT). *Cancer Prev Res (Phila).* 2014;7(9):886–895.

128. Cheung WM, Chu AH, Chu PW, Ip NY. Cloning and expression of a novel nuclear matrix-associated protein that is regulated during the retinoic acid-induced neuronal differentiation. *J Biol Chem.* 2001;276(20):17083–17091.

129. Matthan NR, Giovanni A, Schaefer EJ, Brown BG, Lichtenstein AH. Impact of simvastatin, niacin, and/or antioxidants on cholesterol metabolism in CAD patients with low HDL. *J Lipid Res.* 2003;44(4):800–806.

130. Bertelli AA, Das DK. Grapes, wines, resveratrol and heart health. *J Cardiovasc Pharmacol.* 2009;54:468–476.

131. Penumathsa SV, Maulik N. Resveratrol: A promising agent in promoting cardioprotection against coronary heart disease. *Can J Physiol Pharmacol.* 2009;87(4):275–286.

132. Das S, Das DK. Resveratrol: A therapeutic promise for cardiovascular diseases. *Recent Pat Cardiovasc Drug Discov.* 2007;2(2):133–138.

133. Baur JA, Sinclair DA. Therapeutic potential of resveratrol: The in vivo evidence. *Nat Rev Drug Discov.* 2006;5(6):493–506.

134. Dudley JI, Lekli I, Mukherjee S, Das M, Bertelli AA, Das DK. Does white wine qualify for French paradox? Comparison of the cardioprotective effects of red and white wines and their constituents: Resveratrol, tyrosol, and hydroxytyrosol. *J Agric Food Chem.* 2008;56(20):9362–9373.

135. Xi J, Wang H, Mueller RA, Norfleet EA, Xu Z. Mechanism for resveratrol-induced cardioprotection against reperfusion injury involves glycogen synthase kinase 3beta and mitochondrial permeability transition pore. *Eur J Pharmacol.* 2009;604(1–3):111–116.

136. Yu W, Fu YC, Zhou XH, et al. Effects of resveratrol on H(2)O(2)-induced apoptosis and expression of SIRTs in H9c2 cells. *J Cell Biochem.* 2009;107(4):741–747.

137. Hwang JT, Kwon DY, Park OJ, Kim MS. Resveratrol protects ROS-induced cell death by activating AMPK in H9c2 cardiac muscle cells. *Genes Nutr.* 2008;2(4):323–326.

138. Chen YR, Yi FF, Li XY, et al. Resveratrol attenuates ventricular arrhythmias and improves the long-term survival in rats with myocardial infarction. *Cardiovasc Drugs Ther.* 2008;22(6):479–485.

139. Dudley J, Das S, Mukherjee S, Das DK. Resveratrol, a unique phytoalexin present in red wine, delivers either survival signal or death signal to the ischemic myocardium depending on dose. *J Nutr Biochem.* 2009;20(6):443–452.

140. Chen YJ, Wang JS, Chow SE. Resveratrol protects vascular endothelial cell from ox-LDL-induced reduction in antithrombogenic activity. *Chin J Physiol.* 2007;50(1):22–28.

141. Kaur G, Rao LV, Agrawal A, Pendurthi UR. Effect of wine phenolics on cytokine-induced C-reactive protein expression. *J Thromb Haemost.* 2007;5(6):1309–1317.

142. Wung BS, Hsu MC, Wu CC, Hsieh CW. Resveratrol suppresses IL-6-induced ICAM-1 gene expression in endothelial cells: Effects on the inhibition of STAT3 phosphorylation. *Life Sci.* 2005;78(4):389–397.

143. Stef G, Csiszar A, Lerea K, Ungvari Z, Veress G. Resveratrol inhibits aggregation of platelets from high-risk cardiac patients with aspirin resistance. *J Cardiovasc Pharmacol.* 2006;48(2):1–5.

144. Penumathsa SV, Thirunavukkarasu M, Koneru S, et al. Statin and resveratrol in combination induces cardioprotection against myocardial infarction in hypercholesterolemic rat. *J Mol Cell Cardiol.* 2007;42(3):508–516.

145. Fukuda S, Kaga S, Zhan L, et al. Resveratrol ameliorates myocardial damage by inducing vascular endothelial growth factor-angiogenesis and tyrosine kinase receptor Flk-1. *Cell Biochem Biophys.* 2006;44(1):43–49.

146. Lee JH, O'Keefe JH, Lavie CJ, Harris WS. Omega-3 fatty acids: Cardiovascular benefits, sources, and sustainability. *Nat Rev Cardiol.* 2009;6(12):753.

147. He K. Fish, long-chain omega-3 polyunsaturated fatty acids and prevention of cardiovascular disease—Eat fish or take fish oil supplement? *Prog Cardiovasc Dis.* 2009;52(2):95–114.

148. Marchioli R, Silletta MG, Levantesi G, Pioggiarella R. Omega-3 fatty acids and heart failure. *Curr Atheroscler Rep.* 2009;11(6):440–447.

149. Lavie CJ, Milani RV, Mehra MR, Ventura HO. Omega-3 polyunsaturated fatty acids and cardiovascular diseases. *J Am Coll Cardiol.* 2009;54(7):585–594.

150. Marik PE, Varon J. Omega-3 dietary supplements and the risk of cardiovascular events: A systematic review. *Clin Cardiol.* 2009;32(7):365–372.

151. Holub BJ. Docosahexaenoic acid (DHA) and cardiovascular disease risk factors. *Prostaglandins Leukot Essent Fatty Acids.* 2009;81(2–3):199–204.

152. Jenkins DJ, Josse AR, Dorian P, et al. Heterogeneity in randomized controlled trials of long chain (fish) omega-3 fatty acids in restenosis, secondary prevention and ventricular arrhythmias. *J Am Coll Nutr.* 2008;27(3):367–378.

153. Lombardi F, Terranova P. Anti-arrhythmic properties of N-3 poly-unsaturated fatty acids (n-3 PUFA). *Curr Med Chem.* 2007;14(19):2070–2080.

154. Heidt MC, Vician M, Stracke SK, et al. Beneficial effects of intravenously administered N-3 fatty acids for the prevention of atrial fibrillation after coronary artery bypass surgery: A prospective randomized study. *Thorac Cardiovasc Surg.* 2009;57(5):276–280.

155. Calo L, Bianconi L, Colivicchi F, et al. N-3 Fatty acids for the prevention of atrial fibrillation after coronary artery bypass surgery: A randomized, controlled trial. *J Am Coll Cardiol.* 2005;45(10):1723–1728.

156. Brouwer IA, Raitt MH, Dullemeijer C, et al. Effect of fish oil on ventricular tachyarrhythmia in three studies in patients with implantable cardioverter defibrillators. *Eur Heart J.* 2009;30(7):820–826.

157. Dall TL, Bays H. Addressing lipid treatment targets beyond cholesterol: A role for prescription omega-3 fatty acid therapy. *South Med J.* 2009;102(4):390–396.

158. Davidson MH, Stein EA, Bays HE, et al. Efficacy and tolerability of adding prescription omega-3 fatty acids 4 g/d to simvastatin 40 mg/d in hypertriglyceridemic patients: An 8-week, randomized, double-blind, placebo-controlled study. *Clin Ther.* 2007;29(7):1354–1367.

159. Marchioli R, Levantesi G, Silletta MG, et al. Effect of n-3 polyunsaturated fatty acids and rosuvastatin in patients with heart failure: Results of the GISSI-HF trial. *Expert Rev Cardiovasc Ther.* 2009;7(7):735–748.

160. Mori TA, Burke V, Puddey I, et al. The effects of [omega]3 fatty acids and coenzyme Q10 on blood pressure and heart rate in chronic kidney disease: A randomized controlled trial. *J Hypertens.* 2009;27(9):1863–1872.

161. Cicero AF, Ertek S, Borghi C. Omega-3 polyunsaturated fatty acids: Their potential role in blood pressure prevention and management. *Curr Vasc Pharmacol.* 2009;7(3):330–337.

162. Dimitrow PP, Jawien M. Pleiotropic, cardioprotective effects of omega-3 polyunsaturated fatty acids. *Mini Rev Med Chem.* 2009;9(9):1030–1039.

163. Simopoulos AP. The omega-6/omega-3 fatty acid ratio, genetic variation, and cardiovascular disease. *Asia Pac J Clin Nutr.* 2008;17(Suppl 1):131–134.

164. Bonaa KH, Njolstad I, Ueland PM, et al. Homocysteine lowering and cardiovascular events after acute myocardial infarction. *N Engl J Med.* 2006;354(15):1578–1588.

165. Lonn E, Yusuf S, Arnold MJ, et al. Homocysteine lowering with folic acid and B vitamins in vascular disease. *N Engl J Med.* 2006;354(15):1567–1577.

166. Ray JG, Kearon C, Yi Q, Sheridan P, Lonn E, Heart Outcomes Prevention Evaluation I. Homocysteine-lowering therapy and risk for venous thromboembolism: A randomized trial. *Ann Intern Med.* 2007;146(11):761–767.

167. Toole JF, Malinow MR, Chambless LE, et al. Lowering homocysteine in patients with ischemic stroke to prevent recurrent stroke, myocardial infarction, and death: The Vitamin Intervention for Stroke Prevention (VISP) randomized controlled trial. *JAMA.* 2004;291(5):565–575.

168. Vile GF, Winterbourn CC. Inhibition of adriamycin-promoted microsomal lipid peroxidation by beta-carotene, alpha-tocopherol and retinol at high and low oxygen partial pressures. *FEBS Lett.* 1988;238(2):353–356.

169. Niki E. Interaction of ascorbate and alpha-tocopherol. *Ann N Y Acad Sci.* 1987;498:186–199.

170. Wu H, Kong L, Tan Y, et al. C66 ameliorates diabetic nephropathy in mice by both upregulating NRF2 function via increase in miR-200a and inhibiting miR-21. *Diabetologia.* 2016;59:1558–1568.

171. Itoh K, Chiba T, Takahashi S, et al. An Nrf2/small Maf heterodimer mediates the induction of phase II detoxifying enzyme genes through antioxidant response elements. *Biochem Bioph Res Commun.* 1997;236(2):313–322.

172. Williamson TP, Johnson DA, Johnson JA. Activation of the Nrf2-ARE pathway by siRNA knockdown of Keap1 reduces oxidative stress and provides partial protection from MPTP-mediated neurotoxicity. *Neurotoxicology.* 2012;33(3):272–279.

173. Jaramillo MC, Zhang DD. The emerging role of the Nrf2-Keap1 signaling pathway in cancer. *Genes Dev.* 2013;27(20):2179–2191.

174. Li W, Khor TO, Xu C, et al. Activation of Nrf2-antioxidant signaling attenuates NFkappaB-inflammatory response and elicits apoptosis. *Biochem Pharmacol.* 2008;76(11):1485–1489.

175. Kim J, Cha YN, Surh YJ. A protective role of nuclear factor-erythroid 2-related factor-2 (Nrf2) in inflammatory disorders. *Mutat Res.* 2010;690(1–2):12–23.

176. Suh JH, Shenvi SV, Dixon BM, et al. Decline in transcriptional activity of Nrf2 causes age-related loss of glutathione synthesis, which is reversible with lipoic acid. *P Natl Acad Sci USA.* 2004;101(10):3381–3386.

177. Mozzini C, Fratta Pasini A, Garbin U, et al. Increased endoplasmic reticulum stress and Nrf2 repression in peripheral blood mononuclear cells of patients with stable coronary artery disease. *Free Radic Biol Med.* 2014;68:178–185.

178. Cominacini L, Mozzini C, Garbin U, et al. Endoplasmic reticulum stress and Nrf2 signaling in cardio-vascular diseases. *Free Radic Biol Med*. 2015;88(Pt B):233–242.

179. Chiu PY, Leung HY, Leong PK, et al. Danshen-gegen decoction protects against hypoxia/reoxygenation-induced apoptosis by inhibiting mitochondrial permeability transition via the redox-sensitive ERK/Nrf2 and PKCepsilon/mKATP pathways in H9c2 cardiomyocytes. *Phytomedicine*. 2012;19(2):99–110.

180. Ungvari Z, Bagi Z, Feher A, et al. Resveratrol confers endothelial protection via activation of the anti-oxidant transcription factor Nrf2. *Am J Physiol Heart Circ Physiol*. 2010;299(1):H18–H24.

181. Mostafavi-Pour Z, Ramezani F, Keshavarzi F, Samadi N. The role of quercetin and vitamin C in Nrf2-dependent oxidative stress production in breast cancer cells. *Oncol Lett*. 2017;13(3):1965–1973.

182. Katsuyama Y, Tsuboi T, Taira N, Yoshioka M, Masaki H. 3-O-Laurylglyceryl ascorbate activates the intracellular antioxidant system through the contribution of PPAR-gamma and Nrf2. *J Dermatol Sci*. 2016;82(3):189–196.

183. Xi YD, Yu HL, Ding J, et al. Flavonoids protect cerebrovascular endothelial cells through Nrf2 and PI3K from beta-amyloid peptide-induced oxidative damage. *Current Neurovasc Res*. 2012;9(1):32–41.

184. Choi HK, Pokharel YR, Lim SC, et al. Inhibition of liver fibrosis by solubilized coenzyme Q10: Role of Nrf2 activation in inhibiting transforming growth factor-beta1 expression. *Toxicol Appl Pharmacol*. 2009;240(3):377–384.

185. Ji L, Liu R, Zhang XD, et al. N-acetylcysteine attenuates phosgene-induced acute lung injury via up-regulation of Nrf2 expression. *Inhal Toxicol*. 2010;22(7):535–542.

186. Gao L, Wang J, Sekhar KR, et al. Novel n-3 fatty acid oxidation products activate Nrf2 by destabilizing the association between Keap1 and Cullin3. *J Biol Chem*. 2007;282(4):2529–2537.

187. Saw CL, Yang AY, Guo Y, Kong AN. Astaxanthin and omega-3 fatty acids individually and in combination protect against oxidative stress via the Nrf2-ARE pathway. *Food Chem Toxicol*. 2013;62:869–875.

188. Trujillo J, Chirino YI, Molina-Jijon E, Anderica-Romero AC, Tapia E, Pedraza-Chaverri J. Renoprotective effect of the antioxidant curcumin: Recent findings. *Redox Biol*. 2013;1(1):448–456.

189. Steele ML, Fuller S, Patel M, Kersaitis C, Ooi L, Munch G. Effect of Nrf2 activators on release of glutathi-one, cysteinylglycine and homocysteine by human U373 astroglial cells. *Redox Biol*. 2013;1(1):441–445.

190. Kode A, Rajendrasozhan S, Caito S, Yang SR, Megson IL, Rahman I. Resveratrol induces glutathione synthesis by activation of Nrf2 and protects against cigarette smoke-mediated oxidative stress in human lung epithelial cells. *Am J Physiol Lung Cell Mol Physiol*. 2008;294(3):L478–488.

191. Zambrano S, Blanca AJ, Ruiz-Armenta MV, et al. The renoprotective effect of L-carnitine in hyper-tensive rats is mediated by modulation of oxidative stress-related gene expression. *Eur J Nutr*. 2013;52(6):1649–1659.

192. Eades G, Yang M, Yao Y, Zhang Y, Zhou Q. miR-200a regulates Nrf2 activation by targeting Keap1 mRNA in breast cancer cells. *J Biol Chem*. 2011;286(47):40725–40733.

193. Abate A, Yang G, Dennery PA, Oberle S, Schroder H. Synergistic inhibition of cyclooxygenase-2 expression by vitamin E and aspirin. *Free Radic Biol Med*. 2000;29(11):1135–1142.

194. Fu Y, Zheng S, Lin J, Ryerse J, Chen A. Curcumin protects the rat liver from CCl4-caused injury and fibrogenesis by attenuating oxidative stress and suppressing inflammation. *Mol Pharmacol*. 2008;73(2):399–409.

195. Lee HS, Jung KK, Cho JY, et al. Neuroprotective effect of curcumin is mainly mediated by blockade of microglial cell activation. *Pharmazie*. 2007;62(12):937–942.

196. Rahman S, Bhatia K, Khan AQ, et al. Topically applied vitamin E prevents massive cutaneous inflam-matory and oxidative stress responses induced by double application of 12-O-tetradecanoylphorbol-13-acetate (TPA) in mice. *Chem Biol Interact*. 2008;172(3):195–205.

197. Suzuki YJ, Aggarwal BB, Packer L. Alpha-lipoic acid is a potent inhibitor of NF-kappa B activation in human T cells. *Biochem Biophys Res Commun*. 1992;189(3):1709–1715.

198. Zhu J, Yong W, Wu X, et al. Anti-inflammatory effect of resveratrol on TNF-alpha-induced MCP-1 expression in adipocytes. *Biochem Biophys Res Commun*. 2008;369(2):471–477.

199. Prasad KN. Alpha-tocopheryl succinate exhibits potent anticancer activity: Its interaction with ionizing radiation and chemotherapy effects. In: Reddy VR, Watson RR, ed. *The Encyclopedia of Vitamin E*. London, UK: CAB International; 2007.

200. Triggiani V, Resta F, Guastamacchia E, et al. Role of antioxidants, essential fatty acids, carnitine, vita-mins, phytochemicals, and trace elements in the treatment of diabetes mellitus and its chronic complica-tions. *Endocr Metab Immune Disord Drug Targets*. 2006;6(1):77–93.

201. Patel C, Ghanim H, Ravishankar S, et al. Prolonged reactive oxygen species generation and nuclear fac-tor-kappaB activation after a high-fat, high-carbohydrate meal in the obese. *J Clin Endocrinol Metab*. 2007;92(11):4476–4479.

202. Cotter G, Shemesh E, Zehavi M, et al. Lack of aspirin effect: Aspirin resistance or resistance to taking aspirin? *Am Heart J.* 2004;147(2):293–300.
203. Gum PA, Kottke-Marchant K, Welsh PA, White J, Topol EJ. A prospective, blinded determination of the natural history of aspirin resistance among stable patients with cardiovascular disease. *J Am Coll Cardiol.* 2003;41(6):961–965.
204. Gum PA, Thamilarasan M, Watanabe J, Blackstone EH, Lauer MS. Aspirin use and all-cause mortality among patients being evaluated for known or suspected coronary artery disease: A propensity analysis. *JAMA.* 2001;286(10):1187–1194.
205. Cabungcal JH, Preissmann D, Delseth C, Cuenod M, Do KQ, Schenk F. Transitory glutathione deficit during brain development induces cognitive impairment in juvenile and adult rats: relevance to schizophrenia. *Neurobiol Dis.* 2007;26(3):634–645.
206. Sztriha LK, Sas K, Vecsei L. Aspirin resistance in stroke: 2004. *J Neurol Sci.* 2005;229–230:163–169.

6 Micronutrients in Prevention and Improvement of the Standard Therapy in Diabetes

INTRODUCTION

Diabetes mellitus is a chronic disease characterized by high levels of blood glucose that can result from defects in insulin production, insulin transport and/or utilization, or both. Diabetes can lead to serious complications and premature death if untreated. Diabetes has become a serious health problem throughout the world, including the United States, and has reached epidemic proportions. Despite development of new medications to control glucose and recommendations of losing weight, daily moderate exercise, and a balanced diet, the incidence of diabetes continues to increase in the United States. Severe diabetic-related complications eventually develop in spite of medications. Although the compliance for medications is very good, compliance is not consistent for diet and lifestyle modifications. The analysis of published data suggests that increased oxidative stress and chronic inflammation are associated with the development of all diabetes-related complications. They may also be associated with the initiation and progression of diabetes. Antioxidants are known to reduce oxidative stress and chronic inflammation; therefore, they should be useful in reducing the incidence of diabetes as well as the diabetes-related complications. However, several laboratory and human studies utilizing a single dietary, endogenous antioxidant, certain B-vitamins, omega-3 fatty acids, the mineral chromium, or aspirin alone have been performed to evaluate their efficacy in prevention and improved treatment. The results of these studies showed that different individual agents improved different risk factors and reduced different markers of oxidative stress and chronic inflammation, producing inconsistent results. Antioxidants in combination with standard therapy appear to be more effective than the individual agents.

This chapter describes the incidence, prevalence, cost, and types of diabetes and presents evidence for increased oxidative stress and chronic inflammation in the initiation and progression of diabetes and diabetes-related complications. It describes involvement of microRNAs that regulate the translation of proteins from their respective mRNAs transcripts in the pathogenesis of diabetes. It also presents results of studies on animals, epidemiologic and intervention on the effects of primarily individual micronutrients in prevention and treatment of diabetes, and discusses potential reasons for obtaining inconsistent results varying from no effect to transient benefits on some risk factors. A single micronutrient cannot simultaneously reduce oxidative stress and inflammation that are required for optimal benefits in the prevention and, in combination with standard therapy, improved management of diabetes. In order to accomplish the above goal, it is essential to increase the levels of cytoprotective enzymes including antioxidant enzymes through activation of the Nrf2/ARE pathway, and dietary and endogenous antioxidants. This chapter suggests a mixture of micronutrients that would reduce oxidative stress and chronic inflammation at the same time and thereby would help in reducing the incidence and progression of diabetes.

INCIDENCE, PREVALENCE, AND COST

INCIDENCE

In 2015, an estimated 1.5 million new cases of diabetes among 18 years or older individuals were diagnosed. More than half of them were among 45 to 64 years. Men and women were equally affected. The rate of incidence of new cases is dependent upon ethnicity.

Non-Hispanic whites	5.7 cases/1000 persons
Non-Hispanic blacks	9.0 cases/1000 persons
Hispanics	8.4 cases/1000 persons

The percent of adults with diabetes increases with age. Among aged 65 years and older, it reaches as high as 25.2% of total.

PREVALENCE

In 2015, a total of 30.3 million people in the United States had diabetes, representing 9.4% of the population (23.1 million with diagnosed and 7.2 million with undiagnosed diabetes). In 2010, 19 million had diagnosed and 7 million undiagnosed diabetes (National Diabetes Statistics Reports, 2017). Thus, there is a substantial increase in prevalence of diabetes between 2010 and 2015.

COST

The cost of diabetes and pre-diabetes care in the USA is $322.00 billion per year (American Diabetic Association, 2016).

TYPES OF DIABETES

There are four types of diabetes in humans: type 1 diabetes, type 2 diabetes, gestational diabetes, and other types of diabetes. Pre-diabetic condition and metabolic syndrome are considered high risk for developing type 2 diabetes.

TYPE 1 DIABETES

Type 1 diabetes was previously called insulin-dependent diabetes mellitus, or juvenile-onset diabetes. This form of diabetes develops when the body's immune system destroys pancreatic beta cells that are responsible for synthesizing and releasing insulin, which regulates blood levels of glucose. The type 1 diabetes primarily affects children and young adults, although onset of disease can occur at any age. In adults, type 1 diabetes accounts for 5%–10% of all diagnosed cases of diabetes.[1] Risk factors for type 1 diabetes include autoimmune disease and genetic or environmental factors.

TYPE 2 DIABETES

Type 2 diabetes is previously called non-insulin-dependent diabetes mellitus, or adult-onset diabetes. This form of diabetes develops when cells become resistance to insulin, possibly due to defects in glucose transport protein, or insulin receptors. This forces the beta cells of pancreas to produce more insulin. Pancreas beta cells gradually are damaged leading progressive decrease in insulin production. Type 2 diabetes primarily affects older individuals; however, this form of diabetes is being more frequently diagnosed in children of American Indians, African Americans,

Hispanic/Latino Americans, and Asians/Pacific Islanders.[1] The primary risk factors include older age, obesity, a family history of diabetes, and a history of gestational diabetes, impaired glucose metabolism, physical inactivity, and race/ethnicity.

GESTATIONAL DIABETES

Gestational diabetes is characterized by glucose intolerance that usually develops during pregnancy. This form of diabetes is commonly observed in African Americans, American Indians, and Hispanic/Latino Americans. It is also more common among obese women and women with a family history of diabetes. About 5%–10% of women with gestational diabetes develop type 2 diabetes during the next 5–10 years.[1]

OTHER TYPES OF DIABETES

These forma of diabetes result from genetic defects, surgery, medications, pancreatic disease, and infection that damage pancreas. Such types of diabetes account for 1%–5% of all diagnosed cases.[1]

PRE-DIABETES AND METABOLIC SYNDROME

Pre-diabetes is a condition in which individuals have blood glucose levels higher than normal, but not high enough to be classified as diabetes. Pre-diabetic individuals with fasting blood glucose levels of 100–125 mg per deciliter may be due to an impaired fasting glucose (IFG), or with glucose levels of 140–199 mg per deciliter due to an impaired glucose tolerance (IGT). Individuals with pre-diabetic conditions have an increased risk of developing type 2 diabetes, heart disease, and stroke. The metabolic syndrome is a common and complex health issue combining obesity, abnormal lipid profiles, hypertension, and insulin resistance.

COMPLICATIONS OF DIABETES

There are severe complications associated with diabetes. They include heart disease, stroke, blood pressure, blindness, kidney disease, and impaired function of nerve including peripheral neuropathy, numbness of extremities, erectile dysfunction, amputation, periodontal disease, and birth defects in pregnant women. Adults with diabetes have about two to four times higher heart disease death rates compared to those with no diabetes.[1] The risk of stroke in diabetic individuals is about two to four times higher than the individuals without diabetes. Diabetes is the leading cause of new cases of blindness among US populations of ages 20–74 years. The annual incidence of diabetic retinopathy is about 12,000–24,000 cases. About 60%–70% of diabetic patients have mild to severe forms of damage to the nervous system. Severe forms of diabetic nerve disease are major contributing factors to lower-extremity amputations. Diabetes is the leading cause of kidney failure, accounting for about 44% of new cases in 2005.[1] In the United States, kidney failure requiring dialysis or transplantation among patients with diabetes decreases by about 33% from 2000 to 2014 (CDC's Nov. 3, Mortality and Morbidity reports, 2017). During a 10-year period, the total number of lower limb amputation was 62 cases for women and 71 cases for men with diabetes. These numbers were similar to those found among non-diabetic individuals (79 case for women and 78 cases for men).[2]

EVIDENCE FOR INCREASED OXIDATIVE STRESS IN DIABETES

TYPE 1 DIABETES

Several human and animal studies have suggested that the markers of oxidative stress are elevated in children with type 1 diabetes.[3] The frequency of sister chromatid exchange was evaluated in blood-cell culture from 35 type 1 diabetic patients and 5 healthy age- and sex-matched control.

The results showed that the frequency of sister chromatid exchange was higher in patients with type 1 diabetes compared to controls. It was concluded that hyperglycemia-induced oxidative stress might be primarily responsible for this genetic instability.[4] The levels of protein glycation and oxidative stress parameters in blood and serum from 81 patients with type 1 diabetes (61 patients with long-term poor glycemic control and 20 patients with long-term good glycemic control), and 31 healthy children were evaluated. The results showed that the levels of glycation end products and advanced oxidation protein products in diabetic were higher compared to control; the highest levels were found in patients with poor glycemic control.[5]

The patients with type 1 diabetes eventually develop insulin resistance and other characteristics of type 2 diabetes. The exact mechanisms are unknown. However, it was demonstrated that prolonged exposure of cultured mouse hepatocytes to insulin increased oxidative stress that accounts for the development insulin resistance. The insulin resistance was associated with impaired mitochondrial function, and overexpression of mitochondrial MnSOD prevented insulin-induced insulin resistance.[6] The levels of oxidant/antioxidant defense systems in 20 children with type 1 diabetes, 22 obese children and 16 age-sex-matched controls were evaluated. The results showed that the levels of lipoperoxides and malondialdehyde (MDA) and protein oxidation were significantly higher in both patients with diabetes and obese children compared to control, although the levels of MDA was highest in children with diabetes. In addition, the serum levels of alpha-tocopherol and beta-carotene, red cell glutathione peroxidase activity and reduced glutathione levels in patients with diabetes were lower compared to obese children. It was concluded that oxidative stress is elevated in both children with type 1 diabetes and obesity.[7] Although increased oxidative stress is associated with type 1 diabetes, it is not certain whether increased oxidative stress precedes or merely reflects consequences of the disease. Therefore, the levels of markers of oxidative stress were evaluated in 30 patients with type 1 diabetes (10 without diabetic complications, 10 with retinopathy, and 10 with nephropathy), 36 non-diabetic siblings, 37 non-diabetic parents of type 1 diabetic patients, and 3 control subjects without the familial history of diabetes were evaluated. The results revealed that the levels of MDA in plasma and RBC (red blood cell) were elevated in diabetic patients and their relatives compared to control subjects. However, the levels of reduced glutathione in RBC were lower in diabetic patients. It was concluded that increased oxidative stress occurs in non-diabetic relatives of diabetic patients; therefore, increased oxidative stress may precede type 1 diabetes.[8] In a clinical study involving 59 patients with type 1 diabetes, it was observed that lower plasma vitamin C level was associated with adverse changes in the microcirculation, peripheral arteries, and ventricular repolarization.[9]

In type 1 diabetic patients, especially with poor glycemic control, serum levels of copper were higher and zinc were lower than in non-diabetic subjects. Increased Cu/zinc ration was correlated with enhanced the levels of urinary MDA, and 8-hydroxy-2′-deoxyguanosine in these patients.[10] A meta-analysis of 15 studies involving 1027 diabetes patients (type 1 and type 2 diabetes) suggested that these patients had higher levels of Cu than healthy control subjects.[11] Urinary concentrations of conjugated metabolite of alpha-tocopherol alpha-tocopheronolactone, a novel marker of oxidative stress were elevated in patients with type 1 diabetes.[12] Increased oxidative stress was present in the non-diabetic siblings of type 1 diabetes patients.[13] Shorter telomere length and enhanced oxidative stress were found in both type 1 and type 2 diabetes.[14] This is not surprising, because a previous report suggests that increased oxidative stress contributes to shortening the length of telomeres.[15]

TYPE 2 DIABETES

There are substantial experimental and clinical studies that suggest that increased oxidative stress plays a major role in the pathogenesis of both types of diabetes mellitus.[16–20] In another clinical study, the levels of markers of oxidative stress and DNA damage in 92 subjects with normal glucose tolerance (NGT), 78 patients with impaired glucose tolerance (IGT) and 113 patients with newly diagnosed diabetes were evaluated. The results showed that patients with IGT had reduced erythrocyte SOD activity compared to subjects with normal glucose tolerance; however, the patients with diabetes had higher levels of plasma MDA but lower levels of total antioxidative capacity (TAC) and erythrocyte SOD activity than the subjects with NGT. The damage to DNA was slight in IGT subjects, but the level increased in patients with diabetes.[21] Oxidative stress induces beta-cell dysfunction by activating JNK pathway.[18] Diabetic-related complications such as microalbuminuria, periodontitis, nephropathy, retinopathy, and cardiovascular disease are due to increased oxidative stress induced by hyperglycemia.[22–27]

NAD (P) H oxidases are major sources of reactive oxygen species, and Nox4, one of the ubiquitous of these oxidases, is localized in the mitochondria of many cells and in kidneys of diabetic rats. The expression of mitochondrial Nox4 expression was elevated in the kidney cortex of diabetic rats, suggesting that Nox4 is a major source of ROS in the kidneys during early stages of diabetes.[28,29] Thus, Nox4-derived ROS contribute to renal hypertrophy and increased fibronectin expression in the cell.[29] It has been reported that the exercise capacity and mitochondrial function in skeletal muscles of mice were impaired in type 2 diabetes, which was related to increased oxidative stress.[30]

Since the first edition of this book, additional studies confirming the role of oxidative stress in diabetes have also been published.[31–38] Strongest support for the role of oxidative stress comes from the report that markers of oxidative damage were elevated in pre-diabetic patients[34] and in the parents of diabetic as well as children with type 1 diabetes.[39,40] Increased oxidative stress was also found in the non-diabetic siblings of type 1 diabetes patients.[13]

METABOLIC SYNDROME

Increased oxidative stress also occurs in individuals with metabolic syndrome. Increased levels of insulin and impaired glycemic control were associated with higher levels of oxidized low-density lipid (LDL).[41] This suggests that increased oxidative stress occurs in individuals with metabolic syndrome.

EVIDENCE FOR INCREASED CHRONIC INFLAMMATION IN DIABETES

Increased oxidative damage, if not repaired, can lead to chronic inflammation that releases free radicals, pro-inflammatory cytokines, complement proteins, adhesion molecules and prostaglandins, all of which are toxic to cells. Inflammatory molecules and their transcriptional factor, NF-kappa B, appear to play an important role in diabetes-induced cardiac dysfunction. In diabetic mice, increased NF-kappa B activity was associated with enhanced oxidative stress. Administration of pyrrolidine dithiocarbamates (PDTC), an NF-kappaB inhibitor, reduced oxidative stress and improved mitochondrial dysfunction in diabetic mice.[42] In a rat model of diabetes, elevated levels of IL-1 beta in islet cells promotes cytokines and chemokine expression, leading to the recruitment of innate immune cells. Therefore, IL-1 beta may not produce direct toxic effect on islet beta cells, but may induce tissue inflammation that causes beta cell death and insulin resistance in type 2 diabetes.[43] In a mice model of type 2 diabetes, the interaction between NF-kappa B and TNF-alpha signaling induced the activation of IKK-beta and amplified oxidative stress, leading to endothelial dysfunction.[44]

The histology of islet cells from patients with type 2 diabetes exhibited the presence of inflammatory products such as cytokines, immune cell infiltration, amyloid deposits associated with apoptotic cells and fibrosis.[45] Inflammatory molecules such as IL-beta, interferon-gamma (IFN-gamma) and TNF-alpha contribute to pancreatic beta cell death by activating NF-kappaB activity. This was confirmed by the fact that blocking NF-kappaB activation protected beta cells in culture against IL-beta + IFN-gamma or TNF-alpha + IFN-gamma-induced apoptosis.[46] Thus, activation of NF-kappaB activity appears to be a primary event in progressive loss of beta cells from the pancreas.

In obesity, white adipose tissue is infiltrated by macrophages that release excessive amounts of inflammatory molecules including TNF-alpha and IL-6 that contribute to insulin resistance in type 2 diabetes.[47,48] It has been reported that increased expression of p53 in mice adipose tissue contribute to insulin resistance caused by enhanced inflammatory responses.[49] In a clinical study involving 10 normal-weight and 8 obese subjects, the effects of a high-fat and high-carbohydrate meal on markers of oxidative stress and inflammation after an overnight fast were evaluated. The results showed that high-fat, high-carbohydrate meals induced a significant more prolonged and greater oxidative stress and inflammation compared to normal-weight subjects.[50] This may increase the risk of cardiac disease and insulin resistance.

Additional studies on the role of chronic inflammation in diabetes and diabetic-related complications have been published.[51–58]

Despite advances in medications for controlling blood glucose levels, the disease slowly continues to progress. This may in part be because these medications do not adequately address the issues of increased oxidative stress and chronic inflammation.

MicroRNAs IN DIABETES

Increased oxidative stress and chronic inflammation play a central role in the initiation and progression of diabetes. Previous reviews have revealed that oxidative damage and pro-inflammatory cytokines alter the expression of microRNAs in some neurodegenerative diseases such as Alzheimer's disease (AD)[59] and Parkinson's disease (PD).[60] Therefore, it is likely that they also play an important role in the development of diabetes. Indeed, altered levels of microRNAs were found in the plasma and serum of diabetic patients that have been suggested to be of diagnostic value, and in the cells that may lead to changes that play an important role in the pathogenesis of diabetes.

MicroRNAs

MicroRNAs (miRs) are evolutionarily conserved small noncoding single-stranded RNAs of approximately 22 nucleotides in length, and are present in all living organisms including humans.[61–64] The biogenesis of miRs is very complex and involves multiple biochemical steps. The majority of miRs are transcribed by RNA polymerase II (Pol II), while some are transcribed by RNA polymerase III (Pol III) from the noncoding region of the DNA to produce primary miRs (pri-miRs). Pri-miRs undergo a nuclear cleavage by ribonuclease III Drosa to generate precursor-miRs (pre-miRs) that migrate to the cytoplasm where they are further cleaved by ribonuclease III Dicer to ultimately form mature single-stranded miRs with the help of another protein argonaute (Ago).[63,65–67] Each microRNA binds to its complementary sequences in the 3′-untranslated region (3′-UTR) of the mRNA, promotes degradation of the mRNA transcript, and prevents translation of the message of protein. In this manner, miRs regulate the translation of proapoptotic or antiapoptotic proteins from their respective mRNAs, depending upon whether they receive damaging or protective signal. Damaging signals may include oxidative damage and pro-inflammatory cytokines and protective signals may include antioxidants and phytochemicals.

CIRCULATING MicroRNAs IN DIABETES

Several studies on the levels of circulating microRNAs have been published with a suggestion that their alterations could be of diagnostic value in diabetes. Only the results of a few selected investigations are presented (Table 6.1). The expression of miR-23a, let-7i, miR-486, miR-186, miR-191, miR-192, and miR-146a was lower in patients with type 2 diabetes and pre-diabetes than in normal glucose tolerance control subjects. Furthermore, the expression of miR-23a in the serum of patients with type 2 diabetes was lower than in pre-diabetic patients.[68] Serum concentrations

TABLE 6.1

Serum, Plasma, and Urinary MicroRNAs Levels in Type 1 Diabetes and Type 2 Diabetes

Diabetes Type	Upregulation	Downregulation
Type 2	None	miR-23a, let 7i, miR-486, miR-96, miR-186, miR-191, miR-192, miR-146a
Type 2	miR-101, miR-375, miR-802	None
Type 2	miR-9, miR-29a, miR-30, miR-34a, miR-124, miR-146a, miR-375	None
Type 2	miR-142-3p	miR-126a, miR-30e
Type 2, Obese	miR-486, miR-146b, miR-15b	None
Obese	miR-152, miR-17	miR-138
Type 2 + Obese	None	miR-593
Pre-Type 2	None	miR-126
Type 1	miR-21, miR-210	miR-126
Type 1 Urinary exsosomes	miR-130, miR-145	miR-155, miR-424
Type 2 Urinary exosomes	miR-320c, miR-6068	miR-30d-5p, miR-30e-5p

Note: Alterations in the expression of microRNAs in the blood and urine have suggested to be of diagnostic value.

of miR-101, miR-375, and miR-802 were higher in type 2 diabetic patients compared to normal glucose tolerance control subjects.[69] In serum of newly diagnosed patients with type 2 diabetes, the expression of seven miR-9, miR-29a, miR-30d, miR-34a, miR-124a, miR-146a, and miR-375 was elevated compared with pre-diabetes and type 2 diabetes susceptible individuals with normal glucose tolerance.[70] Plasma and urine levels of miR-21 and miR-210 were unregulated, while urine level of miR-126 was downregulated in patients with type 1 diabetes compared with control subjects; however, plasma level of miR-126 was similar in both groups. Additionally, decreased urine levels of miR-126 were associates with increased levels of A1c.[71] Circulating expression of miR-142-3p was enhanced; while the expression of miR-126a and miR-30e was reduced in type 2 diabetic patients compared with normal glucose tolerance individuals.[72] In streptozotocin-(STZ) induced diabetes mouse model, circulating concentrations of miR-375 were elevated before the onset of hyperglycemia. This was confirmed by experiments in which cytokine- and STZ induced cell death in cultured mouse islets, which was associated with a rise in the extracellular level of miR-375.[73]

The expression of three microRNAs miR-486, miR-146b, and miR-15b was upregulated in the serum of obese children and type 2 diabetic patients. Among these microRNAs, miR-486 was suggested to be involved in enhancing proliferation of pre-adipocyte and myotube glucose intolerance, while miR-146b and miR-15b inhibited glucose-induced pancreatic insulin secretion.[74] Serum levels of miR-152 and miR-17 were increased, whereas, miR-138 level was reduced in obese individuals compared with control subjects, type 2 diabetic patients, or type 2 diabetic patients with obesity. Additionally, serum levels of miR-486 were lower in type 2 diabetic patients and type 2 diabetic patients with obesity compared with controls.[75] Plasma levels of miR-126 were reduced before the onset of diabetes compared with healthy control subjects.[76] Urinary exosomes (miRs packaged in microvesicles of endocytic origin) had elevated levels of miR-130a and miR-145 and reduced levels of miR-155 and miR-424 in type 1 diabetic patients with microalbuminuria.[77] Additionally, in animal model of early experimental diabetic nephropathy, the levels miR-145 in the urinary exosomal and glomeruli were elevated. In the type 2 diabetic patients with nephropathy, the expression of 14 microRNAs (miR-320c, miR-6068, miR-1234, miR-6163, miR-4270, miR-4739, miR-371b-5p, miR-638, miR-572, miR-1227-5p, miR-6126, miR-1913-5p, miR-4778, and miR-2861) in urinary exosomes were enhanced, while the expression of miR-30d-5p and miR-30e-5p were reduced. These results suggest that deregulation of these microRNAs play an important role in the progression of renal disease. Among 14 microRNAs, the levels of miR-320c and miR-6068 in the urinary exosomes were most highly upregulated.[78]

Cellular MicroRNAs in Diabetes (Humans)

Several studies on changes in the expression of microRNAs and their corresponding target proteins play a significant role in the pathogenesis of diabetes. A few selected investigations in human and animal diabetes are presented in Table 6.2. In women with gestational diabetes (GDM), the expression of miR-222 was elevated in omentalsdipode tissue from GDM compared with pregnant women with normal glucose tolerance. The expression of miR-222 was also upregulated in 3T3-L-1 adipocytes in the presence of high concentration of 17β-estrodiol, while the levels of estrogen receptor (ER) protein-α and glucose transporter 4 (GLUT4) protein decreased. These results suggest that miR-222 could be considered a potential regulator of ER-alpha levels in estrogen-induced insulin resistance in GDM.[79] Islet-specific miR-375 was upregulated and downregulated its target protein myotrophin (Mtpn) leading to the suppression of glucose-induced insulin secretion in pancreatic endocrine cells. Inhibition of Mtpn synthesis by a small interfering (siRNA) mimicked the effects of miR-375, suggesting that this microRNA regulated the secretion of insulin.[80] In patients with type 2 diabetes, decreased expression of miR-19-3p increased the levels of its target protein suppressor of cytokine signaling 3 (SOCS3), and these changes were associated with high concentrations of blood glucose in type 2 diabetes. Transfection of β-cells with miR-19-3p enhanced the proliferation and insulin secretion. Additionally. Inhibition of the synthesis of SOCS3 protein

---

TABLE 6.2
Cellular MicroRNAs Levels and Their Associated Proteins in Human and Animal Diabetes

Diabetes Type	Upregulation	Downregulation	Target Proteins
Gestational diabetes	miR-222	None	GLUT4, ER-α
Type 2	miR-375	None	Mtpn
Type 2	None	miR-19a-3p	SOCS3
Type 2	miR-124a	None	Mtpn, FOXA3
Diabetic mouse	None	miR-200b	VEGF, ZEB1, TGF-b1, P300
Diabetic mouse	None	miR-133a	TGF-b1, CTGF, FN1, COL4A1
Diabetic mouse	miR-503	None	cdc25A, CCNE1
Mouse β-cells	miR-483	None	SOCS3
Mouse α-cells	miR-483	None	Glucagon
Diabetic mouse	miR-200	None	Dnajc3, Xiap
Diabetic mouse	miR-9	None	Sirt1
Diabetic mouse	miR-187	None	HIPK3
Diabetic mouse	miR-185	None	SOCS3e

Note: GLUT4, glucose transporter-4; ER-α, estrogen receptor; Mtpn, myotrophin; SOCS3, suppressor of cytokine signaling 3; FOCA3, forkhead box protein A3; VEGF, vascular endothelial growth factor; ZEB1, zinc finger E-box homeobox 1; TGF-1b, transforming growth factor-b1; P300, histone acetyltransferase P300; CTGF, connective tissue growth factor; FN1, fibronectin; SOL4A1, alpha 1 subunit collagen type IV; cdc25A, cell division cycle 25 homolog A; CCNE1, Cyclin E1; Dnajc3, (also known as p581PK); Xiap, X-linked inhibitor of apoptosis protein; Sirt1, NAD-dependent protein deacetylase sirtuin-1.

by siRNA increased cell proliferation and insulin secretion.[81] Overexpression of miR-124a and downregulation of its target proteins Mptn (myotrophin) and FOXa3 (forkhead box protein A3) in MIN6 pseudoislets (insulin-secreting MIN6 cells grown as islet-like clusters), and these changes were associated with reduced glucose-induced insulin secretion.[82]

CELLULAR MicroRNAs IN DIABETES (ANIMAL MODELS)

Downregulation of miR-200b increased the levels of its target proteins VEGF (vascular endothe-lial growth factor), zinc finger-box-binding homebox, TGF-β1 (transforming growth factor-β1), and p300 in the heart of diabetic mice. Overexpression of this microRNA prevented the rise in the levels of these proteins in mouse heart endothelial cells (MHECs), In streptozotocin-induced diabetic mice, reduced expression of miR-133 caused increased levels of its target proteins TGF-β1, connective tissue growth factor (CTGF), fibronectin (FN1), and COL4A1 (alpha 1 subunit of collagen type IV) causing cardiac fibrosis. These effects were decreased in mice overexpression of miR-133a.[83] MiR-503 expression was upregulated in ECc cells growing in the presence of high glu-cose that generates excessive amounts of free radicals and reduced its target proteins cdc25A (Cell Division Cycle 25 Homolog A) and CCNE1 (Cyclin E1).[84] Additionally, deleting the expression of miR-503 improved function of ECs growing under high glucose concentrations. In the β-cells from mouse, overexpression of miR-483 increased insulin secretion by downregulating its target protein SOCS3, while increased expression of this microRNA in α-cells reduced the secretion of glucagon. Additionally, overexpression of miR-483 protected β-cells against pro-inflammatory cytokine-induced apoptosis, and enhanced beta-cells mass in the islets of pre-diabetic (db/db) mice.[85] Overexpression of miR-200 downregulated the levels of its target proteins Dnajc3 (also known as p58IPK) and Xiap, an inhibitor of caspase, and induced apoptosis in the beta cells in diabetic mice. On the other hand, ablation of miR-200 reduced the apoptosis of beta-cells and prevented development of diabetes.[86] The expression of miR-9 was enhanced and its target protein Sirt1 (NSD-dependent protein deacetylase reduced during glucose-dependent insulin secretion in mouse beta-cells secreting insulin. Therefore, miR-9 could be a therapeutic target for diabetes.[87] In type 2 diabetes, increased expression of miR-185 was associated decreased its target protein homeodomain-interacting protein kinase-3 (HIPK3) and decreased glucose-stimulated secretion of insulin (GSIS) in islet cells compared with normal controls. Decreased expression of miR-185 increased its target protein SOCS3 and reduced insulin secretion in mice as well as in humans with diabetes.[88]

The studies discussed above suggest that upregulation and downregulation of microRNAs are involved in the pathogenesis of diabetes. In addition, the results show that one microRNA can prevent the translation of multiple mRNAs transcripts into proteins, and multiple microRNAs can prevent the translation of an mRNA transcript of one protein.

OXIDATIVE STRESS AND PRO-INFLAMMATORY CYTOKINES REGULATE EXPRESSION OF MicroRNAs

We have shown that oxidative stress and pro-inflammatory cytokines regulate the expression of microRNAs and their associated target proteins that cause neurodegeneration in Alzheimer's dis-ease[59] and Parkinson's disease.[60] Since increased oxidative stress and chronic inflammation are involved in the initiation and progression of diabetes, it is not surprising that microRNAs expression is altered in this disease.

ANTIOXIDANTS REGULATE EXPRESSION OF MicroRNAs

Our previous reviews proposed that antioxidants regulate expression of microRNAs that allow translation of only protective proteins from their respective mRNAs transcripts in varieties of cell type and health conditions, such as Alzheimer's disease (AD)[89] and Parkinson's disease (PD).[90]

Since antioxidants protect against some components of diabetes, it is possible that they may also alter the expression of microRNAs that allow translation of cytoprotective proteins for protection against the development of diabetes.

REDUCING OXIDATIVE STRESS AND CHRONIC INFLAMMATION IN DIABETES

Increased oxidative stress and chronic inflammation can damage the pancreas, glucose transporter proteins, and insulin receptors that contribute to hyperglycemia. If the pancreas is producing sufficient amounts of insulin, oxidative damage to the glucose transporter proteins or insulin receptors may cause tissue resistance to insulin leading to hyperglycemia. Since these biochemical defects initiate and promote diabetes and diabetic-related complications, reducing these biochemical defects may be one of the rational choices for the prevention, and in combination with standard treatment, for the improved management of diabetes.

ROLE OF ANTIOXIDANTS AND PHYTOCHEMICALS IN PROTECTING AGAINST DIABETES

Antioxidants and phytochemicals are groups of nontoxic agents that could reduce oxidative stress and chronic inflammation. Therefore they can reduce the risk of developing, and in combination with standard therapy, may improve the management of diabetes, if used on the basis of scientific rationale.

Most animal and human studies have utilized one antioxidant, certain B-vitamins, aspirin, chromium, and omega-3 fatty acids in prevention and improved treatment of diabetes. The results of these studies have been inconsistent with respect to prevention, markers of oxidative stress and inflammation, insulin sensitivity, glycemic index, and diabetic-related complications. The scientific rationale of these inconsistent results is discussed after presenting data on the use of single micronutrient.

Vitamin A (Animal and Human Studies)

There are only limited studies available on the effects of vitamin A. It has been suggested that decreased production of nerve growth factor (NGF) may contribute to diabetic neuropathy; however, administration of exogenous NGF produced only a modest benefit. Retinoic acid (RA), a metabolite of retinol (vitamin A), induced expression of NGF and its receptor. Therefore, it was thought that administration of retinoic acid might be useful in improving some of the symptoms of diabetic retinopathy. Treatment of diabetic rats with RA increased the levels of NGF in serum and nerve cells, and induced nerve cell regeneration[91,92]; however, the levels of plasma glucose did not change, and there was no difference in pain thresholds between treated and untreated groups of diabetic animals.[92] Type 1 diabetes is characterized by inflammation as evidenced by the infiltration of activated T lymphocytes and monocytes into the islet cells of the pancreas resulting into loss of beta-cells. Supplementation with vitamin A (retinyl acetate) through diet caused a marked reduction in inflammatory reaction and loss of beta-cells in diabetic mice.[93]

A review has suggested that vitamin A supplementation may be beneficial in patients with type 2 diabetes who have vitamin A deficiency.[94] Binding of retinol-binding protein to membrane-binding protein suppresses insulin signaling; treatment with all-trans-retinoic acid reversed the above effect, causing increased insulin sensitivity.[95]

Vitamin C (Human Studies)

In a randomized clinical study involving 36 elderly patients with type 2 diabetes, a dose-dependent increase in the cellular levels of reduced glutathione and vitamin E was observed after treatment with vitamin C; however, these changes were not sufficient to reduce LDL susceptibility to per-oxidation.[96] Endothelial dysfunction is associated with hyperglycemia-induced type 2 diabetes, and this may become aggravated in patients with insulin resistance. Both intra-arterial and oral admin-istration of high-dose vitamin C improved plasma vitamin C levels and endothelial dysfunction and insulin resistance in diabetic patients.[97,98] Analysis of 26 observational studies and 12 randomized controlled trials suggested that supplementation with vitamin C alone may reduce fast glucose lev-els, but no HbA1c levels.[99] Review of published studies up to 2013 indicated that prolonged supple-mentation with vitamin C and/or vitamin E may be effective in improving endothelial cell function in nonobese patients with type 2 diabetes.[100]

VITAMIN C (ANIMAL STUDIES)

Treatment of streptozotocin-induced diabetic rats with vitamin C suppressed leukocyte adhesion and endothelial dysfunction and, thus, improved blood flow in the iris microvessels.[101] This suggests that administration of vitamin C could be useful in preventing diabetic retinopathy. Vitamin C treatment of diabetes also prevented diabetic-induced endothelial dysfunction in mesenteric microcirculation in rats.[102] Oxidative stress appears to play an important role in diabetic nephropa-thy. Supplementation with vitamin C in a diabetic rat model reduced number of apoptotic kidney cells, albuminuria, proteinuria, glomerular and tubulointerstitial sclerosis, and renal MDA without changing the level of plasma glucose.[103] This suggests that vitamin C reduces oxidative stress but that it has no role in regulating plasma glucose levels.

VITAMIN D3 (ANIMAL STUDIES)

In a rat model of diabetes, administration of 1alpha-, 25 dihydroxyvitamin D3 [1alpha, 25(OH) 2 VD3] increased plasma insulin levels, normalized the hepatic glycogen concentration, and main-tained the normal plasma glucose level. In addition, treatment with 1alpha, 25(OH) 2VD3 enhanced SOD, catalase, and glutathione peroxidase activities, compared to control diabetic rats. It also reduced lipid peroxidation and toxicity in the liver and kidneys.[104] Vitamin D deficiency may be associated with both type 1 and type 2 diabetes, and it impairs biosynthesis and release of insu-lin in animals and humans with type 2 diabetes. Epidemiologic studies have supported the role of vitamin D deficiency in the etiology of diabetes. In nonobese diabetic mice, supplementation with 1alpha, 25 (OH) 2VD3, or its structural analogs delay the onset of diabetes.[105,106] Therefore, supplementation with vitamin D3 may be one of necessary ingredients of any multiple micronutri-ent preparation for the prevention or improved treatment of diabetes.

VITAMIN E (ANIMAL STUDIES)

It has been reported that an oral administration of vitamin E reduced kidney MDA in both diabetic and control rats.[107] Haptoglobin (Hp) is an antioxidant protein that protects against oxidative dam-age caused by extracorpuscular hemoglobin. There are two alleles at the Hp locus, 1 and 2. Hp-1 is a superior antioxidant compared to Hp-2. The haptoglobin (Hp) 2-2 genotype is associated with increased risk of cardiovascular disease in diabetes. This genotype is also associated with increased risk of diabetic neuropathy and appears to be associated with a more rapid progression to end-stage renal disease. Using transgenic mice, it was demonstrated that vitamin E supplementation provided significant protection against development of functional and histological features of diabetic neu-ropathy in Hp 2-2 mice but not in Hp 1-1 mice.[108] It has been reported that administration of tocotri-enol was more effective in protecting against diabetic neuropathy in streptozotocin-induced diabetic rats than alpha-tocopherol.[109] In a rat model of type 1 diabetes, supplementation with vitamin E reduced the incidence of cardiac failure and myocardial markers of oxidative stress.[110]

VITAMIN E (HUMAN STUDIES)

Vitamin E supplementation decreased the risk of cardiovascular disease in Hp2-2 diabetic patients.[111] This confirms the observation made on the animal model of diabetes with Hp2-2 genotype.[108] Diabetes is associated with increased risk of complications following coronary bypass graft; in which increased oxidative stress and pro-inflammatory markers and adhesion molecules play an important role. The efficacy of vitamin E as an adjunctive therapy on markers of oxidative damage, pro-inflammatory cytokines, and adhesion molecules in diabetic patients with coronary bypass graft were evaluated. The results showed that supplementation with vitamin E reduced oxidative stress, inflammation markers, and adhesion molecules.[112] Memory impairment is observed in patients with type 2 diabetes, and this becomes aggravated after a high-fat meal, possibly due to a generation of excessive amounts of free radicals.

In the Women's Antioxidant Cardiovascular Study involving 8,171 female health professionals with either a history of cardiovascular disease or more cardiovascular risk factors, the efficacy of vitamin C (ascorbic acid, 500 mg every day), vitamin E (RRR-alpha-tocopheryl acetate, 600 IU every other day), beta-carotene (50 mg every other day), or their respective placebos on the risk of developing type 2 was evaluated. The result showed that none of these antioxidants, when used individually, was effective in reducing the risk of type 2 diabetes.[113] Although the selection of the high-risk population of type 2 diabetes was rational, the use of only one dietary antioxidant was not. Inconsistent results with a single antioxidant have been obtained with other chronic diseases including, cancer, heart disease, and neurological diseases. Therefore, the above results were not unexpected. However, these results should not be extrapolated to the potential efficacy of a mixture of micronutrients containing multiple dietary and endogenous antioxidants.

ALPHA-LIPOIC ACID (HUMAN STUDIES)

A review on the role of alpha-lipoic acid in the management of type 2 diabetes has shown that alpha-lipoic acid produced beneficial effects in diabetic patients by improving uptake and utilization of glucose.[114–116] Alpha-lipoic acid also reduced oxidative stress and the formation of advanced glycation end products (AEGs) and improved insulin sensitivity to glucose in skeletal muscle and the liver. The inhibitor of AEG, pyridoxamine (PM), prevented irreversibly protein glycation. In a randomized, double-blind, placebo-controlled trial involving more than 1500 patients with type 1 and type 2 diabetes, the efficacy of supplementation with alpha-lipoic acid on neuropathic symptoms and neuropathic deficits was evaluated. The results showed that supplementation with alpha-lipoic acid (600 mg/day, IV) over a 3-week period significantly improved neuropathic symptoms and neuropathic deficits in diabetic patients with polyneuropathy,[117–119] and autonomic neuropathy in patients with type 1 diabetes.[120] An oral administration of alpha-lipoic acid (600 mg, twice a day, or 600, 1200, or 1800 mg once a day) increased peripheral insulin sensitivity in patients with type 2 diabetes and improved neuropathic symptoms and deficits in patients with diabetic poly-neuropathy.[121–123] Several studies have demonstrated that the combination of enduring exercise and alpha-lipoic acid produced better improvement in insulin sensitivity to glucose in skeletal muscle than either agent alone.[124] In patients with type 1 diabetes receiving insulin therapy, a diet rich in antioxidants, together with alpha-lipoic acid improved endothelial function compared with an antioxidant-rich diet plus placebo.[125]

ALPHA-LIPOIC ACID (ANIMAL STUDIES)

It has been reported that the combination of alpha-lipoic acid and pyridoxamine produced better results in insulin-mediated glucose transport in the soleus muscle of obese Zucker rats with insulin resistance disease.[126] In a diabetic rat model, supplementation with alpha-lipoic acid reduced proteinuria by attenuating expressions of transforming growth factor-beta1 (TGF-beta1) and fibronectin proteins that contribute to diabetic nephropathy.[127] It has been reported that supplementation with alpha-lipoic acid reduced neural tube defects, cardiovascular malformations, and skeletal muscle malformations in the offspring of diabetic mice at term delivery.[128] Lipoic acid synthase is involved in the biosynthesis of alpha-lipoic acid. In the animal model of diabetes type 2, the expression of lipoic acid synthase in tissues is significantly reduced. TNF-alpha and hyperglycemia decreased the alpha-lipoic acid synthase expression in the endothelial cells in culture. Downregulation of alpha-lipoic acid synthase aggravated the inflammatory responses, whereas overexpression of this gene ameliorated the inflammatory responses in the diabetic animals.[129] Supplementation with alpha-lipoic acid delayed development and progression of cataract in streptozotocin-induced diabetic rats.[130]

N-Acetylcysteine (Human Studies)

In a clinical study involving 10 patients with type 2 diabetes and 10 normal subjects, the effect of NAC on the markers of oxidative stress and chronic inflammation after a high-glucose meal was evaluated. The results showed that the levels of 4-hydroxynonenal (HNE) and MDA increased after high-glucose meal consumption in patients with diabetes who did not receive NAC, while the glycemic index, markers of inflammation, and insulinemia remained unchanged. However, in diabetic patients receiving a high-glucose meal after NAC administration, the levels of HNE, MDA, and vascular adhesion molecule-1 (VCAM-1) decreased. The control subjects receiving high-glucose meal before or after NAC administration did not show any significant change on any parameters of oxidative or inflammation markers.[131]

N-Acetylcysteine (Animal Studies)

In a rat model of type 1 diabetes, administration of NAC reduced the levels of hyperglycemia-induced oxidative stress.[132] Increased markers of oxidative stress and inflammation appear to be associated with diabetic retinopathy. Supplementation with NAC reduced the levels of these markers in streptozotocin-induced diabetic rats[133] and, therefore, may reduce the risk of retinopathy. Oxidative stress-mediated activation of membrane bound protein kinase C beta (2) PKC beta (2) in the myocardium is involved in the development of cardiomyopathy associated with diabetes. Supplementation with NAC reduced markers of oxidative stress and prevented hyperglycemia-induced cardiomyocyte hypertrophy in cultured neonatal cardiomyocites.[134] Diabetic encephalopathy caused by hyperglycemia-induced oxidative stress is associated with impaired cognitive function. Supplementation with NAC through drinking water significantly reduced cognitive deficits and oxidative stress in streptozotocin-induced diabetic rats.[135] Diabetes during pregnancy increases the risk for congenital heart disease in the offspring. Administration of NAC together with high concentration of glucose directly into the chick embryos decreased the frequency of heart malformations from 82% to 27%.[136] NAC treatment reduced diabetic myocardial dysfunction by restoring myocardial MnSOD activity.[137] It has been reported that the blood levels of reduced glutathione was significantly decreased in patients with type 1 diabetes; however, supplementation with low levels of cysteine, a precursor of glutathione, failed to restore glutathione levels in patients with poorly controlled type 1 diabetes.[138] This is in contrast to animal studies in which supplementation with high doses of L-cysteine can lower glycemic index and markers of vascular inflammation by preventing the activation of NF-kappaB.[139]

L-Carnitine (Human Studies)

L-carnitine, the L-beta-hydroxy-gamma-N-trimethylaminobutyric acid, is synthesized from lysine and methionine primarily in the liver and kidneys. It plays an important role in lipid metabolism. It acts as an obligatory cofactor for beta-oxidation of fatty acids by transporting the long-chain fatty acids to the mitochondrial membrane as acyl-carnitine esters. Since L-carnitine shuttles acetyl groups from inside to outside the mitochondrial membrane, it plays a key role in glucose metabolism. Any reduction in the transport of fatty acids inside the mitochondria can lead to the cytosolic accumulation of triglycerides, which contributes to insulin resistance. Indeed, it has been reported that L-carnitine and acetyl-L-carnitine improved insulin-mediated glucose metabolism in normal healthy subjects as well as in patients with type 2 diabetes.[140] It has been reported that the accumulation of fatty acyl CoA derivatives/metabolites in muscle inhibited insulin signaling and glucose oxidation. Supplementation with L-carnitine improved insulin-stimulated glucose utilization by reversing abnormalities in lipid metabolism.[141] Diabetes is associated with peripheral neuropathy. A review of two clinical trials involving 1679 diabetes patients revealed that a dose of 2 g daily was well tolerated and caused a reduction in pain scores. One study shows improvements in nerve conduction velocities, while the other did not. Evidence of nerve regeneration was found in some trials.[142,143] The results of these investigations suggest that supplementation with high-dose L-carnitine may reduce some of the symptoms of diabetic peripheral neuropathy. Type 2 diabetes is associated with increased levels of oxidized LDL. In a randomized, placebo-controlled trial involving 81 patients with type 2 diabetes, supplementation with L-carnitine reduced the levels of oxidized LDL.[144] In a randomized clinical trial involving 52 patients with type 2 diabetes, supplementation with L-carnitine and simvastatin lowered serum lipoproteins levels more than that produced by simvastatin treatment alone.[145] Obese subjects with insulin resistance have elevated levels of free fatty acids that contribute to the endothelial dysfunction. In a clinical study involving 7 normal lean subjects, supplementation with L-carnitine improved free fatty acids associated endothelial dysfunction.[146] The role of L-carnitine in diabetes is further supported by the fact that the mean serum-free L-carnitine levels in diabetic patients with complications were almost 25% lower than in diabetic patients without complications.[147]

L-Carnitine (Animal Studies)

Obesity can contribute to glucose intolerance. It has been reported that supplementation with L-carnitine improved insulin-stimulated glucose disposal in genetically-induced diabetic mice and wild-type mice fed a high-fat diet. It increased circulating levels of acetyl-L-carnitine and several medium- and long-chain acyl-carnitine species in both plasma and tissue.[148] Diabetes is known to cause defects in nerve conduction. Using streptozotocin-induced diabetic rats, supplementation with a high dose acetyl-L-carnitine improved nerve conduction velocity of sural nerve; however, a lower dose of acetyl-L-carnitine was less effective.[149] Increased levels of advanced AGE are observed in patients with diabetes. A high-fructose diet induced hyperglycemia and glycation of hemoglobin; however, supplementation with L-carnitine significantly reduced glycation of hemoglobin. The efficacy of L-carnitine in reducing glycation was compared with a well-known anti-glycation agent, aminoguanidine, using bovine serum albumin in vitro. The results showed that L-carnitine was more effective than aminoguanidine in inhibiting glycation in vitro.[150] Streptozotocin-induced diabetes in rats is associated with L-carnitine deficiency, bradycardia, and left ventricular enlargement. An oral supplementation of L-carnitine normalized serum L-carnitine, heart-rate regulation, and left ventricular size.[151] Excessive administration of insulin can cause hypoglycemia, which can induce mitochondrial swelling followed by neuronal death in the brain. Administration of L-carnitine in insulin-induced hypoglycemic rats prevented neuronal damage in the hippocampus by improving mitochondrial function.[152]

Coenzyme Q10 (Human Studies)

In a clinical study involving 28 patients with type 2 diabetes (10 men and 18 women) and 10 healthy individuals with age-and sex-matched controls, the effect of coenzyme Q10 on markers of oxidative stress (MDA in platelet and serum) was evaluated. The levels of MDA in platelet and serum were higher, and the plasma coenzyme Q10 levels were lower in patients with diabetes than in control subjects. There was a negative correlation between plasma coenzyme Q10 concentrations and glyco-sylated hemoglobin. This suggests that the patients with type 2 diabetes have a high internal oxidative environment that may cause impaired glycemic control in diabetic patients.[153]

Maternally inherited diabetes mellitus and deafness (MIDD) is due to a mutation in mitochondrial DNA (mtDNA) 3243 (A-G) and is characterized by progressive insulin secretory defect and neurosensory deafness. In a clinical study involving 28 MIDD patients—7 mutant subjects with impaired glucose tolerance (IGT) and 15 mutant subjects with normal glucose tolerance (NGT)—the efficacy of coenzyme Q10 (150 mg per day for a period of 3 years) on insulin secretory response, hearing disorder, and clinical symptoms of MIDD were evaluated. The results showed that the insulin secretory response in MIDD patients was significantly higher than in control MIDD patients.[154] Coenzyme Q10 treatment also improved hearing loss; however, it did not affect the diabetic complications or other clinical symptoms of MIDD. Furthermore, coenzyme Q10 treatment did not affect insulin secretory response in the mutant IGT or NGT subjects. There were no side effects of coenzyme Q10 during the therapy period of 3 years. In a randomized, double-blind, placebo-controlled 2 × 2 factorial clinical study involving 74 patients with uncomplicated type 2 diabetes and dyslipidemia, an oral supplementation with coenzyme Q10 (100 mg twice a day), 200 mg fenofibrate once a day, or both for 12 weeks showed that coenzyme Q10 improved blood pressure (systolic and diastolic) and long-term glycemic control, whereas fenofibrate, a cholesterol-lowering drug that improve lipid profiles, did not alter blood pressure or glycemic control.[155] An analysis of 7 trials performed up to February 2015 suggests that coenzyme Q10 has no beneficial effects on glycemic control, lipid profiles, or blood pressure in patients with diabetes; however, it may reduce the levels of triglycerides.[156] Thus, coenzyme Q10 supplementation has produced inconsistent results in patients with diabetes. The reasons for this are discussed later in this chapter.

COENZYME Q10 (ANIMAL STUDIES)

Diabetes and obesity can be induced by consumption of excessive dietary fat that increases the levels of markers of oxidative stress and inflammation. It has been reported that supplementation with coenzyme Q10 reduced global hepatic mRNA expressions of inflammatory and metabolic stressor genes without changing the levels of lipid peroxides in mice fed high-fat diet, compared to control mice receiving a high-fat diet alone.[157] This suggests that action of coenzyme Q10 did not involve a reduction in oxidative stress. Treatment of human umbilical vein epithelial cells in culture with coenzyme Q10 prevented hyperglycemia-induced increased oxidative stress and markers of adhesion molecules.[158] This suggests that coenzyme Q10 can protect against hyperglycemia-induced endothelial dysfunction that increases the progression of cardiovascular disease. Neuropathy, a form of disorder of nerve conduction, is associated with type 2 diabetes. Supplementation with coenzyme Q10 improved nerve conduction by sciatic nerve in diabetic rats.[159]

OMEGA-3 FATTY ACIDS (ANIMAL STUDIES)

High dietary intake of omega-3 fatty acids reduced diabetic-related renal disease in diabetic models of rodents.[160] Supplementation with omega-3 fatty acids reduced the levels of MDA and activities of SOD and catalase and decreased the number of cerebral apoptotic neurons that were elevated in diabetic animals.[161] Long-term consumption of diet rich in omega-3 fatty acids improved blood lipids and vascular function in an animal model of insulin resistance and type 2 diabetes; however, only dietary monosaturated fatty acids and alpha linolenic acid enhanced insulin sensitivity and glycemic responses.[162] Increased inflammation in white adipose tissue appears to be associated with obesity and type 2 diabetes. In obese mice with diabetes, omega-3 fatty acids treatment prevented inflammation in white adipose tissue induced by high-fat diet.[163] Dietary intake of low-dose omega-3 fatty acids attenuated leukocyte adhesion and infiltration into tissues of diabetic mice complicated with sepsis.[164] Supplementation with omega-3 fatty acids in pregnant female diabetic rats improved lipid profiles and antioxidant enzyme activities and the levels of antioxidants (vitamins A, C and E) in mothers as well as in their offspring.

OMEGA-3-FATTY ACIDS (EPIDEMIOLOGIC STUDIES)

Epidemiologic studies have suggested that populations consuming large amounts of omega-3 fatty acids (n-3 long-chain polyunsaturated fatty acids) found mainly in fish reduced the incidence of impaired glucose tolerance, type 2 diabetes, and cardiovascular disease. This was not confirmed by a recent epidemiologic study. A large epidemiologic study involving 195,000 US adults (152,700 women and 42,504 men) without pre-existing chronic disease at baseline with a follow-up period of 14–18 years was conducted. The results showed that higher consumption of omega-3 fatty acids and fish was not associated with the reduced risk of type 2 diabetes. Instead, it was modestly associated with increased incidence of the disease.[165] This study suggests that supplementation with omega-3 fatty acids will have no impact on the incidence of type 2 diabetes. However, this suggestion needs to be confirmed by intervention studies before it is accepted.

OMEGA-3-FATTY ACIDS (INTERVENTION STUDIES)

In a randomized intervention study involving 162 healthy individuals, moderate supplementation with fish oil did not affect insulin sensitivity, insulin secretion, beta-cell function, or glucose tolerance.[166] A review of published data showed that supplementation with omega-3 fatty acids in type 2 diabetes has no significant effect on glycemic control or fasting insulin; however, it lowered triglycerides and very low density lipoprotein (VLDL)-cholesterol levels, but it may raise LDL-cholesterol.[167] Several intervention studies to evaluate the efficacy of various doses of omega-3 fatty acids on prevention and diabetic-related complications have produced inconsistent results. A systematic review and meta-analysis of several randomized, placebo-controlled trials involving 1,075 patients with type 2 diabetes, the effects of dietary and non-dietary intake of omega-3 fatty acids on lipid profiles was evaluated. The results revealed that supplementation with omega-3 fatty acids decreased the levels of triglycerides, VLDL-cholesterol, and VLDL-triglycerides, but it slightly enhanced the level of LDL-cholesterol. In addition, it showed improvement in thrombogenesis but had no beneficial effects of cardiovascular disease risk factors such as HDL-cholesterol, LDL particle size, glycemia, insulinemia, inflammatory biomarkers, and blood pressure.[168,169] In a clinical study involving 30 patients with type 2 diabetes and hypertriglyceridemia (16 males and 14 females), it was found that after supplementation with omega-3 fatty acids, the levels of triglycerides, non-HDL-cholesterol, C-reactive protein, and TNF-alpha were decreased, whereas the levels of HDL-cholesterol increased, and there was no change in the levels of IL-6.[170] In a randomized, double-blind, placebo-controlled trial involving 81 patients with type 2 diabetes, the efficacy of omega-3 fatty acids on the levels of homocysteine and MDA was determined. The results revealed that supplementation with omega-3 fatty acids (3 g/day) for a period of 2 months decreased the levels of homocysteine without changing the levels of MDA, fasting blood sugar, and CRP. This study again shows that supplementation with omega-3 fatty acids alone does not reduce glycemic index and some other risk factors associated with cardiovascular disease.[171] Supplementation with omega-3 fatty acids (3 g/day) for a period of two months failed to alter insulin sensitivity in 27 women with type 2 diabetes.[172,173]

ANTIOXIDANT MIXTURES (HUMAN STUDIES)

In a single-blind, controlled clinical study involving 46 patients with type 2 diabetes, 46 subjects with impaired glucose tolerance (IGT), and 46 control subjects, the efficacy of a mixture of antioxidants (vitamin E, vitamin C, and NAC) on the markers of oxidative stress and inflammation was evaluated. The results showed that the plasma levels of markers of oxidative stress (MDA, 4-hydroxynonenal, and oxidized LDL), markers of endothelial function (NO, endothelin-1, and von Willebrand factor [vWF]) and a marker of inflammation, vascular adhesion molecule-1 (VCAM-1), were increased in all groups before supplementation with antioxidants. However, after supplementation, the levels of these markers of oxidative stress and inflammation were reduced.[174] In a clinical study involving 16 patients with type 2 diabetes, supplementation with tablets containing vitamin C 1000 mg and vitamin E 800 IU reduced high-fat-induced memory impairment and markers of oxidative stress.[175] In the Myocardial Infarction and Vitamins Study involving 800 patients with acute myocardial infarction (AMI) in which 122 patients (15%) had confirmed diabetes, the efficacy of vitamin E and vitamin C on mortality was evaluated. The results revealed that supplementation with vitamin E and vitamin C reduced cardiac mortality in patients with AMI and diabetes.[176] In a randomized, double-blind, placebo-controlled trial involving 30 patients with type 2 diabetes, supplementation with chromium (1000 micrograms) alone or in combination with vitamin C (1000 mg) and vitamin E (800 IU) reduced oxidative stress and improved glucose metabolism.[177]

ANTIOXIDANT MIXTURE (ANIMAL STUDIES)

A mixture of vitamin C, vitamin E, and selenium protected the lens of the eye of streptozotocin-induced diabetic rats against oxidative damage by reducing markers of oxidative damage and improving antioxidant defense system.[178]

Treatment of diabetic rats with beta-carotene, pycnogenol, and alpha-lipoic acid alone or in combination, normalized lipid peroxidation in the liver, kidneys, and heart, and elevated hepatic-reduced glutathione levels and cardiac glutathione peroxidase activity, or had no effect on hepatic catalase and SOD activities in all tissues.[179] In streptozotocin-induced diabetic rats, supplementation with curcumin and vitamin C was more effective in reducing blood glucose, glycosylated hemoglobin (HbA1c), dyslipidemia, leukocyte adhesion, and MDA than the individual agents.[180] Combination of vitamin E and magnesium was more effective in improving plasma lipid parameters and blood viscosity in diabetic rats than the individual agents.[181]

The overexpression of CuZn SOD or Mn SOD, together with catalase reduced H_2O_2-induced oxidative stress in islet beta cells in culture.[182] Dexamethasone-induced impairment of beta cells function may be mediated via increased oxidative stress. This is confirmed by the fact that overexpression of catalase prevented dexamethasone-induced toxicity in beta cells in culture.[183]

FOLIC ACID AND THIAMINE (HUMAN STUDIES)

Patients with type 1 diabetes have reduced levels of endothelial progenitor cells with impaired function. Reduced NO and increased oxidative stress contribute to the endothelial progenitor cells dysfunction. The analysis of gene expression profiles of endothelial progenitor cells from patients with type 1 diabetes revealed marked alterations in the expressions of 1591 genes involved in processes regulating development, cell communication, cell adhesion, and localization compared to healthy control subjects. Supplementation with folic acid normalized gene expression profiles in diabetic patients.[184] This is a remarkable observation that treatment of patients with type 1 diabetes with a single micronutrient can restore alterations in gene expression profiles to a normal level.

In the Women's Antioxidants and Folic Acid Cardiovascular Study involving 5,442 female healthy professionals with a history of cardiovascular disease or more cardiovascular disease risk factors, the efficacy of a mixture of 2.5 mg folic acid, 50 mg vitamin B6, and 1 mg vitamin B12 on the risk of type 2 diabetes was evaluated. The results showed that lowering homocysteine levels by B-vitamins in women at high risk for cardiovascular disease did not reduce the risk of type 2 diabetes.[185]

In a clinical study involving 9 patients with type 1 diabetes, the effect of benfotiamine, a lipophilic derivative of thiamine, together with slow-release alpha-lipoic acid on glycemic status was evaluated by measuring hyperglycemia, intracellular AGE formation, hexosamine pathway activity, and prostacyclin. The results showed that the levels of AGE and monocyte hexosamine–modified proteins were increased, whereas the activity of prostacyclin synthase was decreased in diabetic patients. Treatment with benfotiamine together with slow-release alpha-lipoic acid did not affect hyperglycemia, but it normalized the AGE level and the activity of prostacyclin synthase and reduced monocyte hexosamine–modified proteins.[186] Zycose is a new drug released in 2006 for the treatment of diabetes. It contains benfotiamine (150 mg), benzamine (850 mg), a proprietary blend of para-aminobenzoic acid (PABA), vitamin E, and alpha-lipoic acid. Zycose has been shown to improve vascular dysfunction, neuropathy, nephropathy, and nerve function.[187]

Supplementation with B-vitamins and antioxidants enhanced the plasma concentrations of vitamin E and folate, and reduced homocysteine in patients with type 2 diabetes.[188]

FOLIC ACID AND THIAMINE (ANIMAL STUDIES)

Diabetes can lead to thiamine deficiency. Treatment of streptozotocin-induced diabetic mice with benfotiamine, a lipophilic derivative of thiamine, reduced cerebral oxidative stress without affecting the levels of advanced glycation end-product (AGE), protein carbonyl, tissue factor, and TNF-alpha.[189] These results suggest that the primary action of benfotiamine is mediated via antioxidation.

CHROMIUM (HUMAN STUDIES)

A review of 15 published, including 11 randomized, controlled studies on the efficacy of chromium picolinate (Crpic) in improving some of the markers of type 2 diabetes revealed that supplementation with Crpic reduced hyperglycemia, hyperinsulinemia, and requirements for hyperglycemic medication.[190] In a randomized, double-blind, placebo-controlled trial involving patients with metabolic syndrome (obese and non-diabetic), the efficacy of Crpic on insulin sensitivity to glucose was evaluated. The results showed that after 16 weeks of treatment, there was no significant change in insulin sensitivity index, body weight, serum lipids, or markers of oxidative stress and inflammation between the control and treated groups. However, Crpic treatment increased acute insulin response to glucose.[191] This study has no conflict with the above studies, because all the above studies were performed in type 2 patients. It is possible that the mechanisms of action of Crpic in diabetic patients and obese non-diabetic subjects are, in part, different.

Among 25 randomized controlled trials, one study evaluated chromium yeast combined with vitamin C and vitamin E, and two studies examined chromium picolinate plus biotin, and the remaining 22 studies evaluated chromium as a single agent in the treatment of diabetes. The results showed that chromium alone or in combination with other micronutrients improved glycemic control. Supplementation with chromium alone reduced the levels of triglycerides and increase HDL-cholesterol levels.[192]

ANTIOXIDANTS WITH DIABETIC/CARDIOVASCULAR DRUGS AND/OR INSULIN (HUMAN STUDIES)

In a randomized clinical study with 80 patients with type 2 diabetes associated with dyslipidemia, the efficacy of combination treatment with fenofibrate and coenzyme Q10 on endothelial-dependent and -independent vasodilator function of the forearm microcirculation was tested. The results showed that the combination of two agents were more effective in improving vasodilator function of the forearm microcirculation than the individual agents.[193]

In a clinical study involving 34 patients with type 2 diabetes who were treated with anti-diabetic drugs for a month, and then were administered omega-3 fatty acids in combination with anti-diabetic drugs for a period of two months, the effects of omega-3 fatty acids on lipid peroxidation and antioxidant enzyme were evaluated. The results showed that supplementation with omega-3 fatty acids reduced the levels of serum triglycerides, MDA, and increased HDL-cholesterol levels and erythrocytes glutathione peroxidase activity; however, it did not produce significant change in erythrocyte catalase and SOD activities.[194] The addition of 4 g of omega-3 fatty acids to the treatment with a statin improved the lipid profiles better than statin treatment alone.[195,196] In a randomized, placebo-controlled trial involving 24 patients with type 2 diabetes, supplementation with omega-3 fatty acids in combination with a statin and fibrate decreased the risk of cardiovascular disease, and delay the onset and progression of nephropathy in these patients.[197,198] These studies show that supplementation with omega-3 fatty acids in combination with anti-diabetic drugs or heart medications yields better clinical outcomes than supplementation with omega-3 fatty acids alone. In a clinical trial involving 1770 children at increased risk of developing type 1 diabetes, the efficacy of omega-3 fatty acids on the risk of developing islet autoimmunity was evaluated. The results showed that dietary intake of omega-3 fatty acids decreased the risk of developing islet autoimmunity in children at increased risk for type 1 diabetes.[199]

ANTIOXIDANTS WITH DIABETIC/CARDIOVASCULAR DRUGS AND/OR INSULIN (ANIMAL STUDIES)

In a rat model of diabetes, insulin treatment was not as effective in reducing oxidative stress as vitamin A; however the combination of two was more effective in reducing oxidative stress in heart than the individual agents.[200]

In a rat model of insulin resistance induced by feeding 10% glucose for 20 weeks, the increased levels of insulin resistance was associated with a higher production of markers of oxidative stress and systolic blood pressure. Treatment with NAC prevented these alterations, except for systolic blood pressure; however, treatment with ramipril, an inhibitor of an angiotensin I-converting enzyme, did not effectively reduce insulin resistance or oxidative stress.[201]

TREATMENTS OF DIABETES

STANDARD TREATMENTS

Treatments of diabetes are based primarily on control of glycemia. The main classes of oral anti-diabetic medications include stimulators of insulin secretion (rapid-acting secretagogues and sulphanylureas), inhibitors of hepatic glucose production (biguanides), drugs dealing digestion and absorption of intestinal carbohydrate (alpha-glucosidase inhibitors), or stimulators of insulin action (thiazolidinediones). It also involves a combination of diet modification and other anti-diabetic oral medications including metformin, glynides, acarbose, troglitazone, and insulin or its analogs. Other adjunctive therapy may include antihypertensive drugs and cholesterol-lowering medications.[202,203] These standard therapies do not adequately address the issues of increased oxidative stress and increased chronic inflammation that are the primary events in the initiation and progression of diabetes. This is one of the reasons why diabetic complications develop in spite of these multiple medications, although gradually. Therefore, additional approaches should be developed to address these issues. Such approaches would prevent the incidence of diabetes in high-risk populations, improve the efficacy of standard therapy in diabetic patients, and reduce diabetic-related complications.

ASPIRIN (HUMAN STUDIES)

Cardiovascular disease is associated with diabetes. Low-dose aspirin is widely recommended to reduce the risk of cardiac events in patients with cardiovascular disease. Supplementation with aspirin failed to reduce the risk of cardiovascular disease in patients with type 2 diabetes in some major clinical trials.[204–206] Although some studies have suggested minor beneficial effects on cardiac events,[207] its continued use has been suggested by many current diabetic guidelines,[208–210] The role of aspirin in prevention of diabetes has also become controversial. An epidemiologic study involving 22,071 healthy men taking aspirin for a period of 22 years revealed that the incidence of type 2 diabetes decreased by about 14%.[211] Although the decrease in the incidence of type 2 diabetes after aspirin intake is small, the results is very impressive because aspirin, which does not affect oxidative stress, one of the primary events that contribute to the risk of type 2 diabetes, can decrease the incidence of this disease. The small beneficial effects of aspirin could be due to its anti-inflammatory action. In a randomized, double-blind, placebo-controlled trial involving 38,716 women free of clinical diabetes (19,326 received aspirin and 19,390 received placebo) and a follow-up period of 10 years, the efficacy of aspirin treatment on the incidence of type 2 diabetes was evaluated. The results showed that long-term consumption of low-dose aspirin failed to prevent the development of diabetes type 2 in healthy women.[212] A combination of aspirin and statin increased the weight loss in patients with type 2 diabetes.[213] A review of several studies has revealed that aspirin treatment did not lower the risk of diabetic retinopathy.[214]

ASPIRIN RESISTANCE

Although aspirin has become an essential component of the treatment of cardiovascular disease associated with or without type 2 diabetes due to its anti-platelet aggregation activity, the phenomenon of aspirin-resistance has become of great interest because of its implication in increasing cardiac events. A review of studies on aspirin has revealed that about 20%–30% of aspirin treated patients exhibit platelet hyperactivity despite adequate inhibition of cyclooxygenase-1 (COX-1) activity, and several meta-analyses suggested that residual platelet hyperactivity could be a risk factor for the recurrence of ischemic events in aspirin-treated patients.[215–217] The exact reasons for aspirin-resistance are unknown. The suggested mechanisms include genetic polymorphism of cyclooxygenase-1, non-enzymatic formation of prostaglandins responsible for platelet aggregation, and inadequate dose.

ASPIRIN (ANIMAL STUDIES)

Although clinical studies failed to show any beneficial effect of aspirin in prevention of type 2 diabetes, supplementation with aspirin prevented the development of type 2 diabetes by reducing insulin resistance, and elevating the level of fasting insulin and insulin sensitivity in streptozotocin treated rats. It also protected pancreas against streptozotocin-induced damage and maintained near normal level of glucose in diabetic rats.[218] In a rat model of diabetes, treatment with aspirin prevented diabetes-induced tear secretion from lacrimal gland and reduced diabetes-induced degenerative changes in the lacrimal glands.[219] Aspirin treatment protected lacrimal gland against damage produced by increased oxidative stress and inflammation in streptozotocin-induced diabetic rats.[218] Pretreatment with aspirin attenuated cerebral ischemia in diabetic rats and decreased neurological deficits. It also reduced platelet aggregation. However, aspirin treatment did not alter the levels of glucose and insulin in diabetic rats.[220] In diet-induced obese rats, the levels of iNOS and S-nitrosylation of insulin receptor (IR)-beta, IRS-1, and protein kinase B (Akt) were increased. Aspirin treatment not only reduced the levels of above biomarkers of oxidative damage and inflammation but also improved insulin resistance and insulin sensitivity.[221] Thus, in contrast to the results from human intervention studies, aspirin treatment consistently produced beneficial effects in the prevention and progression of diabetes in animals. Hence, the information gained from diabetic animal models cannot readily be extrapolated to human with respect to the efficacy of aspirin in prevention or treatment of diabetes.

POTENTIAL REASONS FOR INCONSISTENT RESULTS WITH INDIVIDUAL MICRONUTRIENTS OR ASPIRIN

The reasons for individual micronutrients or aspirin with or without standard medications produce no effects on the risk factors of diabetes, transient benefits on some markers of diabetes. The exact reasons are not known; however, some potential causes are described here:

(a) antioxidants show differential subcellular distribution and different mechanisms of action; therefore, a single antioxidant cannot protect all parts of the cell; (b) a single antioxidant in a high internal oxidative environment of patients with neurodegenerative diseases is oxidized and can then itself act as a pro-oxidant rather than as an antioxidant; (c) the body protects against oxidative damage by elevating antioxidant enzymes and dietary and endogenous anti-oxidants; (d) antioxidants neutralize free radicals by donating electrons to those molecules with unpaired electron, whereas antioxidant enzymes destroy free radicals by catalysis, con-verting them to harmless molecules such as water and oxygen. Therefore, both of these events need to be enhanced in concert to achieve substantial therapeutic gain against oxidative dam-age; (e) the affinity of different antioxidants for free radicals differs, depending upon their lipophilicity; (f) both the aqueous and lipid compartments of the cell need to be protected together. Water-soluble antioxidants such as vitamin C and glutathione protect molecules in the aqueous environment of the cells, whereas lipid soluble antioxidants such as vitamin A and vitamin E protect molecules in the lipid compartment; (g) vitamin E is more effective in quenching free radicals in a reduced oxygenated cellular environment, whereas vitamin C and alpha-tocopherol are more effective in a higher oxygenated environment of the cells[222]; (h) vitamin C is important for recycling the oxidized form of alpha-tocopherol to the antioxidant form at the lipid/aqueous interface[223]; (i) antioxidants produce cell protective proteins by alter-ing the expression of different microRNAs.[59] For example, some antioxidants can activate Nrf2 by upregulating miR-200a that inhibits its target protein Keap1, whereas others activate Nrf2 by downregulating miR-21 that binds with 3'-UTR Nrf2 mRNA.[224]

Aspirin may reduce chronic inflammation somewhat, but it has no effect on oxidative stress. These studies suggest that use of a single micronutrient in prevention or improved management of human diabetes is not expected to yield any beneficial effects. For this reason, a mixture of micro-nutrients that can simultaneously reduce oxidative stress and inflammation by enhancing the levels of antioxidant enzymes through the activation of Nrf2 pathway together with dietary and endog-enous antioxidants for other chronic diseases, such as Alzheimer's disease and Parkinson's disease has been suggested.[59,89] The same suggestion is proposed for prevention and improved management of diabetes. Oral supplementation can increase the levels of dietary and endogenous antioxidants; however, elevation of the levels of antioxidant enzymes requires an activation of Nrf2. Therefore it is essential to understand the regulation of activation of Nrf2.

REGULATION OF ACTIVATION OF Nrf2

REACTIVE OXYGEN SPECIES (ROS) ACTIVATES Nrf2

Normally, during acute oxidative stress, ROS is needed to activate Nrf2 which then dissociates itself from Keap1-Cul-Rbx1 complex and translocates in the nucleus where it heterodimerizes with a small Maf protein, and binds with the ARE (antioxidant response element) leading to increased expression of target genes coding for several cytoprotective enzymes including antioxidant enzymes.[225-227] In this manner, activation of Nrf2 increases the levels of cytoprotective enzymes including antioxidant enzymes and phase-2-detoxifying enzymes.[228,229]

BINDING OF Nrf2 WITH ARE IN THE NUCLEUS

Activation of Nrf2 alone may not be sufficient to increase the levels of antioxidant enzymes. Activated Nrf2 must bind with antioxidant response element (ARE) in the nucleus for increasing the expression of its target genes. This binding ability of Nrf2 with ARE was impaired in aged rats and this defect was restored by supplementation with alpha-lipoic acid.[230]

EXISTENCE OF ROS-RESISTANT Nrf2 IN DIABETES

The fact that increased oxidative stress and chronic inflammation are present in patients with diabetes suggests that activation of Nrf2 is impaired. The glomeruli of human diabetic nephropathy had elevated levels of Nrf2 in the presence of high oxidative stress.[231] This study suggests that activation of Nrf2 became resistant to ROS during chronic oxidative stress. This is evident by the fact that mice without Nrf2 (–/–) had higher levels of ROS, oxidative DNA damage, and renal injury than those mice with Nrf2 (+/+). In diabetic knockout mice, the levels of superoxide and TNF-alpha increased, while the levels of retinal glutathione decreased compared to wild-type mice. Furthermore, these mice lacking Nrf2 showed early onset of dysfunction of the retina blood-barrier and enhanced neuronal functional defects.[232] It has been proposed that Keap1 protein that binds Nrf2 in the cytoplasm is altered preventing the migration of Nrf2 to the nucleus where it binds with ARE to increase the transcription of cytoprotective enzymes, leading to increased oxidative stress and diabetic retinopathy.[233] In rats with diabetic retinopathy, the binding of Nrf2 with ARE is impaired.[234] In the diabetic type 2 mice model (db/db), Nrf2 expression and its regulated cytoprotective gene transcription were decreased, and myogenic constriction in mesenteric arterioles was greater compared with non-diabetic mice.[235] The wound closure was delayed in stretozotocin-induced diabetic mouse model lacking Nrf2 (–/–) compared with mice with Nrf2 (+/+).[236] Impaired translocation of Nrf2 from the cytoplasm to the nucleus was observed in human fetal endothelial cells obtained patients with gestational diabetes[237] and in the kidney cells of diabetic rats.[238] These changes led to increased oxidative stress due to reduction in the levels of cytoprotective enzymes. The studies described above show that Nrf2 becomes resistant to normal physiological stimulation by ROS due to the defects in Nrf2 levels, Nrf2 activation, and Nrf2 translocation to the nucleus, causing increased oxidative damage and chronic inflammation, which were associated with diabetes and diabetes-related complications, Supplementation with diverse groups of activators and inducers reversed these Nrf2 defects and improved some symptoms of diabetes.

ANTIOXIDANTS AND PHYTOCHEMICALS ACTIVATE ROS-RESISTANT Nrf2

Activation of Nrf2 becomes impaired to ROS. Some dietary antioxidants and phytochemicals can activate Nrf2 without requiring ROS. These include vitamin C[239,240] vitamin E,[241] endogenous antioxidants such as alpha-lipoic acid[230] and coenzyme Q10,[242] synthetic antioxidant N-acetylcysteine (NAC),[243] omega-3-fatty acids,[244,245] and phytochemicals such as curcumin[246] and resveratrol.[247,248]

L-CARNITINE ACTIVATES Nrf2 BY A ROS-DEPENDENT MECHANISM

With L-carnitine activates Nrf2 by a ROS-dependent mechanism,[249] probably by generating transient ROS.

ACTIVATION OF Nrf2 BY MicroRNAs

The complex of Keap1-Nrf2 in the cytoplasm prevents activation of Nrf2. Over-expression of miR-200a reduced Keap-1 levels allowing Nrf2 to migrate to the nucleus where it binds to the ARE that enhanced the transcription of target cytoprotective genes including antioxidant enzymes.[250] Some antioxidants can activate Nrf2 by downregulating miR-21 that binds with 3′-UTR Nrf2 mRNA.[224]

SUPPRESSION OF CHRONIC INFLAMMATION

The activation of Nrf2 also suppresses chronic inflammation.[228,229] Some antioxidant compounds also reduce markers of chronic inflammation.[251–256]

RECOMMENDED MIXTURE OF MICRONUTRIENTS FOR THE PREVENTION OF DIABETES

Based on the studies discussed above, a mixture of micronutrients containing vitamin A, mixed carotenoids, vitamin C, α-tocopheryl acetate, α-tocopheryl succinate, vitamin D3, alpha-lipoic acid, N-acetylcysteine, coenzyme Q10, L-carnitine, omega-3-fatty acids, curcumin, resveratrol, all B-vitamins, selenomethionine, and zinc, but without iron, copper, manganese, or heavy metals such as molybdenum and zirconium for prevention and improved management of diabetes is proposed. The inclusion of iron, copper, or manganese is not suggested because these trace minerals, although essential for many biological reactions, combine with vitamin C and generate excessive amounts of free radicals. Furthermore, these minerals are absorbed from the intestine better in the presence of antioxidants than in their absence that could increase body store of free iron, copper and manganese after a long-term consumption. The body has no significant mechanisms of excretion of these trace minerals. Slight increase in the body store of free forms of these trace minerals can increase the risk of most chronic diseases. Heavy metals such as zirconium and molybdenum were not included because the body has no mechanisms of excretion of these heavy metals. Consequently, their levels in the body would increase after long-term consumption. High levels of these heavy metals could be toxic.

It is expected that the proposed micronutrient mixture would increase the levels of antioxidant enzymes by activating the Nrf2/ARE pathway, and dietary and endogenous antioxidants that would simultaneously reduce oxidative stress and chronic inflammation.

The recommended micronutrient mixture should be taken orally and divided into two doses, half in the morning and the other half in the evening with meal. This is because the biological half-lives of micronutrients are highly variable which can create high levels of fluctuations in the tissue levels of micronutrients. A 2-fold difference in the levels of certain micronutrients such as alpha-tocopheryl succinate causes a marked difference in the expression of gene profiles.[257] In order to maintain relatively steady level of micronutrients in the body, the proposed dose schedule is necessary.

RECOMMENDED CHANGES IN DIET AND LIFESTYLE FOR THE PREVENTION AND IMPROVED MANAGEMENT OF DIABETES

Dietary recommendations include daily consuming of a low-fat and high-fiber diet with plenty of fresh fruits and vegetables, increasing the intake of nuts, avoiding excessive amounts of calories, and minimizing sugar consumption.

Lifestyle-related changes include stopping smoking and chewing tobacco, avoiding exposure to secondhand smoke, maintaining normal weight for your age and height, restricting intake of alcohol, reducing stress by vacation, yoga, or meditation, and performing moderate to vigorous exercise 4–5 times per week.

The efficacy of proposed micronutrient mixture together with diet and lifestyle should be tested by well-designed preclinical and clinical studies. In the meanwhile, the proposed recommendations may be adopted by the individuals in consultation with their physicians or health professionals for reducing the risk and improved management of diabetic-related.

PREVENTION OF DIABETES

Primary Prevention

Primary prevention includes individuals who have not developed any risk biomarkers associated with diabetes. Despite recommendations for diet modifications and lifestyle changes for primary prevention, the incidence of diabetes continues to rise. The proposed mixture of micronutrients together with modifications in the diet and lifestyle may reduce the development of diabetes risk factors by simultaneously reducing oxidative stress and chronic inflammation.

SECONDARY PREVENTION

Individuals with a family history of diabetes, pre-diabetic individuals who are not on diabetic medication, and obese individuals with normal fasting blood glucose levels who have one or more cardiac risk factors are suitable for secondary prevention. The proposed mixture of micronutrients together with modifications in diet and lifestyle may decrease the risk of developing diabetes by simultaneously reducing oxidative stress and chronic inflammation.

IMPROVED MANAGEMENT OF DIABETES

The individuals who have established diabetes and are on one or more diabetic medications are suitable for the study on improved management of diabetes. The proposed mixture of micronutrients and modifications in the diet and lifestyle together with standard treatment may improve the management of diabetes better than standard therapy alone by simultaneously reducing oxidative stress and chronic inflammation. It is expected that the proposed strategy may enhance the effectiveness of standard therapy and may even reduce the drug requirements for maintaining optimal glucose levels.

CONCLUSIONS

Diabetes mellitus is a chronic disease characterized by high levels of blood glucose that result from defects in insulin production, insulin transport and/or utilization, or both. Diabetes leads to serious complications, such as retinopathy, neuropathy, and nephropathy and can cause premature death, if untreated. Diabetes has become a serious health problem throughout the world including the USA. Despite the development of new medications to control glucose and recommendations for diet and lifestyle changes, the incidence of diabetes continues to increase in the USA. Evidence for the involvement of increased oxidative stress and chronic inflammation in the initiation and progression of diabetes as well as in the development of diabetes-related complications were presented. Changes in the circulating and cellular microRNAs in patients with diabetes were described, and their potential significance in the diagnosis and in developing new therapeutic agents was indicated. Antioxidants reduce oxidative stress and inflammation; therefore, they should be useful in reducing the incidence of diabetes as well as the diabetic-related complications. Animals and human studies, using single micronutrients or aspirin in the prevention and improved treatment of diabetes, showed inconsistent results varying from no effects to transient benefits on some risk factors. The potential reasons for these inconsistent results were discussed. A single micronutrient cannot simultaneously reduce oxidative stress and chronic inflammation. In order to achieve this goal, reduction of these two biochemical defects at the same time is required for the prevention and improved management of diabetes. In order to accomplish this, it is essential to enhance the levels of cytoprotective enzymes including antioxidant enzymes by activating the Nrf2/ARE pathway, and dietary and endogenous antioxidants. A mixture of micronutrients that would achieve the above goal is proposed.

REFERENCES

1. Diseases NIoDadaK. National Diabetes Statistics, 2007 fact sheet. In: Services USDoHaH, ed. Bethesda, MD: National Institute of health; 2008.
2. Johannesson A, Larsson GU, Ramstrand N, Turkiewicz A, Wirehn AB, Atroshi I. Incidence of lower-limb amputation in the diabetic and nondiabetic general population: A 10-year population-based cohort study of initial unilateral and contralateral amputations and reamputations. *Diabetes Care.* 2009;32(2):275–280.
3. Martin-Gallan P, Carrascosa A, Gussinye M, Dominguez C. Biomarkers of diabetes-associated oxidative stress and antioxidant status in young diabetic patients with or without subclinical complications. *Free Radic Biol Med.* 2003;34(12):1563–1574.

4. Cinkilic N, Kiyici S, Celikler S, et al. Evaluation of chromosome aberrations, sister chromatid exchange, and micronuclei in patients with type-1 diabetes mellitus. *Mutat Res.* 2009;676(1–2):1–4.

5. Kostolanska J, Jakus V, Barak L. HbA1c and serum levels of advanced glycation and oxidation protein products in poorly and well controlled children and adolescents with type 1 diabetes mellitus. *J Pediatr Endocrinol Metab.* 2009;22(5):433–442.

6. Liu HY, Cao SY, Hong T, Han J, Liu Z, Cao W. Insulin is a stronger inducer of insulin resistance than hyperglycemia in mice with type 1 diabetes mellitus (T1DM). *J Biol Chem.* 2009;284:27090–27100.

7. Codoner-Franch P, Pons-Morales S, Boix-Garcia L, Valls-Belles V. Oxidant/antioxidant status in obese children compared to pediatric patients with type 1 diabetes mellitus. *Pediatr Diabetes.* 2010;11:251–257.

8. Matteucci E, Giampietro O. Oxidative stress in families of type 1 diabetic patients. *Diabetes Care.* 2000;23(8):1182–1186.

9. Odermarsky M, Lykkesfeldt J, Liuba P. Poor vitamin C status is associated with increased carotid intima-media thickness, decreased microvascular function, and delayed myocardial repolarization in young patients with type 1 diabetes. *Am J Clin Nutr.* 2009;90(2):447–452.

10. Lin CC, Huang HH, Hu CW, et al. Trace elements, oxidative stress and glycemic control in young people with type 1 diabetes mellitus. *J Trace Elem Med Biol.* 2014;28(1):18–22.

11. Qiu Q, Zhang F, Zhu W, Wu J, Liang M. Copper in diabetes mellitus: A meta-analysis and systematic review of plasma and serum studies. *Biol Trace Elem Res.* 2017;177(1):53–63.

12. Sharma G, Muller DP, O'Riordan SM, et al. Urinary conjugated alpha-tocopheronolactone: A biomarker of oxidative stress in children with type 1 diabetes. *Free Radic Biol Med.* 2013;55:54–62.

13. Neyestani TR, Ghandchi Z, Eshraghian MR, Kalayi A, Shariatzadeh N, Houshiarrad A. Evidence for augmented oxidative stress in the subjects with type 1 diabetes and their siblings: A possible preventive role for antioxidants. *Eur J Clin Nutr.* 2012;66(9):1054–1058.

14. Ma D, Zhu W, Hu S, Yu X, Yang Y. Association between oxidative stress and telomere length in Type 1 and Type 2 diabetic patients. *J Endocrinol Invest.* 2013;36(11):1032–1037.

15. Prasad KN, Wu M, Bondy SC. Telomere shortening during aging: Attenuation by antioxidants and anti-inflammatory agents. *Mech Ageing Dev.* 2017;164:61–66.

16. Maritim AC, Sanders RA, Watkins JB, 3rd. Diabetes, oxidative stress, and antioxidants: A review. *J Biochem Mol Toxicol.* 2003;17(1):24–38.

17. Kahler WK, kuklinski, b., Ruhlmann, C. Plotz, C., eds. *Diabetes Mellitus-a Free Radical-associated Disease. Effects of Adjuvant Supplementation with Antioxidants.* Frankfurt, Germany: Frnakfurt am Main: pmi Verlag Gruppe; 1993. Gries; FA, Wessel, K. eds., The role of antioxidants in diabetes mellitus: Oxygen radicals and antioxidants in diabetes.

18. Kajimoto Y, Kaneto H. Role of oxidative stress in pancreatic beta-cell dysfunction. *Ann N Y Acad Sci.* 2004;1011:168–176.

19. Osorio JM, Ferreyra C, Perez A, Moreno JM, Osuna A. Prediabetic States, subclinical atheromatosis, and oxidative stress in renal transplant patients. *Transplant Proc.* 2009;41(6):2148–2150.

20. Lodovici M, Bigagli E, Bardini G, Rotella C. Lipoperoxidation and antioxidant capacity in patients with poorly controlled type 2 diabetes. *Toxicol Ind Health.* 2009;25(4–5):337–341.

21. Song F, Jia W, Yao Y, et al. Oxidative stress, antioxidant status and DNA damage in patients with impaired glucose regulation and newly diagnosed Type 2 diabetes. *Clin Sci (Lond).* 2007;112(12):599–606.

22. de Lauzon-Guillain B, Fournier A, Fabre A, et al. Menopausal hormone therapy and new-onset diabetes in the French Etude Epidemiologique de Femmes de la Mutuelle Generale de l'Education Nationale (E3N) cohort. *Diabetologia.* 2009;52(10):2092–2100.

23. Costford SR, Crawford SA, Dent R, McPherson R, Harper ME. Increased susceptibility to oxidative damage in post-diabetic human myotubes. *Diabetologia.* 2009;52(11): 2405–2415.

24. El-Mesallamy H, Hamdy N, Suwailem S, Mostafa S. Oxidative stress and platelet activation: Markers of myocardial infarction in type 2 diabetes mellitus. *Angiology.* 2010;61:14–18.

25. Mellor KM, Ritchie RH, Delbridge LM. Reactive oxygen species and insulin-resistant cardiomyopathy. *Clin Exp Pharmacol Physiol.* 2010;37(2):222–228.

26. Morales-Indiano C, Lauzurica R, Pastor MC, et al. Greater posttransplant inflammation and oxidation are associated with worsening kidney function in patients with pretransplant diabetes mellitus. *Transplant Proc.* 2009;41(6):2126–2128.

27. Allen EM, Matthews JB, O'Connor R, O'Halloran D, Chapple IL. Periodontitis and type 2 diabetes: Is oxidative stress the mechanistic link? *Scott Med J.* 2009;54(2):41–47.

28. Block K, Gorin Y, Abboud HE. Subcellular localization of Nox4 and regulation in diabetes. *Proc Natl Acad Sci U S A.* 2009;106(34):14385–14390.

29. Gorin Y, Block K, Hernandez J, et al. Nox4 NAD(P)H oxidase mediates hypertrophy and fibronectin expression in the diabetic kidney. *J Biol Chem.* 2005;280(47):39616–39626.
30. Yokota T, Kinugawa S, Hirabayashi K, et al. Oxidative stress in skeletal muscle impairs mitochondrial respiration and limits exercise capacity in type 2 diabetic mice. *Am J Physiol Heart Circ Physiol.* 2009;297(3):H1069–H1077.
31. Stefano GB, Challenger S, Kream RM. Hyperglycemia-associated alterations in cellular signaling and dysregulated mitochondrial bioenergetics in human metabolic disorders. *Eur J Nutr.* 2016;55:2339–2345.
32. Yamagishi S, Maeda S, Matsui T, Ueda S, Fukami K, Okuda S. Role of advanced glycation end products (AGEs) and oxidative stress in vascular complications in diabetes. *Biochim Biophys Acta.* 2012;1820(5):663–671.
33. Giovannini C, Piaggi S, Federico G, Scarpato R. High levels of gamma-H2AX foci and cell membrane oxidation in adolescents with type 1 diabetes. *Mutat Res.* 2014;770:128–135.
34. Maschirow L, Khalaf K, Al-Aubaidy HA, Jelinek HF. Inflammation, coagulation, endothelial dysfunction and oxidative stress in prediabetes: Biomarkers as a possible tool for early disease detection for rural screening. *Clin Biochem.* 2015;48(9):581–585.
35. Tatsch E, De Carvalho JA, Hausen BS, et al. Oxidative DNA damage is associated with inflammatory response, insulin resistance and microvascular complications in type 2 diabetes. *Mutat Res.* 2015;782:17–22.
36. Saad MI, Abdelkhalek TM, Saleh MM, et al. Insights into the molecular mechanisms of diabetes-induced endothelial dysfunction: Focus on oxidative stress and endothelial progenitor cells. *Endocrine.* 2015;50(3):537–567.
37. Kowluru RA, Kowluru A, Mishra M, Kumar B. Oxidative stress and epigenetic modifications in the pathogenesis of diabetic retinopathy. *Prog Retin Eye Res.* 2015;48:40–61.
38. Waris S, Winklhofer-Roob BM, Roob JM, et al. Increased DNA dicarbonyl glycation and oxidation markers in patients with type 2 diabetes and link to diabetic nephropathy. *J Diabetes Res.* 2015;2015:915486.
39. Varvarovska J, Racek J, Stozicky F, Soucek J, Trefil L, Pomahacova R. Parameters of oxidative stress in children with Type 1 diabetes mellitus and their relatives. *J Diabetes Complications.* 2003;17(1):7–10.
40. Matteucci E, Rosada J, Pinelli M, Giusti C, Giampietro O. Systolic blood pressure response to exercise in type 1 diabetes families compared with healthy control individuals. *J Hypertens.* 2006;24(9):1745–1751.
41. Holvoet P. Relations between metabolic syndrome, oxidative stress and inflammation and cardiovascular disease. *Verh K Acad Geneeskd Belg.* 2008;70(3):193–219.
42. Mariappan N, Elks CM, Sriramula S, et al. NF-κB -induced oxidative stress contributes to mitochondrial and cardiac dysfunction in type II diabetes. *Cardiovasc Res.* 2010;85:473–483.
43. Ehses JA, Lacraz G, Giroix MH, et al. IL-1 antagonism reduces hyperglycemia and tissue inflammation in the type 2 diabetic GK rat. *Proc Natl Acad Sci U S A.* 2009;106(33):13998–14003.
44. Yang J, Park Y, Zhang H, et al. Feed-forward signaling of TNF-alpha and NF-kappaB via IKK-beta pathway contributes to insulin resistance and coronary arteriolar dysfunction in type 2 diabetic mice. *Am J Physiol Heart Circ Physiol.* 2009;296(6):H1850–H1858.
45. Donath MY, Schumann DM, Faulenbach M, Ellingsgaard H, Perren A, Ehses JA. Islet inflammation in type 2 diabetes: From metabolic stress to therapy. *Diabetes Care.* 2008;31 Suppl 2:S161–S164.
46. Ortis F, Pirot P, Naamane N, et al. Induction of nuclear factor-kappaB and its downstream genes by TNF-alpha and IL-1beta has a pro-apoptotic role in pancreatic beta cells. *Diabetologia.* 2008;51(7):1213–1225.
47. Bastard JP, Maachi M, Lagathu C, et al. Recent advances in the relationship between obesity, inflammation, and insulin resistance. *Eur Cytokine Netw.* 2006;17(1):4–12.
48. Heilbronn LK, Campbell LV. Adipose tissue macrophages, lowgrade inflammation, and insulin resistance in human obesity. *Curr Pharm Des.* 2008;14(12):1225–1230.
49. Minamino T, Orimo M, Shimizu I, et al. A crucial role for adipose tissue p53 in the regulation of insulin resistance. *Nat Med.* 2009;15(9):1082–1087.
50. Patel C, Ghanim H, Ravishankar S, et al. Prolonged reactive oxygen species generation and nuclear factor-kappaB activation after a high-fat, high-carbohydrate meal in the obese. *J Clin Endocrinol Metab.* 2007;92(11):4476–4479.
51. Hussain G, Rizvi SA, Singhal S, Zubair M, Ahmad J. Serum levels of TNF-alpha in peripheral neuropathy patients and its correlation with nerve conduction velocity in type 2 diabetes mellitus. *Diabetes Metab Syndr.* 2013;7(4):238–242.
52. Nishimoto S, Fukuda D, Higashikuni Y, et al. Obesity-induced DNA released from adipocytes stimulates chronic adipose tissue inflammation and insulin resistance. *Sci Adv.* 2016;2(3):e1501332.
53. Reinehr T, Karges B, Meissner T, et al. Inflammatory markers in obese adolescents with type 2 diabetes and their relationship to hepatokines and adipokines. *J Pediatr.* 2016;173:131–135.

54. Barry JC, Shakibakho S, Durrer C, et al. Hyporesponsiveness to the anti-inflammatory action of interleukin-10 in type 2 diabetes. *Sci Rep.* 2016;6:21244.

55. Morettini M, Storm F, Sacchetti M, Cappozzo A, Mazza C. Effects of walking on low-grade inflammation and their implications for type 2 diabetes. *Prev Med Rep.* 2015;2:538–547.

56. Karstoft K, Pedersen BK. Exercise and type 2 diabetes: Focus on metabolism and inflammation. *Immunol Cell Biol.* 2016;94(2):146–150.

57. Singh K, Agrawal NK, Gupta SK, Sinha P, Singh K. Increased expression of TLR9 associated with pro-inflammatory S100A8 and IL-8 in diabetic wounds could lead to unresolved inflammation in type 2 diabetes mellitus (T2DM) cases with impaired wound healing. *J Diabetes Complications.* 2016;30(1):99–108.

58. Perlman AS, Chevalier JM, Wilkinson P, et al. Serum inflammatory and immune mediators are elevated in early stage diabetic nephropathy. *Ann Clin Lab Sci.* Spring 2015;45(3):256–263.

59. Prasad KN. Oxidative stress and pro-inflammatory cytokines may act as one of signals for regulating MicroRNAs expression in Alzheimer's disease. *Mech Ageing Dev.* 2017;162:63–71.

60. Prasad KN. Oxidative stress, pro-inflammatory cytokines, and antioxidants regulate expression levels of MicroRNAs in Parkinson's disease. *Curr Aging Sci.* 2017;10(3):177–184.

61. Lee RC, Feinbaum RL, Ambros V. The C. elegans heterochronic gene lin-4 encodes small RNAs with antisense complementarity to lin-14. *Cell.* 1993;75(5):843–854.

62. Wightman B, Ha I, Ruvkun G. Posttranscriptional regulation of the heterochronic gene lin-14 by lin-4 mediates temporal pattern formation in C. elegans. *Cell.* 1993;75(5):855–862.

63. Macfarlane LA, Murphy PR. MicroRNA: Biogenesis, function and role in cancer. *Curr Genomics.* 2010;11(7):537–561.

64. Londin E, Loher P, Telonis AG, et al. Analysis of 13 cell types reveals evidence for the expression of numerous novel primate- and tissue-specific microRNAs. *Proc Natl Acad Sci U S A.* 2015;112(10):E1106–E1115.

65. Denli AM, Tops BB, Plasterk RH, Ketting RF, Hannon GJ. Processing of primary microRNAs by the Microprocessor complex. *Nature.* 2004;432(7014):231–235.

66. Lee Y, Ahn C, Han J, et al. The nuclear RNase III Drosha initiates microRNA processing. *Nature.* 2003;425(6956):415–419.

67. Hutvagner G, McLachlan J, Pasquinelli AE, Balint E, Tuschl T, Zamore PD. A cellular function for the RNA-interference enzyme Dicer in the maturation of the let-7 small temporal RNA. *Science.* 2001;293(5531):834–838.

68. Yang Z, Chen H, Si H, et al. Serum miR-23a, a potential biomarker for diagnosis of pre-diabetes and type 2 diabetes. *Acta Diabetol.* 2014;51(5):823–831.

69. Higuchi C, Nakatsuka A, Eguchi J, et al. Identification of circulating miR-101, miR-375 and miR-802 as biomarkers for type 2 diabetes. *Metabolism.* 2015;64(4):489–497.

70. Kong L, Zhu J, Han W, et al. Significance of serum microRNAs in pre-diabetes and newly diagnosed type 2 diabetes: A clinical study. *Acta Diabetol.* 2011;48(1):61–69.

71. Osipova J, Fischer DC, Dangwal S, et al. Diabetes-associated microRNAs in pediatric patients with type 1 diabetes mellitus: A cross-sectional cohort study. *J Clin Endocrinol Metab.* 2014;99(9):E1661–E1665.

72. Zhu H, Leung SW. Identification of microRNA biomarkers in type 2 diabetes: A meta-analysis of controlled profiling studies. *Diabetologia.* 2015;58(5):900–911.

73. Erener S, Mojibian M, Fox JK, Denroche HC, Kieffer TJ. Circulating miR-375 as a biomarker of beta-cell death and diabetes in mice. *Endocrinology.* 2013;154(2):603–608.

74. Cui X, You L, Zhu L, et al. Change in circulating microRNA profile of obese children indicates future risk of adult diabetes. *Metabolism.* 2018;78:95–105.

75. Wu L, Dai X, Zhan J, et al. Profiling peripheral microRNAs in obesity and type 2 diabetes mellitus. *APMIS.* 2015;123(7):580–585.

76. Zhang T, Li L, Shang Q, Lv C, Wang C, Su B. Circulating miR-126 is a potential biomarker to predict the onset of type 2 diabetes mellitus in susceptible individuals. *Biochem Biophys Res Commun.* 2015;463(1–2):60–63.

77. Barutta F, Tricarico M, Corbelli A, et al. Urinary exosomal microRNAs in incipient diabetic nephropathy. *PLoS One.* 2013;8(11):e73798.

78. Delic D, Eisele C, Schmid R, et al. Urinary exosomal miRNA signature in type II diabetic nephropathy patients. *PLoS One.* 2016;11(3):e0150154.

79. Shi Z, Zhao C, Guo X, et al. Differential expression of microRNAs in omental adipose tissue from gestational diabetes mellitus subjects reveals miR-222 as a regulator of ERalpha expression in estrogen-induced insulin resistance. *Endocrinology.* 2014;155(5):1982–1990.

80. Poy MN, Eliasson L, Krutzfeldt J, et al. A pancreatic islet-specific microRNA regulates insulin secretion. *Nature.* 2004;432(7014):226–230.
81. Li Y, Luo T, Wang L, Wu J, Guo S. MicroRNA-19a-3p enhances the proliferation and insulin secretion, while it inhibits the apoptosis of pancreatic beta cells via the inhibition of SOCS3. *Int J Mol Med.* 2016;38(5):1515–1524.
82. Sebastiani G, Po A, Miele E, et al. MicroRNA-124a is hyperexpressed in type 2 diabetic human pancreatic islets and negatively regulates insulin secretion. *Acta Diabetol.* 2015;52(3):523–530.
83. Chen S, Puthanveetil P, Feng B, Matkovich SJ, Dorn GW, 2nd, Chakrabarti S. Cardiac miR-133a overexpression prevents early cardiac fibrosis in diabetes. *J Cell Mol Med.* 2014;18(3):415–421.
84. Caporali A, Meloni M, Vollenkle C, et al. Deregulation of microRNA-503 contributes to diabetes mellitus-induced impairment of endothelial function and reparative angiogenesis after limb ischemia. *Circulation.* 2011;123(3):282–291.
85. Mohan R, Mao Y, Zhang S, et al. Differentially expressed MicroRNA-483 confers distinct functions in pancreatic beta- and alpha-Cells. *J Biol Chem.* 2015;290(32):19955–19966.
86. Belgardt BF, Ahmed K, Spranger M, et al. The microRNA-200 family regulates pancreatic beta cell survival in type 2 diabetes. *Nat Med.* 2015;21(6):619–627.
87. Ramachandran D, Roy U, Garg S, Ghosh S, Pathak S, Kolthur-Seetharam U. Sirt1 and mir-9 expression is regulated during glucose-stimulated insulin secretion in pancreatic beta-islets. *FEBS J.* 2011;278(7):1167–1174.
88. Bao L, Fu X, Si M, et al. MicroRNA-185 targets SOCS3 to inhibit beta-cell dysfunction in diabetes. *PLoS One.* 2015;10(2):e0116067.
89. Prasad KN. Simultaneous activation of Nrf2 and elevation of antioxidant compounds for reducing oxidative stress and chronic inflammation in human Alzheimer's disease. *Mech Ageing Dev.* 2016;153:41–47.
90. Prasad KN. Simultaneous activation of Nrf2 and elevation of dietary and endogenous antioxidants for prevention and improved managment of Parkinson's disease. In: Bondy SCC, A., ed. *Inflammation, Aging and Oxidative Stress.* New York: Springer; 2016:277–301.
91. Arrieta O, Garcia-Navarrete R, Zuniga S, et al. Retinoic acid increases tissue and plasma contents of nerve growth factor and prevents neuropathy in diabetic mice. *Eur J Clin Invest.* 2005;35(3):201–207.
92. Hernandez-Pedro N, Ordonez G, Ortiz-Plata A, et al. All-trans retinoic acid induces nerve regeneration and increases serum and nerve contents of neural growth factor in experimental diabetic neuropathy. *Transl Res.* 2008;152(1):31–37.
93. Zumino SJ, Storms DH, Stephensen, CB. Diet rich in polyphenols and vitamin A inhibit the development of type 1autoimmune diabetesin non-obese mice. *J Nutr.* 2007;137:1216–1221.
94. Iqbal S, Naseem I. Role of vitamin A in type 2 diabetes mellitus biology: Effects of intervention therapy in a deficient state. *Nutrition.* 2015;31(7–8):901–907.
95. Dakshinamurti K. Vitamins and their derivatives in the prevention and treatment of metabolic syndrome diseases (diabetes). *Can J Physiol Pharmacol.* 2015;93(5):355–362.
96. Tessier DM, Khalil A, Trottier L, Fulop T. Effects of vitamin C supplementation on antioxidants and lipid peroxidation markers in elderly subjects with type 2 diabetes. *Arch Gerontol Geriatr.* 2009;48(1):67–72.
97. Chen H, Karne RJ, Hall G, et al. High-dose oral vitamin C partially replenishes vitamin C levels in patients with type 2 diabetes and low vitamin C levels but does not improve endothelial dysfunction or insulin resistance. *Am J Physiol Heart Circ Physiol.* 2006;290(1):H137–H145.
98. Anderson RA, Evans LM, Ellis GR, et al. Prolonged deterioration of endothelial dysfunction in response to postprandial lipaemia is attenuated by vitamin C in type 2 diabetes. *Diabet Med.* 2006;23(3):258–264.
99. Tabatabaei, O, Nikfar S, Larijani B, Abdollahi M. Influence of ascorbic acid supplementation on type 2 diabetes mellitus in observational and randomized controlled trials; a systematic review with meta-analysis. *J Pharm Pharm Sci.* 2014;17:554–582.
100. Montero D, Walther G, Stehouwer CD, Houben AJ, Beckman JA, Vinet A. Effect of antioxidant vitamin supplementation on endothelial function in type 2 diabetes mellitus: A systematic review and meta-analysis of randomized controlled trials. *Obes Rev.* 2014;15(2):107–116.
101. Jariyapongskul A, Rungjaroen T, Kasetsuwan N, Patumraj S, Seki J, Niimi H. Long-term effects of oral vitamin C supplementation on the endothelial dysfunction in the iris microvessels of diabetic rats. *Microvasc Res.* 2007;74(1):32–38.
102. Sridulyakul P, Chakraphan D, Patumraj S. Vitamin C supplementation could reverse diabetes-induced endothelial cell dysfunction in mesenteric microcirculation in STZ-rats. *Clin Hemorheol Microcirc.* 2006;34(1–2):315–321.
103. Lee EY, Lee MY, Hong SW, Chung CH, Hong SY. Blockade of oxidative stress by vitamin C ameliorates albuminuria and renal sclerosis in experimental diabetic rats. *Yonsei Med J.* 2007;48(5):847–855.

104. Hamden K, Carreau S, Jamoussi K, et al. 1Alpha, 25 dihydroxyvitamin D3: Therapeutic and preventive effects against oxidative stress, hepatic, pancreatic, and renal injury in alloxan-induced diabetes in rats. *J Nutr Sci Vitaminol (Tokyo).* 2009;55(3):215–222.

105. Mathieu C, Gysemans C, Giulietti A, Bouillon R. Vitamin D and diabetes. *Diabetologia.* 2005;48(7):1247–1257.

106. Palomer X, Gonzalez-Clemente JM, Blanco-Vaca F, Mauricio D. Role of vitamin D in the pathogenesis of type 2 diabetes mellitus. *Diabetes Obes Metab.* 2008;10(3):185–197.

107. Ulusu NN, Sahilli M, Avci A, et al. Pentose phosphate pathway, glutathione-dependent enzymes and antioxidant defense during oxidative stress in diabetic rodent brain and peripheral organs: Effects of stobadine and vitamin E. *Neurochem Res.* 2003;28(6):815–823.

108. Nakhoul FM, Miller-Lotan R, Awad H, et al. Pharmacogenomic effect of vitamin E on kidney structure and function in transgenic mice with the haptoglobin 2-2 genotype and diabetes mellitus. *Am J Physiol Renal Physiol.* 2009;296(4):F830–F838.

109. Kuhad A, Chopra K. Attenuation of diabetic nephropathy by tocotrienol: Involvement of NFkB signaling pathway. *Life Sci.* 2009;84(9–10):296–301.

110. Hamblin M, Smith HM, Hill MF. Dietary supplementation with vitamin E ameliorates cardiac failure in type I diabetic cardiomyopathy by suppressing myocardial generation of 8-iso-prostaglandin F2alpha and oxidized glutathione. *J Card Fail.* 2007;13(10):884–892.

111. Goldenstein H, Levy NS, Lipener YT, Levy AP. Patient selection and vitamin E treatment in diabetes mellitus. *Expert Rev Cardiovasc Ther.* 2013;11(3):319–326.

112. Hamdy NM, Suwailem SM, El-Mesallamy HO. Influence of vitamin E supplementation on endothelial complications in type 2 diabetes mellitus patients who underwent coronary artery bypass graft. *J Diabetes Complications.* 2009;23(3):167–173.

113. Song Y, Cook NR, Albert CM, Van Denburgh M, Manson JE. Effects of vitamins C and E and beta-carotene on the risk of type 2 diabetes in women at high risk of cardiovascular disease: a randomized controlled trial. *Am J Clin Nutr.* 2009;90(2):429–437.

114. Poh Z. A current update on the use of alpha lipoic acid in the management of type 2 diabetes mellitus. *Endocr Metab Immune Disord Drug Targets.* 2009;9(4):392–398.

115. Packer L, Kraemer K, Rimbach G. Molecular aspects of lipoic acid in the prevention of diabetes complications. *Nutrition.* 2001;17(10):888–895.

116. Singh U, Jialal I. Alpha-lipoic acid supplementation and diabetes. *Nutr Rev.* 2008;66(11):646–657.

117. Ziegler D, Nowak H, Kempler P, Vargha P, Low PA. Treatment of symptomatic diabetic polyneuropathy with the antioxidant alpha-lipoic acid: A meta-analysis. *Diabet Med.* 2004;21(2):114–121.

118. Burekovic A, Terzic M, Alajbegovic S, Vukojevic Z, Hadzic N. The role of alpha-lipoic acid in diabetic polyneuropathy treatment. *Bosn J Basic Med Sci.* 2008;8(4):341–345.

119. Liu F, Zhang Y, Yang M, et al. Curative effect of alpha-lipoic acid on peripheral neuropathy in type 2 diabetes: A clinical study. *Zhonghua Yi Xue Za Zhi.* 2007;87(38):2706–2709.

120. Tankova T, Koev D, Dakovska L. Alpha-lipoic acid in the treatment of autonomic diabetic neuropathy (controlled, randomized, open-label study). *Rom J Intern Med.* 2004;42(2):457–464.

121. Kamenova P. Improvement of insulin sensitivity in patients with type 2 diabetes mellitus after oral administration of alpha-lipoic acid. *Hormones (Athens).* 2006;5(4):251–258.

122. Jacob S, Ruus P, Hermann R, et al. Oral administration of RAC-alpha-lipoic acid modulates insulin sensitivity in patients with type-2 diabetes mellitus: A placebo-controlled pilot trial. *Free Radic Biol Med.* 1999;27(3–4):309–314.

123. Ziegler D, Ametov A, Barinov A, et al. Oral treatment with alpha-lipoic acid improves symptomatic diabetic polyneuropathy: The SYDNEY 2 trial. *Diabetes Care.* 2006;29(11):2365–2370.

124. Henriksen EJ. Exercise training and the antioxidant alpha-lipoic acid in the treatment of insulin resistance and type 2 diabetes. *Free Radic Biol Med.* 2006;40(1):3–12.

125. Scaramuzza A, Giani E, Redaelli F, et al. Alpha-lipoic acid and antioxidant diet help to improve endothelial dysfunction in adolescents with type 1 diabetes: A pilot trial. *J Diabetes Res.* 2015;2015:474561.

126. Muellenbach EA, Diehl CJ, Teachey MK, et al. Interactions of the advanced glycation end product inhibitor pyridoxamine and the antioxidant alpha-lipoic acid on insulin resistance in the obese Zucker rat. *Metabolism.* 2008;57(10):1465–1472.

127. Lee SJ, Kang JG, Ryu OH, et al. Effects of alpha-lipoic acid on transforming growth factor beta1-p38 mitogen-activated protein kinase-fibronectin pathway in diabetic nephropathy. *Metabolism.* 2009;58(5):616–623.

128. Sugimura Y, Murase T, Kobayashi K, et al. Alpha-lipoic acid reduces congenital malformations in the offspring of diabetic mice. *Diabetes Metab Res Rev.* 2009;25(3):287–294.

129. Padmalayam I, Hasham S, Saxena U, Pillarisetti S. Lipoic acid synthase (LASY): A novel role in inflammation, mitochondrial function, and insulin resistance. *Diabetes.* 2009;58(3):600–608.

130. Kojima M, Sun L, Hata I, Sakamoto Y, Sasaki H, Sasaki K. Efficacy of alpha-lipoic acid against diabetic cataract in rat. *Jpn J Ophthalmol.* 2007;51(1):10–13.

131. Masha A, Brocato L, Dinatale S, Mascia C, Biasi F, Martina V. N-acetylcysteine is able to reduce the oxidation status and the endothelial activation after a high-glucose content meal in patients with type 2 diabetes mellitus. *J Endocrinol Invest.* 2009;32(4):352–356.

132. Kamboj SS, Chopra K, Sandhir R. Hyperglycemia-induced alterations in synaptosomal membrane fluidity and activity of membrane bound enzymes: Beneficial effect of N-acetylcysteine supplementation. *Neuroscience.* 2009;162(2):349–358.

133. Tsai GY, Cui JZ, Syed H, et al. Effect of N-acetylcysteine on the early expression of inflammatory markers in the retina and plasma of diabetic rats. *Clin Experiment Ophthalmol.* 2009;37(2):223–231.

134. Xia Z, Kuo KH, Nagareddy PR, et al. N-acetylcysteine attenuates PKCbeta2 overexpression and myocardial hypertrophy in streptozotocin-induced diabetic rats. *Cardiovasc Res.* 2007;73(4):770–782.

135. Kamboj SS, Chopra K, Sandhir R. Neuroprotective effect of N-acetylcysteine in the development of diabetic encephalopathy in streptozotocin-induced diabetes. *Metab Brain Dis.* 2008;23(4):427–443.

136. Roest PA, van Iperen L, Vis S, et al. Exposure of neural crest cells to elevated glucose leads to congenital heart defects, an effect that can be prevented by N-acetylcysteine. *Birth Defects Res A Clin Mol Teratol.* 2007;79(3):231–235.

137. Xia Z, Guo Z, Nagareddy PR, Yuen V, Yeung E, McNeill JH. Antioxidant N-acetylcysteine restores myocardial Mn-SOD activity and attenuates myocardial dysfunction in diabetic rats. *Eur J Pharmacol.* 2006;544(1–3):118–125.

138. Darmaun D, Smith SD, Sweeten S, Hartman BK, Welch S, Mauras N. Poorly controlled type 1 diabetes is associated with altered glutathione homeostasis in adolescents: Apparent resistance to N-acetylcysteine supplementation. *Pediatr Diabetes.* 2008;9(6):577–582.

139. Jain SK, Velusamy T, Croad JL, Rains JL, Bull R. L-cysteine supplementation lowers blood glucose, glycated hemoglobin, CRP, MCP-1, and oxidative stress and inhibits NF-kappaB activation in the livers of Zucker diabetic rats. *Free Radic Biol Med.* 2009;46(12):1633–1638.

140. Mingrone G. Carnitine in type 2 diabetes. *Ann N Y Acad Sci.* 2004;1033:99–107.

141. Mynatt RL. Carnitine and type 2 diabetes. *Diabetes Metab Res Rev.* 2009;25 Suppl 1:S45–S49.

142. Evans JD, Jacobs TF, Evans EW. Role of acetyl-L-carnitine in the treatment of diabetic peripheral neuropathy. *Ann Pharmacother.* 2008;42(11):1686–1691.

143. Sima AA. Acetyl-L-carnitine in diabetic polyneuropathy: Experimental and clinical data. *CNS Drugs.* 2007;21 Suppl 1:13–23; discussion 45–16.

144. Malaguarnera M, Vacante M, Avitabile T, Cammalleri L, Motta M. L-Carnitine supplementation reduces oxidized LDL cholesterol in patients with diabetes. *Am J Clin Nutr.* 2009;89(1):71–76.

145. Solfrizzi V, Capurso C, Colacicco AM, et al. Efficacy and tolerability of combined treatment with L-carnitine and simvastatin in lowering lipoprotein(a) serum levels in patients with type 2 diabetes mellitus. *Atherosclerosis.* 2006;188(2):455–461.

146. Shankar SS, Mirzamohammadi B, Walsh JP, Steinberg HO. L-carnitine may attenuate free fatty acid-induced endothelial dysfunction. *Ann N Y Acad Sci.* 2004;1033:189–197.

147. Poorabbas A, Fallah F, Bagdadchi J, et al. Determination of free L-carnitine levels in type II diabetic women with and without complications. *Eur J Clin Nutr.* 2007;61(7):892–895.

148. Power RA, Hulver MW, Zhang JY, et al. Carnitine revisited: Potential use as adjunctive treatment in diabetes. *Diabetologia.* 2007;50(4):824–832.

149. Soneru IL, Khan T, Orfalian Z, Abraira C. Acetyl-L-carnitine effects on nerve conduction and glycemic regulation in experimental diabetes. *Endocr Res.* 1997;23(1–2):27–36.

150. Rajasekar P, Anuradha CV. L-Carnitine inhibits protein glycation *in vitro* and *in vivo*: Evidence for a role in diabetic management. *Acta Diabetol.* 2007;44(2):83–90.

151. Malone JI, Cuthbertson DD, Malone MA, Schocken DD. Cardio-protective effects of carnitine in streptozotocin-induced diabetic rats. *Cardiovasc Diabetol.* 2006;5:2.

152. Hino K, Nishikawa M, Sato E, Inoue M. L-carnitine inhibits hypoglycemia-induced brain damage in the rat. *Brain Res.* 2005;1053(1–2):77–87.

153. El-ghoury EA, Raslan HM, Badawy EA, et al. Malondialdehyde and coenzyme Q10 in platelets and serum in type 2 diabetes mellitus: Correlation with glycemic control. *Blood Coagul Fibrinolysis.* 2009;20(4):248–251.

154. Suzuki S, Hinokio Y, Ohtomo M, et al. The effects of coenzyme Q10 treatment on maternally inherited diabetes mellitus and deafness, and mitochondrial DNA 3243 (A to G) mutation. *Diabetologia.* 1998;41(5):584–588.

155. Hodgson JM, Watts GF, Playford DA, Burke V, Croft KD. Coenzyme Q10 improves blood pressure and glycaemic control: A controlled trial in subjects with type 2 diabetes. *Eur J Clin Nutr.* 2002;56(11):1137–1142.

156. Suksomboon N, Poolsup N, Juanak N. Effects of coenzyme Q10 supplementation on metabolic profile in diabetes: A systematic review and meta-analysis. *J Clin Pharm Ther.* 2015;40(4):413–418.

157. Sohet FM, Neyrinck AM, Pachikian BD, et al. Coenzyme Q10 supplementation lowers hepatic oxidative stress and inflammation associated with diet-induced obesity in mice. *Biochem Pharmacol.* 2009;78(11):1391–400.

158. Tsuneki H, Sekizaki N, Suzuki T, et al. Coenzyme Q10 prevents high glucose-induced oxidative stress in human umbilical vein endothelial cells. *Eur J Pharmacol.* 2007;566(1–3):1–10.

159. Ayaz M, Tuncer S, Okudan N, Gokbel H. Coenzyme Q(10) and alpha-lipoic acid supplementation in diabetic rats: Conduction velocity distributions. *Methods Find Exp Clin Pharmacol.* 2008;30(5):367–374.

160. Garman JH, Mulroney S, Manigrasso M, Flynn E, Maric C. Omega-3 fatty acid rich diet prevents diabetic renal disease. *Am J Physiol Renal Physiol.* 2009;296(2):F306–F316.

161. Cosar M, Songur A, Sahin O, et al. The neuroprotective effect of fish n-3 fatty acids in the hippocampus of diabetic rats. *Nutr Neurosci.* 2008;11(4):161–166.

162. Mustad VA, Demichele S, Huang YS, et al. Differential effects of n-3x polyunsaturated fatty acids on metabolic control and vascular reactivity in the type 2 diabetic ob/ob mouse. *Metabolism.* 2006;55(10):1365–1374.

163. Todoric J, Loffler M, Huber J, et al. Adipose tissue inflammation induced by high-fat diet in obese diabetic mice is prevented by n-3 polyunsaturated fatty acids. *Diabetologia.* 2006;49(9):2109–2119.

164. Chiu WC, Hou YC, Yeh CL, Hu YM, Yeh SL. Effect of dietary fish oil supplementation on cellular adhesion molecule expression and tissue myeloperoxidase activity in diabetic mice with sepsis. *Br J Nutr.* 2007;97(4):685–691.

165. Kaushik M, Mozaffarian D, Spiegelman D, Manson JE, Willett WC, Hu FB. Long-chain omega-3 fatty acids, fish intake, and the risk of type 2 diabetes mellitus. *Am J Clin Nutr.* 2009;90(3):613–620.

166. Giacco R, Cuomo V, Vessby B, et al. Fish oil, insulin sensitivity, insulin secretion, and glucose tolerance in healthy people: Is there any effect of fish oil supplementation in relation to the type of background diet and habitual dietary intake of n-6 and n-3 fatty acids? *Nutr Metab Cardiovasc Dis.* 2007;17(8):572–580.

167. Hartweg J, Perera R, Montori V, Dinneen S, Neil HA, Farmer A. Omega-3 polyunsaturated fatty acids (PUFA) for type 2 diabetes mellitus. *Cochrane Database Syst Rev.* 2008;2008(1):CD003205.

168. Hartweg J, Farmer AJ, Perera R, Holman RR, Neil HA. Meta-analysis of the effects of n-3 polyunsaturated fatty acids on lipoproteins and other emerging lipid cardiovascular risk markers in patients with type 2 diabetes. *Diabetologia.* 2007;50(8):1593–1602.

169. Hartweg J, Farmer AJ, Holman RR, Neil A. Potential impact of omega-3 treatment on cardiovascular disease in type 2 diabetes. *Curr Opin Lipidol.* 2009;20(1):30–38.

170. De Luis DA, Conde R, Aller R, et al. Effect of omega-3 fatty acids on cardiovascular risk factors in patients with type 2 diabetes mellitus and hypertriglyceridemia: An open study. *Eur Rev Med Pharmacol Sci.* 2009;13(1):51–55.

171. Pooya S, Jalali MD, Jazayery AD, Saedisomeolia A, Eshraghian MR, Toorang F. The efficacy of omega-3 fatty acid supplementation on plasma homocysteine and malondialdehyde levels of type 2 diabetic patients. *Nutr Metab Cardiovasc Dis.* 2009;20(5):326–331.

172. Kabir M, Skurnik G, Naour N, et al. Treatment for 2 mo with n 3 polyunsaturated fatty acids reduces adiposity and some atherogenic factors but does not improve insulin sensitivity in women with type 2 diabetes: A randomized controlled study. *Am J Clin Nutr.* 2007;86(6):1670–1679.

173. Mostad IL, Bjerve KS, Lydersen S, Grill V. Effects of marine n-3 fatty acid supplementation on lipoprotein subclasses measured by nuclear magnetic resonance in subjects with type II diabetes. *Eur J Clin Nutr.* 2008;62(3):419–429.

174. Neri S, Signorelli SS, Torrisi B, et al. Effects of antioxidant supplementation on postprandial oxidative stress and endothelial dysfunction: A single-blind, 15-day clinical trial in patients with untreated type 2 diabetes, subjects with impaired glucose tolerance, and healthy controls. *Clin Ther.* 2005;27(11):1764–1773.

175. Chui MH, Greenwood CE. Antioxidant vitamins reduce acute meal-induced memory deficits in adults with type 2 diabetes. *Nutr Res.* 2008;28(7):423–429.
176. Jaxa-Chamiec T, Bednarz B, Herbaczynska-Cedro K, Maciejewski P, Ceremuzynski L. Effects of vitamins C and E on the outcome after acute myocardial infarction in diabetics: A retrospective, hypothesis-generating analysis from the MIVIT study. *Cardiology.* 2009;112(3):219–223.
177. Lai MH. Antioxidant effects and insulin resistance improvement of chromium combined with vitamin C and e supplementation for type 2 diabetes mellitus. *J Clin Biochem Nutr.* 2008;43(3):191–198.
178. Naziroglu M, Dilsiz N, Cay M. Protective role of intraperitoneally administered vitamins C and E and selenium on the levels of lipid peroxidation in the lens of rats made diabetic with streptozotocin. *Biol Trace Elem Res.* 1999;70(3):223–232.
179. Berryman AM, Maritim AC, Sanders RA, Watkins JB, 3rd. Influence of treatment of diabetic rats with combinations of pycnogenol, beta-carotene, and alpha-lipoic acid on parameters of oxidative stress. *J Biochem Mol Toxicol.* 2004;18(6):345–352.
180. Patumraj S, Wongeakin N, Sridulyakul P, Jariyapongskul A, Futrakul N, Bunnag S. Combined effects of curcumin and vitamin C to protect endothelial dysfunction in the iris tissue of STZ-induced diabetic rats. *Clin Hemorheol Microcirc.* 2006;35(4):481–489.
181. Dou M, Ma AG, Wang QZ, et al. Supplementation with magnesium and vitamin E were more effective than magnesium alone to decrease plasma lipids and blood viscosity in diabetic rats. *Nutr Res.* 2009;29(7):519–524.
182. Lortz S, Tiedge M. Sequential inactivation of reactive oxygen species by combined overexpression of SOD isoforms and catalase in insulin-producing cells. *Free Radic Biol Med.* 2003;34(6):683–688.
183. Roma LP, Bosqueiro JR, Cunha DA, et al. Protection of insulin-producing cells against toxicity of dexamethasone by catalase overexpression. *Free Radic Biol Med.* 2009;47(10):1386–1393.
184. van Oostrom O, de Kleijn DP, Fledderus JO, et al. Folic acid supplementation normalizes the endothelial progenitor cell transcriptome of patients with type 1 diabetes: A case-control pilot study. *Cardiovasc Diabetol.* 2009;8:47.
185. Song Y, Cook NR, Albert CM, Van Denburgh M, Manson JE. Effect of homocysteine-lowering treatment with folic acid and B-vitamins on risk of type 2 diabetes in women: A randomized, controlled trial. *Diabetes.* 2009;58(8):1921–1928.
186. Du X, Edelstein D, Brownlee M. Oral benfotiamine plus alpha-lipoic acid normalises complication-causing pathways in type 1 diabetes. *Diabetologia.* 2008;51(10):1930–1932.
187. Stirban A. Drugs for the treatment of diabetes complications. Zycose: A new player in the field? *Drugs Today (Barc).* 2008;44(10):783–796.
188. Gariballa S, Afandi B, Abu Haltem M, Yassin J, Alessa A. Effect of antioxidants and B-group vitamins on risk of infections in patients with type 2 diabetes mellitus. *Nutrients.* 2013;5(3):711–724.
189. Wu S, Ren J. Benfotiamine alleviates diabetes-induced cerebral oxidative damage independent of advanced glycation end-product, tissue factor and TNF-alpha. *Neurosci Lett.* 2006;394(2):158–162.
190. Broadhurst CL, Domenico P. Clinical studies on chromium picolinate supplementation in diabetes mellitus: A review. *Diabetes Technol Ther.* 2006;8(6):677–687.
191. Iqbal N, Cardillo S, Volger S, et al. Chromium picolinate does not improve key features of metabolic syndrome in obese nondiabetic adults. *Metab Syndr Relat Disord.* Summer 2009;7(2):143–150.
192. Suksomboon N, Poolsup N, Yuwanakorn A. Systematic review and meta-analysis of the efficacy and safety of chromium supplementation in diabetes. *J Clin Pharm Ther.* 2014;39(3):292–306.
193. Playford DA, Watts GF, Croft KD, Burke V. Combined effect of coenzyme Q10 and fenofibrate on forearm microcirculatory function in type 2 diabetes. *Atherosclerosis.* 2003;168(1):169–179.
194. Kesavulu MM, Kameswararao B, Apparao C, Kumar EG, Harinarayan CV. Effect of omega-3 fatty acids on lipid peroxidation and antioxidant enzyme status in type 2 diabetic patients. *Diabetes Metab.* 2002;28(1):20–26.
195. Valdivielso P, Rioja J, Garcia-Arias C, Sanchez-Chaparro MA, Gonzalez-Santos P. Omega 3 fatty acids induce a marked reduction of apolipoprotein B48 when added to fluvastatin in patients with type 2 diabetes and mixed hyperlipidemia: A preliminary report. *Cardiovasc Diabetol.* 2009;8:1.
196. Davidson MH, Stein EA, Bays HE, et al. Efficacy and tolerability of adding prescription omega-3 fatty acids 4 g/d to simvastatin 40 mg/d in hypertriglyceridemic patients: An 8-week, randomized, double-blind, placebo-controlled study. *Clin Ther.* 2007;29(7):1354–1367.
197. Zeman M, Zak A, Vecka M, Tvrzicka E, Pisarikova A, Stankova B. N-3 fatty acid supplementation decreases plasma homocysteine in diabetic dyslipidemia treated with statin-fibrate combination. *J Nutr Biochem.* 2006;17(6):379–384.

198. Zeman M, Zak A, Vecka M, Tvrzicka E, Pisarikova A, Stankova B. Effect of n-3 polyunsaturated fatty acids on plasma lipid, LDL lipoperoxidation, homocysteine, and inflammation indicators in diabetic dyslipidemia treated with statin + fibrate combination. *Cas Lek Cesk.* 2005;144(11):737–741.

199. Norris JM, Yin X, Lamb MM, et al. Omega-3 polyunsaturated fatty acid intake and islet autoimmunity in children at increased risk for type 1 diabetes. *JAMA.* 2007;298(12):1420–1428.

200. Zobali F, Avci A, Canbolat O, Karasu C. Effects of vitamin A and insulin on the antioxidative state of diabetic rat heart: A comparison study with combination treatment. *Cell Biochem Funct.* 2002;20(2):75–80.

201. El Midaoui A, Ismael MA, Lu H, Fantus IG, de Champlain J, Couture R. Comparative effects of N-acetyl-L-cysteine and ramipril on arterial hypertension, insulin resistance, and oxidative stress in chronically glucose-fed rats. *Can J Physiol Pharmacol.* 2008;86(11):752–760.

202. Triggiani V, Resta F, Guastamacchia E, et al. Role of antioxidants, essential fatty acids, carnitine, vitamins, phytochemicals and trace elements in the treatment of diabetes mellitus and its chronic complications. *Endocr Metab Immune Disord Drug Targets.* 2006;6(1):77–93.

203. Krentz AJ, Bailey CJ. Oral antidiabetic agents: Current role in type 2 diabetes mellitus. *Drugs.* 2005;65(3):385–411.

204. Price HC, Holman RR. Primary prevention of cardiovascular events in diabetes: Is there a role for aspirin? *Nat Clin Pract Cardiovasc Med.* 2009;6(3):168–169.

205. Ogawa H, Nakayama M, Morimoto T, et al. Low-dose aspirin for primary prevention of atherosclerotic events in patients with type 2 diabetes: A randomized controlled trial. *JAMA.* 2008;300(18):2134–2141.

206. Belch J, MacCuish A, Campbell I, et al. The prevention of progression of arterial disease and diabetes (POPADAD) trial: Factorial randomised placebo controlled trial of aspirin and antioxidants in patients with diabetes and asymptomatic peripheral arterial disease. *BMJ.* 2008;337:a1840.

207. Sacco M, Pellegrini F, Roncaglioni MC, Avanzini F, Tognoni G, Nicolucci A. Primary prevention of cardiovascular events with low-dose aspirin and vitamin E in type 2 diabetic patients: Results of the Primary Prevention Project (PPP) trial. *Diabetes Care.* 2003;26(12):3264–3272.

208. Younis N, Williams S, Soran H. Aspirin therapy and primary prevention of cardiovascular disease in diabetes mellitus. *Diabetes Obes Metab.* 2009;11(11):997–1000.

209. Colwell JA. Antiplatelet agents for the prevention of cardiovascular disease in diabetes mellitus. *Am J Cardiovasc Drugs.* 2004;4(2):87–106.

210. Nobles-James C, James EA, Sowers JR. Prevention of cardiovascular complications of diabetes mellitus by aspirin. *Cardiovasc Drug Rev.* Fall 2004;22(3):215–226.

211. Hayashino Y, Hennekens CH, Kurth T. Aspirin use and risk of type 2 diabetes in apparently healthy men. *Am J Med.* 2009;122(4):374–379.

212. Pradhan AD, Cook NR, Manson JE, Ridker PM, Buring JE. A randomized trial of low-dose aspirin in the prevention of clinical type 2 diabetes in women. *Diabetes Care.* 2009;32(1):3–8.

213. Boaz M, Lisy L, Zandman-Goddard G, Wainstein J. The effect of anti-inflammatory (aspirin and/or statin) therapy on body weight in type 2 diabetic individuals: EAT, a retrospective study. *Diabet Med.* 2009;26(7):708–713.

214. Bergerhoff K, Clar C, Richter B. Aspirin in diabetic retinopathy: A systematic review. *Endocrinol Metab Clin North Am.* 2002;31(3):779–793.

215. Reny JL, Bonvini RF, Barazer I, et al. The concept of aspirin 'resistance': Mechanisms and clinical relevance. *Rev Med Interne.* 2009;30(12):1020–1029.

216. Miyata S, Miyata T, Kada A, Nagatsuka K. Aspirin resistance. *Brain Nerve.* 2008;60(11):1357–1364.

217. Patel D, Moonis M. Clinical implications of aspirin resistance. *Expert Rev Cardiovasc Ther.* 2007;5(5):969–975.

218. Martha S, Devarakonda KR, Anreddy RN, Pantam N. Effect of aspirin treatment in streptozotocin-induced type 2 diabetic rats. *Methods Find Exp Clin Pharmacol.* 2009;31(5):331–335.

219. Jorge AG, Modulo CM, Dias AC, et al. Aspirin prevents diabetic oxidative changes in rat lacrimal gland structure and function. *Endocrine.* 2009;35(2):189–197.

220. Wang T, Fu FH, Han B, Zhu M, Yu X, Zhang LM. Aspirin attenuates cerebral ischemic injury in diabetic rats. *Exp Clin Endocrinol Diabetes.* 2009;117(4):181–185.

221. Carvalho-Filho MA, Ropelle ER, Pauli RJ, et al. Aspirin attenuates insulin resistance in muscle of diet-induced obese rats by inhibiting inducible nitric oxide synthase production and S-nitrosylation of IRbeta/IRS-1, and Akt. *Diabetologia.* 2009;52(11):2425–2434.

222. Vile GF, Winterbourn CC. Inhibition of adriamycin-promoted microsomal lipid peroxidation by beta-carotene, alpha-tocopherol, and retinol at high and low oxygen partial pressures. *FEBS letters.* 1988;238(2):353–356.

223. Niki E. Interaction of ascorbate and alpha-tocopherol. *Ann N Y Acad Sci.* 1987;498:186–199.

224. Wu H, Kong L, Tan Y, et al. C66 ameliorates diabetic nephropathy in mice by both upregulating NRF2 function via increase in miR-200a and inhibiting miR-21. *Diabetologia.* 2016;59:1558–1568.

225. Itoh K, Chiba T, Takahashi S, et al. An Nrf2/small Maf heterodimer mediates the induction of phase II detoxifying enzyme genes through antioxidant response elements. *Biochem Biophys Res Commun.* 1997;236(2):313–322.

226. Williamson TP, Johnson DA, Johnson JA. Activation of the Nrf2-ARE pathway by siRNA knockdown of Keap1 reduces oxidative stress and provides partial protection from MPTP-mediated neurotoxicity. *Neurotoxicology.* 2012;33(3):272–279.

227. Jaramillo MC, Zhang DD. The emerging role of the Nrf2-Keap1 signaling pathway in cancer. *Genes Dev.* 2013;27(20):2179–2191.

228. Li W, Khor TO, Xu C, et al. Activation of Nrf2-antioxidant signaling attenuates NFkappaB-inflammatory response and elicits apoptosis. *Biochem Pharmacol.* 2008;76(11):1485–1489.

229. Kim J, Cha YN, Surh YJ. A protective role of nuclear factor-erythroid 2-related factor-2 (Nrf2) in inflammatory disorders. *Mutat Res.* 2010;690(1–2):12–23.

230. Suh JH, Shenvi SV, Dixon BM, et al. Decline in transcriptional activity of Nrf2 causes age-related loss of glutathione synthesis, which is reversible with lipoic acid. *Proc Natl Acad Sci USA.* 2004;101(10):3381–3386.

231. Jiang T, Huang Z, Lin Y, Zhang Z, Fang D, Zhang DD. The protective role of Nrf2 in streptozotocin-induced diabetic nephropathy. *Diabetes.* 2010;59(4):850–860.

232. Xu Z, Wei Y, Gong J, et al. NRF2 plays a protective role in diabetic retinopathy in mice. *Diabetologia.* 2014;57(1):204–213.

233. Kowluru RA, Mishra M. Epigenetic regulation of redox signaling in diabetic retinopathy: Role of Nrf2. *Free Radic Biol Med.* 2017;103:155–164.

234. Mishra M, Zhong Q, Kowluru RA. Epigenetic modifications of Nrf2-mediated glutamate-cysteine ligase: Implications for the development of diabetic retinopathy and the metabolic memory phenomenon associated with its continued progression. *Free Radic Biol Med.* 2014;75:129–139.

235. Velmurugan GV, Sundaresan NR, Gupta MP, White C. Defective Nrf2-dependent redox signalling contributes to microvascular dysfunction in type 2 diabetes. *Cardiovasc Res.* 2013;100(1):143–150.

236. Long M, Rojo de la Vega M, Wen Q, et al. An essential role of NRF2 in diabetic wound healing. *Diabetes.* 2016;65(3):780–793.

237. Cheng X, Chapple SJ, Patel B, et al. Gestational diabetes mellitus impairs Nrf2-mediated adaptive antioxidant defenses and redox signaling in fetal endothelial cells in utero. *Diabetes.* 2013;62(12):4088–4097.

238. Arellano-Buendia AS, Tostado-Gonzalez M, Garcia-Arroyo FE, et al. Anti-inflammatory therapy modulates Nrf2-keap1 in kidney from rats with diabetes. *Oxid Med Cell Longev.* 2016;2016:4693801.

239. Mostafavi-Pour Z, Ramezani F, Keshavarzi F, Samadi N. The role of quercetin and vitamin C in Nrf2-dependent oxidative stress production in breast cancer cells. *Oncol Lett.* 2017;13(3):1965–1973.

240. Katsuyama Y, Tsuboi T, Taira N, Yoshioka M, Masaki H. 3-O-Laurylglyceryl ascorbate activates the intracellular antioxidant system through the contribution of PPAR-gamma and Nrf2. *J Dermatol Sci.* 2016;82(3):189–196.

241. Xi YD, Yu HL, Ding J, et al. Flavonoids protect cerebrovascular endothelial cells through Nrf2 and PI3K from beta-amyloid peptide-induced oxidative damage. *Curr Neurovasc Res.* 2012;9(1):32–41.

242. Choi HK, Pokharel YR, Lim SC, et al. Inhibition of liver fibrosis by solubilized coenzyme Q10: Role of Nrf2 activation in inhibiting transforming growth factor-beta1 expression. *Toxicol Appl Pharmacol.* 2009;240(3):377–384.

243. Ji L, Liu R, Zhang XD, et al. N-acetylcysteine attenuates phosgene-induced acute lung injury via upregulation of Nrf2 expression. *Inhal Toxicol.* 2010;22(7):535–542.

244. Gao L, Wang J, Sekhar KR, et al. Novel n-3 fatty acid oxidation products activate Nrf2 by destabilizing the association between Keap1 and Cullin3. *J Biol Chem.* 2007;282(4):2529–2537.

245. Saw CL, Yang AY, Guo Y, Kong AN. Astaxanthin and omega-3 fatty acids individually and in combination protect against oxidative stress via the Nrf2-ARE pathway. *Food Chem Toxicol.* 2013;62:869–875.

246. Trujillo J, Chirino YI, Molina-Jijon E, Anderica-Romero AC, Tapia E, Pedraza-Chaverri J. Renoprotective effect of the antioxidant curcumin: Recent findings. *Redox Biol.* 2013;1(1):448–456.

247. Steele ML, Fuller S, Patel M, Kersaitis C, Ooi L, Munch G. Effect of Nrf2 activators on release of glutathione, cysteinylglycine, and homocysteine by human U373 astroglial cells. *Redox Biol.* 2013;1(1):441–445.

248. Kode A, Rajendrasozhan S, Caito S, Yang SR, Megson IL, Rahman I. Resveratrol induces glutathione synthesis by activation of Nrf2 and protects against cigarette smoke-mediated oxidative stress in human lung epithelial cells. *Am J Physiol Lung Cell Mol Physiol.* 2008;294(3):L478–L488.

249. Zambrano S, Blanca AJ, Ruiz-Armenta MV, et al. The renoprotective effect of L-carnitine in hypertensive rats is mediated by modulation of oxidative stress-related gene expression. *Eur J Nutr.* 2013;52(6):1649–1659.

250. Eades G, Yang M, Yao Y, Zhang Y, Zhou Q. miR-200a regulates Nrf2 activation by targeting Keap1 mRNA in breast cancer cells. *J Biol Chem.* 2011;286(47):40725–40733.

251. Abate A, Yang G, Dennery PA, Oberle S, Schroder H. Synergistic inhibition of cyclooxygenase-2 expression by vitamin E and aspirin. *Free Radic Biol Med.* 2000;29(11):1135–1142.

252. Fu Y, Zheng S, Lin J, Ryerse J, Chen A. Curcumin protects the rat liver from CCl4-caused injury and fibrogenesis by attenuating oxidative stress and suppressing inflammation. *Mol Pharmacol.* 2008;73(2):399–409.

253. Lee HS, Jung KK, Cho JY, et al. Neuroprotective effect of curcumin is mainly mediated by blockade of microglial cell activation. *Pharmazie.* 2007;62(12):937–942.

254. Rahman S, Bhatia K, Khan AQ, et al. Topically applied vitamin E prevents massive cutaneous inflammatory and oxidative stress responses induced by double application of 12-O-tetradecanoylphorbol-13-acetate (TPA) in mice. *Chem Biol Interact.* 2008;172(3):195–205.

255. Suzuki YJ, Aggarwal BB, Packer L. Alpha-lipoic acid is a potent inhibitor of NF-kappa B activation in human T cells. *Biochem Biophys Res Commun.* 1992;189(3):1709–1715.

256. Zhu J, Yong W, Wu X, et al. Anti-inflammatory effect of resveratrol on TNF-alpha-induced MCP-1 expression in adipocytes. *Biochem Biophys Res Commun.* 2008;369(2):471–477.

257. Prasad KN. Alpha-tocopheryl succinate exhibits potent anticancer activity: Its interaction with ionizing radiation and chemotherapy effects. In: Reddy VR, and Watson, R.R., eds. *The Encyclopedia of Vitamin E.* London, UK: CAB International; 2007.

7 Micronutrients in Cancer Prevention

INTRODUCTION

Despite extensive basic and clinical research on cancer prevention during the last several decades, the incidence of cancer appears to be on the rise. The number of new cases of cancer rose from 1.1 million in 2002 to 1.689 million in 2017, an increase of about 53.5% in 15 years (CDC, 2017). Despite new advances in early diagnosis and drug treatment, the death from cancer has also increased from 569,490 in 2010 to 600,920 in 2017, a rise of 5.5% in 7 years. Hence, an effective cancer prevention strategy remains one of the best approaches to reduce cancer-related mortality.

It has been estimated that the US diet contributes to about 40% of human cancer, tobacco smoking about 30%, environment about 29%, and familial gene defects about 1%. From these data, it appears that cancer can be considered a preventable disease. Modifying diet and stopping smoking can reduce cancer incidence by about 70%. To address this issue, recommendations of consuming a diet rich in antioxidants, low-fat, high-fiber, and avoiding exposure to potential carcinogens were made. Although these recommendations are very rational, they had no impact in reducing the incidence of cancer. This may be partly because modifications in diet and lifestyle are difficult to implement in humans. Another possibility is that the recommendations themselves may not be sufficient to reduce the incidence of cancer. This issue has been reviewed.[1] To reduce the incidence of cancer, it is essential to identify early and late events that eventually convert dividing normal cells to cancer cells.

Human carcinogenesis is a very complex process with a long latent period (3–30 years) between exposures to carcinogens and clinically detectable cancer. This implies that a preventive strategy can be implemented at any time before cancer detection. The identification of biochemical events that can alter activities of genes responsible for cancer formation during the latent period can help to select agents that can attenuate cancer-causing events. The various proposed hypotheses of human carcinogenesis include (a) chromosomal aberrations, (b) activation of oncogenes, (c) loss of antioncogenes, (d) infection with certain viruses, and (e) overexpression of protooncogenes due to recombinational substitution of strong promoters. These proposed concepts of human carcinogenesis have been critically reviewed.[1,2] Although these concepts are intriguing, none of them alone is sufficient to explain the initial events in human carcinogenesis. For example, chromosomal aberrations that can occur spontaneously or induced by carcinogens can be observed in dividing cells. These cells may or may not transform to cancer cells depending upon the subsequent specific genetic changes. Similarly, overexpression and/or mutation of cellular oncogenes are not sufficient to convert normal cells to cancer cells, nor are the induced expression of antioncogenes sufficient to reverse cancer cells to a normal phenotype. Recently, polymorphism of certain genes appears to be associated with increased risk of cancer.[3–5] Based on the analysis of published studies, we propose that increased oxidative stress and chronic inflammation are early events that initiate and promote human carcinogenesis. The other genetic and chromosomal damage associated with cancer development occur subsequent to increased oxidative stress. Oxidative damage or infection-induced damage, if not repaired, leads to chronic inflammation, which releases additional free radicals and toxic chemicals. Therefore, simultaneous attenuation of oxidative stress and chronic inflammation might be one of the rational choices for reducing the risk of cancer in humans. The evidence for these risk factors is presented later in this chapter.[6]

In order to reduce oxidative stress and chronic inflammation, investigations have utilized primarily single micronutrients or aspirin on cell culture, animals, and humans. The results of these studies have been inconsistent varying from no effect, to some transient beneficial effects, to harmful effects, depending upon the type of antioxidant and type of high-risk population.

Since the first edition of this book, no significant progress on the role of antioxidants and phytochemicals in cancer prevention in humans has been made. The trends of using a single micronutrient in preclinical and clinical studies with inconsistent results continue, despite the failure of such approaches to produce consistent benefits in cancer prevention in humans.

In recent years, microRNAs that prevent the translation of mRNAs transcripts into proteins appear to play an important role in the pathogenesis and diagnosis of chronic diseases; therefore, they may also be involved in the initiation of cancer following exposure to carcinogens and mutagens.

This chapter briefly describes incidence, prevalence, cost, stages of carcinogenesis, environmental, dietary, and lifestyle-related carcinogens, and presents evidence for the involvement of increased oxidative stress and chronic inflammation in the initiation of carcinogenesis following exposure to cancer-causing agents. It describes alterations in the expression of microRNAs in the development of cancer. This chapter also presents results of cell culture, animal, epidemiologic, and intervention studies on the effects of primarily individual micronutrients and aspirin in high-risk populations of developing cancer, and discusses potential reasons for obtaining inconsistent results varying from no effect, to transient beneficial effects, to harmful effects. A single micronutrient cannot simultaneously reduce oxidative stress and inflammation that are required for optimal reduction in cancer incidence. In order to accomplish the above goal, it is essential to increase the levels of cytoprotective enzymes including antioxidant enzymes through activation of the Nrf2/ARE pathway, and dietary and endogenous antioxidants. This chapter discusses the regulation of activation of Nrf2, and suggests a mixture of micronutrients that would reduce oxidative stress and chronic inflammation levels at the same time, and thereby, would help in the prevention of cancer.

INCIDENCE, PREVALENCE, MORTALITY, AND COST

According to the statistics provided by Center for Disease Control and Prevention, 2017, the incidence of new cases of cancer is on the rise.

2002	1.1 million new cases of cancer
2010	1.529 million new cases of cancer
2016	1.685 million new cases of cancer
2017	1.689 million new cases of cancer

In 2014, total number of cancer in the United States was 14, 738, 719 million.

The mortality has slightly increased between 2010 and 2017 in the United States.

2010	569,490 thousands people died of cancer
2014	590,000 thousands people died of cancer
2017	600,920 thousands people died of cancer

American Cancer Society estimated that in 2014, patients spent about $4 billion out of pocket, while the US Healthcare System spent $87.8 billion.

PROPOSED STAGES OF CARCINOGENESIS

TWO-STAGE MODEL OF ANIMAL CARCINOGENESIS

In an effort to develop a model to study carcinogenesis process, carcinogens were applied topically to the skin of animals, and the development of cancer was followed as function of time after treatment. These studies allowed postulation of a two-stage model of carcinogenesis (initiation stage and promotion stage).[7] This model has been useful in identifying carcinogenic and anticarcinogenic substances and characterizing biochemical and genetic changes at each stage. Increased oxidative stress and chronic inflammation play a role at each stage of the animal carcinogenesis following exposure to carcinogens.

SOME EXAMPLES OF TUMOR INITIATORS AND TUMOR PROMOTERS

Human are exposed to several tumor initiators and promoters daily from environmental-, dietary-, and lifestyle-related factors. Tumor initiators at any doses can cause cancer, whereas tumor promoters by themselves do not cause cancer but, in combination with tumor initiators, increase the risk of cancer and may reduce the latent period. There are two types of tumor initiators: direct-acting carcinogens, such as ionizing radiation, and indirect acting carcinogens, such as benzo (a) pyrene, requiring conversion to an active form in the liver. Examples of tumor promoters are phorbol ester, excessive fat consumption, and high estrogen levels in women.

THREE-STAGE MODEL OF HUMAN CARCINOGENESIS

Human carcinogenesis is more complex than animal carcinogenesis because of exposure to marked variations in environmental-, diet-, and lifestyle-related potential cancer-causing agents. Based on the histological progression of cancer formation, we have proposed a three-stage model of human carcinogenesis.[1] A diagrammatic representation of this model is shown below. This model shows that intervention can be made at any time during first- and second-stage of carcinogenesis in order to reduce the risk of cancer. The latent period for each of these stages in humans could vary from a few to several years.

DIAGRAMMATIC REPRESENTATION OF THREE-STAGE MODEL OF HUMAN CARCINOGENESIS

1st Stage

ROS-Induced Mutations in Normal cells

↓

Surviving Mutated cells

↓	**2nd Stage**	**3rd Stage**
Proliferate	**ROS-Induced Mutation**	**ROS-Induced Mutation**
↓	**in differentiation gene**	**in Hyperplastic Cells**
Differentiate	↓	↓
↓	Proliferate	Cancer Cells
Die	↓	
	Hyperplasic Cells	
	(e.g. colon polyp) ↓	

The first stage involves the induction of random mutations in normal dividing cells by ROS generated by exposure to cancer-causing substances associated with the environment, diet, or lifestyle, a deficiency in the natural repair system, or a deficiency in protective substances, such as antioxidants. These mutations can also occur spontaneously due to random errors during replication. The mutated cells may die or survive, depending upon the severity of oxidative damage. The surviving mutated cells continue to divide, differentiate, and die similar to the patterns observed in normal cells that do not have mutations. The mutated cells continue to accumulate additional mutations at a higher rate but continue to divide and differentiate like unmutated normal dividing cells for a long period of time.

The second stage of carcinogenesis involves the induction of mutations in specific genes that are responsible for inducing differentiation in normal cells by ROS. As a result, the mutated cells continue to divide without achieving differentiation and subsequent cell death. Such cells become immortal and form precancerous or benign growths such as polyps in the colon or cyst in the female breast and ovary. They continue to proliferate while accumulating additional mutations for a long period of time.

The third stage of carcinogenesis involves the induction of random mutations in the hyperplastic cells. Most of such mutations play no role in converting hyperplastic cells to cancer cells; however, when mutations occur in specific cellular genes, oncogenes, or antioncogenes, hyperplastic cells become cancerous. This is well demonstrated in colon polyps and female breast and ovarian cysts, which remain noncancerous for a long time, but if not removed, become cancerous. Because mutation occurs randomly, the colon polyp may carry defects in more than one oncogene. The multiple, heterogeneous foci of cancer cells found in the colon polyps are not necessarily clonal with respect to a given oncogene. This heterogeneity may be the reason why, in spite of extensive research in molecular carcinogenesis, it has not been possible to establish any direct relationship between the presence of one defective oncogene or other cellular genes and tumor type or tumor behavior, although some associations between oncogene or anti-oncogene and tumor behavior have been documented.

SOME EXAMPLES OF ENVIRONMENTAL-RELATED CARCINOGENS

There are numerous carcinogens and mutagens in atmospheric and work-related environments. They include ozone, ionizing radiation, ultraviolet radiation from the sun, burning wood in the forest, or buildings that release high levels of polycyclic hydrocarbons, such as benzo (a) pyrene, asbestos, benzene, and vinyl chloride.

SOME EXAMPLES OF DIET-RELATED CARCINOGENS

Human diets contain both cancer-protective and cancer-causing substances.[8] Most of the mutagenic and carcinogenic substances that are present in the diet are naturally occurring; however, small amounts of mutagens have been introduced into the diet by the use of pesticides in agriculture production.[8] The relative ratio of protective and mutagenic substances in a human diet can vary markedly from one individual to another and from one day to another in the same individual. Varying levels of mutagens and carcinogens are formed during storage of food at room temperature (browning of fruits and vegetables), and during cooking process (browning of vegetables and meat). Flame-broiled fatty meat may contain much higher levels of carcinogens like benzo (a) pyrene than those found in grilled meat. Consumption of a nitrite-rich diet (bacon, sausage, cured meat) can form nitrosamine in the stomach at acid pH by the combination of nitrites and secondary amines. Diets rich in meat increased the levels of mutagens in the feces compared to vegetarian diets. Excessively high-caloric diets and the consumption of diets rich in fat can increase the risk of cancer. Epidemiologic studies have reported that acrylamide, which is formed during heating of several foods at very high temperature, was associated with the increased risk of endometrial, ovarian, estrogen-positive breast cancer, and renal cell cancer, but not with lung cancer in men; however, it was inversely associated with lung cancer in women.[9] Aflatoxin alone or in combination with hepatitis B virus can increase the risk of liver cancer.[10]

SOME EXAMPLES OF DIET-RELATED CANCER PROTECTIVE AGENTS

Protective substances in the diets are antioxidants and phytochemicals—the levels and types of which can markedly vary, depending upon the type of food. Generally, fruits and green, red, or yellow vegetables are rich in antioxidants and phytochemicals. Consumption of meat or fish provides endogenous antioxidants (made in the body) that may decrease as a function of aging. Lower intake of nutrients, especially antioxidants and phytochemicals from the diet, can increase the risk of cancer.

In contrast to human diets in the United States, the diet of laboratory rodent is vegetarian and relatively uniform in contents. Therefore, the relative ratio of protective and carcinogenic substances in animal diets may not vary significantly during the study period. The human diet, with respect to cancer-protective and cancer-causing substances, varies markedly from day to day and from one individual to another on the same day. In addition, most rodents, except guinea pigs, make their own vitamin C; humans do not. These differences in rodent and human diets are often ignored while extrapolating the results of micronutrient experiments on rodents to the design of cancer prevention studies in humans. The analysis of animal and human studies with antioxidants has convinced me that the results of investigation on the effects of micronutrients on cancer prevention in animal models should not be extrapolated to the design of human studies with respect to number, type, dose, and dose-schedule of antioxidants.

SOME EXAMPLES OF LIFESTYLE-RELATED CARCINOGENS

ALCOHOL

Several epidemiologic studies have revealed that daily consumption of high amounts of alcohol is associated with increased risk of colorectal cancer, pancreatic cancer, and oral cancer.[11–14] Alcohol intake and overweight were associated with increased risk of breast cancer.[15] Although no intervention studies have been performed to establish a causal relationship between consumption of excessive amounts of alcohol and increased risk of certain cancers, epidemiologic data have been consistent. Therefore, excessive consumption of alcohol should be avoided in the proposed cancer prevention strategy.

CELL PHONE

The cell or mobil phone technology and its use have exploded during last decade throughout the world. It is estimated that about 4–5 billion people use cell phones at this time. The cell phone voices are transmitted over radio waves at frequencies ranging from about 800 to 1,900 MHz (megahertz). The biological effects of the radiofrequencies emitted by the cell phone have been subject of intensive debate, and no firm conclusions on the adverse health effects of this form of radiation can be drawn at this time.

The fact that electromagnetic radiation at radio frequencies from the cell phones can be absorbed into the brain has prompted concerns that regular use of cell phone for a long period of time may increase the risk of acoustic neuroma and other brain tumors. The effects of cell phone use on cancer risk have been investigated using primarily epidemiologic methodologies. The results of these studies on cancer incidence have been inconsistent, varying from no effect to adverse effects.[16] Reviews of several studies on the effect of cell phone use on the risk of brain tumors revealed that regular use of cell phones for a period of 10 years or more was associated with increased risk of acoustic neuroma and glioma.[17] Other epidemiologic studies reported no such association between cell phone use and risk of brain tumor.[18] In another epidemiologic study, regular use of cell phone was associated with increased risk of benign parotid gland tumors.[19] In a Japanese case-control study, the use of cell phone for 20 minutes or more for 5 years was associated with increased risk of acoustic neuroma.[20] A review of epidemiologic study concluded that there was no causal relationship between cell phone use and increased risk of brain cancer.[21]

The laboratory studies with animal and cell culture models are very few. The radiofrequency radiation emitted from a cell phone produced no effect on cancer incidence in mice.[22] Exposure of mammalian cells in culture to 835-MHz radiofrequency radiation electromagnetic field slightly enhanced the levels of chromosomal aberrations induced by a chemical (ethylmethanesulfonate).[23]

At this time, it is not necessary or prudent to recommend any limitation on the use of cell phone in any cancer prevention strategy, but caution should be maintained regarding overuse of this communication technology in the proposed cancer prevention strategy.

SMOKING

Numerous epidemiologic and laboratory studies have confirmed that cigarette smoking is a major human carcinogen. It increases the risk of not only lung cancer but other cancers as well, and contributes to about 30% of all cancers. Passive smoking also increased the risk of cancer. However, some epidemiologic studies with specific cancers have produced inconsistent results. Lifetime exposure to active or passive tobacco smoking was not associated with alterations in breast cancer[24] or esophageal cancer and gastric adenocarcinoma.[25] Other epidemiologic studies revealed that both active and passive tobacco smoking were associated with an increased risk of breast cancer,[26,27] renal carcinoma,[28] and bladder cancer.[29] Despite of some conflicting results, cessation of active and passive tobacco smoking must be included in the proposed cancer prevention strategy.

COFFEE AND CAFFEINE

Epidemiologic studies on the association between coffee or caffeine consumption and the risk of cancer have produced inconsistent results. For example, some studies showed no association between coffee or caffeine consumption and the risk of renal carcinoma.[30] There was no significant association between caffeinated or decaffeinated coffee and tea consumption and the risk of breast cancer; however, a weak inverse association between caffeine-containing beverages and the risk of breast cancer in postmenopausal women was observed.[31] In another study, no association between caffeine consumption and the risk of breast cancer was found[32]; however, in women carrying mutated BRCA1 gene, which increases the risk of breast cancer, an inverse association between coffee consumption and the risk of breast cancer was observed. There was no association between coffee consumption and the risk of ovarian cancer[33]; however, an increased risk of ovarian cancer was associated with heavy consumption of coffee (5 cups or more per day) in postmenopausal women.[34] On the other hand, another study reported an inverse association between caffeine consumption and ovarian cancer risk in women on hormone supplement.[6] An association between coffee and caffeine consumption and an increased risk of bladder cancer was observed,[35] but an inverse association was observed for liver cancer.[36] From these studies, it is difficult to draw any specific conclusions with respect to the impact of coffee, decaffeinated coffee, or caffeine consumption and the risk of overall cancer. In my view, 1–2 cups of coffee or equivalent amount of caffeine-containing beverages may have no effect on the incidence of any type of cancer; however, excessive consumption of caffeine should be avoided in the proposed cancer prevention strategy until definitive data from intervention studies become available.

EVIDENCE FOR INCREASED OXIDATIVE STRESS

Most carcinogens cause cellular damage by generating excessive amounts of free radicals. Evidence for increased oxidative stress comes directly from measurement of markers of oxidative damage following exposure to carcinogens. There are numerous studies and reviews on the role of increased oxidative stress in human carcinogenesis. Only some selected studies with references are described here.

Irrespective of the types of mutagenic or carcinogenic agents, increased oxidative stress[37,38] is associated with human carcinogenesis; and it plays a central role in inducing gene mutations and/or chromosomal changes that initiate carcinogenic changes. Pretreatment with menthol suppressed skin tumor formation and growth following exposure to DMBA (dimethylbenz (a) anthracene) and then TPA (12-O-tetradecanoyalphorbol-13-actate) by reducing oxidative stress and inflammation in female ICR mice.[39] Cadmium-induced gastrointestinal cancer is due to increased oxidative stress, inhibition of DNA damage repair, and apoptosis.[40] Elevated levels of 8-oxo-2-deoxyguanosine (8-OHdG), a marker of oxidative DNA damage, were found in human prostate adenocarcinoma compared to benign prostate cancer. Additionally, the levels of pi-class glutathione S-transferase (GSTP1), a protector against oxidative damage, were lower in adenocarcinoma than in benign tumor of prostate.[41] Silencing GSTP1 in normal human prostate epithelial RWPE1 cells increased production of ROS and increased sensitivity to oxidative stress produced by H_2O_2. Elevated levels of ROS and reactive nitrogen species (RNS) and reduced levels of antioxidants were found in oral pre-cancer and cancer cells.[42] ROS and RNS-induce stabilization of Bcl2 plays a role in the malignant transformation of normal lung epithelial cells following long-term exposure to a carcinogen.[43] Increased oxidative stress is associated with aberrant hypermethylation of tumor suppressor gene promoter regions and global hypomethylation, which play a role malignant transformation, as well as progression of cancer.[44]

EVIDENCE FOR INCREASED CHRONIC INFLAMMATION

When cellular damage induced by physical insults, mutagens, carcinogens, or infective agents is not repaired, chronic inflammation sets in motion, which releases additional ROS, pro-inflammatory cytokines, and other toxic chemicals. There are numerous studies and reviews on the role of chronic inflammation in human carcinogenesis. Only some selected studies with references are described here.

Irrespective of the types of carcinogens, chronic inflammation[45–48] is associated with human carcinogenesis, and it plays an important role in inducing gene mutations and/or chromosomal changes that initiate carcinogenic changes. Chronic inflammation contributes to the development of thyroid cancer,[49] sarcoma,[50] cervical cancer,[51] oral cancer,[52] brain cancer,[53] breast cancer,[54] lung cancer,[55] kidney cancer,[56] and gastric cancer.[57] Activation of nuclear factor-k B (NF-kB), a transcriptional factor, which regulates inflammatory responses, promotes carcinogenesis and progression of cancer.[58] Increased chronic inflammation proportionally enhanced the levels of DNA double-strand breaks, which was correlated with the progression of pre-cancerous lesions to esophageal squamous cell carcinoma.[59] In transgenic mice expressing viral gene HTLV-1βZIP (HBZ), severity of inflammation was correlated with the development of lymphoma. Furthermore, interferon-gamma (IFN-gamma) producing cells increased HBZ-mediated inflammation leading to the formation of lymphoma. This observation is further supported by the fact that silencing IFN-gamma significantly deceased the incidence of dermatitis and lymphoma.[60] Pathogenic bacterial or viral infection caused inflammation, which led to aberrant expression of activation-induced cytidine deaminase (AID), a DNA mutator enzyme, in epithelial cells by activating NF-kB. Increased expression of AID caused accumulation of altered expression of tumor-associated genes, while a deficiency of endogenous AID expression reduced somatic mutations in tumor-related genes and incidence of cancer in a mouse model of inflammation-associated cancer development.[61] Gastric cardia cancer (GCC) is a highly aggressive form of neoplasm associated with chronic inflammation. Analysis of nontumor gastric cardia specimens revealed that the number of dysplastic epithelia with chronic inflammation was higher than that found in nondysplastic tissues. Additionally, the extent of DNA damage increased with the degree of chronic inflammation that correlated with the progression of precancerous lesions to cancer.[62] Pro-inflammatory cytokine interleukin-17 (IL-17) plays an important role in the progression from colon adenoma to colon adenocarcinoma. This is demonstrated by showing that the levels of IL-17A progressively increased from ulcerative colitis, to adenoma, to adenocarcinoma.[63]

> *Since increased oxidative stress and chronic inflammation are involved following exposure to mutagenic and carcinogenic agents, attenuation of these biochemical defects appears to be one of the rationale choices for the prevention of cancer.*

MicroRNAs IN CANCER PREVENTION

Increased oxidative stress and chronic inflammation play a central role in the initiation of carcinogenesis. Previous reviews have revealed that ROS and pro-inflammatory cytokines alter the expression of microRNAs in some neurodegenerative diseases such as Alzheimer's disease (AD)[64] and Parkinson's disease (PD).[65] Therefore, it is likely that they also play an important role in the development of cancer following exposure to carcinogens. Indeed, altered levels of microRNAs were found in various organs of animals after acute and chronic exposure to carcinogens.

MicroRNAs

MicroRNAs (miRs) are evolutionarily conserved small noncoding single-stranded RNAs of approximately 22 nucleotides in length and are present in all living organisms including humans.[66–69] The biogenesis of miRs is very complex and involves multiple biochemical steps. The majority of miRs are transcribed by RNA polymerase II (Pol II), while some are transcribed by RNA polymerase III (Pol III) from the noncoding region of the DNA to produce primary miRs (pri-miRs). Pri-miRs undergo a nuclear cleavage by ribonuclease III Drosa to generate precursor-miRs (pre-miRs) that migrate to the cytoplasm where they are further cleaved by ribonuclease III Dicer to ultimately form mature single-stranded miRs with the help of another protein argonaute (Ago).[68,70–72] Each microRNA binds to its complementary sequences in the 3'-untranslated region (3'-UTR) of the mRNA, promotes degradation of the mRNA transcript, and prevents translation of the message of protein. In this manner, miRs regulate the translation of proapoptotic or antiapoptotic proteins from their respective mRNAs, depending upon whether they receive damaging or protective signal. Damaging signals may include oxidative damage and pro-inflammatory cytokines and protective signals may include antioxidants and phytochemicals.

CHANGES IN MicroRNAs AFTER EXPOSURE TO CHEMICAL CARCINOGENS AND ONCOGENIC VIRUS

Alterations in the expression of microRNAs are observed following exposure to a carcinogen in animals. The expression of miR-34a is upregulated in tissues after chronically or sub-chronically treatment with a carcinogen. The expression level of this microRNA increased 5.5 fold in the spleen of mice one day after treatment with N-ethyl-N-nitrosourea (ENU).[73] Treatment of

GES-1 cells (SV40 transformed human fetal gastric epithelial cell line) with MNNG (N-methyl-N-nitro-N′-nitrosoguanidine) increased the expression of miR-21 in a dose-dependent and time-dependent manner, causing downregulation of its target proteins Fas ligand (FASLG) that plays a role in carconogenesis.[74] Treatment of HepG2 liver cell (cell line derived from a patient with well-differentiated hepatocellular carcinoma) with 4-aminobiphenyl (4-ABP) for a period of 24 h increased the expression of 27 microRNAs, but the expression of miR-513-5p and miR-630 was most significantly enhanced. Overexpression of miR-513-5p and miR-630 downregulated their target proteins FANCG (Fanconi anemia group G protein) and RAD18 (E-3 ubiquitin lagase RAD18 protein).[75] Treatment of HepG2 cells with Fumonisin B, a chemical carcinogen found in maize, downregulated the expression of miR-27b and upregulated the levels of its target protein human cytochrome P450 (CYP1B1).[76]

The expression of miR-93 was elevated in 17 β-estradiol (E2) treated female rat breast tissue and human breast cell line after 8 months of treatment. Treatment with vitamin C reversed estrogen-induced elevation of miR-93. Over expression of miR-93 downregulated the levels of its target protein Nrf2 leading to increased oxidative damage, reduced apoptosis, increased colony formation, and cell migration in breast epithelial cells.[77] Thus, carcinogenic effect of estrogen is mediated via increased expression of miR-93.

Administration of 7,12-dimethylbenz(α)anthracene (DMBA) for a period of 24 hours increased the expression of miR-21, miR-146, and let-7a compared to untreated mice; however, after 7 days of treatment, the expressions of these microRNAs were downregulated.[78] These results suggest that alterations in the expression of miR-21, miR-146, and let-7a might play an important role in DMBA-induced cancer in mice. N-methyl-N-nitrosourea (MNU) decreased the expression of miR-34a and miR-155 in the liver, spleen, and kidneys but increased the expression of miR-21 in the liver of mice at 3 and 6 hours after treatment. On the other hand, DMBA increased the expression of miR-21 in the lungs and kidneys 6 hours after treatment.[79] These results suggest that alterations in certain microRNAs following acute exposure to chemical carcinogens play a role in carcinogenic processes.

Exposure to cigarette smoke (CS) downregulated the expression levels of microRNAs in the lungs of mice and rats. When neonatal mice were exposed to CS at 12 hours after birth and continued for 4 weeks, the expressions of microRNAs including 7 members of the miR-let-7, miR-34b, miR-345, miR-421, miR-450b, miR-466, and miR-469 were reduced. After cessation of exposure to CS, the expression of miR-let-7 returned to normal level; however, the expression of other microRNAs did not fully return to a normal level.[80]

Infection of primary B cells by Epstein-Barr virus (EBV) increased the expression of a tumor suppressor microRNA miR-34a. Inhibition of the expression of this microRNA reduced the growth of EBV-transformed cells.[81] The expression of miR-203 was decreased during early stage of EBV-infection in epithelial cells as well as in nasopharyngeal carcinoma cells. Viral oncoprotein, latent membrane protein 1 (LMP1) induced decreased expression of miR-203. Inhibition of LMP1 protein restored miR-203 expression level. Overexpression of miR-203 reduced EBV-induced S-phase entry and transformation in vivo. These results suggest that EBV initiate carcinogenesis by downregulating miR-203.[82] Long-term exposure to radon downregulated the expression of miR-let-7 and upregulated the expression of K-ras oncogene in rats and human bronchial epithelial (HBE) cells. HBE cells transfected with miR-let-7b-3p and miR-let7a-2-3p decreased the expression of K-ras. These results suggest radon-induced initiation of carcinogenesis involves downregulation of miR-let-7 and upregulation of K-ras oncogene.[83]

The studies discussed above suggest that alterations in the expression of microRNAs initiate carcinogenesis following exposure to carcinogens or oncogenic viruses and cigarette smoke. The results are summarized in Table 7.1.

TABLE 7.1

Alterations in the Expression of MicroRNAs after Exposure to Chemical Carcinogens and Oncogenic Virus

Carcinogens	Upregulation	Downregulation	Target Proteins
ENU	miR-34a	None	Not available
MNNG	miR-021	None	FAS ligand
4-ABP	miR-513-5p, miR-630	None	FANCG, RAD18
Fumonisin	None	miR-27b	Cytochrome 450
Estrogen	miR-93	None	Not available
DMBA	miR-21[a], miR-146, miR-let-7a	miR-21[b], miR-146, miR-let-7a	Not available
MNU	miR-21	miR-34a, miR-155	Not available
EBV	miR-34a	miR-203	Not available
CS		miR-let-7, miR-34b, miR-345, miR-421, miR-450b, miR-466, miR-469	Not available

Note: ENU, N-ethyl-N-nitrosourea; MNNG, N-methyl-N-nitrosoguanidine; 4-ABP, 4-aminobiphenyl; DMBA, 7,12-dimethylbenz (α)anthracene; MNU, N-methyl-N-nitrosourea; EBV, Epstein-Barr virus; FANCG, Fanconi anemia group G; RAD18, E-3 ubiquitin lagase RAD18; CS, cigarette smoke.

[a] 24 hours after treatment.

[b] 7 days after treatment.

FUNCTIONS OF ANTIOXIDANTS RELEVANT TO CANCER PREVENTION

Extensive studies show that antioxidants and phytochemicals can reduce the risk of developing cancer. This issue has been discussed extensively in a review.[1] Antioxidants can neutralize excessive levels of free radicals that increase the risk of cancer. They can prevent the formation of potential carcinogenic substances. For example, vitamin C and vitamin E alone or in combination prevented the formation of nitrosamine in the stomach from nitrites (present in nitrite rich diet) and secondary amines.[84] These dietary antioxidants also reduce the levels of fecal mutagens that are formed during digestion of food.[85] The combination of vitamin C and vitamin E was more effective than the individual antioxidant in reducing the levels of fecal mutagens. High levels of antioxidants can prevent conversion of indirect carcinogen to an active form in the liver that is needed to increase the risk of cancer. Mutation and/or chromosomal damage can increase the risk of cancer. Antioxidants can reduce spontaneous and induced mutations in animals as well as human cells, and thus, could play an important role in cancer prevention. For example, vitamins C and E and beta-carotene reduced chromosomal damage produced by ionizing radiation and chemical carcinogens.[86–88]

They can also inhibit overexpression of oncogenes and mutated oncogenes. A high-fat diet increases the levels of prostaglandins (PGs) in the animal model[89] and may increase the risk of some cancers.[90] Vitamin E and a non-steroidal anti-inflammatory drug (NSAID), aspirin, inhibit the production of PGs more than that produced by the individual agent.

Although the host's immune system may not play a direct role in human carcinogenesis, it could play an important role in allowing or rejecting newly formed cancer cells. The optimally functioning immune cells (natural killer cells) can recognize newly formed cancer cells and kill them. A weak immune system may allow newly formed cancer cells to establish themselves in the host; these cells will then grow and metastasize to distant organs. Antioxidants stimulate humoral and cellular immunity[7,91,92] and thus, can reduce the risk of developing cancer.

ANTIOXIDANTS AND PHYTOCHEMICALS REGULATE EXPRESSION OF MicroRNAs

Our previous reviews proposed that antioxidants regulate expression of microRNAs that allow translation of only protective proteins from their respective mRNAs transcripts in varieties of cell type and health conditions, such as Alzheimer's disease (AD)[93] and Parkinson's disease (PD).[94] Since antioxidants protect against chemical-induced carcinogenesis, it is possible that they may also alter the expression of microRNAs that allow translation of cytoprotective proteins from their respective mRNAs transcripts for protection against the development of cancer. Treatments with phytochemicals protected normal CCD-18Co colon cells against oxidative stress by increasing the activities of antioxidant enzymes and against inflammation by upregulating miR-146a that reduced NFkB activation.[95] Resveratrol treatment prevented dextran sodium sulfate-induced colitis associate carcinogenesis by upregulating the expression of miR-101b and miR-455 that reduced pro-inflammatory cytokines.[96]

REDUCING OXIDATIVE STRESS AND CHRONIC INFLAMMATION IN CANCER PREVENTION

Since antioxidants and phytochemicals are known to reduce oxidative stress and chronic inflammation, several studies used them individually and in combination on cell culture, animal, and high-risk human populations. These studies are described here.

CELL CULTURE MODELS

The availability of primary cultures and immortalized cells of animal and human provides a new opportunity to investigate the mechanisms of action of antioxidants and their derivatives on cancer prevention. In 1982, we identified alpha-tocopheryl succinate (alpha-TS) as the most effective form of vitamin E exhibiting anticancer properties.[97] Alpha-TS, but not alpha-tocopherol or alpha-tocopheryl acetate, reduces the incidence of chemical and ionizing radiation-induced transformation of normal-like murine fibroblasts in culture.[98,99] Beta-carotene also reduced the incidence of chemical- and ionizing radiation-induced transformation of these cells.[100,101] Natural beta-carotene was more effective than synthetic beta-carotene in reducing the incidence of radiation-induced transformation in vitro. N-acetylcysteine (NAC) markedly reduced estrogen-induced transformation of E6 cells (a normal mouse epithelial cell line) in culture.[102] The exact mechanisms of protection of induced carcinogenesis in vitro by these antioxidants are unknown; however, I suggest that antioxidants prevent carcinogen-induced oxidative stress that causes mutagenic changes, which initiate immortalization (pre-neoplastic state). The results of in vitro studies cannot readily be extrapolated to animals or humans with respect to antioxidant type, dose, or dose-schedule.

ANIMAL MODELS

The overwhelming majority of studies performed on the two-stage model of carcinogenesis suggest that the supplementation with high doses of individual antioxidants such as vitamin C,[103] vitamin E,[104] retinoids,[105] and carotenoids[106,107] reduced the risk of chemical-induced tumors. Among various forms of vitamin E, alpha-TS was the most effective form as an anticancer agent.[104] In the Lady transgenic animal model, the combination of vitamin E, selenium, and lycopene was effective in reducing the risk of prostate cancer, whereas the combination of vitamin E and selenium was ineffective.[108] The result of the combined effect of vitamin E and selenium is consistent with the results of the Selenium and Vitamin E Cancer Prevention Trial (SELECT) in which the combination of vitamin E and selenium was found to be ineffective in reducing the risk of prostate cancer.[109]

In p53 knockout pregnant mice, prenatal supplementation with vitamin E (all-rac-alpha-tocopheryl acetate) reduced postnatal malignancies by reducing the levels of DNA oxidation.[110]

Dihydrolipoic acid, a reduced form of alpha-lipoic aid, significantly decreased the tumor incidence and tumor multiplicity in dimethylbenzanthracene (DMBA)/tetrachlorohydroquinone (TCHQ)-induced skin tumor.[111] TCHQ is a tumor promoter, and DMBA is a tumor initiator. Dihydrolipoic acid also markedly inhibited expression of inducible nitric oxide synthase (iNOS) enzyme and cyclooxygenase-2 (COX-2) activity, and reduced the tumor incidence and tumor multiplicity of DMBA/TPA (12-O-tetradecanoylphorbol-13-acetate)-induced skin tumor.[112] Supplementation with alpha-lipoic acid did not affect the incidence of breast cancer in mice overexpressing HER2/neu, an animal model for breast cancer, or of colon cancer in APCmin mice, a model for intestinal cancer.[113] The reasons for these contradictory results between transgenic model of cancer and chemical-induced cancer animal models remain unknown.

The hereditary human disorder ataxia telangiectasia (AT) is characterized by an extremely high incidence of lymphoid malignancy. Supplementation with NAC increased the lifespan and reduced the incidence and tumor multiplicity of lymphoma in AT-deficient mice.[114] However, supplementation with NAC did not change the incidence of liver tumor, but caused a significant decrease in tumor multiplicity in rat treated with DEN/DEDTC (N-diethyl nitrosamine/diethyldithiocarbamate).[115] On the other hand, using the p53 haploinsufficient Tg. AC (v-H-ras) mouse which contains an activated ras oncogene and an inactivated p53 tumor suppressor gene—frequently found in human cancers—it was demonstrated that supplementation with NAC did not affect the incidence of benzo(a)pyrene-induced skin tumor; however, it reduced tumor multiplicity.[116] Supplementation with NAC did not affect DMBA-induced mammary tumor in rodent model.[117] In contrast to DMBA-induced mammary tumor, NAC supplementation reduced the incidence of urethane-induced lung cancer.[118] Vitamin E in combination with NAC was more effective in reducing the incidence of esophageal cancer in esophagogastroduodenal anastomosis (EGDA) rat model than the individual agents.[119] Thus, the effects of NAC in reducing induced cancer in rodent models are variable, depending upon the type of tumor and tumor-inducing agents. Supplementation with coenzyme Q10 reduced azoxymethane-induced aberrant crypt foci and mucin-depleted foci in the colon of male rats.[120] Most studies on animal models have utilized a single dietary or endogenous antioxidant that have yielded inconsistent protective effects against chemical-induced cancer.

A few studies found that certain antioxidants at very high doses when used individually may increase the risk of cancer. For example, vitamin E at very high doses (equivalent of 40 g per person per day) increased the risk of chemical-induced cancer in the small intestine of mice.[121] Vitamin C, in the form of sodium ascorbate, increased the risk of chemical-induced bladder cancer in rats.[122] Increased osmolarity of urine caused chronic irritations in the bladder, which may account for the increased risk of chemical-induced cancer following treatments with a high concentration of sodium ascorbate. The use of such high doses of single antioxidants in cancer prevention studies is not relevant to humans.

Although animal models are useful in identifying potential cancer-protective agents, the results cannot be extrapolating to humans with respect to dose, dose-schedule, and type of antioxidants because the absorption, tissue distribution, biological turnover, and metabolism of various antioxidants in animals are totally different from those found in humans. Unlike humans, rodents except guinea pigs, make their own vitamin C, which could have impact on the dose and efficacy of antioxidants in reducing the risk of chemical-induced cancers.

EPIDEMIOLOGIC STUDIES

Several studies[104,123,124] concluded that diets rich in antioxidants but low in fat and high in fiber were associated with reduced risk of cancer.[125] Consumption of fruits and vegetables and food items rich in carotene and lycopene may reduce the risk of ovarian cancer. A diet low in fat and high in fiber from fruits and vegetables and regular modest consumption of alcohol are associated with reduced risk of benign prostatic hyperplasia (BPH).[109] It has been estimated that eating fruits and vegetables can reduce the risk of cancer by about 30%.[126] Another epidemiologic study showed that eating one or more apple a day was associated with reduced risk of colorectal cancer. This effect was not observed with other fruits.[127] When the risk of cancer was correlated with the level of individual antioxidant in the diet or blood, the inverse association between diet and cancer incidence became weak, nonexistent, or reversed. In a prospective study, the plasma levels of beta-carotene, lycopene, and total carotene were lower in cancer cases compared to controls. The risk of developing breast cancer was inversely proportion to the level of beta-carotene in the plasma.[128] In a similar study, the plasma level of alpha-carotene, but not other carotenoids, was inversely related to the risk of breast cancer.[129,130] In a review of 6 randomized clinical trials and 25 prospective studies, it was concluded that beta-carotene supplementation was not associated with decreased risk of lung cancer.[131] In the VITamines And Lifestyle (VITAL) cohort study, long-term intake of beta-carotene, retinol, and lutein was associated with increased risk of lung cancer.[132] In Brazilian women, dietary intake of folate, vitamin B6, or vitamin B12 had no overall association with breast cancer risk; however, dietary intake of high levels of folate was associated with increased risk of breast cancer in pre-menopausal women and MTR2756GG genotype.[133]

Increased intake of dietary flavonoids was associated with reduced risk of lung cancer[134]; however, another study reported no association between individual or multiple flavonoids intake and the risk of breast, ovarian, colorectal, lung, and endometrial cancer.[135] A study has reported that intake of lycopene and lycopene product through diet was associated with a decreased risk of prostate cancer.[136] In Women's Health Initiative (WHI) involving 133,614 postmenopausal women, dietary intake of antioxidants, carotenoids, and vitamin A was not associated with a reduction in ovarian cancer risk.[137] During 8 years of follow-up involving 56,007 French women, breast cancer risk was inversely associated with alpha-linolenic acid (ALA) intake from fruits, vegetables, and vegetables oil, but it was positively related to ALA intake from nut mixes and processed foods.[138] In addition, it was observed that the risk of breast cancer was inversely associated with intake of omega-3-fatty acids in women having highest levels of omega-6-fatty acids. Thus, epidemiologic studies with dietary intake of antioxidants, fat, fiber, or B-vitamins alone have produced conflicting results.

Experimental designs of any epidemiologic study have several inherent confounding factors that are associated with diet, lifestyle, and environment that could impact cancer incidence. It is very difficult to account for all of them in the data analysis. It should be emphasized that epidemiologic studies, despite the best experimental design and correct data interpretation, can only infer a direct or inverse relationship between single or multiple nutrients and the risk of cancer. The cause-effect relationship between micronutrients intake and cancer risk can only be established by a well-designed intervention trial in high-risk populations.

INTERVENTION STUDIES WITH SINGLE ANTIOXIDANTS (LUNG CANCER)

Most clinical trials have utilized the experimental design of drugs that is based on the concept of single drug-single target effect. In a large randomized, double-blind, placebo-controlled clinical trial, supplementation with synthetic beta-carotene at a dose of 20 mg/day increased the incidence of lung cancer, prostate cancer, and stomach cancer among male heavy tobacco smokers.[139–141] Heavy tobacco smokers are known to have high levels of internal oxidative environment; therefore, this increase in lung cancer incidence could have been predicted, because beta-carotene in a high internal oxidative environment of heavy smokers would be oxidized and then act as a prooxidant rather than as an antioxidant. This was further confirmed by the fact that the same dose of beta-carotene did not affect the incidence of cancer in normal populations who have a lower internal oxidative environment than the heavy tobacco smokers.[142] Supplementation with NAC reduced certain biomarkers associated with lung cancer in smokers,[143] but it remains uncertain whether NAC supplementation alone can affect the incidence of lung cancer.

INTERVENTION STUDIES WITH A SINGLE ANTIOXIDANT (OTHER CANCERS)

Beta-carotene supplementation reduced prostate cancer in patients with a low dietary intake of beta-carotene.[144] High doses of beta-carotene caused regression of leukoplakia (precancerous lesion in mouth).[145,146]

Supplementation with alpha-tocopherol (50 mg/day) reduced prostate cancer and colorectal cancer but increased the incidence of stomach cancer.[139] Supplementation with vitamin E (400 IU) produced no effect on the PSA levels[147]; however, high serum levels of vitamin E was associated with reduced prostate cancer incidence.[148–150] In another study, supplementation with vitamin E 400 IU a day was associated with reduced risk of prostate cancer in tobacco smokers, whereas beta-carotene supplementation was associated with reduced risk of this cancer only in those smokers who have low levels of beta-carotene.[144] Consumption of vitamin E alone increased the incidence of secondary primary cancer or recurrence of the initial tumor after cancer therapy.[151] The causal relationship between vitamin E supplementation and increased mortality as suggested earlier[125] has been contradicted by another statistical analysis.[152] Elevated levels of benzo (a) pyrene (B (a) P)-DNA adducts have been associated with a 3-fold increase in the risk of lung cancer in heavy tobacco smokers,[153] but supplementation with dl-alpha tocopherol (400 IU and vitamin C (500 mg) per day did not reduce the level of B (a) P-DNA adducts in men, but it reduced them in women.[153] Supplementation with individual vitamin C, vitamin E, or beta-carotene had no impact on cancer incidence or cancer mortality.[154] Using the population of Alpha-Tocopherol, Beta-Carotene Cancer Prevention (ATBC) study of male Finnish smokers, it was revealed that higher serum alpha-tocopherol concentrations was associated with reduced risk of pancreatic cancer.[155]

Supplementation with vitamin A at a dose of 300,000 IU/day for 12 months produced an 11% reduction in recurrence of primary non-small cell lung carcinoma,[156] but this high dose cannot be given for a prolonged period of time because of toxicity. Retinoids also caused regression of oral leukoplakia and other cancers.[157]

Supplementation with vitamin A (retinyl palmitate, 300,000 IU daily for one year, and 150,000 IU for the second year) and NAC (600 mg daily for 2 years) alone or in combination produced no benefit with respect to secondary primary tumor.[158] This study has utilized unusually high doses of vitamin A and NAC that could be toxic after a long-term consumption.

INTERVENTION STUDIES WITH MULTIPLE DIETARY ANTIOXIDANTS

Supplementation with multiple dietary antioxidants without endogenous antioxidants may produce inconsistent results in high-risk populations. These studies are described below. The administration of multiple dietary antioxidants vitamin A (40,000 IU), vitamin C (2,000 mg), vitamin E (400 IU), zinc (90 mg), and vitamin B6 (100 mg) per day in combination with BCG (Bacilli bilie de Calmette-Guerin) vaccine caused a 50% reduction in the incidence of recurrence of bladder cancer in 5 years, in comparison to control patients who received multiple vitamins containing RDA levels of nutrients and BCG.[159]

Supplementation with antioxidants (vitamin A, 30,000 IU; vitamin C, 1,000 mg; vitamin E, 70 mg) per day reduced the incidence of recurrence of colon polyps from 36% to 6%[160]; however, consumption of synthetic beta-carotene (25 mg), vitamin C (1,000 mg), and vitamin E (400 mg) per day failed to show any beneficial effects on the recurrence of colon polyps.[161] Daily administration of vitamin C (400 mg) and dl-alpha tocopherol also failed to reduce the incidence of recurrence of colon polyps.[162] In another study, daily supplementation with vitamin C (4,000 mg) and vitamin E (400 mg) also failed to reduce the risk of colon polyps, but when they were combined with a high-fiber diet (more than 12 grams per day), there was significant reduction in the incidence of recurrence of polyps.[163] This study indicated the importance of a high-fiber diet in combination with antioxidants in cancer prevention.

In Linxian General Population, Nutrition Interventional Trial utilized a preparation of multiple dietary antioxidants (beta-carotene, vitamin E, and selenium at doses 2–3 times that of the US RDA) reduced mortality by 10% and cancer incidence by 13%.[164] The beneficial effects of this supplementation on mortality were still evident up to 10 years after the cessation of supplementation and were consistently greater in younger participants.[165]

The combination of vitamins A, C, and E, omega-3 fatty acids, and folic acid significantly reduced recurrence of adenoma in patients after polypectomy.[166] In a clinical study, daily supplementation with vitamin E, selenium, vitamin C, and coenzyme Q10 did not affect serum levels of prostate specific antigen (PSA).[167] In a Selenium and Vitamin E Cancer Prevention Trial (SELECT), selenium (200 mcg/day) or vitamin E (400 IU/day) alone or in combination did not reduce the risk of prostate cancer.[109]

From the intervention studies discussed above, it appears that supplementation with dietary antioxidants alone did not produced consistent reduction in cancer incidence in high-risk populations. Although epidemiologic studies consistently showed inverse relationship between diets rich in antioxidants and risk of developing cancer, this relationship became weak, non-existence, and direct, when the relationship between individual antioxidants in the diet and cancer was evaluated.

INTERVENTION STUDIES WITH VITAMIN D AND CALCIUM

The role of vitamin D alone or in combination with calcium has been evaluated yielding often-inconsistent results. In one study, vitamin D 1000 IU per day reduced colorectal cancer.[168,169] In another study, vitamin D 400 IU and calcium 1000 mg per day produced no effect on colorectal cancer.[170] Administration of vitamin D 400 IU and calcium 1000 mg per day reduced colorectal cancer, but in combination with estrogen increased the risk of this cancer.[171] Analysis of several clinical studies showed that supplementation with elemental calcium may have modest effect in reducing the risk of colorectal cancer; however, this approach was not recommended for reducing the risk of colorectal cancer in general population.[172] Supplementation with elemental calcium 1000 mg and vitamin D 400 IU a day did not reduce the risk of breast cancer.[173] However, in another study, dietary intake of calcium was modestly associated with reduced risk of breast cancer in postmenopausal women.[125] In the Wheat Bran Fiber Trial, higher intake of Ca (1068 mg vs. 690 mg/day) decreased the risk of recurrence of colorectal adenoma by about 45%.[174] A possible effect of this treatment was also noted in women with BRCA mutation. Administration of calcium and vitamin D supplementation together reduced the recurrence of colorectal adenoma.[175]

INTERVENTION STUDIES WITH FOLATE AND B-VITAMINS

Diet rich in folate and vitamins B6 and B12 was associated with reduced risk of breast cancer and colorectal cancer[176–180] but had no association with pancreatic cancer. However, supplementation with folic acid alone did not reduce the incidence of colorectal adenoma and may possibly increase the risk.[181] In other studies,[181,182] consumption of folate did not reduce the incidence of colorectal cancer. In a clinical study on patients with polypectomy, supplementation with 5 mg folate daily reduced recurrence of colonic adenomas.[183] Dietary intake of high amounts of folate and vitamin B12 were independently associated with decreased risk of breast cancer, particularly in postmenopausal women, whereas there was no association between intake of vitamin B6 and breast cancer.[179] An epidemiologic study showed that there may be a nonlinear relationship between folate status and the risk of all-cancer mortality, and thus persons with low serum levels of folate may be at risk of cancer.[184]

INTERVENTION STUDIES WITH FAT AND FIBER

In females, a high-fat, low-fiber, western-style diet appears to be associated with increased levels of plasma and urinary estrogen, which acts as a tumor promoter. An intervention study (The Women's health Initiative Dietary Modification Trial) in which postmenopausal women received a low-fat (40% of calories from fat) or a high-fat (60% of calories from fat) diet showed that a low-fat diet did not reduce the risk of colorectal cancer during 8.1 years follow-up.[170] I am not sure if the diet in which fat contents represent 40% should be considered a low-fat diet. In addition, the protective effect of a low-fat diet alone may be a minor factor; therefore, the cancer protective effect of a low-fat diet alone cannot be assessed in any cancer prevention trial. The mechanisms of cancer protection by high fiber may involve elimination of mutagens and carcinogens formed during digestion through feces, and production of high amounts of butyric acid during fermentation of primarily soluble fibers by probiotic bacteria in the colon.

In the Polyp Prevention Trial, Dietary intervention, supplementation with reduced fat and increased consumption of fruits and vegetables and fiber produced no effect on prostate-specific antigen (PSA) and on the incidence of prostate cancer in normal men.[185] Similarly, adopting a diet low in fat (20% of total calories) and high in fiber (18 g per 1000 kcal) and fruits and vegetables (3.5 serving per 1000 kcal) did not influence the risk of recurrence of colorectal adenomas.[186] A dietary supplement (13.5 g/day vs. 2 g/day) with wheat bran fiber did not protect against recurrence of colorectal adenomas.[187] Supplementation with a diet high in vegetables, fruits, and fiber and low in fat did not reduce additional breast cancer events or mortality during a 7.3 years follow-up period.[188]

INTERVENTION STUDIES WITH NON-STEROIDAL ANTI-INFLAMMATORY DRUGS (NSAIDs)

Aspirin and indomethacin reduced the risk of cancer in animal models.[189] The use of NSAIDs was associated with a small decrease in lung cancer incidence,[190] and other cancers in humans.[191] The use of NSAIDs for a shorter period of time may be more effective in reducing the risk of non-melanoma skin cancer (squamous cell carcinoma and basal cell carcinoma).[192] Since chronic or recurrent prostate inflammation and oxidative stress may be involved in the development of prostate cancer, it has been suggested that a combination of aspirin and antioxidants may be useful in reducing the risk of prostate cancer.[193] These studies have revealed that addition of NSAIDs to a cancer prevention strategy could be useful in reducing the risk of cancer.

POTENTIAL REASONS FOR INCONSISTENT RESULTS WITH INDIVIDUAL MICRONUTRIENTS OR ASPIRIN IN CANCER PREVENTION STUDIES

The reasons for individual micronutrients or aspirin produce no effects, to some transient beneficial effects, to harmful effects on cancer incidence are not known; however, some potential causes are described here: (a) antioxidants show differential subcellular distribution and different mechanisms of action; therefore, a single antioxidant cannot protect all parts of the cell; (b) a single antioxidant in a high internal oxidative environment in high-risk patients is oxidized and can then itself act as a prooxidant rather than as an antioxidant; (c) the body protects against oxidative damage by elevating antioxidant enzymes, and dietary and endogenous antioxidants; (d) antioxidants neutralize free radicals by donating electrons to those molecules with unpaired electron, whereas antioxidant enzymes destroy free radicals by catalysis, converting them to harmless molecules such as water and oxygen. Therefore, both of these agents should be enhanced to achieve substantial protection against oxidative damage; (e) the affinity of different antioxidants for free radicals differs, depending upon their lipophilicity; (f) both the aqueous and lipid compartments of the cell need to be protected together. Water-soluble antioxidants such as vitamin C and glutathione protect molecules in the aqueous environment of the cells, whereas lipid soluble antioxidants such as vitamin A and vitamin

E protect molecules in the lipid compartment; (g) vitamin E is more effective in quenching free radicals in a reduced oxygenated cellular environment, whereas vitamin C and alpha-tocopherol are more effective in a higher oxygenated environment of the cells[194]; (h) vitamin C is important for recycling the oxidized form of alpha-tocopherol to the antioxidant form at the lipid/aqueous interface[195]; (i) antioxidants produce cell protective proteins by altering the expression of different microRNAs.[64] For example, some antioxidants can activate Nrf2 by upregulating miR-200a that inhibits its target protein Keap1, whereas others activate Nrf2 by downregulating miR-21 that binds with 3'-UTR Nrf2 mRNA.[196]

Aspirin may reduce chronic inflammation somewhat, but it has no effect on oxidative stress; therefore, it may not be effective in reducing the risk of cancer consistently.

Thus, the use of a single micronutrient or aspirin is not expected to yield any beneficial effects on cancer prevention. For this reason, a mixture of micronutrients that can simultaneously reduce oxidative stress and inflammation by enhancing the levels of antioxidant enzymes through the activation of Nrf2 pathway together with dietary and endogenous antioxidants for other chronic diseases, such as Alzheimer's disease and Parkinson's disease has been suggested.[64,93] The same suggestion is proposed for prevention of cancer. Oral supplementation can increase the levels of dietary and endogenous antioxidants; however, elevation of the levels of antioxidant enzymes requires an activation of Nrf2. Therefore, it is essential to understand the regulation of activation of Nrf2.

REGULATION OF ACTIVATION OF Nrf2

REACTIVE OXYGEN SPECIES (ROS) ACTIVATES Nrf2

Normally, during acute oxidative stress, ROS is needed to activate Nrf2 which then dissociates itself from Keap1-CuI-Rbx1 complex and translocates in the nucleus where it heterodimerizes with a small Maf protein, and binds with the ARE (antioxidant response element) leading to increased expression of target genes coding for several cytoprotective enzymes including antioxidant enzymes.[197–199] In this manner, activation of Nrf2 increases the levels of cytoprotective enzymes including antioxidant enzymes and phase-2-detoxifying enzymes.[200,201]

BINDING OF Nrf2 WITH ARE IN THE NUCLEUS

Activation of Nrf2 alone may not be sufficient to increase the levels of antioxidant enzymes. Activated Nrf2 must bind with antioxidant response element (ARE) in the nucleus for increasing the expression of its target genes. This binding ability of Nrf2 with ARE was impaired in aged rats and this defect was restored by supplementation with alpha-lipoic acid.[202] It is not known whether the binding ability of Nrf2 with ARE is impaired in cells after exposure to carcinogens.

EXISTENCE OF ROS-RESISTANT Nrf2 IN CELLS FOLLOWING EXPOSURE TO CARCINOGENS

The fact that increased oxidative stress and chronic inflammation occur in the cell following exposure to carcinogens suggest that activation of Nrf2 by ROS is impaired, because these biochemical defects continue to persists despite the presence of Nrf2. Activation of Nrf2 protected the mouse liver against 4ABP, a major human bladder carcinogen from tobacco and other environmental sources, but the levels of N-(deoxyguanosine-8-yl)-4-aminobiphenyl (dG-C8-ABP), a major ABP-DNA adduct in the bladder tissues and cells were higher in Nrf2 (+/+) mice than in Nrf2 lacking (−/−) mice.[203] This suggests that Nrf2 was not activated by ROS, causing increased levels of dG-C8-ABP that initiates carcinogenesis in the bladder. The incidence of bladder cancer was increased more in Nrf2 lacking (−/−) mice than in Nrf2 (+/+) mice. Treatment with oltipraz, a synthetic dithiolrthione, decreased the incidence of bladder cancer in the wild-type mice with Nrf2, but had very little effect in mice lacking Nrf2.[204] This suggests that activation of Nrf2 is essential for protection against a bladder carcinogen.

Exposure to 17β-estradiol increased the expression of miR-93 in the rat breast tissues and human breast cell lines and deceased the levels of its target protein Nrf2, causing increased oxidative stress. Treatment with vitamin C and resveratrol decreased the expression of miR-93 and enhanced the levels of Nrf2 leading to protection against estrogen-induced breast carcinogenesis.[77,205] The response of Nrf2 to inorganic arsenite-generated ROS in arsenic-transformed keratinocytes was weak that might contribute to increased oxidative DNA damage and fixation of mutational DNA damage, which contributes to skin carcinogenesis.[206] Long-term exposure to arsenite causes loss of Keap1 function by hypermethylation of its promoter region leading to accumulation of Nrf2, which is associated with well-established cancer cells.[207] This may account for the high levels of Nrf2 in cancer cells. Using urethane-induced lung cancer mouse model, it was demonstrated dual role of Nrf2: one to prevent cancer development during initiation phase following exposure to carcinogens and the second to facilitates transformation to cancer cells.[208] A curcumin derivative bis (2-hydroxybenzylidene) acetone (BHBA) protected against arsenite-induced lung cancer in human epithelial cells in culture by activating Nrf2.[209] During initiation phase of carcinogenesis following exposure to carcinogens, ROS are generated, but Nrf2 does not either respond to ROS or ROS overwhelms ROS-dependent protective response of Nrf2. Under such scenarios, certain phytochemicals and antioxidants can activate Nrf2. For example, cinnamaldehyde (CA) from the bark of *Cinnamomum aromaticum* suppressed azoxymethane/dextran sulfate sodium-induced colon carcinogenesis by activating Nrf2 in human colorectal epithelial cells in culture. CA-induced protection against chemical-induced colon carcinogenesis was evident in Nrf2 (+/+) mice but not in Nrf2 (−/−) mice.[210] Activation of Nrf2 was also essential for protecting against inflammation-associated colorectal cancer in mice.[211]

ANTIOXIDANTS AND PHYTOCHEMICALS ACTIVATE ROS-RESISTANT Nrf2

Activation of Nrf2 becomes impaired to ROS during chronic oxidative stress. However, some dietary antioxidants and phytochemicals can activate Nrf2 without requiring ROS. These include vitamin C,[212,213] vitamin E,[77] endogenous antioxidants such as alpha-lipoic acid,[202] coenzyme Q10,[214] synthetic antioxidant N-acetylcysteine (NAC),[215] omega-3-fatty acids,[216,217] and phytochemicals such as curcumin[218] and resveratrol.[219,220]

L-CARNITINE ACTIVATES Nrf2 BY A ROS-DEPENDENT MECHANISM

L-carnitine activates Nrf2 by a ROS-dependent mechanism,[221] probably by generating transient ROS.

ACTIVATION OF Nrf2 BY MicroRNAs

The complex of Keap1-Nrf2 in the cytoplasm prevents activation of Nrf2. Overexpression of miR-200a reduced Keap-1 levels, allowing Nrf2 to migrate to the nucleus where it binds to the ARE that enhanced the transcription of target cytoprotective genes, including antioxidant enzymes.[222] Some antioxidants can activate Nrf2 by downregulating miR-21 that binds with 3′-UTR Nrf2 mRNA.[196] Overexpression of miR-141 downregulated the expression of Keap1, causing translocation of Nrf2 from the cytoplasm to the nucleus where it increases the transcription of genes coding for cytoprotective enzymes including antioxidant enzymes. UV radiation-induced ROS reduced the expression of miR-141 that upregulated Keap1 and downregulated Nrf2 resulting cell death in human retinal pigment epithelial cells (RPEs) and retinal ganglion cells (RGSs).[223] Ectopic expression of miR-28 reduced the levels of Nrf2 without affecting the levels of Keap1 protein.[224]

SUPPRESSION OF CHRONIC INFLAMMATION

The activation of Nrf2 also suppresses chronic inflammation.[200,201] Some antioxidant compounds also reduce markers of chronic inflammation.[113,225–229]

RECOMMENDED MIXTURE OF MICRONUTRIENTS FOR THE PREVENTION OF CANCER

Based on the studies discussed above, a mixture of micronutrients containing vitamin A, mixed carotenoids, vitamin C, α-tocopheryl acetate, α-tocopheryl succinate, vitamin D3, alpha-lipoic acid, N-acetylcysteine, coenzyme Q10, L-carnitine, omega-3-fatty acids, curcumin, resveratrol, all B-vitamins, selenomethionine, and zinc, but without iron, copper, manganese, or heavy metals such as molybdenum and zirconium for cancer prevention is proposed. The inclusion of iron, copper, or manganese is not suggested, because these trace minerals, although essential for many biological reactions, combine with vitamin C and generate excessive amounts of free radicals. Furthermore, these minerals are absorbed from the intestine better in the presence of antioxidants than in their absence that could increase body store of free iron, copper, and manganese after long-term consumption. The body has no significant mechanisms of excretion of these trace minerals. Slight increase in the body store of free forms of these trace minerals can increase the risk of most chronic diseases including cancer. Heavy metals such as zirconium and molybdenum were not included because the body has no mechanisms of excretion of these heavy metals. Consequently, their levels in the body would increase after long-term consumption. High levels of these heavy metals could be neurotoxic.

It is expected that the proposed micronutrient mixture would simultaneously increase the levels of antioxidant enzymes by activating the Nrf2/ARE pathway, and dietary and endogenous antioxidants that would reduce oxidative stress and chronic inflammation at the same time, thereby reducing the incidence of cancer.

The recommended micronutrient mixture should be taken orally and divided into two doses, half in the morning and the other half in the evening with meal. This is because the biological half-lives of micronutrients are highly variable which can create high levels of fluctuations in the tissue levels of micronutrients. A 2-fold difference in the levels of certain micronutrients such as alpha-tocopheryl succinate causes a marked difference in the expression of gene profiles.[230] In order to maintain relatively steady level of micronutrients in the body, the proposed dose-schedule is necessary.

RECOMMENDED CHANGES IN DIET AND LIFESTYLE FOR THE PREVENTION OF CANCER

Dietary recommendations include daily consuming of a low-fat and high-fiber diet with plenty of fresh fruits and vegetables, avoiding excessive amounts protein, carbohydrates, or calories, restricting consumption of nitrite-rich cured meat, charcoal-broiled or smoked meat or fish, caffeine-containing beverages (cold or hot), pickled fruits and vegetables, and minimizing sugar consumption.

Lifestyle-related changes include stopping smoking and chewing tobacco, avoiding exposure to secondhand smoke, overexposure to sun and UV light for tanning and hyperbaric therapy for energy, restricting intake of alcohol, maintaining normal weight for your age and height, reducing stress by vacation, yoga, or meditation, and performing moderate exercise 4–5 times a week.

The efficacy of proposed micronutrient mixture together with changes in diet and lifestyle should be tested by well-designed preclinical and clinical studies. In the meanwhile, the proposed recommendations may be adopted by the individuals in consultation with their physicians or health professionals for reducing the risk of cancer

PROPOSED CANCER PREVENTION STRATEGIES

PRIMARY PREVENTION

Primary prevention includes cancer-free normal individuals of all ages and gender. It is expected that the proposed mixture of micronutrients together with modifications in the diet and lifestyle may reduce the development of cancer by simultaneously reducing oxidative stress and chronic inflammation.

SECONDARY PREVENTION

Secondary prevention includes individuals with a family history of cancer, cancer-free persons at high risk of developing cancer such as heavy tobacco smokers and cancer survivors with no sign of detectable cancer. An increased number of cancer patients are surviving because of the advancement in cancer therapy (surgery, chemotherapy, and radiation therapy). However, they exhibit short- and long-term adverse health effects induced by cancer treatment agents. Short-term effects include dementia referred to as *chemo brain*, fatigue, peripheral neuropathy, and increased susceptibility to infection because of impaired immune function. Some of these symptoms can last for a long time. Long-term adverse health effects include recurrence of initial primary tumors and development of secondary new tumors induced by cancer treatment agents. The proposed mixture of micronutrients together with modifications in diet and lifestyle may decrease the risk of the above adverse health effects by simultaneously reducing oxidative stress and chronic inflammation.

CAN CANCER WITH A FAMILY HISTORY BE PREVENTED?

It has been presumed that the genetic basis of cancer cannot be delayed or prevented; therefore, such individuals wait until the tumor appears. A study on the effect of a mixture of dietary and endogenous antioxidants on proton radiation-induced cancer in female *Drosophila melanogaster* suggests that antioxidants can reduce the incidence of genetic basis of cancer. For example, female flies carrying mutant HOP (TUM-1) become very sensitive to developing a leukemia-like cancer. Exposure to proton radiation markedly enhanced the incidence of this cancer. Supplementation with the antioxidant mixture before and after irradiation completely blocked radiation-induced cancer (collaboration with Dr Sharmila Bhattacharya of NASA at Moffat Field, CA). This result obtained from fruit flies cannot be extrapolated to humans, but this study at least suggests that antioxidants have the potential to reduce the risk or delay the appearance of tumors in individuals with a family history of cancer. Clinical studies should be performed to test this possibility.

PROBLEMS ASSOCIATED WITH IMPLEMENTATION OF DIETARY AND LIFESTYLE RECOMMENDATIONS

The reducing exposures to potential carcinogens from diet, environment, and lifestyle appear to be the most effective strategy for reducing the risk of cancer in humans; however, it is the most difficult issue to implement. In some cases, it is counterproductive, if totally eliminated, and in others, it may be difficult to achieve. For example, diagnostic X-rays are commonly used to detect and diagnose disease earlier; therefore, they should not be avoided. Avoiding ultraviolet radiation from sun exposure appears to be the easiest thing to do to reduce the risk of skin cancer, but the beaches in summer are full of sunbathers in spite of repeated warnings. Because of the addictive nature of tobacco smoking, there has been no significant change in the number of smokers in the United States in spite of massive education program and state and federal laws prohibiting smoking in public places. It is difficult to implement the environmental- and lifestyle-related cancer risk factors that contribute to cancer development. Nevertheless, avoiding exposure to potential carcinogens as much as possible must be part of the proposed cancer prevention strategy. Dietary recommendations are difficult to implement, because human behaviors are not easily changed. Nevertheless, the dietary recommendations must be part of proposed cancer preventive strategy for this population.

TOXICITY OF MICRONUTRIENTS

References listed in this section have been described in a review.[231] Antioxidants at doses higher than those that are recommended for the proposed micronutrient preparations have been consumed by the US population for decades without reported toxicity. However, they could be harmful for some individuals at certain high doses when consumed daily for a long period of time. For example, vitamin at doses 10,000 IU or more can cause birth defects in pregnant women, and beta-carotene can produce bronzing of skin at doses 50 mg or more that is reversible on discontinuation. Vitamin C as ascorbic acid at high doses (10 grams or more) can cause diarrhea in some individuals, vitamin E at high doses (2,000 IU or more) can induce clotting defects after long-term consumption, vitamin B6 at high doses may produce peripheral neuropathy, and selenium at doses (400 mcg or more) can cause skin and liver toxicity after long-term consumption. Coenzyme Q10 has no known toxicity, and recommended daily doses are 30–400 mg. N-acetylcysteine doses of 250–1500 mg and alpha-lipoic acid doses of 600 mg are used in humans without toxicity. All ingredients present in the proposed micronutrient preparations are safe and come under category of "food supplement"; therefore, they do not require FDA approval for their use.

CONCLUSIONS

Cancer incidence in the US population appears to be on the rise. Although recommendations for changes in diet and lifestyle appear to have scientific basis for cancer prevention, their implementation is most difficult, because human behaviors are very difficult to change. Therefore, additional cancer prevention strategies are needed. There are substantial data to show that increased oxidative stress and chronic inflammation initiate carcinogenesis following exposure to carcinogens. In addition, alterations in the expression of microRNAs are involved in the initiation of carcinogenic processes. Pro-inflammatory cytokines and ROS mediate their damaging effects by changing the expression of microRNAs, while certain antioxidants mediated their protective effect by altering the expression of microRNAs. Thus, attenuation of oxidative stress and chronic inflammation at the same time appears to be one of the rationale choices for prevention of cancer. To address this issue, several studies primarily using one or more dietary micronutrients, cell culture, animal models, and humans showed inconsistent results varying from no effect, to transient beneficial effects, to harmful effects. The reasons for the inconsistent results are discussed. I have proposed that in order to simultaneously reduce oxidative stress and chronic inflammation, it is essential to increase the levels of cytoprotective enzymes including antioxidant enzymes and dietary and endogenous antioxidant at the same time. The levels of antioxidants can easily be increased by supplementation, but enhancing the levels of cytoprotective enzymes requires activation of Nrf2. During acute stress, activation of Nrf2 requires ROS, however, this response becomes impaired during chronic stress. Certain antioxidants and phytochemicals activate Nrf2 without ROS stimulation. Based on these observations, I have proposed a mixture of micronutrients that would enhance the levels of cytoprotective enzymes including antioxidant enzymes through activation of the Nrf2/ARE pathway, and dietary and endogenous antioxidants. This mixture together with recommendations in changes in diet and lifestyle may reduce the incidence of cancer among individuals belonging to primary or secondary prevention. Preclinical and clinical studies using proposed cancer prevention strategies should be initiated.

REFERENCES

1. Prasad KN, Cole W, Hovland P. Cancer prevention studies: Past, present, and future directions. *Nutrition.* 1998;14(2):197–210; discussion 237–198.
2. Duesberg PH, Schwartz JR. Latent viruses and mutated oncogenes: No evidence for pathogenicity. *Prog Nucleic Acid Res Mol Biol.* 1992;43:135–204.
3. Zhai R, Liu G, Asomaning K, et al. Genetic polymorphisms of VEGF, interactions with cigarette smoking exposure and esophageal adenocarcinoma risk. *Carcinogenesis.* 2008;29(12):2330–2334.
4. Xu T, Zhu Y, Wei QK, et al. A functional polymorphism in the miR-146a gene is associated with the risk for hepatocellular carcinoma. *Carcinogenesis.* 2008;29(11):2126–2131.
5. Zhang Z, Wang S, Wang M, Tong N, Fu G, Zhang Z. Genetic variants in RUNX3 and risk of bladder cancer: A haplotype-based analysis. *Carcinogenesis.* 2008;29(10):1973–1978.
6. Tworoger SS, Gertig DM, Gates MA, Hecht JL, Hankinson SE. Caffeine, alcohol, smoking, and the risk of incident epithelial ovarian cancer. *Cancer.* 2008;112(5):1169–1177.
7. Boutwell R. Biology and biochemistry of two-steps carcinogenesis. In: Meyskens FJ, Prasad, KN, eds. *Modulation and Mediation of Cancer by Vitamins.* Basel, Switzerland: Karger; 1983:2.
8. Ames BN. Dietary carcinogens and anticarcinogens: Oxygen radicals and degenerative diseases. *Science.* 1983;221(4617):1256–1264.
9. Hogervorst JG, Schouten LJ, Konings EJ, Goldbohm RA, van den Brandt PA. Lung cancer risk in relation to dietary acrylamide intake. *J Natl Cancer Inst.* 2009;101(9):651–662.
10. Wogan GN, Hecht SS, Felton JS, Conney AH, Loeb LA. Environmental and chemical carcinogenesis. *Semin Cancer Biol.* 2004;14(6):473–486.
11. Chen YJ, Chang JT, Liao CT, et al. Head and neck cancer in the betel quid chewing area: Recent advances in molecular carcinogenesis. *Cancer Sci.* 2008;99(8):1507–1514.
12. Genkinger JM, Spiegelman D, Anderson KE, et al. Alcohol intake and pancreatic cancer risk: A pooled analysis of fourteen cohort studies. *Cancer Epidemiol Biomarkers Prev.* 2009;18(3):765–776.
13. Crous-Bou M, Porta M, Lopez T, et al. Lifetime history of alcohol consumption and K-ras mutations in pancreatic ductal adenocarcinoma. *Environ Mol Mutagen.* 2009;50(5):421–430.
14. McCullough MJ, Farah CS. The role of alcohol in oral carcinogenesis with particular reference to alcohol-containing mouthwashes. *Aust Dent J.* 2008;53(4):302–305.
15. Lof M, Weiderpass E. Impact of diet on breast cancer risk. *Curr Opin Obstet Gynecol.* 2009;21(1):80–85.
16. Abuzetun JY, Loberiza F, Vose J, et al. The Stanford V regimen is effective in patients with good risk Hodgkin lymphoma but radiotherapy is a necessary component. *Br J Haematol.* 2009;144(4):531–537.
17. Hardell L, Carlberg M, Soderqvist F, Hansson Mild K. Meta-analysis of long-term mobile phone use and the association with brain tumours. *Int J Oncol.* 2008;32(5):1097–1103.
18. Croft RJ, McKenzie RJ, Inyang I, Benke GP, Anderson V, Abramson MJ. Mobile phones and brain tumours: A review of epidemiological research. *Australas Phys Eng Sci Med.* 2008;31(4):255–267.
19. Sadetzki S, Chetrit A, Jarus-Hakak A, et al. Cellular phone use and risk of benign and malignant parotid gland tumors: A nationwide case-control study. *Am J Epidemiol.* 2008;167(4):457–467.
20. Sato Y, Akiba S, Kubo O, Yamaguchi N. A case-case study of mobile phone use and acoustic neuroma risk in Japan. *Bioelectromagnetics.* 2011;32(2):85–93.
21. Lehrer S, Green S, Stock RG. Association between number of cell phone contracts and brain tumor incidence in 19 US states. *J Neurooncol.* 2011;101(3):505–507.
22. Tillmann T, Ernst H, Ebert S, et al. Carcinogenicity study of GSM and DCS wireless communication signals in B6C3F1 mice. *Bioelectromagnetics.* 2007;28(3):173–187.
23. Kim JY, Hong SY, Lee YM, et al. In vitro assessment of clastogenicity of mobile-phone radiation (835 MHz) using the alkaline comet assay and chromosomal aberration test. *Environ Toxicol.* 2008;23(3):319–327.
24. Ahern TP, Lash TL, Egan KM, Baron JA. Lifetime tobacco smoke exposure and breast cancer incidence. *Cancer Causes Control.* 2009;20(10):1837–1844.
25. Hu SY, Duan HF, Li QF, et al. Hepatocyte growth factor protects endothelial cells against gamma ray irradiation-induced damage. *Acta Pharmacol Sin.* 2009;30(10):1415–1420.
26. Calkins MJ, Jakel RJ, Johnson DA, Chan K, Kan YW, Johnson JA. Protection from mitochondrial complex II inhibition in vitro and in vivo by Nrf2-mediated transcription. *Proc Natl Acad Sci U S A.* 2005;102(1):244–249.

27. Kropp S, Chang-Claude J. Active and passive smoking and risk of breast cancer by age 50 years among German women. *Am J Epidemiol.* 2002;156(7):616–626.
28. Theis RP, Dolwick Grieb SM, Burr D, Siddiqui T, Asal NR. Smoking, environmental tobacco smoke, and risk of renal cell cancer: A population-based case-control study. *BMC Cancer.* 2008;8:387.
29. Hemelt M, Yamamoto H, Cheng KK, Zeegers MP. The effect of smoking on the male excess of bladder cancer: A meta-analysis and geographical analyses. *Int J Cancer.* 2009;124(2):412–419.
30. Montella M, Tramacere I, Tavani A, et al. Coffee, decaffeinated coffee, tea intake, and risk of renal cell cancer. *Nutr Cancer.* 2009;61(1):76–80.
31. Ganmaa D, Willett WC, Li TY, et al. Coffee, tea, caffeine and risk of breast cancer: A 22-year follow-up. *Int J Cancer.* 2008;122(9):2071–2076.
32. Ishitani K, Lin J, Manson JE, Buring JE, Zhang SM. Caffeine consumption and the risk of breast cancer in a large prospective cohort of women. *Arch Intern Med.* 2008;168(18):2022–2031.
33. Byun HS, Song JK, Kim YR, et al. Caspase-8 has an essential role in resveratrol-induced apoptosis of rheumatoid fibroblast-like synoviocytes. *Rheumatology (Oxford).* 2008;47(3):301–308.
34. Lueth NA, Anderson KE, Harnack LJ, Fulkerson JA, Robien K. Coffee and caffeine intake and the risk of ovarian cancer: The Iowa Women's Health Study. *Cancer Causes Control.* 2008;19(10):1365–1372.
35. Kurahashi N, Inoue M, Iwasaki M, Sasazuki S, Tsugane S. Coffee, green tea, and caffeine consumption and subsequent risk of bladder cancer in relation to smoking status: A prospective study in Japan. *Cancer Sci.* 2008;100(2):284–291.
36. Larsson SC, Wolk A. Coffee consumption and risk of liver cancer: A meta-analysis. *Gastroenterology.* 2007;132(5):1740–1745.
37. Abdollahi-Roodsaz S, Joosten LA, Koenders MI, van den Brand BT, van de Loo FA, van den Berg WB. Local interleukin-1-driven joint pathology is dependent on toll-like receptor 4 activation. *Am J Pathol.* 2009;175(5):2004–2013.
38. Kim JH, Thimmulappa RK, Kumar V, et al. NRF2-mediated Notch pathway activation enhances hematopoietic reconstitution following myelosuppressive radiation. *The J Clin Invest.* 2014;124(2):730–741.
39. Liu Z, Shen C, Tao Y, et al. Chemopreventive efficacy of menthol on carcinogen-induced cutaneous carcinoma through inhibition of inflammation and oxidative stress in mice. *Food Chem Toxicol.* 2015;82:12–18.
40. Bishak YK, Payahoo L, Osatdrahimi A, Nourazarian A. Mechanisms of cadmium carcinogenicity in the gastrointestinal tract. *Asian Pac J Cancer Prev.* 2015;16(1):9–21.
41. Kanwal R, Pandey M, Bhaskaran N, et al. Protection against oxidative DNA damage and stress in human prostate by glutathione S-transferase P1. *Mol Carcinog.* 2014;53(1):8–18.
42. Choudhari SK, Chaudhary M, Gadbail AR, Sharma A, Tekade S. Oxidative and antioxidative mechanisms in oral cancer and precancer: A review. *Oral Oncol.* 2014;50(1):10–18.
43. Azad N, Iyer A, Vallyathan V, et al. Role of oxidative/nitrosative stress-mediated Bcl-2 regulation in apoptosis and malignant transformation. *Ann N Y Acad Sci.* 2010;1203:1–6.
44. Wu Q, Ni X. ROS-mediated DNA methylation pattern alterations in carcinogenesis. *Curr Drug Targets.* 2015;16(1):13–19.
45. Sugar LM. Inflammation and prostate cancer. *Can J Urol.* 2006;13 Suppl 1:46–47.
46. Walser T, Cui X, Yanagawa J, et al. Smoking and lung cancer: The role of inflammation. *Proc Am Thorac Soc.* 2008;5(8):811–815.
47. Maher SG, Reynolds JV. Basic concepts of inflammation and its role in carcinogenesis. *Recent Results Cancer Res.* 2011;185:1–34.
48. Landskron G, De la Fuente M, Thuwajit P, Thuwajit C, Hermoso MA. Chronic inflammation and cytokines in the tumor microenvironment. *J Immunol Res.* 2014;2014:149185.
49. Cunha LL, Marcello MA, Ward LS. The role of the inflammatory microenvironment in thyroid carcinogenesis. *Endocr Relat Cancer.* 2014;21(3):R85–R103.
50. Radons J. The role of inflammation in sarcoma. *Adv Exp Med Biol.* 2014;816:259–313.
51. Deivendran S, Marzook KH, Radhakrishna Pillai M. The role of inflammation in cervical cancer. *Adv Exp Med Biol.* 2014;816:377–399.
52. Feller L, Altini M, Lemmer J. Inflammation in the context of oral cancer. *Oral Oncol.* 2013;49(9):887–892.
53. Sowers JL, Johnson KM, Conrad C, Patterson JT, Sowers LC. The role of inflammation in brain cancer. *Adv Exp Med Biol.* 2014;816:75–105.
54. Jiang X, Shapiro DJ. The immune system and inflammation in breast cancer. *Mol Cell Endocrinol.* 2014;382(1):673–682.

55. Gomes M, Teixeira AL, Coelho A, Araujo A, Medeiros R. The role of inflammation in lung cancer. *Adv Exp Med Biol.* 2014;816:1–23.

56. de Vivar Chevez AR, Finke J, Bukowski R. The role of inflammation in kidney cancer. *Adv Exp Med Biol.* 2014;816:197–234.

57. Valenzuela MA, Canales J, Corvalan AH, Quest AF. Helicobacter pylori-induced inflammation and epigenetic changes during gastric carcinogenesis. *World J Gastroenterol.* 2015;21(45):12742–12756.

58. Wang H, Cho CH. Effect of NF-kappaB signaling on apoptosis in chronic inflammation-associated carcinogenesis. *Curr Cancer Drug Targets.* 2010;10(6):593–599.

59. Lin R, Zhang C, Zheng J, et al. Chronic inflammation-associated genomic instability paves the way for human esophageal carcinogenesis. *Oncotarget.* 2016;7(17):24564–24571.

60. Mitagami Y, Yasunaga J, Kinosada H, Ohshima K, Matsuoka M. Interferon-gamma promotes inflammation and development of T-cell lymphoma in HTLV-1 bZIP factor transgenic mice. *PLoS Pathog.* 2015;11(8):e1005120.

61. Shimizu T, Marusawa H, Endo Y, Chiba T. Inflammation-mediated genomic instability: Roles of activation-induced cytidine deaminase in carcinogenesis. *Cancer Sci.* 2012;103(7):1201–1206.

62. Lin R, Xiao D, Guo Y, et al. Chronic inflammation-related DNA damage response: A driving force of gastric cardia carcinogenesis. *Oncotarget.* 2015;6(5):2856–2864.

63. Xie Z, Qu Y, Leng Y, et al. Human colon carcinogenesis is associated with increased interleukin-17-driven inflammatory responses. *Drug Des Devel Ther.* 2015;9:1679–1689.

64. Prasad KN. Oxidative stress and pro-inflammatory cytokines may act as one of signals for regulating microRNAs expression in Alzheimer's disease. *Mech Ageing Dev.* 2017;162:63–71.

65. Prasad KN. Oxidative stress, pro-inflammatory cytokines, and antioxidants regulate expression levels of MicroRNAs in Parkinson's Disease. *Curr Aging Sci.* 2017;10(3):177–184.

66. Lee RC, Feinbaum RL, Ambros V. The C. elegans heterochronic gene lin-4 encodes small RNAs with antisense complementarity to lin-14. *Cell.* 1993;75(5):843–854.

67. Wightman B, Ha I, Ruvkun G. Posttranscriptional regulation of the heterochronic gene lin-14 by lin-4 mediates temporal pattern formation in C. elegans. *Cell.* 1993;75(5):855–862.

68. Macfarlane LA, Murphy PR. MicroRNA: Biogenesis, function and role in cancer. *Curr Genomics.* 2010;11(7):537–561.

69. Londin E, Loher P, Telonis AG, et al. Analysis of 13 cell types reveals evidence for the expression of numerous novel primate- and tissue-specific microRNAs. *Proc Natl Acad Sci U S A.* 2015;112 (10):E1106–E1115.

70. Denli AM, Tops BB, Plasterk RH, Ketting RF, Hannon GJ. Processing of primary microRNAs by the Microprocessor complex. *Nature.* 2004;432(7014):231–235.

71. Lee Y, Ahn C, Han J, et al. The nuclear RNase III Drosha initiates microRNA processing. *Nature.* 2003;425(6956):415–419.

72. Hutvagner G, McLachlan J, Pasquinelli AE, Balint E, Tuschl T, Zamore PD. A cellular function for the RNA-interference enzyme Dicer in the maturation of the let-7 small temporal RNA. *Science.* 2001;293(5531):834–838.

73. Chen D, Li Z, Chen T. Increased expression of miR-34a in mouse spleen one day after exposure to N-ethyl-N-nitrosourea. *J Appl Toxicol.* 2011;31(5):496–498.

74. Yang Q, Xu E, Dai J, et al. miR-21 regulates N-methyl-N-nitro-N′-nitrosoguanidine-induced gastric tumorigenesis by targeting FASLG and BTG2. *Toxicol Lett.* 2014;228(3):147–156.

75. Huan LC, Wu JC, Chiou BH, et al. MicroRNA regulation of DNA repair gene expression in 4-aminobiphenyl-treated HepG2 cells. *Toxicology.* 2014;322:69–77.

76. Chuturgoon AA, Phulukdaree A, Moodley D. Fumonisin B(1) modulates expression of human cytochrome P450 1b1 in human hepatoma (Hepg2) cells by repressing Mir-27b. *Toxicol Lett.* 2014;227(1):50–55.

77. Singh B, Ronghe AM, Chatterjee A, Bhat NK, Bhat HK. MicroRNA-93 regulates NRF2 expression and is associated with breast carcinogenesis. *Carcinogenesis.* 2013;34(5):1165–1172.

78. Juhasz K, Gombos K, Szirmai M, et al. DMBA induces deregulation of miRNA expression of let-7, miR-21 and miR-146a in CBA/CA mice. *In Vivo.* 2012;26(1):113–117.

79. Juhasz K, Gombos K, Szirmai M, et al. Very early effect of DMBA and MNU on microRNA expression. *In Vivo.* 2013;27(1):113–117.

80. Izzotti A, Larghero P, Longobardi M, et al. Dose-responsiveness and persistence of microRNA expression alterations induced by cigarette smoke in mouse lung. *Mutat Res.* 2011;717(1–2):9–16.

81. Forte E, Salinas RE, Chang C, et al. The Epstein-Barr virus (EBV)-induced tumor suppressor microRNA MiR-34a is growth promoting in EBV-infected B cells. *J Virol*. 2012;86(12):6889–6898.

82. Yu H, Lu J, Zuo L, et al. Epstein-Barr virus downregulates microRNA 203 through the oncoprotein latent membrane protein 1: A contribution to increased tumor incidence in epithelial cells. *J Virol*. 2012;86(6):3088–3099.

83. Chen Z, Wang D, Gu C, et al. Down-regulation of let-7 microRNA increased K-ras expression in lung damage induced by radon. *Environ Toxicol Pharmacol*. 2015;40(2):541–548.

84. Newmark H, Mergen W. Application of ascorbic acid and tocopherols as inhibitors of nitrosamine formation and oxidation in food. In: Solms J, Hall R, eds. *Criteria of Food Acceptance*. Zurich, Switzerland: Forster Publishing; 1981:379.

85. Dion PW, Bright-See EB, Smith CC, Bruce WR. The effect of dietary ascorbic acid and alpha-tocopherol on fecal mutagenicity. *Mutat Res*. 1982;102(1):27–37.

86. Duthie SJ, Ma A, Ross MA, Collins AR. Antioxidant supplementation decreases oxidative DNA damage in human lymphocytes. *Cancer Res*. 1996;56(6):1291–1295.

87. Sram RJ, Dobias L, Pastorkova A, Rossner P, Janca L. Effect of ascorbic acid prophylaxis on the frequency of chromosome aberrations in the peripheral lymphocytes of coal-tar workers. *Mutat Res*. 1983;120(2–3):181–186.

88. Weitberg AB, Weitzman SA, Clark EP, Stossel TP. Effects of antioxidants on oxidant-induced sister chromatid exchange formation. *J Clin Invest*. 1985;75(6):1835–1841.

89. Zovoilis A, Agbemenyah HY, Agis-Balboa RC, et al. MicroRNA-34c is a novel target to treat dementias. *EMBO J*. 2011;30(20):4299–4308.

90. Reddy BS. Dietary fat, calories, and fiber in colon cancer. *Prev Med*. 1993;22(5):738–749.

91. Delafuente JC, Prendergast JM, Modigh A. Immunologic modulation by vitamin C in the elderly. *Int J Immunopharmacol*. 1986;8(2):205–211.

92. Ringer TV, DeLoof MJ, Winterrowd GE, et al. Beta-carotene's effects on serum lipoproteins and immunologic indices in humans. *Am J Clin Nutr*. 1991;53(3):688–694.

93. Prasad KN. Simultaneous activation of Nrf2 and elevation of antioxidant compounds for reducing oxidative stress and chronic inflammation in human Alzheimer's disease. *Mech Ageing Dev*. 2016;153:41–47.

94. Prasad KN. Simultaneous activation of Nrf2 and elevation of dietary and endogenous antioxidants for prevention and improved managment of Parkinson's disease. In: Bondy SCC, A., ed. *Inflammation, Aging and Oxidative Stress*. New York: Springer; 2016:277–301.

95. Noratto GD, Kim Y, Talcott ST, Mertens-Talcott SU. Flavonol-rich fractions of yaupon holly leaves (Ilex vomitoria, Aquifoliaceae) induce microRNA-146a and have anti-inflammatory and chemopreventive effects in intestinal myofibroblast CCD-18Co cells. *Fitoterapia*. 2011;82(4):557–569.

96. Altamemi I, Murphy EA, Catroppo JF, et al. Role of microRNAs in resveratrol-mediated mitigation of colitis-associated tumorigenesis in Apc(Min/+) mice. *J Pharmacol Exp Ther*. 2014;350(1):99–109.

97. Prasad KN, Edwards-Prasad J. Effects of tocopherol (vitamin E) acid succinate on morphological alterations and growth inhibition in melanoma cells in culture. *Cancer Res*. 1982;42(2):550–555.

98. Radner BS, Kennedy AR. Suppression of X-ray induced transformation by vitamin E in mouse C3H/10T1/2 cells. *Cancer Lett*. 1986;32(1):25–32.

99. Borek C, Ong A, Mason H, Donahue L, Biaglow JE. Selenium and vitamin E inhibit radiogenic and chemically induced transformation in vitro via different mechanisms. *Proc Natl Acad Sci U S A*. 1986;83(5):1490–1494.

100. Pung A, Rundhaug JE, Yoshizawa CN, Bertram JS. Beta-carotene and canthaxanthin inhibit chemically and physically induced neoplastic transformation in 10T1/2 cells. *Carcinogenesis*. 1988;9(9):1533–1539.

101. Kennedy AR, Krinsky NI. Effects of retinoids, beta-carotene, and canthaxanthin on UV- and X-ray-induced transformation of C3H10T1/2 cells in vitro. *Nutr Cancer*. 1994;22(3):219–232.

102. Venugopal D, Zahid M, Mailander PC, et al. Reduction of estrogen-induced transformation of mouse mammary epithelial cells by N-acetylcysteine. *J Steroid Biochem Mol Biol*. 2008;109(1–2):22–30.

103. Cohen M, Bhagavan HN. Ascorbic acid and gastrointestinal cancer. *J Am Coll Nutr*. 1995;14(6):565–578.

104. Prasad KN, Edwards-Prasad J. Vitamin E and cancer prevention: Recent advances and future potentials. *J Am Coll Nutr*. 1992;11(5):487–500.

105. Hill DL, Grubbs CJ. Retinoids as chemopreventive and anticancer agents intact animals (review). *Anticancer Res*. 1982;2(1–2):111–124.

106. Krinsky NI. Antioxidant functions of carotenoids. *Free Radic Biol Med*. 1989;7(6):617–635.

107. Santamaria L, Bianchi, A, Mobilio, G. Cancer prevention by carotenoids. In: Tryfiates GP, KN, ed. *Nutrition, Growth and Cancer*. New York: Alan R Liss; 1988:177.

108. Venkateswaran V, Klotz LH, Ramani M, et al. A combination of micronutrients is beneficial in reducing the incidence of prostate cancer and increasing survival in the Lady transgenic model. *Cancer Prev Res (Phila Pa)*. 2009;2(5):473–483.

109. Lippman SM, Klein EA, Goodman PJ, et al. Effect of selenium and vitamin E on risk of prostate cancer and other cancers: The Selenium and Vitamin E Cancer Prevention Trial (SELECT). *JAMA*. 2009;301(1):39–51.

110. Chen CS, Squire JA, Wells PG. Reduced tumorigenesis in p53 knockout mice exposed in utero to low-dose vitamin E. *Cancer*. 2009;115(7):1563–1575.

111. Chae SW, Kang BY, Hwang O, Choi HJ. Cyclooxygenase-2 is involved in oxidative damage and alpha-synuclein accumulation in dopaminergic cells. *Neurosci Lett*. 2008;436(2):205–209.

112. Aarsland D, Rongve A, Nore SP, et al. Frequency and case identification of dementia with Lewy bodies using the revised consensus criteria. *Dement Geriatr Cogn Disord*. 2008;26(5):445–452.

113. Lee HS, Jung KK, Cho JY, et al. Neuroprotective effect of curcumin is mainly mediated by blockade of microglial cell activation. *Pharmazie*. 2007;62(12):937–942.

114. Reliene R, Schiestl RH. Antioxidant N-acetyl cysteine reduces incidence and multiplicity of lymphoma in Atm deficient mice. *DNA Repair (Amst)*. 2006;5(7):852–859.

115. Balansky RM, Ganchev G, D'Agostini F, De Flora S. Effects of N-acetylcysteine in an esophageal carcinogenesis model in rats treated with diethylnitrosamine and diethyldithiocarbamate. *Int J Cancer*. 2002;98(4):493–497.

116. Martin KR, Trempus C, Saulnier M, Kari FW, Barrett JC, French JE. Dietary N-acetyl-L-cysteine modulates benzo[a]pyrene-induced skin tumors in cancer-prone p53 haploinsufficient Tg. AC (v-Ha-ras) mice. *Carcinogenesis*. 2001;22(9):1373–1378.

117. Lubet RA, Steele VE, Eto I, Juliana MM, Kelloff GJ, Grubbs CJ. Chemopreventive efficacy of anethole trithione, N-acetyl-L-cysteine, miconazole and phenethylisothiocyanate in the DMBA-induced rat mammary cancer model. *Int J Cancer*. 1997;72(1):95–101.

118. De Flora S, Rossi GA, De Flora A. Metabolic, desmutagenic and anticarcinogenic effects of N-acetylcysteine. *Respiration*. 1986;50 Suppl 1:43–49.

119. Hao J, Zhang B, Liu B, et al. Effect of alpha-tocopherol, N-acetylcysteine and omeprazole on esophageal adenocarcinoma formation in a rat surgical model. *Int J Cancer*. 2009;124(6):1270–1275.

120. Sakano K, Takahashi M, Kitano M, Sugimura T, Wakabayashi K. Suppression of azoxymethane-induced colonic premalignant lesion formation by coenzyme Q10 in rats. *Asian Pac J Cancer Prev*. 2006;7(4):599–603.

121. Toth B, Patil K. Enhancing effect of vitamin E on murine intestinal tumorigenesis by 1,2-dimethylhydrazine dihydrochloride. *J Natl Cancer Inst*. 1983;70(6):1107–1111.

122. Fukushima S, Imaida K, Shibata MA, Tamano S, Kurata Y, Shirai T. L-ascorbic acid amplification of second-stage bladder carcinogenesis promotion by NaHCO3. *Cancer Res*. 1988;48(22):6317–6320.

123. Hennekens CH. Antioxidant vitamins and cancer. *Am J Med*. 1994;97(3A):2S–4S; discussion 22S–28S.

124. Buring J, Hennekens, CH. Antioxidant vitamins in cancer: The physician' Health Study and Women's Health Study. In: Prasad K, Santamaria, L, Williams, RM, eds. *Nutrients in Cancer Prevention and Treatment*. Totowa, NJ: Humana Press; 1995:223.

125. Koushik A, Hunter DJ, Spiegelman D, et al. Fruits and vegetables and ovarian cancer risk in a pooled analysis of 12 cohort studies. *Cancer Epidemiol Biomarkers Prev*. 2005;14(9):2160–2167.

126. Rodrigues MJ, Bouyon A, Alexandre J. [Role of antioxidant complements and supplements in oncology in addition to an equilibrate regimen: A systematic review]. *Bull Cancer*. 2009;96(6):677–684.

127. Jedrychowski W, Maugeri U. An apple a day may hold colorectal cancer at bay: Recent evidence from a case-control study. *Rev Environ Health*. 2009;24(1):59–74.

128. Sato R, Helzlsouer KJ, Alberg AJ, Hoffman SC, Norkus EP, Comstock GW. Prospective study of carotenoids, tocopherols, and retinoid concentrations and the risk of breast cancer. *Cancer Epidemiol Biomarkers Prev*. 2002;11(5):451–457.

129. Tamimi RM, Hankinson SE, Campos H, et al. Plasma carotenoids, retinol, and tocopherols and risk of breast cancer. *Am J Epidemiol*. 2005;161(2):153–160.

130. Kabat GC, Kim M, Adams-Campbell LL, et al. Longitudinal study of serum carotenoid, retinol, and tocopherol concentrations in relation to breast cancer risk among postmenopausal women. *Am J Clin Nutr*. 2009;90(1):162–169.

131. Gallicchio L, Boyd K, Matanoski G, et al. Carotenoids and the risk of developing lung cancer: A systematic review. *Am J Clin Nutr.* 2008;88(2):372–383.

132. Satia JA, Littman A, Slatore CG, Galanko JA, White E. Long-term use of beta-carotene, retinol, lycopene, and lutein supplements and lung cancer risk: Results from the VITamins And Lifestyle (VITAL) study. *Am J Epidemiol.* 2009;169(7):815–828.

133. Ma E, Iwasaki M, Junko I, et al. Dietary intake of folate, vitamin B6, and vitamin B12, genetic polymorphism of related enzymes, and risk of breast cancer: A case-control study in Brazilian women. *BMC Cancer.* 2009;9:122.

134. Tang NP, Zhou B, Wang B, Yu RB, Ma J. Flavonoids intake and risk of lung cancer: A meta-analysis. *Jpn J Clin Oncol.* 2009;39(6):352–359.

135. Wang L, Lee IM, Zhang SM, Blumberg JB, Buring JE, Sesso HD. Dietary intake of selected flavonols, flavones, and flavonoid-rich foods and risk of cancer in middle-aged and older women. *Am J Clin Nutr.* 2009;89(3):905–912.

136. Ellinger S, Ellinger J, Muller SC, Stehle P. [Tomatoes and lycopene in prevention and therapy—is there an evidence for prostate diseases?]. *Aktuelle Urol.* 2009;40(1):37–43.

137. Thomson CA, Neuhouser ML, Shikany JM, et al. The role of antioxidants and vitamin A in ovarian cancer: Results from the Women's Health Initiative. *Nutr Cancer.* 2008;60(6):710–719.

138. Thiebaut AC, Chajes V, Gerber M, et al. Dietary intakes of omega-6 and omega-3 polyunsaturated fatty acids and the risk of breast cancer. *Int J Cancer.* 2009;124(4):924–931.

139. Albanes D, Heinonen OP, Huttunen JK, et al. Effects of alpha-tocopherol and beta-carotene supplements on cancer incidence in the Alpha-Tocopherol Beta-Carotene Cancer Prevention Study. *Am J Clin Nutr.* 1995;62(6 Suppl):1427S–1430S.

140. The Alpha-Tocopherol BCCPSG. The effect of vitamin E and beta carotene on the incidence of lung cancer and other cancers in male smokers. *N Engl J Med.* 1994;330(15):1029–1035.

141. Omenn GS, Goodman GE, Thornquist MD, et al. Effects of a combination of beta carotene and vitamin A on lung cancer and cardiovascular disease. *N Engl J Med.* 1996;334(18):1150–1155.

142. Hennekens CH, Buring JE, Manson JE, et al. Lack of effect of long-term supplementation with beta carotene on the incidence of malignant neoplasms and cardiovascular disease. *N Engl J Med.* 1996;334(18):1145–1149.

143. Van Schooten FJ, Besaratinia A, De Flora S, et al. Effects of oral administration of N-acetyl-L-cysteine: A multi-biomarker study in smokers. *Cancer Epidemiol Biomarkers Prev.* 2002;11(2):167–175.

144. Kirsh VA, Hayes RB, Mayne ST, et al. Supplemental and dietary vitamin E, beta-carotene, and vitamin C intakes and prostate cancer risk. *J Natl Cancer Inst.* 2006;98(4):245–254.

145. Benner SE, Winn RJ, Lippman SM, et al. Regression of oral leukoplakia with alpha-tocopherol: A community clinical oncology program chemoprevention study. *J Natl Cancer Inst.* 1993;85(1):44–47.

146. Garewal H. Beta-carotene and antioxidant nutrients in oral cancer prevention. In: Prasad KS, L; Williams, RM, ed. *Nutrients in Cancer Prevention and Treatment.* Totawa, NJ: Humana Press; 1995.

147. Hernaandez J, Syed S, Weiss G, et al. The modulation of prostate cancer risk with alpha-tocopherol: A pilot randomized, controlled clinical trial. *J Urol.* 2005;174(2):519–522.

148. Alkhenizan A, Hafez K. The role of vitamin E in the prevention of cancer: A meta-analysis of randomized controlled trials. *Ann Saudi Med.* 2007;27(6):409–414.

149. Weinstein SJ, Wright ME, Lawson KA, et al. Serum and dietary vitamin E in relation to prostate cancer risk. *Cancer Epidemiol Biomarkers Prev.* 2007;16(6):1253–1259.

150. Weinstein SJ, Wright ME, Pietinen P, et al. Serum alpha-tocopherol and gamma-tocopherol in relation to prostate cancer risk in a prospective study. *J Natl Cancer Inst.* 2005;97(5):396–399.

151. Bairati I, Meyer F, Gelinas M, et al. Randomized trial of antioxidant vitamins to prevent acute adverse effects of radiation therapy in head and neck cancer patients. *J Clin Oncol.* 2005;23(24):5805–5813.

152. Gerss J, Kopcke W. The questionable association of vitamin E supplementation and mortality—inconsistent results of different meta-analytic approaches. *Cell Mol Biol (Noisy-le-grand).* 2009;55 Suppl:OL1111–OL1120.

153. Mooney LA, Madsen AM, Tang D, et al. Antioxidant vitamin supplementation reduces benzo(a) pyrene-DNA adducts and potential cancer risk in female smokers. *Cancer Epidemiol Biomarkers Prev.* 2005;14(1):237–242.

154. Abrahamson EE, Ikonomovic MD, Dixon CE, DeKosky ST. Simvastatin therapy prevents brain trauma-induced increases in beta-amyloid peptide levels. *Ann Neurol.* 2009;66(3):407–414.

155. Stolzenberg-Solomon RZ, Sheffler-Collins S, Weinstein S, et al. Vitamin E intake, alpha-tocopherol status, and pancreatic cancer in a cohort of male smokers. *Am J Clin Nutr.* 2009;89(2):584–591.

156. Pastorino U, Infante M, Maioli M, et al. Adjuvant treatment of stage I lung cancer with high-dose vitamin A. *J Clin Oncol.* 1993;11(7):1216–1222.

157. Meyskens FJ. Role of vitamin A and its derivatives in the treatment of human cancer. In: Prasad KN, Santamaria L, Williams RM, eds. *Nutrients in Cancer Prevention and Treatment.* Totawa, NJ: Humana Oress; 1995.

158. van Zandwijk N, Dalesio O, Pastorino U, de Vries N, van Tinteren H. EUROSCAN, a randomized trial of vitamin A and N-acetylcysteine in patients with head and neck cancer or lung cancer. For the EUropean Organization for Research and Treatment of Cancer Head and Neck and Lung Cancer Cooperative Groups. *J Natl Cancer Inst.* 2000;92(12):977–986.

159. Lamm DL, Riggs DR, Shriver JS, vanGilder PF, Rach JF, DeHaven JI. Megadose vitamins in bladder cancer: A double-blind clinical trial. *J Urol.* 1994;151(1):21–26.

160. Roncucci L, Di Donato P, Carati L, et al. Antioxidant vitamins or lactulose for the prevention of the recurrence of colorectal adenomas. Colorectal Cancer Study Group of the University of Modena and the Health Care District 16. *Dis Colon Rectum.* 1993;36(3):227–234.

161. Greenberg ER, Baron JA, Tosteson TD, et al. A clinical trial of antioxidant vitamins to prevent colorectal adenoma. Polyp Prevention Study Group. *N Engl J Med.* 1994;331(3):141–147.

162. McKeown-Eyssen G, Holloway C, Jazmaji V, Bright-See E, Dion P, Bruce WR. A randomized trial of vitamins C and E in the prevention of recurrence of colorectal polyps. *Cancer Res.* 1988;48(16):4701–4705.

163. DeCosse JJ, Miller HH, Lesser ML. Effect of wheat fiber and vitamins C and E on rectal in patients with a low dietary intake of beta-carotene polyps in patients with familial adenomatous polyposis. *J Natl Cancer Inst.* 1989;81(17):1290–1297.

164. Blot WJ, Li JY, Taylor PR, et al. Nutrition intervention trials in Linxian, China: Supplementation with specific vitamin/mineral combinations, cancer incidence, and disease-specific mortality in the general population. *J Natl Cancer Inst.* 1993;85(18):1483–1492.

165. Qiao YL, Dawsey SM, Kamangar F, et al. Total and cancer mortality after supplementation with vitamins and minerals: Follow-up of the Linxian General Population Nutrition Intervention Trial. *J Natl Cancer Inst.* 2009;101(7):507–518.

166. Biasco G, Paganelli GM. European trials on dietary supplementation for cancer prevention. *Ann N Y Acad Sci.* 1999;889:152–156.

167. Hoenjet KM, Dagnelie PC, Delaere KP, Wijckmans NE, Zambon JV, Oosterhof GO. Effect of a nutritional supplement containing vitamin E, selenium, vitamin c, and coenzyme Q10 on serum PSA in patients with hormonally untreated carcinoma of the prostate: A randomised placebo-controlled study. *Eur Urol.* 2005;47(4):433–439; discussion 439–440.

168. Gorham ED, Garland CF, Garland FC, et al. Vitamin D and prevention of colorectal cancer. *J Steroid Biochem Mol Biol.* 2005;97(1–2):179–194.

169. Gorham ED, Garland CF, Garland FC, et al. Optimal vitamin D status for colorectal cancer prevention: A quantitative meta analysis. *Am J Prev Med.* 2007;32(3):210–216.

170. Wactawski-Wende J, Kotchen JM, Anderson GL, et al. Calcium plus vitamin D supplementation and the risk of colorectal cancer. *N Engl J Med.* 2006;354(7):684–696.

171. Ding EL, Mehta S, Fawzi WW, Giovannucci EL. Interaction of estrogen therapy with calcium and vitamin D supplementation on colorectal cancer risk: Reanalysis of Women's Health Initiative randomized trial. *Int J Cancer.* 2008;122(8):1690–1694.

172. Weingarten MA, Zalmanovici A, Yaphe J. Dietary calcium supplementation for preventing colorectal cancer and adenomatous polyps. *Cochrane Database Syst Rev.* 2008(1):CD003548.

173. Chlebowski RT, Johnson KC, Kooperberg C, et al. Calcium plus vitamin D supplementation and the risk of breast cancer. *J Natl Cancer Inst.* 2008;100(22):1581–1591.

174. Martinez ME, Marshall JR, Sampliner R, Wilkinson J, Alberts DS. Calcium, vitamin D, and risk of adenoma recurrence (United States). *Cancer Causes Control.* 2002;13(3):213–220.

175. Grau MV, Baron JA, Sandler RS, et al. Vitamin D, calcium supplementation, and colorectal adenomas: Results of a randomized trial. *J Natl Cancer Inst.* 2003;95(23):1765–1771.

176. Harnack L, Jacobs DR, Jr., Nicodemus K, Lazovich D, Anderson K, Folsom AR. Relationship of folate, vitamin B6, vitamin B12, and methionine intake to incidence of colorectal cancers. *Nutr Cancer.* 2002;43(2):152–158.

177. Ishihara J, Otani T, Inoue M, Iwasaki M, Sasazuki S, Tsugane S. Low intake of vitamin B6 is associated with increased risk of colorectal cancer in Japanese men. *J Nutr.* 2007;137(7):1808–1814.

178. Kune G, Watson L. Colorectal cancer protective effects and the dietary micronutrients folate, methionine, vitamins B6, B12, C, E, selenium, and lycopene. *Nutr Cancer.* 2006;56(1):11–21.

179. Lajous M, Lazcano-Ponce E, Hernandez-Avila M, Willett W, Romieu I. Folate, vitamin B(6), and vitamin B(12) intake and the risk of breast cancer among Mexican women. *Cancer Epidemiol Biomarkers Prev.* 2006;15(3):443–448.

180. Zhang SM. Role of vitamins in the risk, prevention, and treatment of breast cancer. *Curr Opin Obstet Gynecol.* 2004;16(1):19–25.

181. Cole BF, Baron JA, Sandler RS, et al. Folic acid for the prevention of colorectal adenomas: A randomized clinical trial. *Jama.* 2007;297(21):2351–2359.

182. Logan RF, Grainge MJ, Shepherd VC, Armitage NC, Muir KR. Aspirin and folic acid for the prevention of recurrent colorectal adenomas. *Gastroenterology.* 2008;134(1):29–38.

183. Jaszewski R, Misra S, Tobi M, et al. Folic acid supplementation inhibits recurrence of colorectal adenomas: A randomized chemoprevention trial. *World J Gastroenterol.* 2008;14(28):4492–4498.

184. Yang Q, Bostick RM, Friedman JM, Flanders WD. Serum folate and cancer mortality among U.S. adults: Findings from the Third National Health and Nutritional Examination Survey linked mortality file. *Cancer Epidemiol Biomarkers Prev.* 2009;18(5):1439–1447.

185. Shike M, Latkany L, Riedel E, et al. Lack of effect of a low-fat, high-fruit, -vegetable, and -fiber diet on serum prostate-specific antigen of men without prostate cancer: Results from a randomized trial. *J Clin Oncol.* 2002;20(17):3592–3598.

186. Schatzkin A, Lanza E, Corle D, et al. Lack of effect of a low-fat, high-fiber diet on the recurrence of colorectal adenomas. Polyp Prevention Trial Study Group. *N Engl J Med.* 2000;342(16):1149–1155.

187. Alberts DS, Martinez ME, Roe DJ, et al. Lack of effect of a high-fiber cereal supplement on the recurrence of colorectal adenomas. Phoenix Colon Cancer Prevention Physicians' Network. *N Engl J Med.* 2000;342(16):1156–1162.

188. Thomson CA, Stendell-Hollis NR, Rock CL, Cussler EC, Flatt SW, Pierce JP. Plasma and dietary carotenoids are associated with reduced oxidative stress in women previously treated for breast cancer. *Cancer Epidemiol Biomarkers Prev.* 2007;16(10):2008–2015.

189. Marnett LJ. Aspirin and the potential role of prostaglandins in colon cancer. *Cancer Res.* 1992;52(20):5575–5589.

190. Slatore CG, Au DH, Littman AJ, Satia JA, White E. Association of nonsteroidal anti-inflammatory drugs with lung cancer: Results from a large cohort study. *Cancer Epidemiol Biomarkers Prev.* 2009;18(4):1203–1207.

191. Harris RE, Beebe-Donk J, Doss H, Burr Doss D. Aspirin, ibuprofen, and other non-steroidal anti-inflammatory drugs in cancer prevention: A critical review of non-selective COX-2 blockade (review). *Oncol Rep.* 2005;13(4):559–583.

192. Clouser MC, Roe DJ, Foote JA, Harris RB. Effect of non-steroidal anti-inflammatory drugs on non-melanoma skin cancer incidence in the SKICAP-AK trial. *Pharmacoepidemiol Drug Saf.* 2009;18(4):276–283.

193. Bardia A, Platz EA, Yegnasubramanian S, De Marzo AM, Nelson WG. Anti-inflammatory drugs, antioxidants, and prostate cancer prevention. *Curr Opin Pharmacol.* 2009;9(4):419–426.

194. Vile GF, Winterbourn CC. Inhibition of adriamycin-promoted microsomal lipid peroxidation by beta-carotene, alpha-tocopherol and retinol at high and low oxygen partial pressures. *FEBS letters.* 1988;238(2):353–356.

195. Niki E. Interaction of ascorbate and alpha-tocopherol. *Ann N Y Acad Sci.* 1987;498:186–199.

196. Wu H, Kong L, Tan Y, et al. C66 ameliorates diabetic nephropathy in mice by both upregulating NRF2 function via increase in miR-200a and inhibiting miR-21. *Diabetologia.* 2016;59:1558–1568.

197. Itoh K, Chiba T, Takahashi S, et al. An Nrf2/small Maf heterodimer mediates the induction of phase II detoxifying enzyme genes through antioxidant response elements. *Biochem Biophys Res Commun.* 1997;236(2):313–322.

198. Williamson TP, Johnson DA, Johnson JA. Activation of the Nrf2-ARE pathway by siRNA knockdown of Keap1 reduces oxidative stress and provides partial protection from MPTP-mediated neurotoxicity. *Neurotoxicology.* 2012;33(3):272–279.

199. Jaramillo MC, Zhang DD. The emerging role of the Nrf2-Keap1 signaling pathway in cancer. *Genes Dev.* 2013;27(20):2179–2191.

200. Li W, Khor TO, Xu C, et al. Activation of Nrf2-antioxidant signaling attenuates NFkappaB-inflammatory response and elicits apoptosis. *Biochem Pharmacol.* 2008;76(11):1485–1489.

201. Kim J, Cha YN, Surh YJ. A protective role of nuclear factor-erythroid 2-related factor-2 (Nrf2) in inflammatory disorders. *Mutat Res.* 2010;690(1–2):12–23.

202. Suh JH, Shenvi SV, Dixon BM, et al. Decline in transcriptional activity of Nrf2 causes age-related loss of glutathione synthesis, which is reversible with lipoic acid. *Proc Natl Acad Sci U S A.* 2004;101(10):3381–3386.

203. Paonessa JD, Ding Y, Randall KL, et al. Identification of an unintended consequence of Nrf2-directed cytoprotection against a key tobacco carcinogen plus a counteracting chemopreventive intervention. *Cancer Res.* 2011;71(11):3904–3911.

204. Iida K, Itoh K, Kumagai Y, et al. Nrf2 is essential for the chemopreventive efficacy of oltipraz against urinary bladder carcinogenesis. *Cancer Res.* 2004;64(18):6424–6431.

205. Singh B, Shoulson R, Chatterjee A, et al. Resveratrol inhibits estrogen-induced breast carcinogenesis through induction of NRF2-mediated protective pathways. *Carcinogenesis.* 2014;35(8):1872–1880.

206. Pi J, Diwan BA, Sun Y, et al. Arsenic-induced malignant transformation of human keratinocytes: Involvement of Nrf2. *Free Radic Biol Med.* 2008;45(5):651–658.

207. Wang D, Ma Y, Yang X, et al. Hypermethylation of the Keap1 gene inactivates its function, promotes Nrf2 nuclear accumulation, and is involved in arsenite-induced human keratinocyte transformation. *Free Radic Biol Med.* 2015;89:209–219.

208. Satoh H, Moriguchi T, Takai J, Ebina M, Yamamoto M. Nrf2 prevents initiation but accelerates progression through the Kras signaling pathway during lung carcinogenesis. *Cancer Res.* 2013;73(13):4158–4168.

209. Shen T, Jiang T, Long M, et al. A curcumin derivative that inhibits vinyl carbamate-induced lung carcinogenesis via activation of the Nrf2 protective response. *Antioxid Redox Signal.* 2015;23(8):651–664.

210. Long M, Tao S, Rojo de la Vega M, et al. Nrf2-dependent suppression of azoxymethane/dextran sulfate sodium-induced colon carcinogenesis by the cinnamon-derived dietary factor cinnamaldehyde. *Cancer Prev Res (Phila).* 2015;8(5):444–454.

211. Khor TO, Huang MT, Prawan A, et al. Increased susceptibility of Nrf2 knockout mice to colitis-associated colorectal cancer. *Cancer Prev Res (Phila).* 2008;1(3):187–191.

212. Mostafavi-Pour Z, Ramezani F, Keshavarzi F, Samadi N. The role of quercetin and vitamin C in Nrf2-dependent oxidative stress production in breast cancer cells. *Oncol Lett.* 2017;13(3):1965–1973.

213. Katsuyama Y, Tsuboi T, Taira N, Yoshioka M, Masaki H. 3-O-Laurylglyceryl ascorbate activates the intracellular antioxidant system through the contribution of PPAR-gamma and Nrf2. *J Dermatol Sci.* 2016;82(3):189–196.

214. Choi HK, Pokharel YR, Lim SC, et al. Inhibition of liver fibrosis by solubilized coenzyme Q10: Role of Nrf2 activation in inhibiting transforming growth factor-beta1 expression. *Toxicol Appl Pharmacol.* 2009;240(3):377–384.

215. Ji L, Liu R, Zhang XD, et al. N-acetylcysteine attenuates phosgene-induced acute lung injury via upregulation of Nrf2 expression. *Inhal Toxicol.* 2010;22(7):535–542.

216. Gao L, Wang J, Sekhar KR, et al. Novel n-3 fatty acid oxidation products activate Nrf2 by destabilizing the association between Keap1 and Cullin3. *J Biol Chem.* 2007;282(4):2529–2537.

217. Saw CL, Yang AY, Guo Y, Kong AN. Astaxanthin and omega-3 fatty acids individually and in combination protect against oxidative stress via the Nrf2-ARE pathway. *Food Chem Toxicol.* 2013;62:869–875.

218. Trujillo J, Chirino YI, Molina-Jijon E, Anderica-Romero AC, Tapia E, Pedraza-Chaverri J. Renoprotective effect of the antioxidant curcumin: Recent findings. *Redox Biol.* 2013;1(1):448–456.

219. Steele ML, Fuller S, Patel M, Kersaitis C, Ooi L, Munch G. Effect of Nrf2 activators on release of glutathione, cysteinylglycine and homocysteine by human U373 astroglial cells. *Redox Biol.* 2013;1(1):441–445.

220. Kode A, Rajendrasozhan S, Caito S, Yang SR, Megson IL, Rahman I. Resveratrol induces glutathione synthesis by activation of Nrf2 and protects against cigarette smoke-mediated oxidative stress in human lung epithelial cells. *Am J Physiol Lung Cell Mol Physiol.* 2008;294(3):L478–488.

221. Zambrano S, Blanca AJ, Ruiz-Armenta MV, et al. The renoprotective effect of L-carnitine in hypertensive rats is mediated by modulation of oxidative stress-related gene expression. *Eur J Nutr.* 2013;52(6):1649–1659.

222. Eades G, Yang M, Yao Y, Zhang Y, Zhou Q. miR-200a regulates Nrf2 activation by targeting Keap1 mRNA in breast cancer cells. *J Biol Chem.* 2011;286(47):40725–40733.

223. Cheng LB, Li KR, Yi N, et al. miRNA-141 attenuates UV-induced oxidative stress via activating Keap1-Nrf2 signaling in human retinal pigment epithelium cells and retinal ganglion cells. *Oncotarget.* 2017;8(8):13186–13194.

224. Yang M, Yao Y, Eades G, Zhang Y, Zhou Q. MiR-28 regulates Nrf2 expression through a Keap1-independent mechanism. *Breast Cancer Res Treat.* 2011;129(3):983–991.

225. Abate A, Yang G, Dennery PA, Oberle S, Schroder H. Synergistic inhibition of cyclooxygenase-2 expression by vitamin E and aspirin. *Free Radic Biol Med.* 2000;29(11):1135–1142.

226. Fu Y, Zheng S, Lin J, Ryerse J, Chen A. Curcumin protects the rat liver from CCl4-caused injury and fibrogenesis by attenuating oxidative stress and suppressing inflammation. *Mol Pharmacol.* 2008;73(2):399–409.

227. Rahman S, Bhatia K, Khan AQ, et al. Topically applied vitamin E prevents massive cutaneous inflammatory and oxidative stress responses induced by double application of 12-O-tetradecanoylphorbol-13-acetate (TPA) in mice. *Chem Biol Interact.* 2008;172(3):195–205.

228. Suzuki YJ, Aggarwal BB, Packer L. Alpha-lipoic acid is a potent inhibitor of NF-kappa B activation in human T cells. *Biochem Biophys Res Commun.* 1992;189(3):1709–1715.

229. Zhu J, Yong W, Wu X, et al. Anti-inflammatory effect of resveratrol on TNF-alpha-induced MCP-1 expression in adipocytes. *Biochem Biophys Res Commun.* 2008;369(2):471–477.

230. Prasad KN. Alpha-tocopheryl succinate exhibits potent anticancer activity: Its interaction with ionizing radiation and chemotherapy effects. In: Reddy VR, and Watson, R.R., ed. *The Encyclopedia of Vitamin E.* London, UK: CAB International; 2007.

231. Prasad KN, Hovland AR, Cole WC, et al. Multiple antioxidants in the prevention and treatment of Alzheimer disease: Analysis of biologic rationale. *Clin Neuropharmacol.* 2000;23(1):2–13.

8 Micronutrients in Improvement of the Standard Therapy in Cancer

INTRODUCTION

Most human cancers are polyclonal, which makes them heterogeneous with respect to their response to treatment agents. The extent of heterogeneity differs from one cancer type to another and even within the same tumor, depending upon the stage of tumor. Cancer cells surviving after standard therapy have increased levels of heterogeneity that makes them difficult to treat. Despite recent advances in chemotherapy, radiation therapy, surgery (for solid tumors), hyperthermia, gene therapy, and immunotherapy alone or in combination, the mortality has increased from 569,490 in 2010 to 600,920 in 2017 in the United States, an increase of about 5.5% in 7 years. In 2014, the total number of patients with cancer in the United States was 14,738 million. The direct annual cost of treatment of cancer was $4 billion from patients and about $87 billion from the US Health Care System.

There are no effective strategies to reduce the side effects of radiation therapy and/or chemotherapy, because they damage both cancer cells and normal cells, and in some instances, such damage becomes the limiting factor for the continuation of therapy. Despite short-term and long-term toxicity of standard therapy, it has increased cure rates in certain tumors including Hodgkin's disease, childhood leukemia, and teratocarcinoma, and prolonged survival time of other types of tumors. However, the risk of recurrence of the primary tumor and the development of a new cancer and non-neoplastic diseases exist. At present, there are no effective approaches to decrease the risk of these late adverse effects.

Therefore, additional approaches should be developed and tested: (a) to improve the efficacy of standard therapy in terms of killing more cancer cells while protecting the normal cells, (b) to improve the quality of life and survival time of those patients who become unresponsive to all standard and experimental cancer therapies for as long as possible, and (c) to decrease the risk of recurrence of the primary tumor and the development of a second new cancer and noncancerous diseases.

In recent years, the role of microRNAs and their target proteins in the pathogenesis and suppression of cancer has been extensively studied, and suggestions were made that they can be used as targets for developing new cancer treatment drugs and as biomarkers of cancer. The detailed studies are discussed later in this chapter.

The role of antioxidants in the treatment of cancer has become a controversial issue. On one hand, oncologists prevent patients from taking antioxidant supplements during radiation therapy or chemotherapy because of fear that they might protect cancer cells from free radicals generated by the therapeutic agents. On the other hand, patients take commercially sold multivitamins containing low doses of antioxidants without knowing that they may stimulate the growth of cancer cells and may reduce the effectiveness of therapy.

Analysis of 49 studies in which individual or multiple antioxidants used during standard therapy suggests that no conclusions can be made with respect to its efficacy in improving treatment outcomes or in reducing adverse side effects.[1] One of the reasons for these inconclusive results could have been due to use of low or preventive doses of antioxidants. Studies discussed later in this chapter show that preventive doses of antioxidants stimulate the growth of cancer cells and protect both normal and cancer cells against damage produced by therapeutic agents. In contrast to the effect of low doses of antioxidants, therapeutic doses of antioxidants selectively inhibit the growth of several tumor cells, while protecting normal cells in cell culture and animal models. Therapeutic doses of antioxidants also enhance the cell-killing effects of radiation therapy and chemotherapy in cancer cells, while they protect normal cells against their toxicity.

Cancer cells constitutively express high levels of Nrf2 that allow cell proliferation, migration, and invasion and prevent apoptosis by elevating cytoprotective enzymes including antioxidant enzymes. Elevated levels of Nrf2 also make cancer cells resistant to cancer drugs and radiation therapy. Therapeutic doses of antioxidant activate Nrf2 and reduce growth of cancer cells. How can one explain growth-inhibitory effects of antioxidants on cancer cells in the presence high levels of Nrf2? Studies discussed later in this chapter show that therapeutic doses of antioxidants bypass the protective effect of Nrf2 and induce apoptosis by enhancing the expression of apoptotic signaling pathways, reducing the levels or interfering with the function of Nrf2, and altering the expression of microRNAs and their respective target proteins that cause growth inhibition.

This chapter describes (a) the role of microRNAs in the pathogenesis of various types of human tumor; (b) discusses the role of Nrf2 that is constitutively expressed in cancer cells in preventing apoptosis and making tumor cells radiation-resistant and chemo-resistant; (c) presents results on the growth-inhibitory effects of antioxidants alone or in combination with standard therapy on cancer cells; (d) presents studies that support the hypothesis that therapeutic doses antioxidants inhibit the growth of cancer cells by bypassing the protective effects of Nrf2 and by inducing pro-apoptotic signaling pathways; (e) proposes a mixture of therapeutic doses of multiple antioxidants to be administered orally before and during the entire treatment period in order to enhance their effects on apoptosis and reduce migration and invasion of cancer cells, while protecting normal cells; (f) the same mixture of antioxidants may improve the survival time and quality of life among those who have become unresponsive to all therapies; and (g) proposes a mixture of preventive doses of antioxidants for reducing the risk of long-term adverse effects of therapy among survivors.

MicroRNAs IN CANCER CELLS

MicroRNAs

MicroRNAs (miRs) are evolutionarily conserved small non-coding single-stranded RNAs of approximately 22 nucleotides in length, and are present in all living organisms including humans.[2–5] The biogenesis of miRs is very complex and involves multiple biochemical steps. The majority of miRs are transcribed by RNA polymerase II (Pol II), while some are transcribed by RNA polymerase III (Pol III) from the noncoding region of the DNA to produce primary miRs (pri-miRs). Pri-miRs undergo a nuclear cleavage by ribonuclease III Drosa to generate precursor-miRs (pre-miRs) that migrate to the cytoplasm where they are further cleaved by ribonuclease III Dicer to ultimately form mature single-stranded miRs with the help of another protein argonaute (Ago).[4,6–8] Each microRNA binds to its complementary sequences in the 3'-untranslated region (3'-UTR) of the mRNA, promotes degradation of the mRNA transcript, and prevents translation of the message of protein. In this manner, miRs regulate the translation of proapoptotic or antiapoptotic proteins from their respective mRNAs, depending upon whether they receive damaging or protective signal. Damaging signals may include oxidative damage and pro-inflammatory cytokines and protective signals may include antioxidants and phytochemicals.

Overexpression of certain microRNAs and reduced levels of their respective proteins may act as tumor suppressors or antioncogenes, whereas overexpression of some other microRNAs behaves as oncogene. There are extensive publications on these issues. Only a few studies on the changes in the expression of microRNAs and their respective proteins in selected tumors are described here.

MicroRNAs ACTING AS TUMOR SUPPRESSORS OR ANTI-ONCOGENES

COLON CANCER

The expression miR-15 was lower in colon cancer cells. Transfection-induced overexpression of miR-15 increased the levels of 5-fluorouracil (5-FU)- and oxaliplatin (OX)-induce apoptosis in HCT116 colon cancer cells. This effect of miR-15 was mediated by inhibiting NFkB that includes their two antiapoptotic targets proteins Bcl2 and Bcl-xL.[9] The expression of miR-506 was low in colorectal cancer (CRC) tissue. Low tissue expression of this microRNA was associated with lower 5-year overall survival (OS) and lower relapse free survival (RFS) than the high miR-506 expression group. Overexpression of miR-506 inhibited growth and increased oxaliplatin-induced apoptosis by inhibiting MDR1/p-gp (multidrug resistance protein1/P-glycoprotein) via downregulation of Wnt/β-catenin pathway in HCT116 cells.[10] The expression of miR-26b was downregulated in colon cancer cell lines, while its target protein lymphoid enhancer factor (LEF1) was elevated. Normal human colon cell lines had high expression of miR-26b and low levels of LEF1.[11] MiR-497 expression was low and the level of its target protein IGF1 receptor (IGF1-R) was high in CRC lines. Overexpression of miR-497 suppressed the growth by inhibiting its target protein IGF1-R and increased sensitivity of the cells to 5-FU and cisplatin.[12] Expression of miR-128 was downregulated and the level of its target protein insulin receptor substrate1 (IRS1) was increased in colon cancer cell lines. Low expression was miR-128 in tumor tissue was negatively correlated with Tumor, Node Metastasis (TNM) stage and lymph node metastasis in patients with CRC. Overexpression of miR-128 reduced proliferation, colony formation, migration, and invasion, and promoted apoptosis in cells in culture, and inhibited the growth of CRC tumor growing in athymic mice.[13] Expression of miR-874 was downregulated and the level of its target protein X-linked inhibitor of apoptosis protein was increased in colon cancer tissues and cell lines. Low expression was miR-874 in tumor tissue was negatively correlated with Tumor, Node Metastasis (TNM) stage and lymph node metastasis in patients with CRC. Overexpression of miR-128 reduced proliferation, colony formation, increased apoptosis, and enhanced 5-FU-induced cell death in CRC cells.[14] These results suggest that the expressions of at least 6 microRNAs are downregulated each of which has different target proteins that are enhanced in tumor tissues and cell lines of CRC. The results are summarized in Table 8.1.

GASTRIC CANCER CELLS

Gastric cancer cells have low expression of miR-133a, miR-128b, miR-9, miR-126, and miR-124, but have high levels of their respective proteins TAGLN2 (transgelin 2), A2bR (adenosine A2b receptor), TNFAIP8 (TNF-alpha-induced protein 8), Crk (vsrc sarcoma virus CT10 oncogene homolog), and ROCK1 (Rho-associated protein kinase 1) compared to normal tissues. These elevated levels of proteins play a role in cell proliferation, migration, and invasion. Overexpression of these microRNAs inhibited their respective target proteins and reduced the growth, migration, and invasion of tumor cells in culture.[15–19] The results are summarized in Table 8.1.

NON-SMALL CELL LUNG CANCER (NSCLC)

Lung cancer cells have reduced expression of miR-140 and miR-99a and have elevated levels of their respective proteins IGF1-R and ATK1. Overexpression of these microRNAs inhibited their respective target proteins and reduced the growth, migration, and invasion of tumor cells in culture. The results are summarized in Table 8.1.

TABLE 8.1

Low Expression of MicroRNAs in Various Cancers and Their Respective Elevated Levels of Target Proteins

Cancer Type	Downregulation	Increased Levels of Proteins
Colon Cancer Cells	miR-15	NF-kB
Colon Cancer Cells	miR-506	MDR1/R-gp
Colon Cancer Cells	miR-26b	LEF1
Colon Cancer Cells	miR-497	IGFI-R
Colon Cancer Cells	miR-128	IRS1
Colon Cancer Cells	miR-874	XIAP
Gastric Cancer Cells	miR-133a	TAGLN2
Gastric Cancer Cells	miR-128b	A2bR
Gastric Cancer Cells	miR-9	TNFAIP8
Gastric Cancer Cells	miR-126	Crk
Gastric Cancer Cells	miR-124	ROCK1
Non-small Cell lung cancer	miR-140	IGF1R
Non-small Cell lung cancer	miR-99a	AKT1

Note: NF-kB, nuclear factor kappa-light-chain-enhancer activated B-cells; MDR1/ R-gp, multidrug resistance protein1/P-glycoprotein; LEF1, lymphoid enhancer binding factor-1; IGF1-R, insulin growth factor1-receptor; IRS1, insulin receptor substrate-1; XIAP, X-linked inhibitor of apoptosis protein; TAGLN2, Transgelin-2; A2bR, Adenosine A2b receptor; TNFATP8, TNF-alpha-induced protein 8; Crk-v-src sarcoma virus CT10 oncogene homolog; ROCK1, Rho-associated protein kinase1; AKT1, serine-threonine protein kinase 1. All elevated proteins inhibit proliferation, migration, invasion, metastasis, and induced apoptosis in athymic mice carrying human cancer cells.

RETINOBLASTOMA

Retinoblastoma cells and tissues have lower expression of miR-183 and miR-124 but have higher levels of their respective proteins LRP 6 and STAT3 than noncancerous cells and tissues. Overexpression of these microRNAs inhibited their respective target proteins and reduced the growth, migration, and invasion of tumor cells in culture.[20,21] Thus, elevated expression of miR-183 and miR-124 acts as tumor suppressors. The results are summarized in Table 8.2.

BREAST CANCER CELLS

Breast cancer cells (MDA-MB-231 and MCF-7) and tissues have lower expression of miR-137, miR-15a, and miR-16 but have higher levels of their respective proteins EFF-α, CCNE, and cyclin D and Bcl2 than noncancerous cells and tissues. Overexpression of these microRNAs inhibited their respective target proteins, and reduced the growth, migration, and invasion of tumor cells in culture and induced apoptosis.[22–24] Normal breast epithelial cells have elevated expression of miR-135 and miR-203 and undetectable levels of its target protein Runx2 (runt-related transcription factor-2). Overexpression of these microRNAs in MDA-MB-231-luv cells reduced the tumor growth and bone metastasis by reducing the levels of Runx2-regulated IL-11 (interleukin-11), MMP-13 (Matrix metallopeptidase-13), and PTHrP (parathyroid hormone-related peptide).[25] Thus, elevated expression of miR-137, miR-15a, miR-16, miR-135, and miR-203 may act as tumor suppressors. The results are summarized in Table 8.2.

TABLE 8.2

Low Expression of MicroRNAs in Various Cancers and Their Elevated Levels of Their Respective Target Protein

Cancer Type	Downregulation	Increased Levels of Proteins
Retinoblastoma	miR-183	LRP6
Retinoblastoma	miR-124	STAT3
Breast Cancer	miR-137	ERR-alpha
Breast Cancer	miR-15a	CCNE
Breast cancer	miR-16	Cyclin D, Bcl2
Breast Cancer	miR-135, miR-203	Runx2
Ovarian Cancer	miR-145	C-Myc
Liver Cancer	miR-122, miR-145	ADAM 17
Bladder Cancer	miR-320	CDK6
Bladder Cancer	miR-449a	CDK6, CDC25a
Cervical Cancer	miR-491-5p	hTERT
Cervical Cancer	miR-135b	FOXO1

Note: LRP6, Low-density lipoprotein receptor-related protein 6 precursor; STAT3, signal transducer and activator of transcriptional 3; ERR-alpha, estrogen-related receptor alpha; CCNE1, Cyclin E; Runx2, Runt-related transcriptional factor-2; C-myc, a oncogene; ADAM17, A disintegrin and metalloproteinase 17; CDK6, cyclin-dependent kinase 6; CDC25a, cell division cycle 25 homolog A; hTERT, human telomere reverse transcriptase; FOXO1, forkhead box protein O1. All elevated proteins inhibit proliferation, migration, invasion, metastasis, and induced apoptosis in athymic mice carrying human cancer cells.

HEPATOCELLULAR CARCINOMA

Liver cancer cells with intrahepatic metastasis have lower expression of miR-122 and miR-145 and higher levels of their common target protein ADAM17 (a disintegrin and metalloproteinase 17) than normal cells. Ectopic overexpression of these microRNAs reduced the levels of their target protein ADAD17 and suppressed tumor growth migration, invasion, angiogenesis, and metastasis.[26,27] The results are summarized in Table 8.2.

BLADDER CANCER

The expression of miR-320c and miR-449a was downregulated and the levels of its target protein CDK6 (cyclin-dependent kinase 6), and CDC25a, cell division cycle 25 homolog A, are increased in the bladder cancer cells lines. Overexpression of these microRNAs inhibited their respective target proteins and inhibited tumor growth, migration, and invasion in bladder cancer cells.[28,29] The results are summarized in Table 8.2.

CERVICAL CANCER

Cervical cancer cells have reduced expression of miR-491-5p and miR-135b elevated levels of their target proteins hTERT (human telomere reverse transcription) and FOXO1. Overexpression of these microRNAs and reduction in the levels of their respective target proteins inhibited cell proliferation, migration, and invasion and induced apoptosis.[30,31] The results are summarized in Table 8.2.

The studies discussed suggest that either elevating the expression of microRNAs or decreasing the levels of their respective target proteins could be used as substrates for developing new cancer therapeutic agents. This could be difficult because multiple microRNAs are downregulated and the levels of their respective target proteins are elevated in the same tumor.

MicroRNAs ACTING AS ONCOGENES

BLADDER CANCER

Overexpression of miR-19a and its reduced target protein PTEN (phosphatase and tension homolog) is related to aggressive behavior of bladder cancer.[32] The oncogenic role of miR-19a was dependent on targeting PTEN.

LUNG CANCER

Specific protein1 (SP1), a transcriptional factor, enhanced the expression of miR-182 that inhibited its target protein, PTEN, and promoted growth and reduced metastasis of cancer cells. In the late stage of cancer, the expression of SP1 and miR-182 decreased and the levels of FOXO3 enhanced, leading to lung metastasis.[33] Lung cancer tissues and lung cancer cell lines have higher expression of miR-5100 and lower levels of its target protein Rab6 (Ras-related protein Rab6A) than normal tissues. Overexpression of this microRNA and reduced levels of its target protein Rab6 promoted growth of cancer in nude mice and enhanced the proliferation in cancer cell lines.[34]

NON-SMALL-CELL LUNG CANCER

Overexpression of miR-106a, miR-205, and miR-92a and reduced levels of their common target protein PTEN increased tumor growth, migration, and invasion in tumor cell lines.[35–37]

PROSTATE CANCER, GASTRIC CANCER, AND ESOPHAGEAL CANCER

Prostate cancer cells have higher expression of miR-183 and lower levels of its target proteins DKK-3 (Dickkopf-related protein3) and SMAD4 (Mothers against decapentaplegic 4) than normal prostate tissue, these changes in the expression of this microRNA and its target proteins were associated with increased levels prostate-specific antigen and shorter overall survival.[38]

Overexpression of miR-296-5p and reduced levels of its target protein CDX1 (Caudal-related homebox 1) were associated with increased proliferation, tumor growth, and reduced apoptosis in gastric cancer cells.[39]

The expression of miR-374a was upregulated and the levels of its target protein Axin2 (Axin-related protein) were reduced in esophageal tumor tissues and cell lines; these changes promoted tumor growth.[40]

CERVICAL CANCER, COLORECTAL CANCER, AND BREAST CANCER

Cervical cancer has increased expression of miR-590 and reduced levels of its target protein CHL1 (Cell adhesion molecule L1), and these changes in the expression of this microRNA and its target protein CHL1 were associated with tumor growth, cell cycle progression, and invasion.[41]

Overexpression of miR-181a and reduced levels of its target protein WIF1 (Wnt inhibitory factoe-1) were associated with increased cell proliferation, migration, invasion, and metastasis in colorectal cancer cells.[42]

Upregulation of miR-203 and reduced levels of its target protein SOCS3 (suppressor of cytokine signaling 3) promoted tumor growth in several cell lines of ER-positive breast cancer.[43]

The studies discussed suggest that either suppressing the expression of microRNAs or increasing the levels of their respective target proteins could be used as substrates for developing new cancer therapeutic agents. This could be difficult because multiple microRNAs are upregulated and the

TABLE 8.3

High Expression of MicroRNAs in Various Cancers and Their Reduced Levels of Their Respective Target Proteins

Tumor Type	Upregulation	Reduced Protein Levels
Bladder Cancer	miR-19a	PTEN
Lung Cancer	miR-182	FOXO3
Lung Cancer	miR-5100	Rab6
Non-Small Cell Lung Cancer	miR-106a, miR-205, miR-92a	PTEN
Prostate Cancer	miR-183	DKK3, SMDA4
Gastric Cancer	miR-296-5p	CDX1
Esophageal Cancer	miR-374a	Axin
Cervical Cancer	miR-590	CHL1
Colorectal Cancer	miR-181	WIF1
Breast Cancer	miR-203	SOCS3

Note: PTEN, Phosphatase and tension homolog; FOXO3, forkhead box protein 3; Rab6, Ras-related protein Rab6A; DKK3, Dickkopf-related protein 3; SMDA4, mothers against decapentaplegic 4; CDX1, caudal type homeobox 1; WiF1, Wnt inhibitory factor-1.

levels of their respective target proteins are decreased in the same tumor. The changes in the expression of microRNAs and their respective target proteins are presented in Table 8.3.

Nrf2 IN CANCER CELLS

NORMAL CELL RESPONSE TO ACTIVATED Nrf2

In normal cells, during acute oxidative stress, reactive oxygen species (ROS) is needed to activate Nrf2 which then dissociates itself from Keap1-Cul-Rbx1 complex and translocates in the nucleus where it heterodimerizes with a small Maf protein, and binds with the ARE (antioxidant response element) leading to increased expression of target genes coding for several cytoprotective enzymes including antioxidant enzymes.[44–46] In this manner, activation of Nrf2 increases the levels of cytoprotective enzymes including antioxidant enzymes and phase-2-detoxifying enzymes.[47,48]

The role of Nrf2 in proliferation, and resistant to chemotherapy and radiation therapy has been extensively studied in various cancer cells in culture and animal models. Only a few selected studies to demonstrate the relationship between cancer cells and Nrf2 are described here.

HIGH EXPRESSION OF Nrf2 PROMOTES CANCER GROWTH AND DRUG-RESISTANT

Cancer cells have constitutively expressed Nrf2 leading to enhanced levels of antioxidant enzymes that protect against oxidative damage and inflammation, allow continued proliferation and inhibit apoptosis. An elevation of Nrf2 in cancer cells makes them resistant to standard therapeutic agents.[49,50]

The expression of Nrf2 was elevated in mammosphere of breast cancer cell lines enriched in cancer stem cells were highly tumorigenic and resistant to taxol. Brusatol, an inhibitor of the Nrf2 pathway, enhanced ROS level; reduced Nrf2-mediated cytoprotective enzymes levels, and restored sensitivity of these cells to taxol.[51] In A549 xenografts (human adenocarcinoma of alveolar basal epithelial cell growing in athymic mice), coadministration with brusatol and cisplatin induced apoptosis, and reduced cell proliferation and tumor growth more than those produced by cisplatin alone.[52] Genetic ablation of Nrf2 enhanced drug-induced cell death in cervical cancer cells in culture (CaSki cells).[53] Thus, development of nontoxic inhibitors of Nrf2 would help in improving the management of cancer.

Nrf2 is highly expressed in non-small-cell lung cancer cells (NSCLCs) and plays an important role in proliferation and chemoresistance. This effect of Nrf2 is mediated via upregulated levels of epidermal growth factor receptor (EGFR) signaling, which inhibits the levels of Keap1.[54]

Persistent elevation of Nrf2 in NSCLCs due to mutation in Nrf2 and/or loss of or mutation in Keap1 is associated with tumorgenicity and chemoresistance. Stable knockdown of Keap1 caused increased sensitization to multiple chemotherapeutic agents, even though the levels of Nrf2 were moderately elevated. Furthermore, silencing Keap1 enhanced the expression of peroxisome proliferator-activated receptor y (PPARy) and genes associated with differentiation, including E-cadherin and gelsolin.[55] Nrf2 is constitutively overexpressed in pancreatic cancer cell line and ductal adenocarcinoma and this makes them chemoresistant.[56]

Trastuzumab and Pertuzumab are monoclonal antibodies used in combination to treat breast cancer with human epidermal growth factor receptor 2 (HER2) positive cells. Treatment of ovarian cancer cells with these antibodies reduced the growth, level and function of Nrf2, and glutathione, and increased the amounts of ROS. Combination of antibodies produces increased methylation at the Nrf2 promoter that impaired its function.[57]

INDIVIDUAL ANTIOXIDANTS INHIBIT CANCER GROWTH IN THE PRESENCE OF ELEVATED LEVELS OF Nrf2

LUTEOLIN

Luteolin (3',4',5,7-tetrahydroxyflavone), a common flavonoid (also called phytochemical) found in fruits, vegetable, and medicinal herbs exhibits antioxidant and anti-inflammation activity, inhibited the expression of Nrf2 and reduce the growth of human non-small-cell lung cancer cell line A549 and in athymic mice carrying A549 tumor cells.[58] Procyanidins from Cinnamomi cortex promotes proteasome-independent degradation of Nrf2 through phosphorylation of insulin-like growth factor 1 receptor reduces levels of Nrf2 led to decreased levels of cytoprotective enzymes, causing growth inhibition in several cancer cells, which have high levels of constitutively expressed Nrf2.[59]

PTEROSTILBENE

Pterostilbene (Pter, a dimethoxylated analog of resveratrol) that exhibits antioxidant and anti-inflammation activities reduce Nrf2 activity and Nrf2-dependent antioxidant defense system such as cytoprotective enzymes leading to apoptosis of melanoma cells in vivo and in human pancreatic cancer cells growing in athymic mice. These effects of Pter are associated with decreased production of glucocorticoid. Treatment of melanoma cells with corticosterone or genetically induced overexpression of Nrf2 abolished the Pter-induced growth-inhibition and reduction in antioxidant defense system.[60]

ANTIOXIDANTS ACTIVATE ROS-RESISTANT Nrf2

Some antioxidants can activate Nrf2 without requiring ROS. These include vitamin C,[61,62] vitamin E,[63] endogenous antioxidants such as alpha-lipoic acid,[64] coenzyme Q10,[65] synthetic antioxidant N-acetylcysteine (NAC),[66] omega-3-fatty acids,[67,68] curcumin,[69] and resveratrol.[70,71] These antioxidants at therapeutic doses also reduce growth of cancer cells.

Synthetic Triterpenoid RTA 405

The therapeutic doses of antioxidants and phytochemicals activate Nrf2 and inhibit the growth of tumor cells at the same time and enhance the growth-inhibitory effects of therapeutic agents. In order to explain this paradoxical effects of antioxidants synthetic triterpenoid RTA 405, which exhibits antioxidant and anti-inflammation activities and prevents the ability of Keap1 to promote degradation of Nrf2 via proteasome complex leading to increased Nrf2 levels. Increased levels of Nrf2 lead to increased levels of cytoprotective enzymes, which reduce oxidative stress and inflammation, and thereby inhibit apoptosis. On the other hand, this triterpenoid reduced the proliferation and metastasis of tumor cells by increasing Nrf2 activity in the tumor microenvironment and by increasing oncogenic signaling pathways. It appears that loss of Keap1 or mutation in Keap1 causes increased activity of Nrf2 that promote growth of cancer and increase chemoresistant as well as increased the levels of oncogenic proteins, such as IKKβ and Bcl2. The levels of Nrf2 and oncoproteins IKKβ and Bcl2 were elevated in murine fibroblasts lacking Keap1 (–/–), and the rates of proliferation and colony formation were higher than in the wild-type fibroblasts. On the other hand, in the tumor cells with functional Keap1, treatment with RTA 405 enhanced the levels of Nrf2 but not the levels of IKKβ and Bcl2. Pretreatment with RTA 405 did not protect tumor cells from doxorubicin- or cisplain-induced growth inhibition.[72] Activation of Nrf2 in the microenvironment of tumors by a synthetic tritepennoid RTA408 causes reversal of tumor-mediated evasion of immune function and inhibits tumor growth and metastasis. It also enhanced the levels of oncogenic proteins IKKβ and Bcl2. The growth-inhibitory effect of RTA 408 was due to increased caspase activity in tumor cells but not in normal primary human cells.[73] Thus, RTA408 reduced the growth of cancer cells by increasing pro-apoptotic protein, by bypassing protective effects of activated Nrf2.

Curcumin

Overexpression of Flap endonuclease 1 (Fen1), a DNA repair-specific nuclease, appears to be involved in the development of breast cancer. Curcumin, which exhibits antioxidant and anti-inflammation activities, decreased the growth of breast cancer cells (MCF-7) in the presence of activated Nrf2. This effect of curcumin is mediated by reduced level of Fen1.[74] Thus, curcumin can inhibit the growth of cancer cells in the presence of activated Nrf2 by enhancing the levels of proteins in apoptotic pathways.

Tert-Butylhydroquinone

Treatment of mouse hepatoma cells with an antioxidant tert-butylhydroquinone activated Nrf2 and increased the levels of Bcl-xL (B-cell lymphoid-extra large, a member of antiapoptotic Bcl2 family). Inhibition of Nrf2 decreased the expression of Bcl-xL. Nrf2-mediated elevation of Bcl-xL led to reduced expression of Bax and decreased activity of caspase 3/7 activity and increased survival of tumor cells.[75]

These results suggest that therapeutic doses of antioxidants or phytochemicals inhibit the growth of cancer cells by bypassing Nrf2-mediated elevation of cytoprotective enzymes and by increasing the levels of proapoptotic pathways. Some of them inhibit cancer growth by inhibiting Nrf2 function, while tert-butylhydroquinone increases the survival of cancer cells. Additional studies on growth-inhibitory effects of individual antioxidants and their potential mechanisms are described here.

Vitamin E Succinate

In 1982, I discovered that alpha-tocopheryl succinate (alpha-TS) induced differentiation, growth inhibition, and cell death in murine melanoma cells in culture, depending upon the

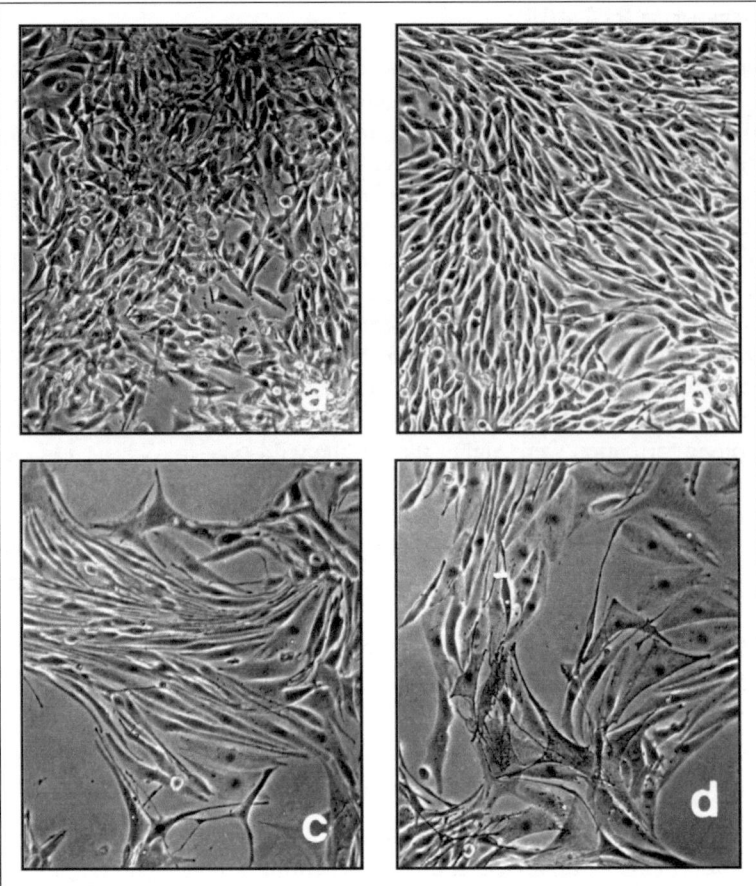

FIGURE 8.1   Melanoma cells (10^5) were plated in tissue culture dishes (60 mm), and *d*-alpha-tocopheryl succinate (alpha-TS) and sodium succinate plus ethanol were added to separate cultures 24 h after plating. Drugs and medium were changed at 2 and 3 d after treatment. Photomicrographs were taken 4 d after treatment. Control cultures showed fibroblastic cells as well as round cells in clumps (a); cultures treated with ethanol (1%) and sodium succinate (5–6 μg/mL) also exhibited fibroblastic morphology with fewer round cells (b); alpha-TS-treated cultures 6 μg/mL (c); and 8 μg/mL (d) showed a dramatic change in morphology, Mag. X 300. (From Prasad, K.N. and Edwards-Prasad, J., *Cancer Res.*, 42, 550–555, 1982.)

dose and period of treatment (Figure 8.1), whereas alpha-tocopherol, alpha-tocopheryl acetate, and alpha-tocopheryl nicotinate were ineffective.[76] Since then, numerous studies showed that alpha-TS selectively inhibited the growth of cancer cells without affecting the growth of normal cells.[77,78] Alpha-TS also inhibited androgen receptor expression in prostate cancer cells, but not in normal prostate epithelial cells in culture.[79] It also reduced the expression of prostate-specific antigen (PSA) by acting at both transcription and translation levels.[80] Treatment of hormone-resistance human breast cancer cells in culture with alpha-TS makes them sensitive to hormone treatment.[81]

VITAMIN C

The therapeutic doses of vitamin C inhibited the growth and migration of several animal and human cancer cell in culture.[82–84]

Vitamin A and Carotenoids

Several studies show that vitamin A and its derivatives, retinoids, and carotenoids at therapeutic doses induced differentiation, apoptosis, and growth inhibition on several human and rodent cancer cells in culture without affecting the growth of normal cells.[85,86] Retinoic acid at therapeutic doses inhibited cell proliferation of human squamous cell carcinoma cells in culture by decreasing ERK1 (extracellular signal-related kinase 1, a serine/threonine kinase) activation.[87]

Carotenoids, including alpha- and beta-carotene, lycopene, and canthaxanthin reduced the growth of prostate cancer cells and colon cancer cells in culture.[88,89]

Selenium

Therapeutic doses of selenium compounds (sodium selenite or seleno-L-methionine) inhibited the growth of several human and rodent cancer cells, including breast cancer and prostate cancer in vitro and in animal models without affecting the growth of normal cells.[90,91] Selenium treatment at therapeutic doses markedly reduced androgen signaling and androgen-receptor (AR)-mediated gene expression, including prostate-specific antigen (PSA) in human prostate cancer cells in culture,[92] and estrogen receptor alpha (ERalpha) expression in breast tumor cells in culture.[93]

N-Acetylcysteine (NAC) and Alpha-Lipoic Acid

NAC at therapeutic doses reduced the growth of several rodent and human cancer cells in culture by inducing apoptosis.[94,95] Apoptosis was preceded by increased production of reactive oxygen species (ROS), activation of tumor suppressor gene, increased expression of Bax, release of cytochrome C from mitochondria, caspase activation, induction of pro-apoptotic signaling (i.e., JNK), and inhibition of anti-apoptotic signaling (i.e. PKB/Akt) pathways.[95] Therapeutic doses of NAC treatment inhibited tumor growth by increasing the expressions of TNF-alpha in T-cell lymphocytes and TNF-RI and TNF-RII on tumor cells and on T-cell lymphocytes.[96] NAC treatment also reduced incidence and multiplicity of lymphoma in Atm (AT-mutated) deficient mice, and increased their lifespan.[97] It has been reported that NAC treatment for 8 weeks induced anti-angiogenesis by increasing the production of angiostatin that resulted in endothelial apoptosis and vascular collapse in the tumor.[98] Others have also reported that NAC treatment inhibited angiogenesis and reduced growth of tumor cells in vitro and in animal models.[99]

Alpha-lipoic acid at therapeutic doses induced apoptosis in several types of cancer cells in culture without affecting the normal cells.[100,101] The mechanisms of apoptosis involve increased generation of ROS, inhibition of TNF-alpha-induced activation of NF-kappaB, induction of proapoptotic signaling, and inhibition of antiapoptotic signaling.

ANTIOXIDANT-INDUCED CHANGES IN GENE EXPRESSION PROFILES IN CANCER CELLS

Therapeutic doses of antioxidants inhibited the expression of genes. For example, vitamin E succinate inhibited the expression of c-myc, H-ras,[102] N-myc,[103] mutated p53,[104] the activity of protein kinase C activity,[105] caspase,[106] tumor necrosis factor,[107] transcriptional factor E2F.[108]

Marked changes in gene expression have been observed as early as 30 min after treatment of neuroblastoma cells with a therapeutic dose of alpha-TS (Figure 8.2). The above changes in gene expression may be one of the major factors that account for the growth-inhibitory effect of alpha-TS on cancer cells. Alpha-TS at therapeutic doses inhibited the growth of tumor cells in vivo without affecting the normal cells. It has been reported that NAC at therapeutic doses also induced anti-angiogenesis.[98] Others have also reported that NAC treatment inhibited angiogenesis and reduced growth of tumor cells in animal models.[99]

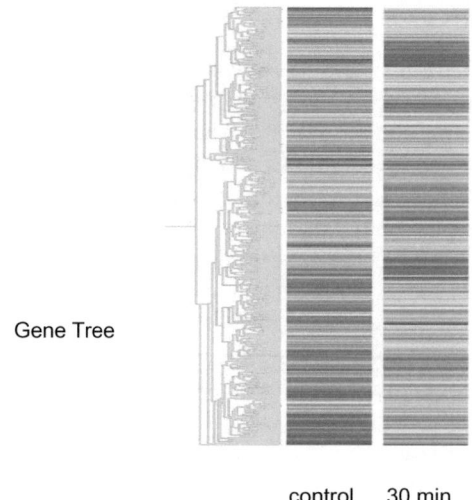

Gene Tree

control   30 min

FIGURE 8.2 Hierarchical clustering analysis of gene array data 30 min after treatment with α-TS shows a marked alteration in the levels of gene expression. Black color indicates high gene expression, faint black color medium expression, and gray color low expression.

EFFECTS OF THERAPEUTIC DOSES OF INDIVIDUAL ANTIOXIDANTS IN COMBINATION WITH RADIATION THERAPY ON CANCER CELLS AND NORMAL CELLS

CELL CULTURE STUDIES

Therapeutic doses of antioxidants or their derivatives enhanced the growth-inhibitory-effects of ionizing radiation selectively on cancer cells, while protecting normal cells against radiation damage or having no effects on normal cells. Retinoic acid enhanced the effect of X-irradiation on tumor cells by inhibiting the repair of potential lethal damage in cancer cells more effectively than that produced in normal fibroblasts.[109] Retinoic acid in combination with interferon alpha-2a enhanced radiation-induced damage on neck and head squamous cell carcinoma cells in culture.[110]

We have reported that therapeutic doses of vitamin E (alpha-TS) given before and/or after irradiation enhanced the levels of radiation-induced decrease in mitotic accumulation[111] and chromosomal damage[112] in human cervical cancer cells in culture (Figure 8.3). On the other hand, the same dose of alpha-TS did not modify the effect of irradiation on mitotic accumulation in normal cells,[111] but it protected normal cells against radiation-induced chromosomal damage.[112] In another study, we have reported that an aqueous form of vitamin E (alpha-tocopherol) and alpha-TS enhanced the level of radiation-induced growth inhibition in neuroblastoma (NB) cells (Figure 8.4).[77] Alpha-TS enhanced the growth-inhibitory effects of gamma-radiation in Ehrlich ascites cells, and human cervical and breast cancer cells in culture.[113] Vitamin C increased the growth-inhibitory effects of irradiation on NB cells, but not on glioma cells in culture.[76]

Selenomethionine at therapeutic doses enhanced the cell-killing effect of ionizing radiation on two human lung cancer cell lines, but not on human diploid lung fibroblasts in culture.[114]

ANIMAL STUDIES

Vitamin A (retinyl palmitate) or beta-carotene at therapeutic doses given daily through dietary supplement before X-irradiation and throughout the experimental period enhanced the levels of

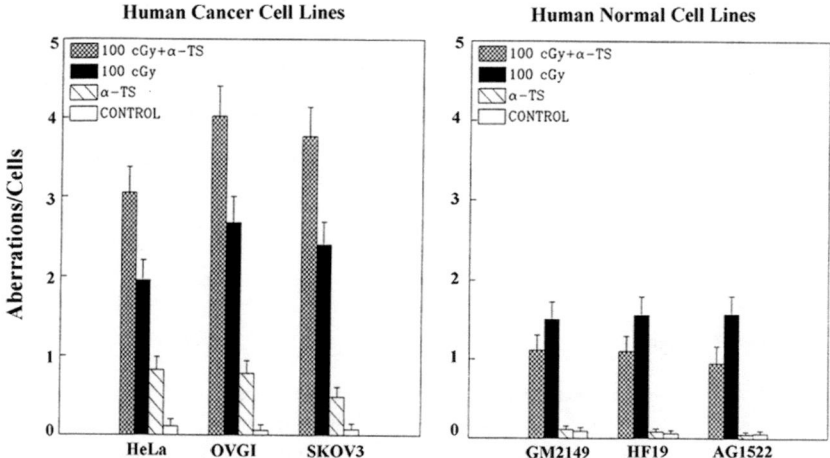

FIGURE 8.3 Effect of *d*-alpha-tocopheryl succinate (alpha-TS) on the level of radiation-induced chromosomal damage in human cervical cancer (HeLa cells), ovarian carcinoma cell lines (OVG1 and SKOV3), and in human normal skin fibroblasts (GM2149, HF19 and AG1522). Alpha-TS treatment alone increased chromosomal damage in all three cancer cell lines, but not in any normal cell lines. Alpha-TS treatment also enhanced the levels of radiation-induced chromosomal damage in cancer cells but it protected normal cells against such damage. The bar is standard error of the mean; and the difference between control and experimental groups in cancer cells, and between control (irradiation alone) and experimental groups (irradiation plus alpha-TS) is significant at P < 0.05. (From Chandrashekara, S. et al., *J. Assoc. Physicians. India*, 50, 225–227, 2002.)

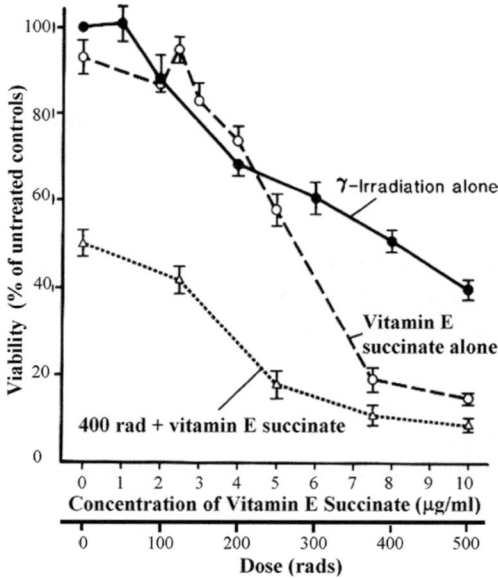

FIGURE 8.4 Neuroblastoma cells (NBP2) were plated in tissue culture dishes (60 mm), and the cells were gamma-irradiated 24 h after plating. Vitamin E succinate or the solvent (ethanol 0.25% and sodium succinate 5 mg/mL) was added immediately before irradiation. The drugs and medium were changed after 2 d of treatment. The number of cells per dish was determined after 3 d of treatment. Each experiment was repeated at least twice involving 3 samples per treatment. The average value (172 ± 7 × 104) of untreated control NB cells was considered 100%, and the growth in treated cultures was expressed as a % of untreated controls. The bar at each point is standard error of the mean. (From Hanson, A.J. et al., *J. Neurosci. Res.*, 74, 148–159, 2003.)

TABLE 8.4

Effect of Vitamin A, Beta-carotene and Local X-irradiation on Survival of Mice with Transplanted Breast Adenocarcinoma

Treatments	No. of Mice	One Year Survival (No. of Mice)
Control	24	0
3,000 rads, single dose	24	0
Vitamin A	24	0
Beta-carotene	24	0
Vitamin A Plus X-ray	24	22
Beta-Carotene Plus X-ray	24	22

Data were summarized from a previous study. (From Seifter, E. et al., Vitamin A and ß-carotene as adjunctive therapy to tumor excision, radiation therapy and chemotherapy. In: Prasad KN, ed. *Vitamins, Nutrition and Cancer.* Basel, Switzerland, Karger, 1–19, 1984.) Diets were supplemented with vitamin A (3,000 IU/mouse) and beta-carotene (270 µg/mouse), and these doses were about 10 times greater than the RDA for a mouse.

radiation damage on transplanted breast adenocarcinoma in mice and protected normal tissue against some of the toxicity of local irradiation (Table 8.4).[115] The administration of vitamin C through drinking water before and after X-irradiation decreased the survival of ascites tumor cells in mice without causing a similar effect on normal cells.[116] The administration of multiple antioxidant micronutrients (vitamins A, C and E) protected normal cells against damage produced by radio-immunotherapy in mice without protecting cancer cells.[117]

HUMAN STUDIES

Analysis of 49 studies in which antioxidants used during standard therapy (chemotherapy and/or radiation therapy) suggests that no conclusions can be with respect to its efficacy in improving treatment outcomes or in reducing adverse side effects.[1]

EFFECTS OF THERAPEUTIC DOSES OF INDIVIDUAL ANTIOXIDANTS IN COMBINATION WITH CHEMOTHERAPEUTIC ON CANCER CELLS AND NORMAL CELLS

CELL CULTURE STUDIES

Several studies have revealed that vitamin C, alpha-TS, alpha-TA, vitamin A (including retinoids), and polar carotenoids including beta-carotene at therapeutic doses enhanced the growth-inhibitory effects of most chemotherapeutic agents on some cancer cells in culture.[118] Chemotherapeutic agents used in these studies include 5-FU, vincristine, Adriamycin, bleomycin, 5-(3, 3-dimethyl-1-triazeno)-imidazole-4-carboximide (DTIC), cisplatin, tamoxifen, cyclophosphamide, mutamycin, chlorozotocin, and carmustine. The extent of this enhancement depends on dose and form of antioxidant, treatment schedule, dose and type of chemotherapeutic agent and type of tumor cell. Some examples of antioxidant-induced enhancement of the effect of chemotherapeutic agents are described below.

Vitamin C at therapeutic doses enhanced the effect of 5-fluouracil (5-FU) on neuroblastoma cells in culture[119] (Figure 8.5). Vitamin C at therapeutic doses increased the anti-tumor activity of doxorubicin, cisplatin, and paclitaxel in human breast cancer cells in culture.[120] Vitamin C also increased

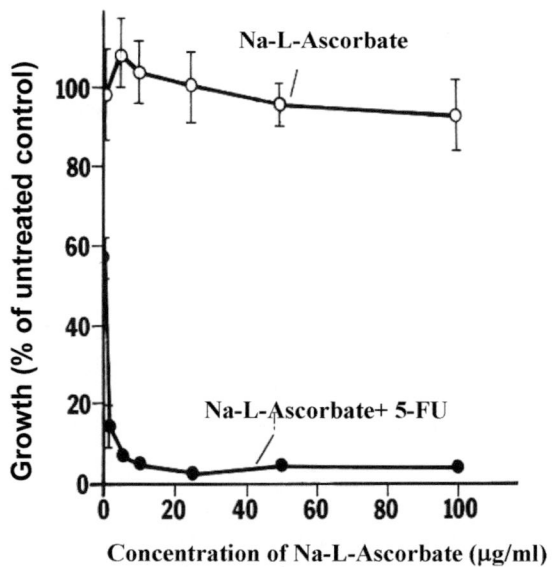

FIGURE 8.5   Neuroblastoma cells (50,000 per dish) were plated in tissue culture dishes (60 mm), and 5-Fluorouracil (5-FU) (0.08 mg/mL) plus sodium ascorbate or sodium ascorbate alone was added 24 h after plating. The drug and medium were changed every day, and the number of cells per dish was determined 3 d after treatment. Each value represents the mean of six to nine samples ± standard deviation. (From Prasad, K.N., *Experientia.*, 35, 906–908, 1979.)

drug accumulation and reversed vincristine resistance of human non-small-cell lung carcinoma cells.[121]Vitamin C at therapeutic doses enhanced antitumor activity of 5-FU and cisplatin in esophageal cancer cells in culture by inhibiting translocation of NF-kappaB and AP-1 {Abdel-Latif, 2005 #321}.

An aqueous form of vitamin E, alpha-tocopheryl acetate, at therapeutic doses enhanced the effect of vincristine on neuroblastoma cells in culture {Prasad, 1999 #244}. Alpha-TS increased the effect of Adriamycin on human prostate carcinoma cells in culture.[122] Recently, we have found that alpha-TS increased the effect of Adriamycin on human cervical cancer cells (HeLa) without modifying the effect of Adriamycin on normal human fibroblasts in culture (Table 8.5). Alpha-TS also enhanced the effect of carmustine on rat glioma cells in culture. Alpha-tocopherol protected cisplatin-induced toxicity without interfering with its anti-tumor activity in human melanoma transplanted in athymic mice.[123]

Beta-carotene and lycopene at therapeutic doses also enhanced the growth-inhibitory effect of docetaxel on human ER+ MCF-7 breast cancer cells in culture.[124] Sodium selenite and selenous acid induced growth inhibition in 5-FU-resistant cell lines.[125] Supplementation with selenium enhanced growth-inhibitory effects of taxol and doxorubicin in several tumor cell lines in culture.[126] Selenium nanoparticles enhanced the efficacy of Adriamycin on tumor cells.[127]

A mixture of antioxidants containing retinoic acid, vitamin C, alpha-TS, and polar carotenoids in combination with DTIC, tamoxifen, cisplatin, or interferon-alpha-2a inhibited the proliferation of human melanoma cells in culture more than the growth-inhibition produced by the individual agents[128] (Table 8.6). A mixture of dietary antioxidants (vitamin C, 100 μg/mL; alpha-tocopherol, 10 μg/mL and beta-carotene, 10 μg/mL) in combination carboplatin and paclitaxel enhanced the apoptotic effect of paclitaxel and carboplatin.[129] The most pronounced effect was observed when antioxidant mixture was given before treatment with chemotherapeutic agents, followed by paclitaxel treatment for 24 hours and then followed by carboplatin treatment for 24 hours (Table 8.7).

TABLE 8.5

Modification of Adriamycin Effect on Human Cervical Cancer Cells (HeLa) and Human Normal Skin Fibroblasts in Culture by *d*-Alpha-Tocopheryl Succinate

Treatment	HeLa Cells	Normal Fibroblasts
Solvent Control	99 ± 2.6	104 ± 3.4
Adriamycin (0.1 µg/mL)	57 ± 6.2	77 ± 2.4
Alpha-TS (10 µg/mL)	99 ± 1.6	101 ± 3.7
Adramycin (0.1 µg/mL) Plus alpha-TS	20 ± 7.9	77 ± 1.7
Adriamycin (0.25 µg/mL)	14 ± 2.9	68 ± 1.0
Adriamycin (0.25 µg/mL) Plus alpha-TS	5 ± 0.8	62 ± 1.8

Note: Cells (20,000) were plated in 24-well chamber and Adriamycin and alpha-tocopheryl succinate (alpha-TS) were added one after another at the same time. Drug, alpha-TS and fresh growth medium were changed at 2 days after treatment and the viability of cells was determined by MTT assay. Growth in experimental groups was expressed % of untreated control. Each experiment was repeated at least twice, and each value represents an average of 6–9 samples ± SEM (our unpublished observation).

TABLE 8.6

Enhancement of the Effect of Certain Chemotherapeutic Agents by a Mixture of Four Antioxidants on Human Melanoma Cells in Culture

Treatments	Cell Number (% of Controls)
Solvent	101 ± 4[a]
Cis-platin (1 mg/mL)	67 ± 4
Antioxidant mixture	56 ± 3
Cisplatin + Antioxidant mixture	38 ± 2
Tamoxifen (2 mg/mL)	81 ± 3
Tamoxifen + Antioxidant mixture	30 ± 2
DTIC (100 mg/mL)	71 ± 2
DTIC + Antioxidant mixture	38 ± 2
Interferon-alpha2b	82 ± 5
Interferon-alpha2b + Antioxidant mixture	29 ± 1

Data were summarized from a previous publication. (From Kentroti, S. et al., *Brain Res.*, 651, 1–6, 1994.)

Polar carotenoids were originally referred as beta-carotene. (From Jha, M.N. et al., *Nutr. Cancer.*, 35, 189–194, 1999.)

Vitamin C, 50 mg/mL; polar carotenoids, 10 mg/mL; alpha-tocopheryl succinate, 10 mg/mL and 13-cis-retinoic acid, 7.5 mg/mL were added simultaneously.

[a] Standard error of the mean.

TABLE 8.7

Flow-Cytometric Analysis of the Effect of Combination of the Agents (Paclitaxel, Carboplatin and Antioxidant Mixture) on Apoptosis in H520 Cells

| Serial No. | Treatment of Cells | | | | Apoptosis (% Cells) (Mean ± SE[a]) |
	Day 1	Day 2	Day 3	Day 4	(Day 5)
1	Cells plated	—	—	—	20.6 ± 1.2
2	Cells plated	Paclitaxel + Carboplatin	—	—	40.3 ± 3.1
3	Cells plated	Paclitaxel	Carboplatin	—	54.3 ± 2.2
4	Cells plated	Vitamins + Paclitaxel	Carboplatin	—	70.11 ± 3.7
5	Cells plated	Vitamins	Paclitaxel	Carboplatin	89.15 ± 4.3

Cells were plated on Day 1 and flow-cytometry was performed on Day 5. Control = Serial no. 1. Doses: Paclitaxel: 0.05 μmol/mL, Carboplatin: 0.5 μg/mL, Vitamin C: 100 μg/mL, Vitamin E: 10 μg/mL, beta-carotene: 10 μg/mL. (From Pathak, A.K. et al. Role of vitamins along with chemotherapy in non-small-cell lung cancer. Paper presented at: *International Conference on Nutrition and Cancer*, Montevideo-Uruguay, 2002.)

[a] SE = Standard error. Results are of three separate experiments, each performed in duplicate.

ANIMAL STUDIES

Therapeutic doses of selenium compounds (sodium selenite and selenosulfate) reduced cisplatin-induced toxicity without compromising its efficacy on the growth of tumor cells in animal models; however, selenosulfate appeared to be less toxic. In addition, supplementation with selenosulfate and cisplatin produced a cure rate of 87.5% compared to 25% cure rate observed in cisplatin treated group in a highly malignant cancer cell animal model.[100] However, organic selenium at therapeutic doses dose (0.2 mg/mouse/day or 10 mg/kg of body weight/day) enhanced the treatment efficacy of some chemotherapeutic agents in athymic mice bearing human squamous cell carcinoma of head and neck.[130]

Vitamin A (retinyl palmitate) or synthetic beta-carotene at therapeutic doses which were 10-fold higher than the RDA for these micronutrients, in combination with cyclophosphamide, increased the cure rate from 0 to more than 90% in mice with transplanted adenocarcinoma of the breast.[115] The synthetic retinoid (fenretinide) was effective against a human ovarian carcinoma xenograft and potentiated cisplatin activity.[131]

Intraperitoneal administration of NAC (200 mg/kg of body weight) enhanced the cytotoxic effects of 5-FU in athymic mice carrying human colon cancer cells without increasing the toxicity.[132] A study has reported that NAC at a therapeutic dose of 1 g/kg of body weight delivered IP in combination with doxorubicin reduced tumorigenicity and metastasis following transplantation of B-16 murine melanoma cells in mice.[133]

HUMAN STUDIES

Analysis of 49 studies in which antioxidants were used during standard therapy (chemotherapy and/or radiation therapy) suggests that no conclusions can be made with respect to its efficacy in improving treatment outcomes or in reducing adverse side effects.[1]

REASONS FOR GROWTH-INHIBITORY EFFECTS ANTIOXIDANTS IN THE PRESENCE OF ELEVATED LEVELS OF Nrf2

The growth-inhibitory effects of high doses antioxidants in the presence of elevated levels of Nrf2 on cancer cell can be explained by the following observations: (a) they bypass protective effect of Nrf2 and induce apoptosis by inducing proapoptotic signaling pathways; (b) they directly reduce the expression of Nrf2 as well as interfere with its function leading to decreased cytoprotective enzymes that cause apoptosis; and (c) they alter the expression of microRNAs and their respective enzymes leading to apoptosis.

PREVENTIVE DOSES OF INDIVIDUAL ANTIOXIDANTS REDUCE THE EFFICACY OF THERAPEUTIC AGENTS

Several studies have shown that preventive doses of antioxidants that do not affect the proliferation of cancer cells, when administered only one time shortly before cancer therapeutic agents, reduced the efficacy of therapeutic agents. Vitamin E (alpha-tocopherol), vitamin C, or N-acetylcysteine (NAC), when given in a single low preventive dose shortly before X-irradiation, reduced the effectiveness of irradiation on cancer cells culture and in vivo models.[134,135] Preventive doses of antioxidants used in these studies do not affect the growth of cancer cells. Alpha-lipoic acid at preventive doses reduced the effectiveness of doxorubicin in murine leukemia.[136] N-Acetylcysteine at a preventive dose reduced cisplatin-induced apoptosis from about 31% to about 11% in bladder cancer cells.[137]

EFFECTS OF THERAPEUTIC DOSES OF INDIVIDUAL ANTIOXIDANTS IN COMBINATION WITH EXPERIMENTAL THERAPIES ON CANCER CELLS

HYPERTHERMIA

Hyperthermia (43°C–45°C) alone, or in combination with radiation, is primarily used in the management of local tumors when all other therapeutic modalities have failed. This approach has not been effective for the long-term management of tumors. Therefore, the current treatment approaches must be altered from local hyperthermia at higher temperatures to whole-body hyperthermia at fever range temperatures that could be tolerated without side effects. In addition, non-toxic therapeutic doses of antioxidants could be used to enhance the efficacy of hyperthermia on cancer cells. We have reported that alpha-TS markedly increased the growth-inhibitory effect of low temperature (41°C) and high temperature (43°C) hyperthermia on neuroblastoma cells in culture[138] (Table 8.8). Administration of vitamin C locally markedly enhanced the efficacy of hyperthermia in

TABLE 8.8
Effect of Alpha Tocopheryl Succinate (α-TS) on Hyperthermia-Induced Growth Inhibition in Neuroblastoma Cells in Culture

Treatments	Cell Number (% of Controls)
Solvent (Ethanol 0.25%) + Sodium Succinate (5 mg/mL)	102 ± 3
A-TS (5 mg/mL)	50 ± 3
43°C (20 min)	43 ± 1
α-TS + 43°C	9 ± 1
41°C (45 min)	56 ± 3
α-TS + 41°C	21 ± 2
40°C (8 hr)	55 ± 2
α-TS + 40°C	30 ± 2

Data were summarized from a previous publication Values are mean + SEM. (From Rama, B.N. and Prasad, K.N., *Life Sci.*, 34, 2089–2097, 1984.)

reducing the growth of Lewis tumor in mice.[139] Therapeutic doses of vitamin C in combination with hyperthermia increased the survival time of mice carrying Ehrlich ascites tumor cells compared to untreated controls.[140] Bioflavonoid quercetin, in combination with hyperthermia, caused synergistic apoptosis in lymphoid cancer cells in culture.[141] Quercetin and tamoxifen together enhanced hyperthermia-induced apoptosis in a synergistic manner in human melanoma cells in culture.[142] Quercetin may also be useful in increasing the tumor responses to hyperthermia in combination chemotherapy.[143,144] The proposed micronutrient mixture may also enhance the efficacy of hyperthermia (local or whole-body in the management of human cancer). A clinical study can be initiated to test the safety and effectiveness of this approach.

SODIUM BUTYRATE AND INTERFERON-ALPHA2B

Anticancer property of butyric acid, a 4-carbon fatty acid, was accidently discovered when sodium butyrate was added as a control for the effect of dibutyryl adenosine 3′-5′-cyclic monophosphate (dibutyryl cAMP) on differentiation of neuroblastoma cells in culture. Dibutyryl cAMP induced irreversible morphological differentiation and growth inhibition; however, sodium butyrate reduced only growth of neuroblastoma cells.[145] Sodium butyrate, a potent inhibitor of histone deacetylase[119,146] or its analog, phenylbutyrate[147,148] induced apoptosis and inhibition of cell proliferation on several rodent and human tumor cell lines in culture. However, clinical studies with these agents produced minimal benefits in cancer patients.[149] Therefore, any agents that can enhance the effect of sodium butyrate or phenylbutyrate would enhance the value of these agents in clinical studies. We have reported that alpha-TS at therapeutic doses enhanced the growth-inhibitory effect of sodium butyrate on certain tumor cells in culture (Figure 8.6).[150] Retinoic acid increased the effect of phenylbutyrate on human prostate cancer cell growth and angiogenesis in athymic mice.[151] Retinoic acid in combination with sodium butyrate also caused a synergistic effects on cell differentiation in poorly differentiated thyroid carcinoma cells in culture; however, in athymic mice carrying the

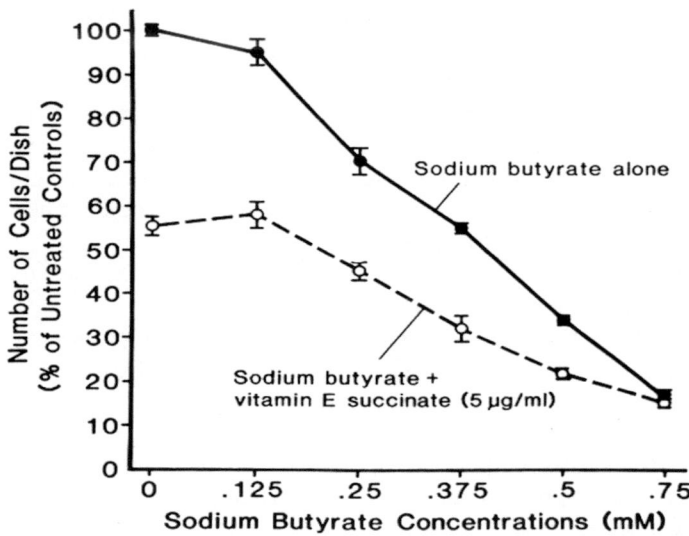

FIGURE 8.6 Effect of d-α-tocopheryl succinate (vitamin E succinate) in combination with sodium butyrate on the growth of neuroblastoma cells in culture. Cells (50,000 cells/60 mm dish) were plated in tissue culture dishes, and vitamin E succinate and sodium butyrate were added one after another 24 hours later. Fresh growth medium and agents were changed at two days after treatment and growth was determined at three days after treatment. Each value represents an average of six samples. The bar at each point is SEM. (From Cosar, M. et al., *Nutr. Neurosci.*, 11, 161–166, 2008.)

same tumor, the combination of two agents did not reduce the growth of tumor more than that produced by retinoic acid treatment alone[152] Antioxidants such as quercetin, curcumin, and ferulic acid enhanced sodium butyrate–induced apoptosis in human erythroleukemic cells in culture.[153] Since these studies, 6,276 new studies and reviews on the effect of sodium butyrate on inhibition of cancer growth have been published (PubMed).

α-TS[128] and retinoids[110] also enhance the effect of interferon in cell culture and in vivo, respectively. Although treatment of squamous cell carcinoma of head and neck in culture with retinoic acid, interferon-alpha2a, and alpha-tocopherol individually or in combination of two produced varying degree of growth inhibition, the combination of three was most effective.[154] The combination of 13-cis retinoic acid and interferon-alpha2a enhanced radiation-induced growth inhibition in human cervical carcinoma cells in culture.[155]

IMMUNOTHERAPY AND GENE THERAPY

Immunotherapy appears to be one of the most effective way of selective killing of cancer cells. Drugs that can stimulate immune function to kill cancer are being used with some success. Because of polyclonal nature of most tumors, effective gene therapy may be difficult to develop. It is uncertain whether antioxidants would have any significant impact on the effectiveness of any of these treatment modalities.

PROPOSED MIXTURE THERAPEUTIC DOSES OF ANTIOXIDANTS DURING CANCER THERAPY

Based on the data obtained from cell culture and animal models, I propose a mixture of micronutrients containing vitamin A 25,000 IU, beta-carotene 100 mg, vitamin C 10 grams, *d*-alpha-tocopheryl succinate 1600 IU, selenium 300 mcg, coenzyme Q10 600 mg, omega-3 fatty acids 4 grams, glutamine 5 grams, vitamin D3 10,000 IU, B-vitamins (2–3 times higher than RDA), curcumin 500 mg, and resveratrol 500 mg. This micronutrient mixture can be administered orally in two divided doses, one-half dose in the morning and one-half dose in the evening. The rationale for taking antioxidants twice a day is that the biological half-lives of micronutrients markedly vary. This micronutrient mixture can be started at 3 days prior to standard or experimental therapy and should be continued for one month after completion of therapy. This micronutrient mixture is expected to improve the efficacy of radiation therapy and chemotherapy by increasing tumor response and decreasing toxicity. This micronutrient mixture should not be used before surgery, because high dose of vitamin E may interfere with the clotting mechanism; however, it can be started 3 days after surgery in order to stimulate the healing processes.

This micronutrient mixture can also be used for those patients who have become refractory to all therapies in order to improve the survival time and quality of life.

A phase-1 study is needed in order to determine the safety of the proposed micronutrient mixture, followed by a well-designed clinical study. The results obtained from these studies would settle the current controversies, and if positive, may markedly enhance the efficacy of cancer therapies and reduce their toxicities.

The micronutrients and diet modifications proposed for cancer prevention in Chapter 7 would be the same for cancer survivors who are at risk of developing recurrence of primary tumor or new cancer and noncancerous diseases.

CONCLUSIONS

Despite recent advances in chemotherapy, radiation therapy, surgery (for solid tumors), hyperthermia, gene therapy, and immunotherapy alone or in combination, mortality has increased in the United States by about 5.5% in 7 years. Effective strategies to reduce the toxicity of cancer therapy are lacking. Despite short-term and long-term toxicity of standard therapy, it has increased cure rates in certain tumors and prolonging survival time of others. The risk of recurrence of the primary tumor, and the development of a new cancer and non-neoplastic diseases continues among cancer survivors. At present, there are no effective approaches to decrease the risk of these adverse effects.

Studies showed that microRNAs act either as oncogenes or antioncogenes; therefore, suggestions have been made that they can be used as targets for developing new cancer treatment drugs or as biomarkers of cancer.

Analysis of published studies showed that individual or multiple antioxidants administered during standard therapy did not significantly and consistently improve treatment outcomes or reduce adverse side effects. One of the reasons for these for inconclusive results could be that most human studies with antioxidant have administered low or preventive doses of antioxidants. Preventive doses of antioxidants stimulate the growth of cancer cells, and protect both normal and cancer cells during standard therapy.

Cancer cells constitutively express high levels of Nrf2 that allow cell proliferation, migration, and invasion, and prevent apoptosis by elevating cytoprotective enzymes including antioxidant enzymes. Elevated levels of Nrf2 also make cancer cells resistant to cancer drugs and radiation therapy. Antioxidants activate Nrf2 and at same time inhibit the growth of cancer cells. This paradoxical effect of therapeutic doses of antioxidants on cancer cells is explained by the studies in which antioxidants bypass the protective effects of Nrf2 and cause apoptosis by enhancing the expression of apoptotic signaling pathways, reducing the levels or interfere with the function of Nrf2, and by changing the expression of microRNAs and their target proteins that induce growth inhibition.

A mixture of micronutrients containing therapeutic doses of antioxidants to be administered orally before and after standard therapy is proposed. The efficacy and safety of this mixture should be tested by a well-designed clinical study.

REFERENCES

1. Yasueda A, Urushima H, Ito T. Efficacy and interaction of antioxidant supplements as adjuvant therapy in cancer treatment: A systematic review. *Integr Cancer Ther.* 2016;15(1):17–39.
2. Lee RC, Feinbaum RL, Ambros V. The C. elegans heterochronic gene lin-4 encodes small RNAs with antisense complementarity to lin-14. *Cell.* 1993;75(5):843–854.
3. Wightman B, Ha I, Ruvkun G. Posttranscriptional regulation of the heterochronic gene lin-14 by lin-4 mediates temporal pattern formation in C. elegans. *Cell.* 1993;75(5):855–862.
4. Macfarlane LA, Murphy PR. MicroRNA: Biogenesis, function and role in cancer. *Curr Genomics.* 2010;11(7):537–561.
5. Londin E, Loher P, Telonis AG, et al. Analysis of 13 cell types reveals evidence for the expression of numerous novel primate- and tissue-specific microRNAs. *Proc Natl Acad Sci U S A.* 2015;112(10):E1106–1115.
6. Denli AM, Tops BB, Plasterk RH, Ketting RF, Hannon GJ. Processing of primary microRNAs by the microprocessor complex. *Nature.* 2004;432(7014):231–235.
7. Lee Y, Ahn C, Han J, et al. The nuclear RNase III Drosha initiates microRNA processing. *Nature.* 2003;425(6956):415–419.
8. Hutvagner G, McLachlan J, Pasquinelli AE, Balint E, Tuschl T, Zamore PD. A cellular function for the RNA-interference enzyme Dicer in the maturation of the let-7 small temporal RNA. *Science.* 2001;293(5531):834–838.
9. Liu L, Wang D, Qiu Y, Dong H, Zhan X. Overexpression of microRNA-15 increases the chemosensitivity of colon cancer cells to 5-fluorouracil and oxaliplatin by inhibiting the nuclear factor-kappaB signalling pathway and inducing apoptosis. *Exp Ther Med.* 2018;15(3):2655–2660.
10. Zhou H, Lin C, Zhang Y, et al. miR-506 enhances the sensitivity of human colorectal cancer cells to oxaliplatin by suppressing MDR1/P-gp expression. *Cell Prolif.* 2017;50(3):e12341.
11. Zhang Z, Kim K, Li X, et al. MicroRNA-26b represses colon cancer cell proliferation by inhibiting lymphoid enhancer factor 1 expression. *Mol Cancer Ther.* 2014;13(7):1942–1951.
12. Guo ST, Jiang CC, Wang GP, et al. MicroRNA-497 targets insulin-like growth factor 1 receptor and has a tumour suppressive role in human colorectal cancer. *Oncogene.* 2013;32(15):1910–1920.

13. Wu L, Shi B, Huang K, Fan G. MicroRNA-128 suppresses cell growth and metastasis in colorectal carcinoma by targeting IRS1. *Oncol Rep*. 2015;34(5):2797–2805.

14. Han J, Liu Z, Wang N, Pan W. MicroRNA-874 inhibits growth, induces apoptosis and reverses chemoresistance in colorectal cancer by targeting X-linked inhibitor of apoptosis protein. *Oncol Rep*. 2016;36(1):542–550.

15. Xu XC, Zhang YH, Zhang WB, Li T, Gao H, Wang YH. MicroRNA-133a functions as a tumor suppressor in gastric cancer. *J Biol Regul Homeost Agents*. 2014;28(4):615–624.

16. Wang P, Guo X, Zong W, Song B, Liu G, He S. MicroRNA-128b suppresses tumor growth and promotes apoptosis by targeting A2bR in gastric cancer. *Biochem Biophys Res Commun*. 2015;467(4):798–804.

17. Gao HY, Huo FC, Wang HY, Pei DS. MicroRNA-9 inhibits the gastric cancer cell proliferation by targeting TNFAIP8. *Cell Prolif*. 2017;50(2):e12331.

18. Li X, Wang F, Qi Y. MiR-126 inhibits the invasion of gastric cancer cell in part by targeting Crk. *Eur Rev Med Pharmacol Sci*. 2014;18(14):2031–2037.

19. Hu CB, Li QL, Hu JF, Zhang Q, Xie JP, Deng L. miR-124 inhibits growth and invasion of gastric cancer by targeting ROCK1. *Asian Pac J Cancer Prev*. 2014;15(16):6543–6546.

20. Wang J, Wang X, Li Z, Liu H, Teng Y. MicroRNA-183 suppresses retinoblastoma cell growth, invasion and migration by targeting LRP6. *FEBS J*. 2014;281(5):1355–1365.

21. Liu S, Hu C, Wang Y, Shi G, Li Y, Wu H. miR-124 inhibits proliferation and invasion of human retinoblastoma cells by targeting STAT3. *Oncol Rep*. 2016;36(4):2398–2404.

22. Zhao Y, Li Y, Lou G, et al. MiR-137 targets estrogen-related receptor alpha and impairs the proliferative and migratory capacity of breast cancer cells. *PLoS One*. 2012;7(6):e39102.

23. Luo Q, Li X, Li J, et al. MiR-15a is underexpressed and inhibits the cell cycle by targeting CCNE1 in breast cancer. *Int J Oncol*. 2013;43(4):1212–1218.

24. Mobarra N, Shafiee A, Rad SM, et al. Overexpression of microRNA-16 declines cellular growth, proliferation and induces apoptosis in human breast cancer cells. *In Vitro Cell Dev Biol Anim*. 2015;51(6):604–611.

25. Taipaleenmaki H, Browne G, Akech J, et al. Targeting of Runx2 by miR-135 and miR-203 impairs progression of breast cancer and metastatic bone disease. *Cancer Res*. 2015;75(7):1433–1444.

26. Tsai WC, Hsu PW, Lai TC, et al. MicroRNA-122, a tumor suppressor microRNA that regulates intrahepatic metastasis of hepatocellular carcinoma. *Hepatology*. 2009;49(5):1571–1582.

27. Liu Y, Wu C, Wang Y, et al. MicroRNA-145 inhibits cell proliferation by directly targeting ADAM17 in hepatocellular carcinoma. *Oncol Rep*. 2014;32(5):1923–1930.

28. Wang X, Wu J, Lin Y, et al. MicroRNA-320c inhibits tumorous behaviors of bladder cancer by targeting Cyclin-dependent kinase 6. *J Exp Clin Cancer Res*. 2014;33:69.

29. Chen H, Lin YW, Mao YQ, et al. MicroRNA-449a acts as a tumor suppressor in human bladder cancer through the regulation of pocket proteins. *Cancer Lett*. 2012;320(1):40–47.

30. Zhao Q, Zhai YX, Liu HQ, Shi YA, Li XB. MicroRNA-491-5p suppresses cervical cancer cell growth by targeting hTERT. *Oncol Rep*. 2015;34(2):979–986.

31. Xu Y, Zhao S, Cui M, Wang Q. Down-regulation of microRNA-135b inhibited growth of cervical cancer cells by targeting FOXO1. *Int J Clin Exp Pathol*. 2015;8(9):10294–10304.

32. Feng Y, Liu J, Kang Y, et al. miR-19a acts as an oncogenic microRNA and is up-regulated in bladder cancer. *J Exp Clin Cancer Res*. 2014;33:67.

33. Yang WB, Chen PH, Hsu Ts, et al. Sp1-mediated microRNA-182 expression regulates lung cancer progression. *Oncotarget*. 2014;5(3):740–753.

34. Huang H, Jiang Y, Wang Y, et al. miR-5100 promotes tumor growth in lung cancer by targeting Rab6. *Cancer Lett*. 2015;362(1):15–24.

35. Xie X, Liu HT, Mei J, et al. miR-106a promotes growth and metastasis of non-small cell lung cancer by targeting PTEN. *Int J Clin Exp Pathol*. 2015;8(4):3827–3834.

36. Lei L, Huang Y, Gong W. miR-205 promotes the growth, metastasis and chemoresistance of NSCLC cells by targeting PTEN. *Oncol Rep*. 2013;30(6):2897–2902.

37. Ren P, Gong F, Zhang Y, Jiang J, Zhang H. MicroRNA-92a promotes growth, metastasis, and chemoresistance in non-small cell lung cancer cells by targeting PTEN. *Tumor Biol*. 2016;37(3):3215–3225.

38. Ueno K, Hirata H, Shahryari V, et al. microRNA-183 is an oncogene targeting Dkk-3 and SMAD4 in prostate cancer. *Br J Cancer*. 2013;108(8):1659–1667.

39. Li T, Lu YY, Zhao XD, et al. MicroRNA-296-5p increases proliferation in gastric cancer through repression of Caudal-related homeobox 1. *Oncogene*. 2014;33(6):783–793.

40. Bao L, Fu X, Si M, et al. MicroRNA-185 targets SOCS3 to inhibit beta-cell dysfunction in diabetes. *PLoS One*. 2015;10(2):e0116067.

41. Chu Y, Ouyang Y, Wang F, et al. MicroRNA-590 promotes cervical cancer cell growth and invasion by targeting CHL1. *J Cell Biochem*. 2014;115(5):847–853.

42. Ji D, Chen Z, Li M, et al. MicroRNA-181a promotes tumor growth and liver metastasis in colorectal cancer by targeting the tumor suppressor WIF-1. *Mol Cancer*. 2014;13:86.

43. Muhammad N, Bhattacharya S, Steele R, Ray RB. Anti-miR-203 suppresses ER-positive breast cancer growth and stemness by targeting SOCS3. *Oncotarget*. 2016;7(36):58595–58605.

44. Itoh K, Chiba T, Takahashi S, et al. An Nrf2/small Maf heterodimer mediates the induction of phase II detoxifying enzyme genes through antioxidant response elements. *Biochem Biophy Res Co*. 1997;236(2):313–322.

45. Williamson TP, Johnson DA, Johnson JA. Activation of the Nrf2-ARE pathway by siRNA knockdown of Keap1 reduces oxidative stress and provides partial protection from MPTP-mediated neurotoxicity. *Neurotoxicology*. 2012;33(3):272–279.

46. Jaramillo MC, Zhang DD. The emerging role of the Nrf2-Keap1 signaling pathway in cancer. *Genes Dev*. 2013;27(20):2179–2191.

47. Li W, Khor TO, Xu C, et al. Activation of Nrf2-antioxidant signaling attenuates NFkappaB-inflammatory response and elicits apoptosis. *Biochem Pharmacol*. 2008;76(11):1485–1489.

48. Kim J, Cha YN, Surh YJ. A protective role of nuclear factor-erythroid 2-related factor-2 (Nrf2) in inflammatory disorders. *Mutat Res*. 2010;690(1–2):12–23.

49. Furfaro AL, Traverso N, Domenicotti C, et al. The Nrf2/HO-1 axis in cancer cell growth and chemoresistance. *Oxid Med Cell Longev*. 2016;2016:1958174.

50. Leinonen HM, Kansanen E, Polonen P, Heinaniemi M, Levonen AL. Dysregulation of the Keap1-Nrf2 pathway in cancer. *Biochem Soc Trans*. 2015;43(4):645–649.

51. Wu T, Harder BG, Wong PK, Lang JE, Zhang DD. Oxidative stress, mammospheres and Nrf2-new implication for breast cancer therapy? *Mol Carcinog*. 2015;54(11):1494–1502.

52. Ren D, Villeneuve NF, Jiang T, et al. Brusatol enhances the efficacy of chemotherapy by inhibiting the Nrf2-mediated defense mechanism. *Proc Natl Acad Sci U S A*. 2011;108(4):1433–1438.

53. Ma X, Zhang J, Liu S, Huang Y, Chen B, Wang D. Nrf2 knockdown by shRNA inhibits tumor growth and increases efficacy of chemotherapy in cervical cancer. *Cancer Chemother Pharmacol*. 2012;69(2):485–494.

54. Yamadori T, Ishii Y, Homma S, et al. Molecular mechanisms for the regulation of Nrf2-mediated cell proliferation in non-small-cell lung cancers. *Oncogene*. 2012;31(45):4768–4777.

55. Zhan L, Zhang H, Zhang Q, et al. Regulatory role of KEAP1 and NRF2 in PPARgamma expression and chemoresistance in human non-small-cell lung carcinoma cells. *Free Radic Biol Med*. 2012;53(4):758–768.

56. Lister A, Nedjadi T, Kitteringham NR, et al. Nrf2 is overexpressed in pancreatic cancer: Implications for cell proliferation and therapy. *Mol Cancer*. 2011;10:37.

57. Khalil HS, Langdon SP, Goltsov A, et al. A novel mechanism of action of HER2 targeted immunotherapy is explained by inhibition of NRF2 function in ovarian cancer cells. *Oncotarget*. 2016;7(46):75874–75901.

58. Chian S, Thapa R, Chi Z, Wang XJ, Tang X. Luteolin inhibits the Nrf2 signaling pathway and tumor growth in vivo. *Biochem Biophys Res Commun*. 2014;447(4):602–608.

59. Ohnuma T, Anzai E, Suzuki Y, et al. Selective antagonization of activated Nrf2 and inhibition of cancer cell proliferation by procyanidins from Cinnamomi Cortex extract. *Arch Biochem Biophys*. 2015;585:17–24.

60. Benlloch M, Obrador E, Valles SL, et al. Pterostilbene decreases the antioxidant defenses of aggressive cancer cells in vivo: A physiological glucocorticoids- and Nrf2-Dependent mechanism. *Antioxid Redox Signal*. 2016;24(17):974–990.

61. Mostafavi-Pour Z, Ramezani F, Keshavarzi F, Samadi N. The role of quercetin and vitamin C in Nrf2-dependent oxidative stress production in breast cancer cells. *Oncol Lett*. 2017;13(3):1965–1973.

62. Katsuyama Y, Tsuboi T, Taira N, Yoshioka M, Masaki H. 3-O-Laurylglyceryl ascorbate activates the intracellular antioxidant system through the contribution of PPAR-gamma and Nrf2. *J Dermatol Sci*. 2016;82(3):189–196.

63. Singh B, Ronghe AM, Chatterjee A, Bhat NK, Bhat HK. MicroRNA-93 regulates NRF2 expression and is associated with breast carcinogenesis. *Carcinogenesis*. 2013;34(5):1165–1172.

64. Suh JH, Shenvi SV, Dixon BM, et al. Decline in transcriptional activity of Nrf2 causes age-related loss of glutathione synthesis, which is reversible with lipoic acid. *Proc Natl Acad Sci U S A*. 2004;101(10):3381–3386.

65. Choi HK, Pokharel YR, Lim SC, et al. Inhibition of liver fibrosis by solubilized coenzyme Q10: Role of Nrf2 activation in inhibiting transforming growth factor-beta1 expression. *Toxicol Appl Pharm*. 2009;240(3):377–384.

66. Ji L, Liu R, Zhang XD, et al. N-acetylcysteine attenuates phosgene-induced acute lung injury via up-regulation of Nrf2 expression. *Inhal Toxicol.* 2010;22(7):535–542.

67. Gao L, Wang J, Sekhar KR, et al. Novel n-3 fatty acid oxidation products activate Nrf2 by destabilizing the association between Keap1 and Cullin3. *J Biol Chem.* 2007;282(4):2529–2537.

68. Saw CL, Yang AY, Guo Y, Kong AN. Astaxanthin and omega-3 fatty acids individually and in combination protect against oxidative stress via the Nrf2-ARE pathway. *Food Chem Toxicol.* 2013;62:869–875.

69. Trujillo J, Chirino YI, Molina-Jijon E, Anderica-Romero AC, Tapia E, Pedraza-Chaverri J. Renoprotective effect of the antioxidant curcumin: Recent findings. *Redox Biol.* 2013;1(1):448–456.

70. Steele ML, Fuller S, Patel M, Kersaitis C, Ooi L, Munch G. Effect of Nrf2 activators on release of glutathione, cysteinylglycine, and homocysteine by human U373 astroglial cells. *Redox biology.* 2013;1(1):441–445.

71. Kode A, Rajendrasozhan S, Caito S, Yang SR, Megson IL, Rahman I. Resveratrol induces glutathione synthesis by activation of Nrf2 and protects against cigarette smoke-mediated oxidative stress in human lung epithelial cells. *Am J Physiol Lung Cell Mol Physiol.* 2008;294(3):L478–L488.

72. Probst BL, McCauley L, Trevino I, Wigley WC, Ferguson DA. Cancer cell growth is differentially affected by constitutive activation of NRF2 by KEAP1 deletion and pharmacological activation of NRF2 by the synthetic triterpenoid, RTA 405. *PLoS One.* 2015;10(8):e0135257.

73. Probst BL, Trevino I, McCauley L, et al. RTA 408, A novel synthetic triterpenoid with broad anticancer and anti-inflammatory activity. *PLoS One.* 2015;10(4):e0122942.

74. Chen B, Zhang Y, Wang Y, Rao J, Jiang X, Xu Z. Curcumin inhibits proliferation of breast cancer cells through Nrf2-mediated downregulation of Fen1 expression. *J Steroid Biochem Mol Biol.* 2014;143:11–18.

75. Niture SK, Jaiswal AK. Nrf2-induced antiapoptotic Bcl-xL protein enhances cell survival and drug resistance. *Free Radic Biol Med.* 2013;57:119–131.

76. Prasad KN, Edwards-Prasad J. Effects of tocopherol (vitamin E) acid succinate on morphological alterations and growth inhibition in melanoma cells in culture. *Cancer Res.* 1982;42(2):550–555.

77. Hanson AJ, Prasad JE, Nahreini P, et al. Overexpression of amyloid precursor protein is associated with degeneration, decreased viability, and increased damage caused by neurotoxins (prostaglandins A1 and E2, hydrogen peroxide, and nitric oxide) in differentiated neuroblastoma cells. *J Neurosci Res.* 2003;74(1):148–159.

78. Kline K, Yu W, Sanders BG. Vitamin E: Mechanisms of action as tumor cell growth inhibitors. *J Nutr.* 2001;131(1):161S–163S.

79. Chiu TM, Huang CC, Lin TJ, Fang JY, Wu NL, Hung CF. In vitro and in vivo anti-photoaging effects of an isoflavone extract from soybean cake. *J Ethnopharmacol.* 2009;126(1):108–113.

80. Frost G, Sleeth ML, Sahuri-Arisoylu M, et al. The short-chain fatty acid acetate reduces appetite via a central homeostatic mechanism. *Nat Commun.* 2014;5:3611.

81. Ciechanover A, Orian A, Schwartz AL. The ubiquitin-mediated proteolytic pathway: Mode of action and clinical implications. *J Cell Biochem Suppl.* 2000;34:40–51.

82. Aerts AM, Zabrocki P, Govaert G, et al. Mitochondrial dysfunction leads to reduced chronological lifespan and increased apoptosis in yeast. *FEBS Lett.* 2008;583(1):113–117.

83. Wybieralska E, Koza M, Sroka J, Czyz J, Madeja Z. Ascorbic acid inhibits the migration of Walker 256 carcinosarcoma cells. *Cell Mol Biol Lett.* 2008;13(1):103–111.

84. Prasad KN. Effect of sodium butyrate in combination with X-irradiation, chemotherapeutic and cyclic AMP stimulating agents on neuroblastoma cells in culture. *Experientia.* 1979;35(7):906–908.

85. Garewal H. Beta-carotene and antioxidant nutrients in oral cancer prevention. In: Prasad KS, Santamaria L, Williams RM, ed. *Nutrients in Cancer Prevention and Treatment.* Totawa, NJ: Humana Press; 1995.

86. Simeone AM, Tari AM. How retinoids regulate breast cancer cell proliferation and apoptosis. *Cell Mol Life Sci.* 2004;61(12):1475–1484.

87. Crowe DL, Kim R, Chandraratna RA. Retinoic acid differentially regulates cancer cell proliferation via dose-dependent modulation of the mitogen-activated protein kinase pathway. *Mol Cancer Res.* 2003;1(7):532–540.

88. Hwang ES, Bowen PE. Cell cycle arrest and induction of apoptosis by lycopene in LNCaP human prostate cancer cells. *J Med Food.* 2004;7(3):284–289.

89. van Breemen RB, Pajkovic N. Multitargeted therapy of cancer by lycopene. *Cancer Lett.* 2008;269(2):339–351.

90. Rooprai HK, Kyriazis I, Nuttall RK, et al. Inhibition of invasion and induction of apoptosis by selenium in human malignant brain tumour cells in vitro. *Int J Oncol.* 2007;30(5):1263–1271.

91. Husbeck B, Nonn L, Peehl DM, Knox SJ. Tumor-selective killing by selenite in patient-matched pairs of normal and malignant prostate cells. *Prostate.* 2006;66(2):218–225.

92. Chen YJ, Chang JT, Liao CT, et al. Head and neck cancer in the betel quid chewing area: Recent advances in molecular carcinogenesis. *Cancer Sci.* 2008;99(8):1507–1514.

93. Shah YM, Kaul A, Dong Y, Ip C, Rowan BG. Attenuation of estrogen receptor alpha (ERalpha) signaling by selenium in breast cancer cells via downregulation of ERalpha gene expression. *Breast Cancer Res Treat.* 2005;92(3):239–250.

94. Aarsland D, Rongve A, Nore SP, et al. Frequency and case identification of dementia with Lewy bodies using the revised consensus criteria. *Dement Geriatr Cogn Disord.* 2008;26(5):445–452.

95. Simbula G, Columbano A, Ledda-Columbano GM, et al. Increased ROS generation and p53 activation in alpha-lipoic acid-induced apoptosis of hepatoma cells. *Apoptosis.* 2007;12(1):113–123.

96. Delneste Y, Jeannin P, Potier L, Romero P, Bonnefoy JY. N-Acetyl-L-cysteine exhibits antitumoral activity by increasing tumor necrosis factor alpha-dependent T-cell cytotoxicity. *Blood.* 1997;90(3):1124–1132.

97. Reliene R, Schiestl RH. Antioxidant N-acetyl cysteine reduces incidence and multiplicity of lymphoma in Atm deficient mice. *DNA Repair (Amst).* 2006;5(7):852–859.

98. Agarwal A, Munoz-Najar U, Klueh U, Shih SC, Claffey KP. N-acetylcysteine promotes angiostatin production and vascular collapse in an orthotopic model of breast cancer. *Am J Pathol.* 2004;164(5):1683–1696.

99. Albini A, Morini M, D'Agostini F, et al. Inhibition of angiogenesis-driven Kaposi's sarcoma tumor growth in nude mice by oral N-acetylcysteine. *Cancer Res.* 2001;61(22):8171–8178.

100. 1994–2004 TDoDs. *Lessons Learned and New Challenges: Workshop.* Washington, DC: National Academic Press; 2008.

101. Wenzel U, Nickel A, Daniel H. Alpha-Lipoic acid induces apoptosis in human colon cancer cells by increasing mitochondrial respiration with a concomitant O2-*-generation. *Apoptosis.* 2005;10(2):359–368.

102. Hazuka MB, Edwards-Prasad J, Newman F, Kinzie JJ, Prasad KN. Beta-carotene induces morphological differentiation and decreases adenylate cyclase activity in melanoma cells in culture. *J Am Coll Nutr.* 1990;9(2):143–149.

103. Thiele CJ, Reynolds CP, Israel MA. Decreased expression of N-myc precedes retinoic acid-induced morphological differentiation of human neuroblastoma. *Nature.* 1985;313(6001):404–406.

104. Schwartz JL. Molecular and biochemical control of tumor growth following treatment with carotenoids or tocopherols. In: Prasad KN, Santamaria L, Williams RM, eds. *Nutrients in Cancer Prevention and Treatment.* Totowa, NJ: Humana Press; 1995:287–316.

105. Gopalakrishna R, Gundimeda U, Chen Z. Vitamin E succinate inhibits protein Kinase C: Correlation with its unique inhibitory effects on cell growth and transformation. In: Prasad KN, Santamaria L, Williams RM, eds. *Nutrients in Cancer Prevention and Treatment.* Totowa, NJ: Humana Press; 1995:21–37.

106. Neuzil J, Svensson I, Weber T, Weber C, Brunk UT. Alpha-tocopheryl succinate-induced apoptosis in Jurkat T cells involves caspase-3 activation, and both lysosomal and mitochondrial destabilisation. *FEBS Lett.* 1999;445(2–3):295–300.

107. Hishiki T, Nimura Y, Isogai E, et al. Glial cell line-derived neurotrophic factor/neurturin-induced differentiation and its enhancement by retinoic acid in primary human neuroblastomas expressing c-Ret, GFR alpha-1, and GFR alpha-2. *Cancer Res.* 1998;58(10):2158–2165.

108. Turley JM, Fu T, Ruscetti FW, Mikovits JA, Bertolette 3rd DC, Birchenall-Roberts MC. Vitamin E succinate induces fas-mediated apoptosis in estrogen receptor-negative human breast cancer cells. *Cancer Res.* 1997;57(5):881–890.

109. Rutz HP, Little JB. Modification of radiosensitivity and recovery from X ray damage in vitro by retinoic acid. *Int J Radiat Oncol Biol Phys.* 1989;16(5):1285–1288.

110. Lippman SM, Kavanagh JJ, Paredes-Espinoza M, et al. 13-cis-retinoic acid plus interferon alpha-2a: Highly active systemic therapy for squamous cell carcinoma of the cervix. *J Natl Cancer I.* 1992;84(4):241–245.

111. Jha MN, Bedford JS, Cole WC, Edward-Prasad J, Prasad KN. Vitamin E (d-alpha-tocopheryl succinate) decreases mitotic accumulation in gamma-irradiated human tumor, but not in normal, cells. *Nutr Cancer.* 1999;35(2):189–194.

112. Chandrashekara S, Anilkumar T, Jamuna S. Complementary and alternative drug therapy in arthritis. *J Assoc Physicians India.* 2002;50:225–227.

113. Girdhani S, Bhosle SM, Thulsidas SA, Kumar A, Mishra KP. Potential of radiosensitizing agents in cancer chemo-radiotherapy. *J Cancer Res Ther.* 2005;1(3):129–131.

114. Coleman CN, Hrdina C, Bader JL, et al. Medical response to a radiologic/nuclear event: Integrated plan from the Office of the Assistant Secretary for Preparedness and Response, Department of Health and Human Services. *Ann Emerg Med.* 2009;53(2):213–222.

115. Seifter E, Rettura A, Padawar J, Levenson SM. Vitamin A and ß-carotene as adjunctive therapy to tumor excision, radiation therapy and chemotherapy. In: Prasad KN, ed. *Vitamins, Nutrition and Cancer.* Basel, Switzerland: Karger; 1984:1–19.

116. Tewfik FA, Tewfik HH, Riley EF. The influence of ascorbic acid on the growth of solid tumors in mice and on tumor control by X-irradiation. *Int J Vitam Nutr Res Suppl.* 1982;23:257–263.

117. Blumenthal RD, Lew W, Reising A, et al. Anti-oxidant vitamins reduce normal tissue toxicity induced by radio-immunotherapy. *Int J Cancer.* 2000;86(2):276–280.

118. Hovland AR, La Rosa FG, Hovland PG, et al. Cyclosporin A regulates the levels of cyclophilin A in neuroblastoma cells in culture. *Neurochem Int.* 1999;35(3):229–235.

119. Chang JH, Prasad KN. Differentiation of mouse neuroblastoma cells in vitro and in vivo induced by cyclic adenosine monophosphate (cAMP). *J Pediatr Surg.* 1976;11(5):847–858.

120. Kurbacher CM, Wagner U, Kolster B, Andreotti PE, Krebs D, Bruckner HW. Ascorbic acid (vitamin C) improves the antineoplastic activity of doxorubicin, cisplatin, and paclitaxel in human breast carcinoma cells in vitro. *Cancer Lett.* 1996;103(2):183–189.

121. Chiang CD, Song EJ, Yang VC, Chao CC. Ascorbic acid increases drug accumulation and reverses vincristine resistance of human non-small-cell lung-cancer cells. *Biochem J.* 1994;301 (Pt 3):759–764.

122. Ripoll EA, Rama BN, Webber MM. Vitamin E enhances the chemotherapeutic effects of adriamycin on human prostatic carcinoma cells in vitro. *J Urol.* 1986;136(2):529–531.

123. Leonetti C, Biroccio A, Gabellini C, et al. Alpha-tocopherol protects against cisplatin-induced toxicity without interfering with antitumor efficacy. *Int J Cancer.* 2003;104(2):243–250.

124. Czeczuga-Semeniuk E, Lemancewicz D, Wolczynski S. Can vitamin A modify the activity of docetaxel in MCF-7 breast cancer cells? *Folia Histochem Cytobiol.* 2007;45(Suppl 1):S169–174.

125. Thant AA, Wu Y, Lee J, et al. Role of caspases in 5-FU and selenium-induced growth inhibition of colorectal cancer cells. *Anticancer Res.* 2008;28(6A):3579–3592.

126. Vadgama JV, Wu Y, Shen D, Hsia S, Block J. Effect of selenium in combination with Adriamycin or Taxol on several different cancer cells. *Anticancer Res.* 2000;20(3A):1391–1414.

127. Tan L, Jia X, Jiang X, et al. In vitro study on the individual and synergistic cytotoxicity of adriamycin and selenium nanoparticles against Bel7402 cells with a quartz crystal microbalance. *Biosens Bioelectron.* 2009;24(7):2268–2272.

128. Kentroti S, Prasad KN, Carvalho E, Vernadakis A. Differential regulation of phenotypic expression in a pluripotential neuroblastoma cell line. *Brain Res.* 1994;651(1–2):1–6.

129. Pathak AK, Signh N, Guleria R, et al. Role of vitamins along with chemotherapy in non-small-cell lung cancer. Paper presented at: *International Conference on Nutrition and Cancer*; October 3–5, 2002; Montevideo-Uruguay.

130. Cao S, Durrani FA, Rustum YM. Selective modulation of the therapeutic efficacy of anticancer drugs by selenium containing compounds against human tumor xenografts. *Clin Cancer Res.* 2004;10(7):2561–2569.

131. Formelli F, Cleris L. Synthetic retinoid fenretinide is effective against a human ovarian carcinoma xenograft and potentiates cisplatin activity. *Cancer Res.* 1993;53(22):5374–5376.

132. Dreher F, Maibach H. Protective effects of topical antioxidants in humans. *Curr Probl Dermatol.* 2001;29:157–164.

133. De Flora S, D'Agostini F, Masiello L, Giunciuglio D, Albini A. Synergism between N-acetylcysteine and doxorubicin in the prevention of tumorigenicity and metastasis in murine models. *Int J Cancer.* 1996;67(6):842–848.

134. Prasad KN, Kumar S, Carvalho E, et al. Characterization of human and rat immortalized clones parotid acinar cells with respect to specific proteins and their mRNAs, and receptor-linked adenylate cyclase. *In Vitro Cell Dev Biol Anim.* 1995;31(10):767–772.

135. Salganik RI, Albright CD, Rodgers J, et al. Dietary antioxidant depletion: Enhancement of tumor apoptosis and inhibition of brain tumor growth in transgenic mice. *Carcinogenesis.* 2000;21(5):909–914.

136. Dovinova I, Novotny L, Rauko P, Kvasnicka P. Combined effect of lipoic acid and doxorubicin in murine leukemia. *Neoplasma*. 1999;46(4):237–241.
137. Miyajima A, Nakashima J, Tachibana M, Nakamura K, Hayakawa M, Murai M. N-acetylcysteine modifies cis-dichlorodiammineplatinum-induced effects in bladder cancer cells. *Jpn J Cancer Res*. 1999;90(5):565–570.
138. Rama BN, Prasad KN. Effect of hyperthermia in combination with vitamin E and cyclic AMP on neuroblastoma cells in culture. *Life Sci*. 1984;34(21):2089–2097.
139. Bae SC, Jung WJ, Lee EJ, Yu R, Sung MK. Effects of antioxidant supplements intervention on the level of plasma inflammatory molecules and disease severity of rheumatoid arthritis patients. *J Am Coll Nutr*. 2009;28(1):56–62.
140. Kageyama K, Onoyama Y, Otani S, Matsui-Yuasa I, Nagao N, Miwa N. Enhanced inhibitory effects of hyperthermia combined with ascorbic acid on DNA synthesis in Ehrlich ascites tumor cells grown at a low cell density. *Cancer Biochem Biophys*. 1995;14(4):273–280.
141. Fujita M, Nagai M, Murata M, Kawakami K, Irino S, Takahara J. Synergistic cytotoxic effect of quercetin and heat treatment in a lymphoid cell line (OZ) with low HSP70 expression. *Leuk Res*. 1997;21(2):139–145.
142. Piantelli M, Tatone D, Castrilli G, et al. Quercetin and tamoxifen sensitize human melanoma cells to hyperthermia. *Melanoma Res*. 2001;11(5):469–476.
143. Debes A, Oerding M, Willers R, Gobel U, Wessalowski R. Sensitization of human Ewing's tumor cells to chemotherapy and heat treatment by the bioflavonoid quercetin. *Anticancer Res*. 2003;23(4):3359–3366.
144. Shen J, Zhang W, Wu J, Zhu Y. The synergistic reversal effect of multidrug resistance by quercetin and hyperthermia in doxorubicin-resistant human myelogenous leukemia cells. *Int J Hyperthermia*. 2008;24(2):151–159.
145. Prasad KN, Hsie AW. Morphologic differentiation of mouse neuroblastoma cells induced in vitro by dibutyryl adenosine 3′:5′-cyclic monophosphate. *Nat New Biol*. 1971;233(39):141–142.
146. Aabdallah DM, Eid NI. Possible neuroprotective effects of lecithin and alpha-tocopherol alone or in combination against ischemia/reperfusion insult in rat brain. *J Biochem Mol Toxic*. 2004;18(5):273–278.
147. Samid D, Shack S, Sherman LT. Phenylacetate: A novel nontoxic inducer of tumor cell differentiation. *Cancer Res*. 1992;52(7):1988–1992.
148. Melchior SW, Brown LG, Figg WD, et al. Effects of phenylbutyrate on proliferation and apoptosis in human prostate cancer cells in vitro and in vivo. *Int J Oncol*. 1999;14(3):501–508.
149. Thibault A, Samid D, Cooper MR, et al. Phase I study of phenylacetate administered twice daily to patients with cancer. *Cancer*. 1995;75(12):2932–2938.
150. Grundke-Iqbal I, Iqbal K, Tung YC, Quinlan M, Wisniewski HM, Binder LI. Abnormal phosphorylation of the microtubule-associated protein tau (tau) in Alzheimer cytoskeletal pathology. *Proc Natl Acad Sci USA*. 1986;83(13):4913–4917.
151. Pili R, Kruszewski MP, Hager BW, Lantz J, Carducci MA. Combination of phenylbutyrate and 13-cis retinoic acid inhibits prostate tumor growth and angiogenesis. *Cancer Res*. 2001;61(4):1477–1485.
152. Massart C, Denais A, Gibassier J. Effect of all-trans retinoic acid and sodium butyrate in vitro and in vivo on thyroid carcinoma xenografts. *Colloq Inse*. 2006;17(5):559–563.
153. Indap MA, Barkume MS. Efficacies of plant phenolic compounds on sodium butyrate induced antitumor activity. *Indian J Exp Biol*. 2003;41(8):861–864.
154. Epperly M, Jin S, Nie S, et al. Ethyl pyruvate, a potentially effective mitigator of damage after total-body irradiation. *Radiat Res*. 2007;168(5):552–559.
155. Ryu S, Kim OB, Kim SH, He SQ, Kim JH. In vitro radiosensitization of human cervical carcinoma cells by combined use of 13-cis-retinoic acid and interferon-alpha2a. *Int J Radiat Oncol Biol Phys*. 1998;41(4):869–873.
156. Cosar M, Songur A, Sahin O, et al. The neuroprotective effect of fish n-3 fatty acids in the hippocampus of diabetic rats. *Nutr Neurosci*. 2008;11(4):161–166.

9 Micronutrients in the Prevention and Improvement of the Standard Therapy for Alzheimer's Disease

INTRODUCTION

Alzheimer's disease (AD) is a progressive neurodegenerative disease characterized by the gradual loss of cognitive function and death of cortical neurons in the brain. The development of AD has been divided into two stages: mild cognitive impairment (MCI) and established AD. Approximately, 15%–20% of Americans 65 years or older have MCI. AD remains the major cause of dementia and accounts for 50%–70% of cases. The main features of dementia include difficulty with memory, language, and solving problems. More than 90% of AD is acquired and only about 5%–10% is inherited from parents.

AD is the 5th leading cause of death in the United States. In 2017, it was estimated that every 66 seconds Americans develop AD, and by 2050, someone would develop AD every 33 seconds.[1] This disturbing trend will continue until evidence-based prevention and improved management strategies are developed and implemented. In order to achieve this goal, it would be essential to identify early cellular or genetic defects that initiate the development of AD.

Extensive basic studies have identified several cellular and genetic defects that contribute to the initiation, progressive degeneration, and death of neurons in AD. They include: (a) increased oxidative stress,[2–5] (b) chronic inflammation,[6–8] (c) mitochondrial dysfunction,[9–11] (d) Aβ1-42 peptides generated from the cleavage of amyloid precursor protein (APP),[12,13] (e) proteasome inhibition,[14] (f) high cholesterol levels,[15,16] (g) heritable mutations in APP, presenilin-1 and presenilin-2 genes,[17–20] and (h) hyperphosphorylated tau protein.[21–23]

Analysis of published studies suggests that increased oxidative damage precedes other biochemical and genetic defects in AD.[24] Oxidative damage, if not repaired, leads to chronic inflammation. Chronic inflammation releases additional free radicals, pro-inflammatory cytokines, complement proteins, and adhesion molecules, all of which contribute to the initiation and progression of AD. Therefore, attenuation of oxidative stress and chronic inflammation may reduce the risk of developing AD, and in combination with standard therapy, may improve the management of this disease.

In order to reduce oxidative stress and chronic inflammation, investigations have utilized primarily single micronutrients or aspirin in cell culture and animal models as well as in human AD. The results of these studies have been inconsistent. Most showed no effect of a single agent in human AD. A few studies revealed some improvement in cognitive function.

Since the first edition of this book, no significant progress on the role of micronutrients in the prevention of human AD has occurred. We have published two reviews emphasizing the need for using multiple antioxidants for reducing oxidative stress and inflammation.[25,26] However, the trends of using a single micronutrient in preclinical and clinical studies with inconsistent results continue, despite the failure of such approaches. Recently, we have proposed that simultaneous elevation of the levels of antioxidant enzymes and dietary and endogenous antioxidants is essential for optimally reducing oxidative stress and chronic inflammation.[27] No studies have been performed using this concept.

Analysis of previous studies suggests that microRNAs, which prevent the translation of mRNAs transcripts into proteins, appear to play an important role in the pathogenesis of AD.[28]

Current AD drug therapy is based on the symptoms rather than the causes of the disease. Commonly used drugs include acetylcholinesterase inhibitors to improve cognitive function by increasing acetylcholine levels in the surviving cholinergic neurons and antagonists of glutamate receptor N-methyl-D-aspartate (NMDA) to reduce anxiety and fear associated with AD. These drugs produce modest short-term beneficial effects on these symptoms; however, they also produce unpleasant side effects. None of these drugs have any effect on oxidative stress or chronic inflammation; therefore, the neurons continue to die despite drug treatments. Since the effectiveness of drugs depends upon the viability of neurons, the beneficial effects on cognitive function lasts only a short period of time.

This chapter briefly discusses following topics:

- Prevalence, incidence, and cost of AD
- Etiology and neuropathology of AD
- MicroRNAs in the pathogenesis of AD
- Increased oxidative stress and chronic inflammation precede other cellular defects in AD
- Studies with individual antioxidants and reasons for inconsistent results in AD
- Increase the levels of cytoprotective enzymes through activation of the Nrf2/ARE pathway, and dietary and endogenous antioxidants for reducing oxidative stress and chronic inflammation in AD
- Activation of Nrf2 for increasing the levels of cytoprotective enzymes in AD
- Proposes a mixture of micronutrients that would prevent AD by simultaneously reducing oxidative stress and chronic inflammation levels, and in combination of standard therapy, improve the management of AD
- Role of non-steroidal anti-inflammatory drugs in prevention and treatment of AD
- Primary prevention of AD by proposed micronutrient mixture
- Secondary prevention of AD by proposed micronutrient mixture
- Improved management of AD by proposed micronutrient mixture in combination of standard therapy

PREVALENCE, INCIDENCE, AND COST OF AD

Despite extensive basic and clinical research, the prevalence of AD increased from 5.3 million in 2013 to 5.5 million in 2017 (5.3 million 65 years or older and 0.2 million under the age of 65 years). Women age 65 or older have 2/3rd higher incidence of AD than men, and African Americans have a 2-fold higher incidence than white Americans.

The incidence of AD depends upon the age of the individuals. In 2017, 64,000 Americans age 65 years or older developed AD, 173,000 age 75–84 years, and 243,000 age 85 and older. It is the 10th leading cause of death in the United States. The incidence of AD and other dementia doubles every 5 years after the age of 65 years.[1] About 50% of the US population who are 85 years or older have symptoms of AD.[29] In view of the fact that about 33 million Americans are of age 65 and older at this time, and this number is predicted to increase to 51 million by the year 2025.[29] Thus, AD remains a major medical concern now and will continue in future.

ESTIMATED COST OF TREATMENT OF AD

The total cost of treatment of AD increased from \$203 billion in 2013 to \$259 billion in 2017 as presented here.[1]

Sources of payment	2013	2017
Medicare	\$107 billion	\$131 billion
Medicaid	\$35 billion	\$44 billion
Out-of-pocket cost	\$34 billion	\$56 billion
Other sources (private insurance, health organizations, managed care organizations, and uncompensated care)	\$27 billion	\$28 billion
Total	\$203 billion	\$259 billion

ETIOLOGY OF AD

In order to develop an effective strategy for the prevention and improved management of AD, it is essential to identify environmental-, dietary, and lifestyle-related factors that increase the risk of developing AD. It is equally important to identify early biochemical defects that initiate and promote AD. Among environmental factors, high consumption of aluminum from drinking water may increase the risk of developing dementia.[30] High dietary intake of vitamin C and vitamin E may reduce the risk of AD, and higher intake of beta-carotene and flavonoids may also decrease the risk of AD among current smokers.[31] Vitamin D deficiency appears to be associated with both AD and Parkinson's disease.[32]

The major biochemical defects that increase the risk of AD include increased oxidative stress and chronic inflammatory. Even beta-amyloid fragments that play a dominant role in the pathogenesis of AD mediate their toxic effect via free radicals.[33–35] Other biochemical etiological factors that increase the risk of dementia include high levels of cholesterol,[15,16] hyperphosphorylated tau protein,[21–23] and proteosome inhibition.[14,36]

NEUROPATHOLOGY OF AD

The diagnosis of AD is made by postmortem analysis of the brains of patients with dementia. The presence of intracellular neurofibrillary tangles (NFTs) containing hyperphosphorylated tau protein and apolipoprotein E,[37–39] and extracellular senile (neuritic) plaques containing many proteins, including alpha-synuclein, beta-amyloids, ubiquitin, apolipoprotein E, presenilins, and alpha anti-chymotrypsin, are considered hallmarks of AD.[12,13,40–43] NFTs are insoluble and difficult to degrade by proteolytic enzymes. They are commonly found in cortical neurons. Senile plaques are focal and spherical, and their size ranges from 20 to 200 microns in diameter. Microglia and reactive astrocytes are present at their periphery, suggesting that senile plaques serve as continuous source of inflammation. Lewy bodies that are characteristics of Parkinson's disease are also present in the brains of about 60% of AD cases.[44] The mechanisms of formation and dissolution of these cytoplasmic inclusions are under extensive investigation in order to develop novel drugs for the treatment of AD.

MicroRNAs IN THE PATHOGENESIS OF AD

MicroRNAs

MicroRNAs (miRs) are evolutionarily conserved small noncoding single-stranded RNAs of approximately 22 nucleotides in length, and are present in all living organisms including humans.[45–48] The biogenesis of miRs is very complex and involves multiple biochemical steps. The majority of miRs are transcribed by RNA polymerase II (Pol II), while some are transcribed by RNA poly-merase III (Pol III) from the noncoding region of the DNA to produce primary miRs (pri-miRs). Pri-miRs undergo a nuclear cleavage by ribonuclease III Drosa to generate precursor-miRs (pre-miRs) that migrate to the cytoplasm where they are further cleaved by ribonuclease III Dicer to ultimately form mature single-stranded miRs with the help of another protein argonaute (Ago).[47,49–51] Each microRNA binds to its complimentary sequences in the 3′-untranslated region (3′-UTR) of the mRNA, promotes degradation of the mRNA transcript, and prevents translation of the message of protein. In this manner, miRs regulate the translation of proapoptotic or antiapoptotic proteins from their respective mRNAs, depending upon whether the DNA receives damaging or protective signals. The binding site of the mRNA for a microRNA is only about 6–8 base pairs; therefore, one miRNA may target as many as 100 different mRNAs,[47,52] altering the levels of the proteins to regulate cellular functions. On the other hand, individual mRNA contains multiple binding sites for different microRNAs.

CHANGES IN THE EXPRESSIONS OF MicroRNAS IN HUMAN AD

Several studies show that the expressions of microRNAs and their target proteins are altered in the autopsied brain tissue of AD patients. These studies are briefly described here.

ELEVATED EXPRESSIONS OF MicroRNAs

Elevated expression of miR-26b was found in the autopsied brain tissue of AD patients.[53] Overexpression of miR-26b in rat primary post-mitotic neurons leads to hyperphosphorylation of tau protein that decreased the levels of its target retinoblastoma protein that eventually led to activation of a major kinase cdk5, which caused hyperphosphorylation of tau protein. Increased expression of miR-138 and its reduced target protein retinoic acid receptor-alpha (EARA) that activated glycogen synthase kinase-3β leading to phosphorylation of tau protein was found in the autopsied brain tissues of AD patients.[54] The expressions of miR-9, miR-125b miR-146a were enhanced while their target proteins synapsin protein and compliment factor H (CFH) were inhib-ited in the autopsied temporal lobe neocortex tissue of AD patients, but not in other neurological disorders.[55]

Transfection of neuronal cells (Neuro-2a) with miR-202 enhanced oxidative stress-induced apoptosis by inhibiting the levels of Oct1/Pou2f1, a transcriptional factor that regulate stress responses. Silencing the expression of miR-202 by treatment with an antigomir (a synthetic small RNA complimentary to miR-202) prevented the effects of miR-202 on oxidative stress-induced cell death.[56]

Overexpressions of miR-144 and miR-451 decreased the levels of their target protein α-secretase ADAM-10 (a disintegrin metalloprotease-10) was found in the autopsied brain tissue of older pri-mate and AD patients.[57] Reduction in the activity of α-secretase ADAM-10 decreases the production of α-APPs, allowing the accumulation of more APP that would then produce of more beta-amyloids by BACE1 (a β-site APP-cleaving enzyme 1).

Elevated expression of miR-125b and reduced levels of its two target proteins phosphatases DUSP6 (dual specificity phosphatase 6) and PPP1CA (protein phosphatase1 catalytic subunit alpha) was found in the autopsied brain tissue of patients with AD.[58] In the primary neurons in culture, overexpression of miR-125b caused hyperphosphorylation of tau protein. These results suggest that miR-125b increases the phosphorylation of tau protein by decreasing the phospha-tases activities.

Elevated expression of miR-34c and reduced levels of its protein SIRT1 responsible for memory function was found in the autopsied brain tissue of AD patients as well as in the mouse AD model.[59] Reducing the expression of miR-34c improved cognitive function by increasing the levels of SIRT1 in mouse AD model.[59]

TABLE 9.1

Upregulated and Downregulated MicroRNAs and Their Respective Target Proteins in Alzheimer's Disease

Upregulated MicroRNAs	Target Proteins
miR-9, miR-26b, miR-34c, miR-125b, miR-144, miR-146a, miR-202, miR-451	α-secretase, SIRT1, Rb1, BACE1, phosphatises
Downregulated MicroRNAs	
miR-23a, miR-23b, miR-34a, miR-29c, miR-107	APP, BACE1, IL-1RAK1
miR-132, miR-132-3p, miR-212, miR-219, miR-339-5p, miR-512	tau protein, NFkB, SIRT1

Note: Rb1-Retinoblastoma 1 APP-Amyloid precursor protein Retinoblastoma 1; APP, amyloid precursor protein; BACE1, beta-site APP-cleaving enzyme 1, also called beta-secretase; IL-1RAK1, IL-1 receptor-associated kinase 1; NF-kB, nuclear factor kappaB; SIRT1, a member of the sirtuin family.

Downregulation of microRNAs may be results of their rapid degradation, reduced rate of transcription or decreased processing by Dorsa and Dicer in the nucleus and cytoplasm, respectively, whereas upregulation of microRNAs may be result of changes opposite to those with downregulation in patients with Alzheimer's disease.

Table 9.1 showed that 8 microRNAs were upregulated affecting reduced levels of only 5 proteins, suggesting that more than one microRNAs bind with the same 3′-UTR mRNA.

DECREASED EXPRESSIONS OF MicroRNAs

The expressions of miR-132 and miR-212 were decreased in the autopsied brain tissues of AD patients.[60] Decreased expressions of miR-107 and miR-339-5p and increased levels of its target protein BACE1 led to increased production of Aβ peptides, while the levels of neuritic plaque and NFT in the adjacent tissue were enhanced in the autopsied brain cortex of AD patients.[61–63] Overexpressions of miR-107 or miR-339-5p reduced the levels of BACE1, whereas silencing miR-339-5p significantly increased the levels of BACE1.[61] The expression of miR-107 was decreased in the autopsied brain tissues of patients with MCI and AD.[63]

Downregulation of miR-29c was associated with increased levels of BACE1 and Aβ peptides in the autopsied brain tissue of sporadic AD patients.[64] Overexpression of miR-29c reduced the levels of BACE1 and Aβ peptides in human neuroblastoma cells (SH-SY5Y) in culture. Decreased expression of miR-29c was associated with the increased levels of human β-secretase (hBACE1) in the autopsied brain tissue of AD patients.[65] Downregulation of miR-132-3P and miR-512 was associated with hyperphosphorylated tau protein in the autopsied samples of AD brain.[66,67]

Decreased expression of miR-219 and increased levels of its target protein tau was found in the autopsied brain tissue of patients with AD.[68] It has been demonstrated that upregulation of miR-34a reduced the level of tau protein by binding to its 3′-UTR mRNA.[69] Reduction of the levels of tau protein could be of neuroprotective value.

Mutation in presenilin-2 (PS-2) that causes autosomal dominant AD increases the pro-inflammatory responses of microglia cells in culture. The expression of miR-146 was downregulated, whereas the levels of its target proteins IL-1 receptor-associated kinase-1 (IL1-RAK1) and NF-kB increased in microglia cells of PS-2 knockout mice.[70]

The expressions of miR-212, miR-132, miR-23a, and miR-23b were downregulated in the autopsied tissue of frontal cortex of patients with amnestic mild cognitive impairment (aMCI).[71] In neuronal cells in culture, downregulation of miR-212 and miR-23a enhanced the levels of SIRT1 protein and protected neurons from Aβ peptide-induced toxicity. Since the toxicity of beta-amyloids is mediated by free radicals,[34,72,73] these microRNAs may protect neurons by reducing oxidative stress.

Table 9.1 showed that 11 microRNAs were downregulated affecting the levels of 6 proteins suggesting that more than one microRNAs bind with the same 3′-UTR mRNA.

CHANGES IN MicroRNAs IN ANIMAL AND CELL CULTURE AD MODELS

ELEVATED EXPRESSIONS OF MicroRNAs

Overexpression of miR-26b in rat primary neuronal culture increased phosphorylation of tau protein by complex mechanisms leading to neuronal death.[53] This microRNA has multiple target proteins including retinoblastoma peotein1 (Rb1), a tumor suppressor. Increased expression of miR-138 was found in animal models as well as in cell culture models of AD (N2a/APP and HEK293 tau cells).[54] It was further demonstrated that overexpression of miR-138 activated glycogen synthase kinase-3 beta (GSK-3beta) and enhanced tau phosphorylation in HEK293 tau cells. Elevated expression of miR-181 and reduced levels of its target proteins c-Fos and SIRT-1 proteins were found in the hippocampal region of the brain of transgenic mice (3xTg-AD) with AD pathology.[74] In young AD mouse model (APPswe/PS∇E9), increased expression of miR-29c was associated with decreased levels of its target protein neuron navigator 3 (NAV3).[75]

The expression of miR-34c was upregulated in transgenic mouse AD model and patients with AD. Treatments of AD mouse model with Aβ peptides upregulated the expressions of miR-34c and miR-106b and downregulated the levels of their target protein VAMP2 (vesicle associated membrane protein 2).[76] Silencing miR-34c expression increased the levels of VAMP2, and thereby, restored the synaptic function, and learning and memory deficits induced by the treatment with Aβ peptides.

Expressions of miR-99b-5p and miR-100-5p were elevated at late stages in the brain of double transgenic mice (APP/PS1) when compared to wild-type animals.[77] Treatment of neuronal culture with Aβ peptides that generate ROS also increased expressions of these microRNAs, and induced apoptosis by inhibiting rapamycin, a phosphoinositide 3-kinase-related protein kinase, responsible for survival, synaptic plasticity, and long-term memory.

DECREASED EXPRESSION OF MicroRNAs

Reduced expressions of miR-132 and miR-212 induced apoptosis in rat primary neuronal culture, whereas their overexpression protected neurons from oxidative stress.[60] Deficiency of miR-132 and miR-212 increased the levels of phosphorylation and aggregation of tau proteins that induced degeneration of neurons in AD mice. Treatment of AD mice with miR-132 mimics reduced tau phosphorylation and improved memory.[78]

Reduced expression of miR-153 was found in the mouse model of AD[79] and in the autopsied brain samples of subset of AD patients with moderate AD pathology.[80] In neuronal cell line, overexpression of miR-153 inhibited the expressions of amyloid precursor protein (APP) and amyloid precursor-like protein-2 (APLP-2), which are involved in the pathogenesis of AD.[79]

Increased levels of ceramide and its rate-limiting enzyme serine palmitoyltransferase were found in sporadic AD.[81,82] Using AD mouse model (TgCRND8), it was demonstrated that the expressions of miR-137, miR-181c, miR-9, and miR-29a/b were downregulated that allowed increased levels of serine palmitoyltransferase and Aβ peptides. Inhibition of this enzyme by L-cycloserine reduced the levels of Aβ peptides and hyperphosphorylated tau protein in the cortex of AD mouse model.[81]

Chronic brain hypoperfusion (CBH) downregulated the expression of miR-195 in the rat cortex and the hippocampus and the plasma of patients with dementia. Since APP and BACE1 are targets for miR-195, reduction in the expression of this microRNA would enhance the levels of APP and BACE1.[83]

In neuronal cell culture (N2a) and mouse fibroblasts, decreased expressions of miR-298 and miR-328 and elevated levels of their target protein BACE1 that would to increased production of Aβ peptides.[84]

Expression of miR-106b was downregulated and the levels of its target protein transforming growth factor-β (TGF-β) were increased in a double transgenic mouse model (APPswe/PS∇E9).[85] An elevation of TGF-β plays a role in the pathogenesis of AD.

Treatment of hippocampal cell culture with Aβ peptides downregulated the expressions of miR-9 and miR-181c and increased the levels of their target proteins TGF-beta1, TREM2 (triggering receptor expressed on myeloid cells 2), SIRT1 (silent information regulator 1), and BTBD3 (BTB/POZ domain-containing protein 3).[86]

In senescence accelerated mouse-prone 8 (SAMP8), a model for age-related dementia, the expression of miR-195 was decreased and the level of its target protein BACE1 was increased leading to increased production of Aβ peptides.[87] In SAMP8 mouse, the expression of miR-216 was downregulated and the levels of its target protein APP were elevated.[88]

ROS AND PRO-INFLAMMATORY CYTOKINES
REGULATE THE EXPRESSIONS OF MicroRNAs

ROS UPREGULATES THE EXPRESSIONS OF MicroRNAs CAUSING NEURODEGENERATION

Increased oxidative stress is one of the earliest biochemical defects that initiate AD.[24] Therefore, it may act as one of the signals to enhance the expressions of certain specific microRNAs. For example, treatment of human neurons in culture with H_2O_2 (hydrogen peroxide) or parquet caused degeneration of neurons by increasing oxidative stress. These treatments elevated the expression of miR-153 that decreased the level of Nrf2. Reduction in Nrf2 level would increase oxidative stress due to a decrease in the levels of antioxidant enzymes.[89] Mutation in miR-153, anti-miR-153 or Nrf2 c DNA devoid of 3'-UTR site protected neurons from parquet- or H_2O_2-induced oxidative stress by increasing the levels of Nrf2-mediated elevation of the levels of antioxidant enzymes.

Treatment of rat spinal cord neurons with H_2O_2 unregulated the expressions of miR-146a, miR-21, and miR-150, and caused neurodegeneration by inhibiting its target protein Nrf2. Silencing miR-21 expression reduced H_2O_2-induced cell death by increasing the levels of Nrf2. These results suggest that only decreased expression of miR-21 expression leads to reduced oxidative stress.[90]

Treatment of primary hippocampal neurons or different strains of accelerated aging model of mice with H_2O_2 upregulated the expressions of miR-329, miR-193b, miR-20a, miR-296, and miR-130b.[91] Increased oxidative stress also upregulated expressions of miR-135b, and miR-708 in the primary culture of mouse hippocampal neurons,[92] causing neurodegeneration. Oxidative stress induces premature aging in the aging animal model. Oxidative stress-induced upregulated miR-24 and decreased the levels of its target protein DNA totpisomerase-1 (TOP1), an enzyme controlling DNA topology. Reduction in the levels of TOP1 caused senescence in the fibroblasts.[93] This is further supported by the fact that knocking down TOP1 induced senescence in the fibroblasts.

Treatment of primary neuronal culture with soluble Aβ peptides that generates ROS[34,72,73] upregulated the expressions of miR-134, miR-145 and miR-210, and this effect of Aβ peptides was reversed by NMDA receptor inhibitors.[94] These results suggest that ROS acts as one of the signals for upregulating these microRNAs, and that glutamate may be involved in neurodegeneration. The target proteins of these microRNAs were not identified.

The expression of miR-342-5p was elevated and the levels of its target protein Ankyrin G (AnkG) decreased that can lead to AD axonopathy in AD mouse model.[95]

TABLE 9.2

Reactive Oxygen Species (ROS) and Pro-inflammatory Cytokine Regulated MicroRNAs Expressions

ROS-Induced Upregulated MicroRNAs	Target Proteins
miR-20a, miR-24, miR-130b, miR-134, miR-135b,	Nrf2, TOP1, Ankg
miR-145, miR-146a, miR-150, miR-153, miR-185,	Histone deacetylase
miR-193b, miR-210, miR-296, miR-329, miR-342-5p, miR-708	
ROS-Induced Downregulated MicroRNAs	
miR-743a	Malate dehydrogenase
Pro-inflammatory Cytokine-Induced Upregulated MicroRNAs	
miR-7, miR-9, miR-34a, miR-125b, miR-146a,	IRK1, Complement
miR-155	Factor H

Note: Nrf2, Nuclear transcriptional factor-2; TOP1, DNA topoisomerase 1; Ankg, AnkyrinG; IRK1, Interleukin1-receptor associated kinase.
The table was reproduced from a previous publication.[27]

Table 9.2 showed that oxidative stress is one of the signals that upregulated 16 specific microRNAs leading to the events causing neurodegeneration. Only three proteins were targets for these microRNAs, suggesting that more than one microRNAs target the same protein.

ROS DOWNREGULATES THE EXPRESSIONS OF MicroRNAs CAUSING NEURODEGENERATION

The levels of mitochondrial enzymes malate dehydrogenase (MDH) are elevated in the autopsied brain tissue of patients with AD. Using a mouse hippocampal cell line (HT22), it was demonstrated that oxidative stress decreased the expression of miR-743a and enhanced the levels of MDH[96] (Table 9.2).

PRO-INFLAMMATORY CYTOKINES UPREGULATE THE EXPRESSIONS OF MicroRNAs CAUSING NEURODEGENERATION

Since chronic inflammation plays an important role in the development of AD,[24] it is possible that pro-inflammatory cytokines may be one of the signals that increase the expressions of microRNAs. Indeed, elevated levels of pro-inflammatory cytokines and the expressions of miR-125b and miR-146a were elevated in patients with AD, suggesting their role in neurodegeneration. Treatment of human astroglial cells in culture with the donors of ROS and NFkB (the combination of iron and aluminum sulfate) upregulated the expressions of miR-125b and miR-146a. The results suggest that both ROS and NF-kB act as signals for increasing the expressions of these microRNAs.[97] Phenylbutyl nitrone, an antioxidant, and curcumin, an inhibitor of NF-kB, prevented the upregulation of miR-125b and miR-146a astroglial cells treated with the donors of ROS and NFkB.[97] Another study reported that increased expression of miR-146a was associated with the reduced levels of IRK1 in the autopsied samples of hippocampus and neocortex regions of the AD brain.[98] Treatment of human astroglial cells in culture with IL-1β, a pro-inflammatory cytokine, or Aβ42, a generator of ROS,[34,72,73] elevated the expression of miR-146a, causing cell death. Treatment of neuron-glial cells with NF-kB upregulated the expressions of miR-7, miR-9, miR-34a, miR-125b, miR-146a, and miR-155. These microRNAs were elevated in the autopsied brain tissue of AD patients, and in human neuronal-glial cultured cells treated with TNF-α, IL-1β, or Aβ42 peptides.[99]

Another study reported increased expressions of miR-146a and miR-155 in the autopsied brain tissue of AD patients, and in human primary neurons in culture treated with TNF-α or Aβ42 peptides.[100] Addition of the condition medium containing miR-146a and miR-155 to the normal neurons in culture induced changes in gene expressions characteristics of AD. These results suggest that upregulation of these two microRNAs play an important role in the pathogenesis of AD. Upregulated miR-9, miR-125b, miR-146a, and miR-155 were found in the temporal lobe neocortex of the autopsied brain tissue of AD patients.[55]

Human primary neural cells (a co-culture of neurons and astroglia) stressed by the treatment with amyloid peptides (Aβ42) or IL-1β upregulated NF-kB that mediated increased expressions of miR-125b and miR-146a.[101]

Table 9.2 showed that pro-inflammatory cytokines increased the expressions of 6 microRNAs that contribute to the degeneration of neurons in AD. Only two target proteins of these microRNAs were identified, suggesting that more than one microRNAs may target the same protein.

MICRONUTRIENTS REGULATE THE EXPRESSIONS OF MicroRNAs

A previous review has discussed the role of antioxidant in protecting neurons against damage produced by increased oxidative stress and chronic inflammation in AD[24]; therefore, they may mediate their neuroprotective effects by altering the expressions of certain microRNAs and their respective target proteins. Although most studies on the effects of antioxidants on the expressions of micro-RNAs have been studied on various types of cancer cells, they do show potential of regulating the expression of microRNAs in other cell types including neurons. These studies are described here.

RESVERATROL ENHANCES THE EXPRESSIONS OF MicroRNAs

Treatment with resveratrol increased the expression of miR-328 and reduced its target protein metalloproteinase-2 (MMP-2) in osteosarcoma cells.[102] Resveratrol treatment also enhanced the expression of miR-137 and inhibited the levels of its target protein polycomb protein histone methyltransferase EZH2 (enhancer of Zest 2 polycomb repressive complex 2 subunit) in neuroblastoma cells.[103] Treatment of human colon cancer cells with resveratrol upregulated the expression of miR-663 and decreased the levels of its target proteins program cell death protein 4 (PDCD4), phosphatase and tensin homolog (PTEN) and transforming growth factor (TGF).[104] Resveratrol treatment also increased the expression of miR-622 and reduced its target protein K-Ras in transformed human bronchial epithelial cells (16HBE-T).[105]

RESVERATROL DECREASES THE EXPRESSIONS OF MicroRNAs

Resveratrol treatment of mice decreased the expressions of miR-134 and miR-124, and enhanced their target protein CREB (cyclic-AMP response binding protein, a nuclear transcriptional factor), leading to enhance synthesis of BDNF (brain-derived neurotrophic factor).[106] Resveratrol treatment reduced the expression of miR-21 in several types of cancers cells in culture.[107–110] Resveratrol treatment decreased the expressions of miR-33a and miR-122 in liver cells in culture.[111] Grapeseed extract attenuated the expression of miR-27a and increased the levels of its target protein forkhead box protein O1 (FOXO1).[112]

ISOFLAVONE INCREASES THE EXPRESSIONS OF MicroRNAs

Isoflavone treatment enhanced the expressions of miR-200b, miR-200c, miR-let-7b, miR-let-7c, miR-let-7d, and miR-let-7e and reduced the levels of their target proteins ZEB1 (zinc finger E-box-binding homeobox 1) and vimentin in pancreatic cancer cells.[113] The natural products, such as enoxolone (or glycyrrhetinic acid), a major component of licorice, and magnolol, a major part of the bark of *Magnolia officinalis*, enhanced the expression of miR-200c and decreased the levels of its target protein ZEB1 in breast cancer cells.[114]

GENISTEIN DECREASES THE EXPRESSIONS OF MicroRNAs

Treatment with genistein decreased the expressions of miR-223 and miR-34a and enhanced the levels of their target proteins Fbw7 (F-box and WD repeat domain-containing 7) and Notch-1 Type 1 transmembrane protein in pancreatic cancer cells.[115,116]

QUERCETIN ENHANCES THE EXPRESSIONS OF MicroRNAs

Treatment with quercetin enhanced the expression of miR-146a and reduced the growth of breast cancer cells in culture.[117] Treatment with quercetin also increased the expressions of miR-122 and miR-125b and inhibited the levels of inflammatory proteins in the liver cells.[118]

CURCUMIN DECREASES THE EXPRESSIONS OF MicroRNAs

Treatment of cells with a donor of ROS and NF-kB (a combination of iron and aluminum sulfate) increased the expressions of miR-125b and miR-146a.[97] Curcumin treatment attenuated ROS and NF-kB-induced upregulation of miR-125b and miR-146a in human astroglial cells.[97] Treatment with a pro-inflammatory cytokine IL-1β enhanced the expression of miR-146a; however, treatment with curcumin prevented IL-1β-induced increase in the expression of miR-146a in human primary culture of neuronal-glial cells.[119] Curcumin treatment inhibited the expression of miR-21 and enhanced its target protein PTEN (phosphatase and tensin homolog) in human non-small-cell lung carcinoma.[120]

CURCUMIN ENHANCES THE EXPRESSIONS OF MicroRNAs

Treatment with curcumin increased the expression of miR-22 and reduced the levels of its target protein transcription factor-1 (SP-1) in human pancreatic cancer cells.[121] Silencing the expression of miR-22 increased the levels of SP-1. Curcumin treatment enhanced the expression of miR-203 and decreased the levels of its target proteins protein kinase B (Akt2) and Src tyrosine protein kinase in bladder cancer cells.[122] Curcumin treatment also upregulated the expression of miR-7 and decreased the level of its target protein SET8 histone lysine methyltransferase. Breast cancer cells treated with curcumin showed increased expression of miR-181b and decreased level of its target protein in CXCL-1 (chemokine (C-X-C Motif) ligand-1).[123] Treatment with curcumin upregulated the expressions of miR-15a and miR-16-1 and downregulated the levels of its target protein WT1 (Wilm's tumor protein-1) in leukemic cells and primary acute myeloid leukemia cells.[124]

COENZYME Q10 REGULATES THE EXPRESSIONS OF MicroRNAs

Coenzyme Q10 treatment reduced lipopolysaccharide (LPS)-induced elevation of the expression of miR-146a and reduced its target protein IL-1 receptor associated kinase-1 (ILRAL-1) in the primary culture of umbilical vein endothelial cells.[125] Supplementation with coenzyme Q10 increased the expressions of miR-15a, miR-21, and miR-33a, and decreased the levels of its target protein alkaline phosphatase, and inhibited apoptosis and inflammatory pathways in the liver cells (HepG2 cell line).[126]

VITAMIN D3 REGULATES THE EXPRESSIONS OF MicroRNAs

Supplementation with vitamin D3 upregulated the expressions of miR-100 and miR-125b and reduced the growth of prostate cancer cells by decreasing their target protein E2F3, a family of transcriptional factor, responsible for proliferation and differentiation, which is highly expressed in prostate cancer cells.[127] Treatment of primary cultures of human osteoblasts (HOBs) with vitamin D3 enhanced the expressions of miR-637 and miR-1228 and suppressed their target proteins type iv collagen (COL4A1) and bone morphogenic protein-2 kinase (BMP2K). Silencing the expression of miR-1228 prevented vitamin D3-induced suppression of BMP2K.[128] Treatment of androgen-sensitive human prostate cancer cells (LNCaP) with vitamin D3 increased expression of miR-98 and decreased the levels of its target protein cyclin J (CCNJ) that controls mitosis, and inhibited growth of cancer cells.[129] Overexpression of miR-98 reduced the growth of tumor cells, whereas silencing the expression of miR-98 abolished the anti-tumor effects of vitamin D3.[129]

Supplementation with vitamin D3 upregulated miR-498, reduced the levels of its target protein human telomerase reverse transcriptase, and inhibited the growth of human ovarian cancer cells.[130] Expression of miR-22 was lower in most human colon cancer. Treatment of cancer with vitamin D3 upregulated miR-22 and downregulated its multiple protein targets, such as NELL2 (neural epidermal growth factor-like 2), RERE (arginine-glutamic acid dipeptide repeats) and OGN (osteoglycin), and reduced the growth of colon cancer cells.[131]

Vitamin D3 enhanced the expression of miR-32, reduced the levels of its target pro-apoptotic protein Bim, and induced differentiation in human acute myeloid leukemia (AML) cells.[132] Suppression of the expression of miR-32 upregulated the levels of Bim, whereas overexpression of miR-32 downregulated the levels of Bim and increased vitamin D3-induced differentiation of myeloid leukemia cells.[132]

NICOTINAMIDE (VITAMIN-B3) REGULATES THE EXPRESSIONS OF MicroRNAs

Treatment with nicotinamide mononucleotide enhanced expression of miR-34a reduced the levels of its target protein NAPT (nicotinamide phosphoribosyltransferase, a rate-limiting enzyme in the biosynthesis of NAD+ in the liver of obese individuals.[133] Increased expression of miR-34a leads to reduction in the levels of SIRT1, a NAD+-dependent deacetylase. Reduction in SIRT1 activity enhanced the transcription of its target proteins, such as PGC-1 alpha, NF-kB, and SREBP-1c (sterol Regulatory Element-Binding Transcriptional Factor-1).

SELENIUM REGULATES THE EXPRESSIONS OF MicroRNAs

Treatment of kidney cells (LLC-PK1 cells) derived from the kidney of a normal healthy male pig with selenium reduced cadmium-induced apoptosis, increased the expressions of miR-125a and miR-125b, and enhanced the levels of the antiapoptotic protein Bcl2 and decreased the levels of pro-apoptotic proteins Bax and Bak.[134]

VITAMIN E AND DELTA-TOCOTRIENOL REGULATE THE EXPRESSIONS OF MicroRNAs

Vitamin E deficiency reduced the expressions of miR-122a and miR-125b that are involved in lipid metabolism (miR-122a) in cancer and inflammation (miR-125b) in the rat liver cells[135]; therefore, sufficiency of vitamin E would enhance the expression of these microRNAs. Treatment of non-small-cell lung carcinoma cells with delta-tocotrienol upregulated expression of miR-34a and reduced its target proteins Notch-1, Hes-1, cyclin D1, surviving and Bcl2, inhibited growth and invasiveness of cancer cells, and induced apoptosis.[136]

VITAMIN A (RETINOIC ACID) REGULATES THE EXPRESSIONS OF MicroRNAs

Retinoic acid treatment of mouse embryonic stem cells (mESCs) induced differentiation by downregulating the expressions of miR-200b and miR-200c and increasing the levels of ectodermal marker gene nestin.[137] The Level of miR-10a was lower in freshly obtained breast cancer tissues after surgery; however, after treatment with retinoic acid the expression of miR-10a was increased.[138]

Treatment of acute myeloid leukemia cells (HL-60) with retinoic acid up-regulated six micro-RNAs (miR-663, miR-494, miR-145, miR-22, miR-363, and miR-223) and downregulated three microRNAs (miR-10a, miR-181, miR-612).[139] Transfection of HL-60 leukemia cells with miR-663 induced differentiation. Thus, retinoic acid-induced differentiation of leukemic cells is mediated by upregulation of the expression of miR-663. Retinoic acid treatment of leukemic cells induced differentiation by upregulating the expressions of miR-15a and miR-16-1.[140] The patients with acute myeloid leukemia who were in a complete remission also exhibited increased expressions of miR-15a and miR-16-1; and those who relapsed showed decreased expression of these microRNAs.

VITAMIN C REGULATES THE EXPRESSION OF A MicroRNA

Vitamin C supplementation downregulated the level of miR-153, improved lipid profiles, and enhanced anti-inflammation and anti-senescence effects of HDL in young subjects who were nonsmokers and smokers.[141]

Tables 9.3 and 9.4 describe the effects of antioxidants, B-vitamins, and mineral on the expression of microRNAs in cancer cells.

TABLE 9.3
Effects of Antioxidant Compounds on the Expressions of MicroRNAs in Mammalian Cells

Antioxidants	Upregulation	Downregulation
Resveratrol	miR-21, miR-30c2, miR-34a, miR-137, miR-155, miR-181b, miR-328, miR-622, miR-663	miR-21, miR-27a, miR-33a, miR-122, miR-124, miR-134
Curcumin	miR-7, miR-22, miR-181b, miR-203, miR-15a, miR-16-1	miR-21, miR-125b miR-146a
Isoflavone	miR-let-7b, miR-let-7c, miR-let-7d miR-let-7e, miR-200b, miR-200c	None
Genistein	None	miR-34a, miR-223
Quercetin	miR-122, miR-125b, miR-146a	None
Coenzyme Q10	miR-15a, miR-21, miR-33a	miR-146a

Note: Antioxidant-induced up- and downregulation of microRNAs could be due to alterations in their transcription, processing by Drosa in the nucleus and Dicer in the cytoplasm or stability.
The table was reproduced from a previous publication.[27]

TABLE 9.4
Effect of Vitamins on the Expression of MicroRNAs in Mammalian Cells

Vitamin Type	Upregulation	Downregulation
Vitamin D3	miR-100, miR-125b, miR-637, miR-1228, miR-98, miR-498, miR-22, miR-32	
Nicotinamide	None	miR-34a
Selenium	miR-125a, miR-125b	None
Vitamin E and Delta-tocotrienol	miR-122a, miR-125b, miR-34a	None
Retinoic acid	miR-10a, miR-663, miR-494, miR-145, miR-22, miR-363, miR-223, miR-15a, miR-16-1	miR-200b, miR-200c, miR-146, miR-10a, miR-181, miR-612
Vitamin C	None	miR-153

Note: Antioxidant-induced upregulation and downregulation of microRNAs could be due to alterations in their transcription, processing by Drosa in the nucleus and Dicer in the cytoplasm or stability.

SOURCES OF FREE RADICALS IN THE NORMAL BRAIN

Before discussing the role of increased oxidative stress in AD, it is essential to describe briefly sources of free radicals in the normal brain. The brain utilizes about 25% of respired oxygen even though it represents only 5% of the body weight. Free radicals are generated in the brain during the normal intake of oxygen, during infection, and during normal oxidative metabolism of certain substrates. During normal aerobic respiration, the mitochondria of one rat nerve cell will process about 10^{12} oxygen molecules and reduce them to water. During this process, superoxide anion ($O_2^{\cdot-}$), hydrogen peroxide (H_2O_2), and hydroxyl ($OH^{\cdot}$) are produced. In addition, partially reduced oxygen, which represents about 2% of consumed oxygen, leaks out from the mitochondria and generates about 20 billion molecules of $O_2^{-\cdot}$ and H_2O_2 per cell per day.[142,143]

Some brain enzymes, such as monoamine oxidase (MAO), tyrosine hydroxylase, and L-amino acid oxidase produce H_2O_2 as a normal byproduct of their activity.[144] Furthermore, auto-oxidation of ascorbate and catecholamines generates H_2O_2.[145] Oxidative stress can also be generated by Ca^{2+}-mediated activation of glutamate receptors. The Ca^{2+}-dependent activation of phospholipase A_2 by N-methyl-D-aspartate (NMDA) releases arachidonic acid, which then liberates $O_2^{-\cdot}$ during the biosynthesis of eicosanoids.[146] Another radical, NO, is formed by nitric oxide synthase stimulated by Ca^{2+}. NO can react with $O_2^{-\cdot}$ to form peroxynitrite anions. NMDA receptor stimulation produces marked elevations in $O_2^{-\cdot}$ and $OH^{\cdot}$ levels.[147] Some enzymes such as xanthine oxidase and flavoprotein oxidase (e.g., aldehyde oxidase) also form superoxide anions during metabolism of their respective substrates.

Free iron and copper can increase the levels of free radicals.[148] These studies suggest that the brain is exposed to high levels of reactive oxygen species (ROS) and reactive nitrogen species (RNS) every day. In addition, the brain has the highest levels of unsaturated fatty acids, which are easily oxidizable by free radicals. Paradoxically, the brain is least prepared to handle this excessive load of free radicals. It has low levels of both antioxidant enzyme systems and antioxidants. These inherent biological features make brain very vulnerable to increased oxidative damage. Despite this, clinical symptoms of AD appear only when a significant number of neurons are lost, suggesting the value of plasticity of the neurons in maintaining normal brain function.

EVIDENCE FOR INCREASED OXIDATIVE STRESS AS AN EARLY EVENT IN THE INITIATION OF AD

Analysis of previous studies reveals that increased oxidative stress is found in the autopsied brain samples of AD patients.[149] However, it is difficult to conclude whether increased oxidative stress is the cause or the consequence of the disease. Strongest support for the support of the hypothesis that increased oxidative stress initiates AD comes from three sources, the cell culture model of AD, asymptomatic transgenic animal model of AD, and from asymptomatic individuals carrying AD specific mutated genes.

STUDIES ON CELL CULTURE MODEL OF AD

The levels of markers of oxidative stress, such as protein carbonyl-4-hydroxynonenal (4-HNE) and 3-nitrotyrosine (3-NT) were elevated in nerve cells obtained from the transgenic mice expressing mutated APP and mutated presenilin-1, compared to those found in nerve cells from the wild type mice.[150] This study suggested that increased oxidative stress occurs in neurons of transgenic AD mice.

The relation between early increased oxidative stress and later enhanced production of amyloid peptides production is demonstrated by the observation that treatment of human neuroblastoma cells in culture with hydrogen peroxide (H_2O_2) significantly increased Aβ production by enhancing the expression of beta- and gamma-secretases responsible for the cleavage of APP to Aβ peptides.[151]

Treatment of nerve cells with H_2O_2 also induced hyperacetylation of histone by downregulating histone deacetylase that causes increased expression of APP-cleaving enzymes beta- and gamma-secretases. These results suggest that increased oxidative stress produces more beta-amyloids, which cause damage to the nerve cells by generating free radicals.

Primary culture of neurons obtained from transgenic mice expressing both mutated APP and mutated preseninlin-1 exhibited increased oxidative stress and enhanced sensitivity to oxidative stress induced by Aβ1-42, H_2O_2, and kainic acid, which contribute to neuronal death.[18] These results also suggest that mutations in preseninlin-1 and APP may cause neurodegeneration in familial AD by further increasing oxidative stress, which may progressively participate in the damage and ultimately loss of neurons in D.

STUDIES ON ANIMAL MODELS OF AD

Using a transgenic mouse model of AD (APP23 mice), increased protein oxidation and reduced energy metabolism occur in the cortex of asymptomatic mice, suggesting that these markers of oxidative stress occur prior to the development of other biochemical defects and amyloidogenic phenotype.[152] Using an imaging technique on the brain of transgenic mouse AD model, it was shown that oxidative stress was markedly elevated in neuritis near plaques, propagated to cell bodies, and preceded caspase activation, which led to death of neurons within 24 hours.[4] The results suggest that local increase in oxidative stress surrounding plaques may initiate neurodegeneration and death of neuron in that area.

Transgenic A mice (tau 3xTg) exhibited cognitive dysfunction and fear conditioning. Pretreatment with the SOD/catalase mimetic, EUK-207 prevented cognitive dysfunction and fear conditioning, and reduced the levels of Aβ1-42, tau and hyperphosphorylated tau, oxidized nucleic acid, and lipid peroxidation in the amygdala and hippocampus.[153] The above studies on animal models of AD suggest that increased oxidative stress occur prior to other biochemical defects associated with neurodegeneration in AD. This is further supported by the fact that administration of antioxidants in these transgenic AD model mice prevented memory loss.

STUDIES ON ASYMPTOMATIC INDIVIDUALS CARRYING MUTATED AD SPECIFIC GENES

Increased levels of oxidized proteins were found in the blood of both AD patients and their relatives when compared with non-AD controls.[154] In a study on individuals carrying mutated preseninline-1 or APP the plasma levels of oxidative damage markers, such as methionine sulfoxide, an oxidation product of methionine, were elevated compared to relatives with no mutated genes.[155] These studies provides the strongest support in support of a hypothesis that increased oxidative stress is one of the earliest biochemical defects that initiate damage to the nerve cells in the brain of AD patients.

STUDIES ON INCREASED OXIDATIVE STRESS IN AN EARLY PHASE OF AD

The presence of mild cognitive impairment (MCI) can be considered an early phase of AD. Several investigations show that increased oxidative stress occurs in patients with MCI, implying that increased oxidative damage is an early event, which also participates in the progression of AD. Biliverdin reductase-A (BVR-A) is considered a pleiotropic enzyme, which protects neurons against oxidative damage. In patients with AD as well as in patients with MCI, a significant increase in oxidized and nitrated BVR-A was found in the hippocampal region, but not in the cerebellum.[156] Thus, nitrosylative stress in the hippocampus may be an early event in the pathogenesis of AD. Analysis of serum levels of markers of oxidative stress in 101 patients with AD, 134 patients with MCI suggested that increased levels of serum hydroperoxides were independently associated with the increased risk of developing MCI as well as AD, whereas low levels of serum total antioxidant capacity were associated with the increased risk of developing MCI.[157] In a clinical study involving 33 patients with

MCI, 29 patients with mild probably AD and 26 healthy age-matched subjects, it was demonstrated that plasma levels of malondialdehyde (MDA) were higher in patients with MCI and AD than in control subjects, whereas glutathione reductase activity in RBC was lower in patients with MCI and AD than in control subjects.[158] A study has reported that peripheral lymphocytes obtained from the patients with AD as well as from the patients with MCI exhibited mitochondrial dysfunction as evidenced by decreased mitochondrial membrane potential and enhanced sensitivity to different inhibitors of respiratory chain complexes.[159] Further studies revealed that an early increase in markers of oxidative stress, such as nitric oxide synthase and NADPH-oxidases, which could impair the mitochondrial function by reducing activities of chain complexes VI and V was associated with AD. In addition, reduction in the levels of uncoupling protein (UCP) and peroxisome-proliferator activated receptor (PPAR), which protect the neurons, further aggravates oxidative stress-induced damage.[160] These results suggest that increased oxidative stress and reduced energy metabolism occur in early phase of AD.

STUDIES ON INCREASED OXIDATIVE STRESS IN ESTABLISHED HUMAN AD (AUTOPSIED BRAIN TISSUE)

A review showed that markers of oxidative stress, such as protein nitrotyrosine, carbonyls in proteins, lipid oxidation products, and oxidized DNA bases were elevated in the autopsied brain tissue of patients with AD.[5] A number of observations substantiate the presence of high levels of oxidative stress in patients with AD. For example, (a) higher expression of heme oxygenase-1 is found in the brains of AD patients[161]; (b) increased consumption of oxygen is found in AD patients[162]; (c) increased activity of glucose-6-phosphate dehydrogenase is found in the AD brain[3]; and (d) activation of calcium-dependent neural proteinase (calpain) is found in AD brains,[163] which may trigger events leading to the formation of free radicals.[164]

Additional evidence for the increased oxidative stress in the AD brain include the following: (a) homogenates of frontal cortex from AD brains obtained at autopsy revealed a 22% higher production of free radicals and, in the presence of iron, a 50% higher production of free radicals than those from age-matched normal controls[165]; (b) peroxynitrite also exacerbates the pathogenesis of AD[166]; (c) increased neuronal nitric oxide synthase (nNOS) expression in reactive astrocytes correlated with apoptosis in hippocampal neurons of the AD brains[167]; (d) the activity of glutamine synthetase decreased in the AD brains[166]; and (e) the level of glutathione transferase is decreased in ventricular CSF and in the AD brains compared to that in the brains from age-matched controls.[168] Analysis of 50 patients with AD and 100 control subjects revealed that deletion of glutathione-S-transferase T1 increased the risk of AD by 2.47 times.[169] Taken together, these data strongly suggest that increased oxidative stress represents one of the major cellular defects that play an important role in the progression of AD.

STUDIES ON INCREASED OXIDATIVE STRESS IN ESTABLISHED HUMAN AD (PERIPHERAL TISSUE)

The fibroblasts obtained from familial AD patients were more sensitive to oxidative stress than those obtained from age-matched normal controls.[170] In another study using fibroblasts from patients with AD and normal subjects, it was shown that treatment with hydrogen peroxide altered the expression of 215 genes and their associated pathways that may be responsible for cell death.[171] The serum levels of vitamins A, vitamin E, and beta-carotene were lower in patients with AD (who were well nourished) than in control patients.[172] In a clinical study involving 12 patients with AD, 13 patients with non-AD dementia, 14 age-matched subjects, and 14 young adult controls, red blood cells (RBC) had elevated levels of markers of oxidative stress (H_2O_2 and organic hydroperoxides) that were associated with age-related dementia, whereas decreased activity of glutathione peroxidase was associated with AD.[173] None of these markers can be considered reliable predictor of MCI or AD.

MITOCHONDRIAL DYSFUNCTION

Most free radicals are produced in the mitochondria, although some are also produced in the cytoplasm by oxidases. Mitochondria may be one of the most sensitive primary targets of oxidative damage in adult neurons.[11] This may be due to the fact that mitochondrial DNA (mtDNA) does not encode for any repair enzymes, and, unlike nuclear DNA, it is not shielded by protective histones. In addition, mtDNA is in close proximity to the site where free radicals are generated during oxidative phosphorylation.[11] Indeed, an increased frequency of mutations in mtDNA has been found in the autopsied samples of the AD brains.[10] Several studies have implicated other types of mitochondrial defects in the pathogenesis of AD.[10,174,175] A defect in energy production may also increase the sensitivity of neurons to excitatory amino acids such as glutamate.[176] Impaired mitochondria may alter metabolism of amyloid precursor protein (APP) leading to increased generation of Aβ1-42 peptides.[177] These studies suggest that mitochondrial dysfunctions may be more important for the development of AD in patients who carry APOE4 allele than in those who do not.

Several oxidized mitochondrial proteins in the brain were detected by using proteomics assay. In addition, decreased energy metabolism was detected in patients with AD exhibiting a mild cognitive dysfunction.[178] In another review, it was shown that decreased energy production preceded the development of clinical symptoms of AD.[179] In addition, reduced energy production can lead to hyperphosphorylation of tau protein and increased production of Aβ1-42 peptides.

PROCESSES OF GENERATING BETA-AMYLOID FRAGMENTS (Aβ1-42) AND THEIR TOXICITY

It is now established that beta-amyloid fragments (Aβ1-42) generated by the cleavage of APP play a central role in the pathogenesis of AD.[12,13,40,180] There are two pathways of processing of APP in the neurons. The predominant pathway of APP processing consists of successive cleavages by alpha- and gamma-secretases, whereas the other pathway involves sequential cleavage of APP by beta- and gamma-secretases. It is the latter pathway that generates neurotoxic beta-amyloids. Normally, alpha-secretase cleaves inside beta-amyloid sequence of APP, releasing the soluble N-terminal domain of APP that exhibit neurotrophic and neuroprotective properties. In patients with AD, a decrease in alpha-secretase-mediated processing of APP has been found in the autopsied brain samples.[181] This process would allow accumulation of APPs, which are cleaved by beta- and gamma-secretase to produce beta-amyloids.

It has been shown that aggregates of beta-amyloid fragments are toxic to neurons in culture[35,182,183] and can cause cell death by apoptosis[184] or necrosis.[33] Several agents can enhance the aggregation of beta-amyloids. They include excess amounts of free Zn and Cu,[185] iron and aluminium,[186] and complement proteins.[187] The aggregated form of beta-amyloids participates in the formation of senile plaque, which can serve as a chronic source of inflammatory reactions, the products of which can enhance the progression of degeneration in nerve cells.

OXIDATIVE STRESS INCREASES PRODUCTION OF BETA AMYLOIDS (Aβ1-42 PEPTIDES)

Increased oxidative stress increases the production and accumulation of β-amyloids in neurons. Indeed, it has been reported that increased oxidative events can accelerate the intracellular buildup of β-amyloids in neurons.[188] Studies showed that membranes containing oxidatively damaged phospholipids accumulated of β-amyloids faster than membranes containing only unoxidized saturated phospholipids.[189] The rate of cleavage of APP to Aβ1-42 was increased in a transgenic AD mouse model lacking cytoplasmic superoxide dismutase-1 (SOD-1) relative to control mice, implying that increased oxidative events can promote the production of Aβ1-42 peptides.[190] Furthermore, 4-hydroxynonenal (HNE), a product of lipid peroxidation, increased γ-secretase activity and

Aβ1-42 assembly in neurons.[191] HNE modified the γ-secretase substrate receptor, nicastrin, in neurons from patients with AD. Such modification of nicastrin heightened its binding to the γ-secretase substrate APP. The levels of HNE-nicastrin were associated with increased γ-secretase activity and Aβ plaque deposition.[191,192]

Aβ1-42 PEPTIDES CAUSE NEURONAL DEGENERATION BY INDUCING FREE RADICALS

Since vitamin E is protective against β-amyloid-induced injury of neuronal cells in culture,[72] it has been proposed that β-amyloid-induced neurotoxicity is facilitated by free radicals.[33–35] Methionine in the 35 position of the beta-amyloid peptide may be a key site relating to the generation of free radicals.[73,193] Binding of erythrocytes with Aβ peptides triggers increased formation of free radicals that could impair delivery of oxygen to the brain tissue.[192] These data suggest that Aβ-induced neuronal death may be partially mediated by way of free radicals. These studies together imply that elevated prooxidant events are likely to participate in the progression of AD.

MUTATIONS IN AD SPECIFIC GENES INCREASES THE PRODUCTION OF BETA-AMYLOIDS

Mutations in specific genes are associated with familial AD. Mutations in APP, presenilin-1, presenilin-2, and γ-secretase increased production of beta-amyloids leading to neuronal death. Mutation in presenilin-1 gene increased the activity of γ-secretase that increased the production of β-amyloids.[194] Mutation of the γ-secretase gene also increases the formation of β-amyloids.[195] Thus, mutation in AD specific genes may cause neuronal damage at least in part by generating excessive amounts of free radicals via elevation of the levels of β-amyloids.

OXIDATIVE STRESS INCREASES HYPERPHOSPHORYLATED TAU (P-TAU) PROTEIN IN AD

Tau is a microtubule-binding protein found within neurofibrillary tangles (NFT). Increased levels of β-amyloids in AD precede the development of tau pathology, namely the hyperphosphorylation of tau and formation of NFTs in the frontal cortex.[196] This suggest that tau pathology, which requires at least two steps, hyperphosphorylation and hyperphosphorylated tau, occurs later than increased generation of beta-amyloid fragments, Antioxidants prevent hyperphosphorylation of tau in transgenic AD mice (Tg2576),[22] suggesting involvement of free radicals in hyperphosphorylation of tau protein. Proteasome inhibition may also reduce degradation of hyperphosphorylated tau proteins causing to slowly accumulate and lead to the formation of NFTs within the cells. It has been reported that intraneuronal tau inclusions appear decades before the deposition of Aβ plaques. However, in the cerebrospinal fluid, altered levels of Aβ peptides occur before the elevation of phosphorylated tau, which only becomes apparent in the later progression of AD.[21] In addition to hyperphosphorylation of tau, acetylation of tau is also markedly elevated at the advanced stage of the disease and may also participate in the progression of AD.[197]

OXIDATIVE STRESS INHIBITS PROTEASOME ACTIVITY IN AD

Proteasomes play an important role in regulating certain transcriptional factors by splicing inactive peptide fragments into active ones. Proteasomes also play a crucial role in the degradation of ubiquitin-conjugated abnormal proteins that could be toxic to neurons. Therefore, inhibition of proteasome in neurons can cause neurodegeneration. Indeed, the role of proteasome inhibition has been proposed for the degeneration of neurons in AD brains.[14,198] In our study, inhibition of proteasome activity by lactacystin causes rapid degeneration and death neurons in culture.[199] Several factors can inhibit proteasome activity. They include increased oxidative stress, defects in ubiquitin conjugation enzymes,[36] mutation in ubiquitin,[200] and beta-amyloid.[198]

EVIDENCE FOR INCREASED LEVELS OF MARKERS OF CHRONIC INFLAMMATION IN AD

Dr. Alois Alzheimer was the first to observe the evidence for chronic inflammation in the autopsied brain tissue of patients with AD. The role of chronic inflammation in AD pathogenesis is supported by the epidemiologic studies that show that rheumatoid arthritis patients, who were on high doses of non-steroidal anti-inflammatory drugs (NSAIDs), had a reduced incidence of AD.[201–204] The direct evidence came from the studies in which it was demonstrated that the mediators and products of inflammatory reaction, such as cytokines,[205,206] complement proteins,[187,207–209] free radicals,[210–213] adhesion molecules,[214–216] and prostaglandins[217,218] were toxic in experimental models of neurons.

Increased levels of pro-inflammatory cytokines such as IL-1 beta and TNF-alpha are found in autopsied samples of brains of AD patients.[7] There appears to be close interaction between beta-amyloids and pro-inflammatory cytokines with respect to production and levels of beta-amyloids and beta-amyloid-induced neurotoxicity. Beta-amyloid-induced inflammatory responses and vascular disruption in AD brain are mediated through TNF-alpha and IL-1 beta.[6,8] In wild type mice, the levels of beta-amyloids can be enhanced by INF-gamma and TNF-alpha through suppression of degradation of beta-amyloids. TNF-alpha also enhanced the levels of beta-amyloids by stimulating the activity of beta-secretase, a rate-limiting enzyme in the production of beta-amyloids.[8] The combination of INF- gamma and TNF-alpha increased the production of beta-amyloids, and reduce the secretion of non-toxic soluble APP fragments in human neuronal cells in culture.[219] Beta-amyloid-induced toxicity can be enhanced by IL-1beta and TNF-alpha.[6,220] Interferon-gamma, IL-1beta, and TNF-alpha increase the gamma-secretase activity and production of beta-amyloids via JNK-dependent mitogen-activated protein kinase pathway.[221]

Both beta-amyloid and NMDA interact with each other in causing neuronal damage. Individually, beta-amyloid and NMDA produced neuronal damage, whereas IL-6, a pro-inflammatory cytokines, did not.[222] The combination of beta-amyloid and NMDA was more effective than the individual agents. However, the combination of 3 (beta-amyloid, NMDA, and IL-6) was most effective in causing damage to neurons.[222] It appears that the combination of beta-amyloid and NMDA causes increased production ROS in cortical neurons through activation of NADPH oxidase,[223] suggesting the involvement of NMDA receptor subtype in the mechanisms of damage produced by beta-amyloids.

The role of inflammatory reactions in AD pathogenesis was further supported by clinical studies in which administration of NSAIDs reduced the rate of deterioration of cognitive function in moderate to advanced AD patients.[224–227] However, a clinical study with new NSAIDs (celecoxib or naproxen) in men and women age 70 years or older with a familial history of AD revealed that these drugs did not improve cognitive function, but a detrimental effect of naproxen was observed.[228] In another clinical trial, the effect of ibuprofen on sources of resting electroencephalographic (EEG) rhythms in mild AD patients was evaluated. The results showed that in the placebo group, amplitude of delta sources was globally greater at follow-up than baseline; however, amplitude of delta sources remained stable or decreased in the majority of patients receiving ibuprofen.[229] It has been reported that NSAIDs such as ibuprofen, aspirin, indomethacin, and naproxen inhibit to a varying degree formation of beta-amyloid fibrils from beta-amyloids and destabilize preformed beta-amyloid fibrils in vitro.[230] Ibuprofen reduced the levels of beta-amyloids and hyperphosphorylated tau protein and improved memory deficits in AD transgenic mice.[231]

There appears to be strong evidence to suggest that increased oxidative stress and chronic inflammation play an important role in the pathogenesis of idiopathic AD; however, in familial

AD, chronic inflammation may play a minor role in the progression of AD. This is due to the fact that mutations in APP, PS-1, or PS-2 that are found in familial AD increase production of beta-amyloids, which mediate their action through free radicals.[17–19,194,195,232,233] Most studies with NSAID on patients with idiopathic AD reported beneficial effects.[224–227,229] However, another study with NSAIDs on patients with familial AD reported no beneficial effect.[228] This result may not be surprising, because in familial AD, excessive production of beta-amyloid fragments that mediate their action through free radicals causes neurodegeneration. Therefore, the data obtained from the use of NSAID in familial AD should not be extrapolated to idiopathic AD. It is possible that the use of free radical scavengers such as antioxidants would have been more useful in reducing the progression of familial AD patients than NSAIDs alone. The combination of two may be more effective than the individual agents.

CHOLESTEROL-INDUCED GENERATION OF BETA-AMYLOIDS

Epidemiologic studies have found that hypercholesterolemia may be a risk factor in the development of AD.[15,16] This was confirmed in the transgenic animal model of AD.[16] This study revealed that high dietary cholesterol increases beta-amyloid accumulation and, thereby, accelerates AD-related pathology in animals.[234] The accumulation of beta-amyloid fragments was reversed by removing cholesterol from the rabbit's diet.[234] Inhibitors of HMG CoA reductase decreased production of beta-amyloids in rabbit[16] and in fetal rat hippocampal neurons in culture.[235] An epidemiologic study has shown that lovastatin, an inhibitor of HMG CoA reductase, reduced the risk of AD in hypercholesterolemic patients.[236] In another epidemiologic study, the use of statins, but not of non-statin cholesterol-lowering drugs, was associated with a reduced incidence of AD in comparison to those who never took statins.[237] These results suggest that lower levels of cholesterol may reduce the risk of AD and that some of the effects of high cholesterol levels are primarily mediated via beta-amyloids.

Statins (cholesterol-lowering drugs) can be divided into two distinct groups, those with a closed-ring structure (lovastatin, Simvastatin, mevastatin) and those with an open-ring structure (pravastatin and Fluvastatin). Statins with a closed-ring structure are metabolized in vivo to an open-ring structure, which then inhibits HMG CoA reductase activity. However, a small amount of the drug could be maintained in a closed-ring structure, which can inhibit proteasome activity.[238] We have demonstrated that mevastatin with a closed-ring structure caused rapid degeneration of differentiated neuroblastoma (NB) cells in culture, whereas, pravastatin with an open-ring structure did not.[239] Mevastatin inhibited proteasome activity in differentiated NB; whereas pravastatin did not. Differentiated NB cells did not convert any portion of mevastatin into an open-ring structure. This is in sharp contrast to the observation made in vivo, where most mevastatin is converted to an open-ring structure by the liver enzyme. These results suggest that mevastatin-induced degeneration of differentiated NB cells may be related to inhibition of proteasome activity.[239] The studies discussed in this section reveal that lowering cholesterol levels could reduce the risk of AD, whereas the presence of increased amounts of unmetabolized statin with a closed-ring structure could increase the risk of AD. A careful study on the effects of statins with a closed-ring and an open-ring structure on neuroprotection and neurodegeneration should be evaluated by laboratory experiments and epidemiologic studies before their relevance in AD can be determined.

GENETIC DEFECTS IN IDIOPATHIC AD

There is no solid evidence for nuclear gene defects, which increase the risk of idiopathic AD, although varying degrees of association between certain gene defects and onset of this disease exist. Several studies have suggested that persons who are homozygous for the apolipoprotein E (APOE), e4 allele, develop AD 10–20 years earlier than those who have e2 or e3 alleles.[240,241] Even persons, who are heterozygous for e4 allele, develop AD 5–10 years earlier than those who have e2 or e3 alleles.[242] About 40% of idiopathic AD is associated with the presence of e4 allele, and it is present in the senile plaque.[37,242] These data suggest that the presence of e4 allele could be an important risk factor for AD. However, it has been shown that this allele is neither essential nor specific for the development of AD.[242] Thus, the role of this APOE allele in neurodegeneration remains uncertain. It has been reported that e4 allele binds to NFTs and beta-amyloid.[37] This property of APOE e4 is not sufficient to have any direct role in neurodegeneration associated with AD. However, a clinical study has reported that in patients who carry ApoE4, the Clinical Dementia Rating was correlated better with decreased alpha-ketoglutarate dehydrogenase complex, a mitochondrial enzyme, than with the plaques or NFTs.[9] This suggests that in some cases of AD, ApoE4 may have some role in the propagation of degenerative processes. A study has reported that mutation in alpha2-macroglobulin gene is present in about 30% of idiopathic AD[243]; however, another study found no such association between alpha$_2$-macroglobulin mutation and risk of AD.[244] A few studies have identified two gene defects in idiopathic AD. Mutation in the ubiquitin gene and downregulation of PS-2 were observed in AD brains.[245,246] We have shown that differentiated neuronal cells in culture overexpressing human APP become sensitive to neurotoxin including oxidative stress.[247]

The genetic polymorphisms play an important role in determining the risk of AD in some populations.[248,249] The levels of beta-secretase, a rate-limiting enzyme in formation of beta-amyloids, were elevated in the autopsied samples of AD brain.[250,251] It appears that amyloid plaque induces beta-secretase in surrounding neurons. In addition, transforming growth factor-beta (TGF-beta) enhances beta-amyloid production in human astrocytes, but not in neurons.[252] This could contribute to the formation of NFTs.

MUTATED AD GENES INDUCE NEURODEGENERATION BY PRODUCING OF BETA-AMYLOIDS

In some familial AD, mutations (about 7) in the APP gene have been reported, all of which increase the production of beta-amyloids[19]; however, this accounts for less than 1% of all familial AD. Mutations (about 50) in presenilin-I gene have been found in about 50% of familial AD[19]; whereas mutations in presenilin-II have been observed in less than 1% of familial AD.[19,232] Presenilin-I is present in senile plaques and NTFs of AD brains.[19] Mutations in APP and presenilin-1 (PS-1) increases the production of beta-amyloid1-42 that causes neuronal death via increasing oxidative stress in primary neuronal cultures obtained from knock-in mice expressing mutant human APP and PS-1 compared to those obtained from wild-type mice.[18] The levels of oxidative damage as a function of age was more pronounced in knock-in mice expressing mutant human APP and PS-1 genes compared to those observed in wild-type mice.[17] This effect was independent of dietary cholesterol.[233] It has been reported that mutations in PS-1 may increase neuronal sensitivity to apoptosis by decreasing the levels of beta-catenin, which is involved in regulation of apoptosis.[20] In addition, PS-1 mutation may also impair proteolytic release and nuclear translocation of Notch-1 intracellular domain, an essential step in activating Notch-1 signaling.[253] Mutation in PS-1 increased the activity of gamma-secretase that increases the production of beta-amyloids.[194]

Mutation in gamma-secretase results in rare forms of early onset of AD due to production of increased amounts of beta-amyloids.[195] The activity of gamma secretase increases, as a function of age in female mice[195] and that may be, in part, responsible for the relatively increased incidence of AD commonly observed in women.

The nature of the interaction between APP and presenilins in causing neuronal damage is not well understood. It has been postulated[41] that APP interacts specifically and transcellularly with either PS-1 or PS-2. This complex is incorporated into intracellular vesicles, which fuse with multivesicular bodies that contain proteases. Beta-amyloid is then produced by proteolysis of APP and released by the usual intracellular traffic between the lysosomal compartment and the plasma membrane into the extracellular spaces where it forms senile (neuritic) plaques.

These studies suggest that mutations in both APP and PS-1 increase the rate of production of beta-amyloids. Excessive production of beta-amyloids can generate more free radicals, inhibit proteasome activity, and contribute to the formation of senile plaques, all of which contribute to progressive neurodegeneration in the AD brain.

NEUROGLOBIN IN AD

Neuroglobin (Ngb) is O_2-binding heme protein related to hemoglobin and myoglobin. It is widely and specifically located in neurons of central and peripheral nervous system of vertebrates. It reversibly binds with oxygen with a high affinity. Expression of Ngb increases in response to neuronal hypoxia and protect neurons caused by hypoxia in vitro and in vivo.[254–256] It also protects the brain from experimental stroke in vivo.[257] Age-dependent loss of Ngb was found in rat cerebral neocortex, hippocampus, caudate-putamen, and cerebellum.[258,259]

Overexpression of wild type of Ngb, but not mutant Ngb, in neuronal cells in culture (PC-12 cell line) decreased H_2O_2-induced free radical accumulation and lipid peroxidation without changing the levels of antioxidant enzymes.[260] It also reduced H_2O_2-induced mitochondrial dysfunction and improved the survival of cells. It has been reported that Ngb also protected neurons against beta-amyloid-induced toxicity in PC-12 neuronal cell line[261] and in murine cortical neurons in culture.[262] Ngb also attenuates the AD phenotype of transgenic mice.[263] These studies suggest that Ngb reduces oxidative stress in neurons by acting as an antioxidant. It has been observed that Ngb expression is reduced with increasing age, and it is lower in women than in men.[263] The latter may, in part, may account for the increased risk of AD in women. Furthermore, the expression of Ngb is upregulated in the autopsied samples of temporal lobe of AD patients, which may be a protective response to the disease process. Therefore, it is possible that the decreased levels of Ngb may increase the risk of AD.

LABORATORY AND CLINICAL STUDIES WITH INDIVIDUAL MICRONUTRIENTS IN AD

The studies with individual micronutrients are described here.

ALPHA-LIPOIC ACID

In an open-label study involving 43 patients with mild to moderate AD receiving standard therapy and follow-up period of 48 months, it was observed that the addition of alpha-lipoic acid to the treatment protocol reduced the progression of the disease.[264] This effect was more pronounced in patients with mild AD than those with moderate AD. The fibroblasts from AD patients exhibited the highest levels of oxidative damage markers in comparison to fibroblasts from age-matched and young control; however, treatment with alpha-lipoic acid and N-acetylcysteine individually reduced the levels of markers of oxidative damage, but the combination of two was more effective than the individual agents.[265] Alpha-lipoic acid also reduced beta-amyloid-induced toxicity on neuronal cells in culture.[266] Natural form of alpha-lipoic acid (R-LA) is more effective than the synthetic form (Rac-LA).[267] Orally administered alpha-lipoic acid does cross blood brain barrier in rats.[268] In a mouse model of AD, administration of R-LA through diet reduced oxidative damage, but did not improve cognitive performance or the levels of beta-amyloids.[269] Chronic administration of alpha-lipoic acid through diet reduced hippocampal-dependent memory deficits of a transgenic mice model of cerebral amyloidosis associated with AD.[270] Dietary supplementation with a combination of alpha-lipoic acid, acetyl-L-carnitine, glycerophosphocoline, docosahexaenoic acid, and phosphatidylserine reduced oxidative damage to the murine brain and improves cognitive performance.[271] These studies suggest that treatment with alpha-lipoic acid alone does not produce consistent results in patients with AD.

Coenzyme Q10

Coenzyme Q10 reduced overproduction of beta-amyloids and intracellular deposit of beta-amyloid in the cortex of the AD transgenic mice.[272] In addition, coenzyme Q10 treatment decreased malondialdehyde (MDA) level and enhanced the activity of superoxide dismutase in these mice. Coenzyme Q10 also prevented the formation beta-amyloid fibrils and destabilized preformed beta-amyloid fibrils.[273] It decreased beta-amyloid-induced mitochondrial dysfunction in vitro.[274] Serum levels of coenzyme Q10 did not change in patients with AD.[275] It has been reported that supplementation with both coenzyme Q10 and alpha-tocopheryl acetate improved age-related learning deficits in mice.[276]

Melatonin

Melatonin treatment increased the levels of thiobarbituric acid-reactive substances (TBARS), superoxide dismutase activity, decreased glutathione levels, and upregulated apoptotic-related factors such as BAX, caspase-3, prostate apoptosis response-4 (Par-4) in AD transgenic mice.[277] Long-term melatonin treatment improves cognitive function in AD transgenic mice. The mechanisms of this protection by melatonin involve preventing aggregation of beta-amyloids, and reducing the levels of pro-inflammatory cytokines and oxidative stress.[278] Patients with AD often exhibit both agitated behavior and poor sleep patterns. In a clinical study, supplementation with melatonin failed to affect these abnormal symptoms in AD patients compared to placebo group.[279] However, melatonin in combination with standard therapy produced beneficial effects on cognitive function and depression test more than that produced by standard therapy alone.[280] These studies suggest that treatment with melatonin alone does not produce consistent results in patients with AD.

Nicotinamide (Vitamin B3)

Histone deacetylase inhibitors increase histone acetylation and enhance memory and neuronal plasticity. Nicotinamide, a competitive inhibitor of histone deacetylase activity, restored memory deficits in AD transgenic mice.[281] In addition, it selectively reduced a specific phospho-species of tau protein (Thr231) that is associated with microtubule depolymerization. The overexpression of a Thr231-phospho-mimic tau in neuronal cells in culture increased clearance and decreased accumulation of tau compared with wild-type tau. Nicotinamide, a precursor of NAD^+ also attenuated glutamate-induced toxicity and preserve cellular levels of NAD+ to support the activity of SIRT-1.[282] These preclinical data suggest that oral supplementation with nicotinamide may be safe and useful in the treatment of AD and other taupathies. Caloric restriction upregulated NAD^+-dependent SIRT1 in the mouse brain[282] and this may be one of the mechanisms of protection against amyloid neuropathology.[283] A 30% caloric restriction reduced the levels of beta-amyloids but increased the levels of SIRT1 in the brain of squirrel monkeys.[284]

Vitamin A, Vitamin E, and Vitamin C

Vitamin A and beta-carotene inhibited formation of beta-amyloid fibrils in a dose-dependent manner. They also destabilized preformed beta-amyloid fibrils in vitro.[285] Retinoic acid treatment decreased activation of microglia and astrocytes, reduced degeneration of neurons, and improved spatial learning and memory in AD transgenic mice compared with the vehicle-control.[286] It also downregulated the activity of cyclin-dependent kinase 5, a major kinase, involved in both APP and tau phosphorylation.

Vitamin E treatment protected cortical synaptosomal membranes and hippocampal neurons[193] and other neurons[72] in culture against beta-amyloid-induced toxicity. Vitamin E and pycnogenol protected neuronal cells in culture against beta-amyloid-induced apoptosis by attenuating caspase-3 activation, DNA fragmentation, and cleavage of poly (ADP-ribose) polymerase (PARP).[287]

Analysis of clinical studies revealed that vitamin E alone might not be useful in the prevention or treatment of AD.[288] However, a controlled clinical trial with *dl*-alpha-tocopherol (synthetic form; 2,000 IU/day) in patients with moderately severe impairment from AD showed some beneficial effects with respect to the rate of deterioration of cognitive function.[289] In certain counties of North Carolina, analysis of older African American and white individuals during 1986–2000 revealed that the supplemental use of vitamins was low; however, supplementation with vitamin C and/or vitamin E did not delay the incidence of AD or dementia in these populations.[290] In a prospective cohort study performed by Group Health Cooperative, Seattle, Washington, it was found that supplementation with vitamin E and vitamin C individually or in combination did not reduce the risk of AD or overall dementia over 5.5 years of observation period.[291] In a cross-sectional and prospective study in elderly (65 years or older) patients with dementia, it was found that use of vitamin C and vitamin E in combination was associated with reduced prevalence and incidence of AD.[292] In AD transgenic mice, it was shown that vitamin E supplementation reduced the levels and deposits of amyloids in the brain; however, vitamin E supplementation was ineffective in decreasing the levels and deposit of amyloids in older mice.[293] In a transgenic model of Down syndrome, supplementation with vitamin E alone delays onset of cognitive dysfunction and pathological changes in the basal forebrain.[294] These studies suggest that treatment with one or two antioxidant alone does not produce consistent results in AD.

SERUM LEVELS OF ANTIOXIDANTS

To determine the antioxidant status in patients with AD, serum and cerebrospinal fluid (CSF) levels of antioxidants were analyzed. The results showed that serum levels of vitamin E and beta-carotene were lower in patients with AD and multi-infarct dementia compared to controls.[172] In another study, serum levels of beta-carotene and vitamin A were lower in AD patients compared to control; however the level of alpha-carotene did not change.[295] The average CSF and serum level of vitamin E was lower in patients with AD than controls.[296] The plasma levels of dietary antioxidants (vitamin C, vitamin A, vitamin E, and carotenoids including beta-carotene, alpha-carotene, lutein, zeaxanthin, and lycopene, SOD, and glutathione peroxidase) were lower in patients with AD as well as in elderly subjects with mild cognitive impairment compared to control subjects.[297] In another study, plasma vitamin C levels were lowered in subjects with dementia compared to controls, which was not explained by their dietary intake of vitamin C.[298]

B-VITAMINS

In most studies, the serum levels of vitamin B12 in AD patients were significantly lower than controls.[299,300] Indeed, vitamin B12 supplementation increased choline acetyl transferase activity in cholinergic neurons of cats[301] and improved cognitive functions in AD patients.[302] Analysis of published data revealed that there was no benefit from folic acid supplementation with or without vitamin B12 on cognitive function or mood of healthy elderly people[303]; however, in a group of healthy elderly people with high homocysteine levels, supplementation with folic acid for a period of three years was associated with significant improvement in global functioning, memory storage, and information processing speed. In a pilot study, it was observed that supplementation with folic improved the efficacy of cholinesterase inhibitor in patients with AD.[303] In another multicenter clinical study, supplementation with folic acid, vitamin B6, and vitamin B12 did not show any beneficial effects on cognitive function decline in individuals with mild to moderate AD.[304] Supplementation with vitamin B12 alone did not benefit cognitive or psychiatric symptoms in vast majority of elderly patients with dementia having low serum vitamin-12 levels.[305] These studies suggest that treatment with one or more B-vitamins alone does not produce consistent results in patients with AD.

CURCUMIN

Curcumin inhibited formation of beta-amyloid fibrils and destabilized preformed beta-amyloid fibrils in vitro in a dose-dependent manner.[285]

RESVERATROL

Epidemiologic studies suggest that the moderate consumption of red wine is associated with a lower incidence of AD and dementia in general population, and that resveratrol, a major polyphenol in red wine, exhibits neuroprotective effects in vitro and in animal models of AD.[306,307] Consumption of 3 serving of wine daily was associated with a lower risk of AD in elderly individuals without the APOE epsilon-4-allele.[308] Resveratrol protects neuronal cells in culture against beta-amyloid-induced toxicity. This effect is mediated through enhancing the intracellular levels of glutathione, an important antioxidant within the cells.[309] It also lowered intracellular levels of beta-amyloids in different neuronal cell lines.[310] This effect of resveratrol was due to increased degradation of beta-amyloids by proteasome. This mechanism of resveratrol was supported by the fact that resveratrol-induced decrease in beta-amyloid was prevented by several selective inhibitors of proteasome and by siRNA-directed silencing of proteasome subunit beta5 activity.[310] Resveratrol treatment upregulated the expression of SIRT1 gene that attenuated degeneration and death of neurons in an animal model of AD.[311,312]

GINKGO BILOBA AND OMEGA-3 FATTY ACIDS

In a randomized, double-blind, placebo-controlled clinical trial in community volunteers aged 75 years or older with normal cognition revealed that administration of *Ginkgo biloba* was not effective in reducing the incidence of AD or overall dementia.[313] Long-term consumption of *Ginkgo biloba* extract through diet lowered human APP levels by 50% compared to controls in the cortex but not in the hippocampal regions of the brain of AD transgenic mice.[314]

In a similarly designed study in patients with mild to moderate AD, supplementation with omega-3 fatty acid (1.7 g of docosahexaenoic acid and 0.6 g of eicosapentaenoic acid) did not delay the rate of cognitive decline; however, beneficial effects were observed in a small group of patients with very mild AD.[315] Analysis of published observational studies and clinical trials suggest that omega-3 fatty acids may slow down cognitive decline in elderly individuals without dementia, but it was ineffective in reducing the incidence of AD or dementia.[316] In the Canadian Study of Health and Aging (CSHA), there was no association between omega-3 fatty acids and the risk of dementia.[317] In a randomized, double-blind, placebo-controlled trial, supplementation with omega-3 fatty acids showed significant improvement in Alzheimer's Disease Assessment scale (ADAS-cog) compared to placebo control in individuals with MCI; however, there was no significant difference in patients with AD.[318] These studies suggest that treatment with *Ginkgo biloba* or omega-3 fatty acids alone does not produce consistent results in patients with AD.

GREEN TEA EPIGALLOCATECHIN-3-GALLATE (EGCG) AND CAFFEINE

Treatment of AD transgenic mice with Green tea epigallocatechin-3-gallate (EGCG) improved cognitive function and reduced the levels of beta-amyloids and phosphorylated tau isoforms.[319] Long-term caffeine consumption decreased the production of beta-amyloids and improved cognitive function in AD transgenic mice; therefore, it was suggested that daily moderate consumption of caffeine might reduce the risk of AD.[320] These studies are not sufficient to recommend either EGCG or caffeine for reduction in the risk of developing AD.

NON-STEROIDAL ANTI-INFLAMMATORY DRUGS (NSAIDs) IN AD

Since chronic inflammation represents one of the major factors that initiate and promote neurodegeneration in AD brain, the use of NSAIDs in the prevention and treatment of AD appears rational. Epidemiological studies revealed that rheumatoid arthritis patients, who are on high doses of NSAIDs), have a reduced incidence of AD.[201–204,321–323] NSAIDs also reduce the rate of deterioration of cognitive functions in AD patients.[225–227,324] However, administration of prednisone, a powerful anti-inflammatory agent, was not useful in patients with AD.[325] Treatment with a mixed Cox-1/Cox-2 inhibitor and a PGE2 analog failed to produce any significant benefit on cognitive function.[326] A specific inhibitor of Cox-2 was also not useful in improving cognitive function.[327] These results suggest that inflammatory drugs alone do not produce consistent benefits on cognitive function.

POTENTIAL REASONS FOR INCONSISTENT RESULTS WITH INDIVIDUAL MICRONUTRIENTS OR ASPIRIN IN AD

The reasons for individual micronutrients or aspirin producing no effects to some transient beneficial effects on AD are not known; however, some potentials causes are described here: (a) antioxidants show differential subcellular distribution and different mechanisms of action; therefore, a single antioxidant cannot protect all parts of the cell; (b) a single antioxidant in a high internal oxidative environment in high-risk patients is oxidized and can then itself act as a prooxidant rather than as an antioxidant; (c) the body protects against oxidative damage by elevating antioxidant enzymes, and dietary and endogenous antioxidants; therefore a single antioxidant cannot achieve this goal; (d) antioxidants neutralize free radicals by donating electrons to those molecules with unpaired electron, whereas antioxidant enzymes destroy free radicals by catalysis; therefore, the levels of both antioxidant enzymes and dietary and endogenous antioxidants should be enhanced for substantial protection against oxidative damage and inflammation; (e) the affinity of different antioxidants for free radicals differs, depending upon their solubility; (f) both the aqueous and lipid compartments of the cell need to be protected together. Water-soluble antioxidants such as vitamin C and glutathione protect molecules in the aqueous environment of the cells, whereas lipid soluble antioxidants such as vitamin A and vitamin E protect molecules in the lipid compartment; therefore, a single antioxidant cannot protect molecules in both aqueous and lipid environment; (g) vitamin E is more effective in quenching free radicals in a reduced oxygenated cellular environment, whereas vitamin C and alpha-tocopherol are more effective in a higher oxygenated environment of the cells[328]; (h) vitamin C is important for recycling the oxidized form of alpha-tocopherol to the antioxidant form at the lipid/aqueous interface[329]; (i) different antioxidants produce cell protective proteins by altering the expression of different microRNAs.[28] For example, some antioxidants can activate Nrf2 by upregulating miR-200a that inhibits its target protein Keap1, whereas others activate Nrf2 by downregulating miR-21 that binds with 3'-UTR Nrf2 mRNA[330]; therefore, a single antioxidant cannot achieve this effect.

Aspirin may reduce chronic inflammation somewhat, but it has no effect on oxidative stress; therefore, it may not be effective in reducing the risk of AD consistently.

The studies discussed above show that a single micronutrient or aspirin is not expected to yield any consistent beneficial effects on AD prevention. For this reason, a mixture of micronutrients that can simultaneously reduce oxidative stress and inflammation by enhancing the levels of antioxidant enzymes through the activation of Nrf2 pathway together with dietary and endogenous antioxidants for Alzheimer's disease and Parkinson's disease has been suggested.[27,28] Oral supplementation can increase the levels of dietary and endogenous antioxidants; however, elevation of the levels of antioxidant enzymes requires an activation of Nrf2. Therefore, it is essential to understand about activation of Nrf2.

ACTIVATION OF Nrf2 (NUCLEAR FACTOR-ERYTHROID-2-RELATED FACTOR 2)

Nrf2

The nuclear transcriptional factor, Nrf2 belongs to the Cap 'n' Collar (CNC) family that contains a conserved basic leucine zipper (bZIP) transcriptional factor.[331] Under physiological condition, Nrf2 is associated with Kelch-like ECH associated protein 1 (Keap1), which acts as an inhibitor of Nrf2.[332] Keap1 protein serves as an adaptor to link Nrf2 to the ubiquitin ligase CuI-Rbx1 complex for degradation by proteasomes and maintains the steady levels of Nrf2 in the cytoplasm. Nrf2-keap1 complex is primarily located in the cytoplasm. Keap1 acts as a sensor for ROS/electrophilic stress.

ROS Activates Nrf2

Normally, ROS is needed to activate Nrf2 which then dissociates itself from Keap1-CuI-Rbx1 complex and translocates in the nucleus where it heterodimerizes with a small Maf protein, binds with ARE, leading to increased expression of target genes coding for several cytoprotective enzymes including antioxidant enzymes.[333–335]

ROS-Resistant Nrf2

In contrast to acute oxidative stress, Nrf2 becomes resistant to ROS during chronic oxidative stress,[336–338] suggesting that activation of Nrf2 by a ROS-independent mechanism exists. This is evidenced by the fact that increased chronic oxidative stress occurs in the presence of Nrf2 in neurodegenerative diseases such as AD. The question arises as to how to activate ROS-resistant Nrf2 in AD.

Antioxidants Activate ROS-Resistant Nrf2

Some examples are vitamin E and genistein,[339] alpha-lipoic acid,[340] curcumin,[341] resveratrol,[342,343] omega-3-fatty acids,[344,345] glutathione,[346] NAC,[347] and coenzyme Q10.[348] Several plant-derived phytochemicals, such as epigallocatechin-3-gallate, carestol, kahweol, cinnamonyl-based compounds, zerumbone, lycopene and carnosol,[331,349,350] genistein,[339] allicin, a major organosulfur compound found in garlic,[351] sulforaphane, a organosulfur compound, found in cruciferous vegetables,[352] and kavalactones (methysticin, kavain, and yangonin).[353] The reasons for the activation of Nrf2 without ROS by antioxidant compounds are not known.

BINDING OF Nrf2 WITH ARE IN THE NUCLEUS

An activation of Nrf2 alone is not sufficient to increase the levels of antioxidant enzymes. Activated Nrf2 must bind with ARE in the nucleus for increasing the expression of target genes coding for antioxidant enzymes. This binding ability of Nrf2 with ARE was impaired in aged rats and this defect was restored by supplementation with alpha-lipoic acid.[340] It is unknown whether the binding ability of Nrf2 with ARE is impaired in AD.

SUPPRESSION OF CHRONIC INFLAMMATION

Activation of Nrf2 also suppresses inflammation.[354,355] Some individual antioxidants also reduce chronic inflammation.[356–363]

Nrf2 in AD

The activation of Nrf2 becomes unresponsive to ROS during chronic oxidative stress found in AD. The levels of Nrf2 decreased in the hippocampal neurons from patients with AD and

Lewy body variant of AD compared to normal hippocampal neurons.[336] Treatment with tert-butylhydroquinone, an inducer of Nrf2, or with adenoviral Nrf2 gene transfer, protected neurons against Aβ-induced toxicity in transgenic mouse model of AD.[364] Other agents that induce Nrf2 include Pierisformoside B (PFB) (isolated from Rhododendron brachycarpum)[365] and Cudraflavone B, a prenylated flavone, isolated from Cudrania triscuspidata.[366] Agmatine treatment inhibited the accumulation of beta-amyloids, and enhanced insulin signal transduction, and improved cognitive function via the Nrf2/ARE pathway in streptomycin-induced AD rat model.[367] These inducers of Nrf2 reduced markers of oxidative damage and chronic inflammation in the hippocampal neurons.

Treatment of primary culture of hippocampal neurons with Puerarin, a major flavonoid from the root of Pueraria lobata, reduced beta-amyloid-induced oxidative stress by activating the Nrf2-ARE pathway.[368] Genistein, a flavonoid, and vitamin E reduced oxidative damage produced by beta-amyloids (Aβ25-35) in transformed cerebrovascular mouse endothelial cells by enhancing the Nrf2-regulated antioxidant genes.[339]

Genetic deletion of Nrf2 in APP/PS1 transgenic AD mice increased chronic inflammation, intracellular levels of APP, Aβ1-41 and Aβ1-40.[369] The insoluble fractions of APP and Aβ as well as poly-ubiquitin conjugated proteins were elevated in these mice. Furthermore, neurons from the genetic deleted APP/PS1 mice showed accumulation of multivesicular bodies, endosomes, and lysosomes. Overexpression of Nrf2 prevented Aβ1-41-induced toxicity and reduction in proliferation of neural stem cells.[370] Activation of Nrf2 decreased the levels of phosphorylated tau protein by inducing an autophagy adaptor protein NDP52 in neurons. The NDP52 has three AREs in its promoter region, and its overexpression removes phosphorylated tau in the presence of an autophagy enhancer. In Nrf2 knockout mice, the levels of NDP52 decreased and the levels of phosphorylated tau increased in the brain.[371] These data suggest that activation of Nrf2 is one of essential features of reducing oxidative stress and chronic inflammation. Other feature that must be elevated includes dietary and endogenous antioxidants.

PROPOSED MICRONUTRIENT MIXTURE FOR OPTIMALLY REDUCING OXIDATIVE STRESS AND CHRONIC INFLAMMATION IN AD

In order to reduce the risk and improve the management of AD, I propose a micronutrient mixture containing multiple dietary antioxidants (vitamin A, beta-carotene, vitamin C, vitamin E acetate, vitamin E succinate, curcumin, resveratrol, and selenomethionine), endogenous antioxidants (alpha-lipoic acid, L-carnitine, and coenzyme Q10), a synthetic antioxidant N-acetylcysteine (NAC), vitamin D3, all B-vitamins with high doses of vitamin B3, zinc, and omega-3-fatty acids. This micronutrient mixture may optimally reduce oxidative stress by simultaneously enhancing the levels of antioxidant enzymes through activation of the Nrf2/ARE pathway and dietary and endogenous antioxidants. Animal and limited human studies suggest that the micronutrients in the mixture can cross blood-brain barrier at varying levels. This is supported by the observations described earlier in which supplementation with these micronutrients individually improved some neurological symptoms in animal models of AD and human AD.

PROPOSED MICRONUTRIENT STRATEGIES FOR PREVENTION OF AD

PRIMARY PREVENTION FOR AD

The purpose of primary prevention is to protect healthy individuals from developing AD. Individuals 50 years or older, individuals carrying APOE-epsilon-4-alle, and individuals with a family history of AD, who have not developed any clinical symptoms of AD, are suitable for the primary prevention studies. It is expected that supplementation with the proposed micronutrient mixture may reduce the incidence of AD in high-risk populations.

The recommended multiple micronutrient preparation should be taken orally and divided into two doses, half in the morning and the other half in the evening with meal. This is because the biological half-lives of micronutrients in the mixture are highly variable; this can create high levels of fluctuations in the tissue levels of micronutrients. A 2-fold difference in the levels of certain micronutrients such as alpha-TS can cause a marked difference in the expression of gene profiles. In order to maintain relatively consistent levels of micronutrients in the brain, the proposed micronutrients must be taken twice a day.

CAN AD SYMPTOMS BE PREVENTED OR DELAYED IN INDIVIDUALS CARRYING MUTATED GENE?

At present, there are no strategies to prevent or delay the onset of symptoms of AD in individuals carrying mutated AD genes, but has not developed any symptoms. Since high levels of oxidative stress and chronic inflammation are detected in asymptomatic individuals carrying mutated AD gene; the proposed mixture of micronutrients would be equally effective in reducing these biochemical defects, and thereby, preventing or delaying the onset of symptoms of AD. This possibility is indirectly supported by another line of experimental evidence described here.

The gene HOP (TUM-1) is essential for the development of *Drosophila melanogaster* (fruit fly). A mutation in this gene markedly increases the risk of developing a leukemia-like tumor in female flies. In collaboration with Dr Bhattacharya of NASA Moffat Field, CA, we observed that whole-body irradiation of these flies with proton radiation dramatically increased the incidence of cancer compared to that observed in unirradiated flies. Treatment with an antioxidant mixture before and after irradiation blocked the proton radiation-induced cancer in fruit flies.[149] This finding suggests that consequences of heritable mutation in specific gene can be prevented by treatment with a mixture of antioxidants at least in fruit flies. However, the results from this study cannot be extrapolated to humans.

SECONDARY PREVENTION FOR AD

The purpose of secondary prevention is to stop or slow the progression of AD. Individuals who exhibit early sign of AD, but are not taking any medication, can be included in secondary prevention studies. The micronutrient mixture recommended for the primary prevention is also recommended for the secondary prevention. It is expected that this strategy would slow the progression of the disease, and may prolong the time period before the drugs are needed.

PROPOSED MICRONUTRIENT MIXTURE FOR IMPROVING THE MANAGEMENT OF AD

CURRENT DRUG THERAPY FOR AD

Current drug treatments of AD primarily include acetylcholinesterase inhibitors donepezil, galantamine, and rivastigmine. These drugs increase the levels of acetylcholine in the surviving cholinergic neurons. These treatments improve cognitive function, behavior and activities of daily living in most individuals for a limited period of time, but have failed to stop the progression of the AD. In a recent study, treatment with donepezil failed to produce any benefit in ethnically diverse AD patients. The reasons for this contradictory results between the previous studies and the present study are unknown. The beneficial effects of acetylcholinesterase inhibitors are due to improved function of cholinergic neurons. Thus, it appears that the effectiveness of AD drugs depends upon the viability of surviving cholinergic neurons; therefore, their effects in improving the cognitive function only last as long as the cholinergic neurons are viable. None of the drugs reduce the underlying oxidative stress or chronic inflammation responsible for degeneration and death of neurons. Consequently, neurons continue to die despite the drug treatments.

PROPOSED MICRONUTRIENT MIXTURE IN COMBINATION WITH DRUG THERAPY FOR AD

The proposed micronutrient mixture recommended for the primary prevention is also suggested in combination with drug therapy. This strategy may reduce the progression and prolong the beneficial effects of current drugs in patients with dementia with or without AD by protecting surviving neurons from oxidative damage and chronic inflammation. The effectiveness of this micronutrient mixture in combination with drugs should be tested by well-designed clinical studies in the management of AD.

DIET AND LIFESTYLE RECOMMENDATIONS FOR AD

Dietary recommendations include minimizing the intake of saturated fat and trans-fatty acids and exposure to aluminum, increased consumption of vegetables, legumes, fruits, high fibers, and low fat. Lifestyle recommendations include physical and mental exercises, and relaxation through meditation, yoga, and vacation, in addition to stopping cigarette smoking and all tobacco-related products.

CONCLUSIONS

Alzheimer's disease (AD) is a slow, progressive, degenerative disease characterized by the gradual loss of cognitive function and death of cortical neurons in the brain. The development of AD has been divided into two stages: mild cognitive impairment (MCI) and established AD. AD is the 5th leading cause of death in the United States. The incidence of AD continues to rise. Extensive basic studies have identified several cellular and genetic defects that contribute to the initiation, progressive degeneration, and death of neurons in AD. They include: (a) increased oxidative stress, (b) chronic inflammation, (c) mitochondrial dysfunction, (d) $A\beta1$-42 peptides generated from the cleavage of amyloid precursor protein (APP), (e) proteasome inhibition, (f) high cholesterol levels, (g) hyperphosphorylated tau protein, and (h) heritable mutations in APP, presenilin-1, and presenilin-2 genes. Analysis of published studies suggests that increased oxidative damage precedes other biochemical and genetic defects in AD.[24] Oxidative damage, if not repaired, leads to chronic inflammation. Therefore, attenuation of oxidative stress and chronic inflammation may reduce the risk of developing AD, and in combination with standard therapy, may improve the management of this disease. Alterations in the expressions of microRNAs play an important role in the pathogenesis of AD. Reactive oxygen species (ROS) and pro-inflammatory cytokines regulate the expression of microRNAs and their target proteins that cause neurodegeneration. Antioxidants also regulate the expression of microRNAs and their target proteins that protects neurons against damaging agents. Studies on the effects of micronutrients in experimental models and human AD have produced inconsistent results varying from no effect to some transient effects on the symptoms of AD. The reasons for the inconsistent results are discussed. In order to reduce oxidative stress and chronic inflammation, elevation of the antioxidant enzymes, and the dietary and endogenous antioxidants, is essential. A mixture of micronutrients that would achieve this goal is proposed for primary and secondary prevention, and in combination with standard therapy, for improved management of AD.

REFERENCES

1. Alzheimer's Association. Alzheimer's disease. Facts and figures. *Alzheimer's Dementia.* 2017;13:325–373.
2. Koppal T, Drake, J., Yatin, et al., Peroxynitrites-mediated damage to brain membrane proteins and lipids: Anoter oxidative pathway for membrane alterations in Alzheimer's disease (AD). *Soc Neurosci.* 1998;24:1217a.
3. Martins RN, Harper CG, Stokes GB, Masters CL. Increased cerebral glucose-6-phosphate dehydrogenase activity in Alzheimer's disease may reflect oxidative stress. *J Neurochem.* 1986;46(4):1042–1045.
4. Xie H, Hou S, Jiang J, Sekutowicz M, Kelly J, Bacskai BJ. Rapid cell death is preceded by amyloid plaque-mediated oxidative stress. *Proc Natl Acad Sci U S A.* 2013;110(19):7904–7909.
5. Sultana R, Perluigi M, Butterfield DA. Protein oxidation and lipid peroxidation in brain of subjects with Alzheimer's disease: Insights into mechanism of neurodegeneration from redox proteomics. *Antioxid Redox Signal.* 2006;8(11–12):2021–2037.
6. Ramirez G, Rey S, von Bernhardi R. Proinflammatory stimuli are needed for induction of microglial cell-mediated AbetaPP_{244-C} and Abeta-neurotoxicity in hippocampal cultures. *J Alzheimers Dis.* 2008;15(1):45–59.
7. Sutton ET, Thomas T, Bryant MW, Landon CS, Newton CA, Rhodin JA. Amyloid-beta peptide induced inflammatory reaction is mediated by the cytokines tumor necrosis factor and interleukin-1. *J Submicrosc Cytol Pathol.* 1999;31(3):313–323.
8. Yamamoto M, Kiyota T, Horiba M, et al. Interferon-gamma and tumor necrosis factor-alpha regulate amyloid-beta plaque deposition and beta-secretase expression in Swedish mutant APP transgenic mice. *Am J Pathol.* 2007;170(2):680–692.
9. Gibson GE, Haroutunian V, Zhang H, et al. Mitochondrial damage in Alzheimer's disease varies with apolipoprotein E genotype. *Ann Neurol.* 2000;48(3):297–303.
10. Shoffner JM, Brown MD, Torroni A, et al. Mitochondrial DNA variants observed in Alzheimer disease and Parkinson disease patients. *Genomics.* 1993;17(1):171–184.
11. Wallace DC. Mitochondrial genetics: A paradigm for aging and degenerative diseases? *Science.* 1992;256(5057):628–632.
12. Selkoe DJ. Cell biology of the amyloid beta-protein precursor and the mechanism of Alzheimer's disease. *Annu Rev Cell Biol.* 1994;10:373–403.
13. Yankner BA, Mesulam MM. Seminars in medicine of the Beth Israel Hospital, Boston. beta-Amyloid and the pathogenesis of Alzheimer's disease. *N Engl J Med.* 1991;325(26):1849–1857.
14. Checler F, da Costa CA, Ancolio K, Chevallier N, Lopez-Perez E, Marambaud P. Role of the proteasome in Alzheimer's disease. *Biochim Biophys Acta.* 2000;1502(1):133–138.
15. Wolozin B, Kellman W, Ruosseau P, Celesia GG, Siegel G. Decreased prevalence of Alzheimer disease associated with 3-hydroxy-3-methyglutaryl coenzyme A reductase inhibitors. *Arch Neurol.* 2000;57(10):1439–1443.
16. Sparks DL, Martin TA, Gross DR, Hunsaker JC, 3rd. Link between heart disease, cholesterol, and Alzheimer's disease: A review. *Microsc Res Tech.* 2000;50(4):287–290.
17. Abdul HM, Sultana R, St Clair DK, Markesbery WR, Butterfield DA. Oxidative damage in brain from human mutant APP/PS-1 double knock-in mice as a function of age. *Free Radic Biol Med.* 2008;45(10):1420–1425.
18. Mohmmad Abdul H, Sultana R, Keller JN, St Clair DK, Markesbery WR, Butterfield DA. Mutations in amyloid precursor protein and presenilin-1 genes increase the basal oxidative stress in murine neuronal cells and lead to increased sensitivity to oxidative stress mediated by amyloid beta-peptide (1–42), HO and kainic acid: Implications for Alzheimer's disease. *J Neurochem.* 2006;96(5):1322–1335.
19. Sherrington R, Rogaev EI, Liang Y, et al. Cloning of a gene bearing missense mutations in early-onset familial Alzheimer's disease. *Nature.* 1995;375(6534):754–760.
20. Zhang Z, Hartmann H, Do VM, et al. Destabilization of beta-catenin by mutations in presenilin-1 potentiates neuronal apoptosis. *Nature.* 1998;395(6703):698–702.
21. Braak H, Zetterberg H, Del Tredici K, Blennow K. Intraneuronal tau aggregation precedes diffuse plaque deposition, but amyloid-beta changes occur before increases of tau in cerebrospinal fluid. *Acta Neuropathol.* 2013;126(5):631–641.
22. Melov S, Adlard PA, Morten K, et al. Mitochondrial oxidative stress causes hyperphosphorylation of tau. *PLoS ONE.* 2007;2(6):e536.

23. Tai HC, Serrano-Pozo A, Hashimoto T, Frosch MP, Spires-Jones TL, Hyman BT. The synaptic accumulation of hyperphosphorylated tau oligomers in Alzheimer disease is associated with dysfunction of the ubiquitin-proteasome system. *Am J Pathol.* 2012;181(4):1426–1435.
24. Prasad KN, Bondy SC. Inhibition of early upstream events in prodromal Alzheimer's disease by use of targeted antioxidants. *Curr Aging Sci.* 2014;7(2):77–90.
25. Prasad KN, Hovland AR, Cole WC, et al. Multiple antioxidants in the prevention and treatment of Alzheimer disease: Analysis of biologic rationale. *Clin Neuropharmacol.* 2000;23(1):2–13.
26. Prasad KN, Cole WC, Prasad KC. Risk factors for Alzheimer's disease: Role of multiple antioxidants, non-steroidal anti-inflammatory, and cholinergic agents alone or in combination in prevention and treatment. *J Am Coll Nutr.* 2002;21(6):506–522.
27. Prasad KN. Simultaneous activation of Nrf2 and elevation of antioxidant compounds for reducing oxidative stress and chronic inflammation in human Alzheimer's disease. *Mech Ageing Dev.* 2016;153:41–47.
28. Prasad KN. Oxidative stress and pro-inflammatory cytokines may act as one of signals for regulating MicroRNAs expression in Alzheimer's disease. *Mech Ageing Dev.* 2017;162:63–71.
29. NIA. *Progress Report on Alzheimer's Disease.* Bethesda, MD: National Institute of Health; 1997.
30. Rondeau V, Jacqmin-Gadda H, Commenges D, Helmer C, Dartigues JF. Aluminum and silica in drinking water and the risk of Alzheimer's disease or cognitive decline: Findings from 15-year follow-up of the PAQUID cohort. *Am J Epidemiol.* 2009;169(4):489–496.
31. Engelhart MJ, Geerlings MI, Ruitenberg A, et al. Dietary intake of antioxidants and risk of Alzheimer disease. *JAMA.* 2002;287(24):3223–3229.
32. Evatt ML, Delong MR, Khazai N, Rosen A, Triche S, Tangpricha V. Prevalence of vitamin d insufficiency in patients with Parkinson disease and Alzheimer disease. *Arch Neurol.* 2008;65(10):1348–1352.
33. Behl C, Davis JB, Lesley R, Schubert D. Hydrogen peroxide mediates amyloid beta protein toxicity. *Cell.* 1994;77(6):817–827.
34. Butterfield DA, Hensley K, Harris M, Mattson M, Carney J. beta-Amyloid peptide free radical fragments initiate synaptosomal lipoperoxidation in a sequence-specific fashion: Implications to Alzheimer's disease. *Biochem Biophys Res Commun.* 1994;200(2):710–715.
35. Schubert D, Behl C, Lesley R, et al. Amyloid peptides are toxic via a common oxidative mechanism. *Proc Natl Acad Sci U S A.* 1995;92(6):1989–1993.
36. Lopez Salon M, Morelli L, Castano EM, Soto EF, Pasquini JM. Defective ubiquitination of cerebral proteins in Alzheimer's disease. *J Neurosci Res.* 2000;62(2):302–310.
37. Martin JB. Molecular basis of the neurodegenerative disorders. *N Engl J Med.* 1999;340(25):1970–1980.
38. Goedert M, Jakes R, Crowther RA, et al. The abnormal phosphorylation of tau protein at Ser-202 in Alzheimer disease recapitulates phosphorylation during development. *Proc Natl Acad Sci U S A.* 1993;90(11):5066–5070.
39. Grundke-Iqbal I, Iqbal K, Tung YC, Quinlan M, Wisniewski HM, Binder LI. Abnormal phosphorylation of the microtubule-associated protein tau (tau) in Alzheimer cytoskeletal pathology. *Proc Natl Acad Sci U S A.* 1986;83(13):4913–4917.
40. Hardy J, Allsop D. Amyloid deposition as the central event in the aetiology of Alzheimer's disease. *Trends Pharmacol Sci.* 1991;12(10):383–388.
41. Dewji NN, Singer SJ. Genetic clues to Alzheimer's disease. *Science.* 1996;271(5246):159–160.
42. Wang GP, Khatoon S, Iqbal K, Grundke-Iqbal I. Brain ubiquitin is markedly elevated in Alzheimer disease. *Brain Res.* 1991;566(1–2):146–151.
43. Kudo T, Iqbal K, Ravid R, Swaab DF, Grundke-Iqbal I. Alzheimer disease: Correlation of cerebrospinal fluid and brain ubiquitin levels. *Brain Res.* 1994;639(1):1–7.
44. Hamilton RL. Lewy bodies in Alzheimer's disease: A neuropathological review of 145 cases using alpha-synuclein immunohistochemistry. *Brain Pathol.* 2000;10(3):378–384.
45. Lee RC, Feinbaum RL, Ambros V. The C. elegans heterochronic gene lin-4 encodes small RNAs with antisense complementarity to lin-14. *Cell.* 1993;75(5):843–854.
46. Wightman B, Ha I, Ruvkun G. Posttranscriptional regulation of the heterochronic gene lin-14 by lin-4 mediates temporal pattern formation in C. elegans. *Cell.* 1993;75(5):855–862.
47. Macfarlane LA, Murphy PR. MicroRNA: Biogenesis, function and role in cancer. *Curr Genomics.* 2010;11(7):537–561.
48. Londin E, Loher P, Telonis AG, et al. Analysis of 13 cell types reveals evidence for the expression of numerous novel primate- and tissue-specific microRNAs. *Proc Natl Acad Sci U S A.* 2015;112(10):E1106–1115.
49. Denli AM, Tops BB, Plasterk RH, Ketting RF, Hannon GJ. Processing of primary microRNAs by the Microprocessor complex. *Nature.* 2004;432(7014):231–235.

50. Lee Y, Ahn C, Han J, et al. The nuclear RNase III Drosha initiates microRNA processing. *Nature.* 2003;425(6956):415–419.

51. Hutvagner G, McLachlan J, Pasquinelli AE, Balint E, Tuschl T, Zamore PD. A cellular function for the RNA-interference enzyme Dicer in the maturation of the let-7 small temporal RNA. *Science.* 2001;293(5531):834–838.

52. Bartel DP. MicroRNAs: Aenomics, biogenesis, mechanism, and function. *Cell.* 2004;116(2):281–297.

53. Absalon S, Kochanek DM, Raghavan V, Krichevsky AM. MiR-26b, upregulated in Alzheimer's disease, activates cell cycle entry, tau-phosphorylation, and apoptosis in postmitotic neurons. *J Neurosci: The Official Journal of the Society for Neuroscience.* 2013;33(37):14645–14659.

54. Wang X, Tan L, Lu Y, et al. MicroRNA-138 promotes tau phosphorylation by targeting retinoic acid receptor alpha. *FEBS Lett.* 2015;589(6):726–729.

55. Sethi P, Lukiw WJ. Micro-RNA abundance and stability in human brain: Specific alterations in Alzheimer's disease temporal lobe neocortex. *Neurosci Lett.* 2009;459(2):100–104.

56. Lee ST, Chu K, Jung KH, et al. Altered expression of miR-202 in cerebellum of multiple-system atrophy. *Mol Neurobiol.* 2015;51(1):180–186.

57. Cheng C, Li W, Zhang Z, et al. MicroRNA-144 is regulated by activator protein-1 (AP-1) and decreases expression of Alzheimer disease-related a disintegrin and metalloprotease 10 (ADAM10). *J Biol Chem.* 2013;288(19):13748–13761.

58. Banzhaf-Strathmann J, Benito E, May S, et al. MicroRNA-125b induces tau hyperphosphorylation and cognitive deficits in Alzheimer's disease. *EMBO J.* 2014;33(15):1667–1680.

59. Zovoilis A, Agbemenyah HY, Agis-Balboa RC, et al. MicroRNA-34c is a novel target to treat dementias. *EMBO J.* 2011;30(20):4299–4308.

60. Wong HK, Veremeyko T, Patel N, et al. De-repression of FOXO3a death axis by microRNA-132 and -212 causes neuronal apoptosis in Alzheimer's disease. *Hum Mol Genet.* 2013;22(15):3077–3092.

61. Long JM, Ray B, Lahiri DK. MicroRNA-339–5p down-regulates protein expression of beta-site amyloid precursor protein-cleaving enzyme 1 (BACE1) in human primary brain cultures and is reduced in brain tissue specimens of Alzheimer disease subjects. *J Biol Chem.* 2014;289(8):5184–5198.

62. Nelson PT, Wang WX. MiR-107 is reduced in Alzheimer's disease brain neocortex: Validation study. *J Alzheimers Dis.* 2010;21(1):75–79.

63. Wang WX, Rajeev BW, Stromberg AJ, et al. The expression of microRNA miR-107 decreases early in Alzheimer's disease and may accelerate disease progression through regulation of beta-site amyloid precursor protein-cleaving enzyme 1. *J Neurosci: The Official Journal of the Society for Neuroscience.* 2008;28(5):1213–1223.

64. Lei X, Lei L, Zhang Z, Zhang Z, Cheng Y. Downregulated miR-29c correlates with increased BACE1 expression in sporadic Alzheimer's disease. *Int J Clin Exp Pathol.* 2015;8(2):1565–1574.

65. Pereira PA, Tomas JF, Queiroz JA, Figueiras AR, Sousa F. Recombinant pre-miR-29b for Alzheimer s disease therapeutics. *Sci Rep.* 2016;6:19946.

66. Lau P, Bossers K, Janky R, et al. Alteration of the microRNA network during the progression of Alzheimer's disease. *EMBO Mol Med.* 2013;5(10):1613–1634.

67. Mezache L, Mikhail M, Garofalo M, Nuovo GJ. Reduced miR-512 and the elevated expression of its targets cFLIP and MCL1 localize to neurons with hyperphosphorylated tau protein in Alzheimer disease. *Appl Immunohistochem Mol Morphol.* 2015;23(9):615–623.

68. Santa-Maria I, Alaniz ME, Renwick N, et al. Dysregulation of microRNA-219 promotes neurodegeneration through post-transcriptional regulation of tau. *J Clin Invest.* 2015;125(2):681–686.

69. Dickson JR, Kruse C, Montagna DR, Finsen B, Wolfe MS. Alternative polyadenylation and miR-34 family members regulate tau expression. *J Neurochem.* 2013;127(6):739–749.

70. Jayadev S, Case A, Alajajian B, Eastman AJ, Moller T, Garden GA. Presenilin 2 influences miR146 level and activity in microglia. *J Neurochem.* 2013;127(5):592–599.

71. Weinberg RB, Mufson EJ, Counts SE. Evidence for a neuroprotective microRNA pathway in amnestic mild cognitive impairment. *Front Neurosci.* 2015;9:430.

72. Behl C, Davis J, Cole GM, Schubert D. Vitamin E protects nerve cells from amyloid beta protein toxicity. *Biochem Biophys Res Commun.* 1992;186(2):944–950.

73. Butterfield DA, Bush AI. Alzheimer's amyloid beta-peptide (1–42): Involvement of methionine residue 35 in the oxidative stress and neurotoxicity properties of this peptide. *Neurobiol Aging.* 2004;25(5):563–568.

74. Rodriguez-Ortiz CJ, Baglietto-Vargas D, Martinez-Coria H, LaFerla FM, Kitazawa M. Upregulation of miR-181 decreases c-Fos and SIRT-1 in the hippocampus of 3xTg-AD mice. *J Alzheimers Dis.* 2014;42(4):1229–1238.

75. Zong Y, Yu P, Cheng H, et al. miR-29c regulates NAV3 protein expression in a transgenic mouse model of Alzheimer's disease. *Brain Res*. 2015;1624:95–102.

76. Hu S, Wang H, Chen K, et al. MicroRNA-34c downregulation ameliorates amyloid-beta-induced synaptic failure and memory deficits by targeting VAMP2. *J Alzheimers Dis*. 2015;48(3):673–686.

77. Ye X, Luo H, Chen Y, et al. MicroRNAs 99b-5p/100–5p regulated by endoplasmic reticulum stress are involved in abeta-induced pathologies. *Front Aging Neurosci*. 2015;7:210.

78. Smith PY, Hernandez-Rapp J, Jolivette F, et al. miR-132/212 deficiency impairs tau metabolism and promotes pathological aggregation in vivo. *Hum Mol Genet*. 2015;24(23):6721–6735.

79. Liang C, Zhu H, Xu Y, et al. MicroRNA-153 negatively regulates the expression of amyloid precursor protein and amyloid precursor-like protein 2. *Brain Res*. 2012;1455:103–113.

80. Long JM, Ray B, Lahiri DK. MicroRNA-153 physiologically inhibits expression of amyloid-beta precursor protein in cultured human fetal brain cells and is dysregulated in a subset of Alzheimer disease patients. *J Biol Chem*. 2012;287(37):31298–31310.

81. Geekiyanage H, Upadhye A, Chan C. Inhibition of serine palmitoyltransferase reduces Abeta and tau hyperphosphorylation in a murine model: A safe therapeutic strategy for Alzheimer's disease. *Neurobiol Aging*. 2013;34(8):2037–2051.

82. Geekiyanage H, Chan C. MicroRNA-137/181c regulates serine palmitoyltransferase and in turn amyloid beta, novel targets in sporadic Alzheimer's disease. *J Neurosci: The Official Journal of the Society for Neuroscience*. 2011;31(41):14820–14830.

83. Ai J, Sun LH, Che H, et al. MicroRNA-195 protects against dementia induced by chronic brain hypoperfusion via its anti-amyloidogenic effect in rats. *J Neurosci: The Official Journal of the Society for Neuroscience*. 2013;33(9):3989–4001.

84. Boissonneault V, Plante I, Rivest S, Provost P. MicroRNA-298 and microRNA-328 regulate expression of mouse beta-amyloid precursor protein-converting enzyme 1. *J Biol Chem*. 2009;284(4):1971–1981.

85. Wang H, Liu J, Zong Y, et al. miR-106b aberrantly expressed in a double transgenic mouse model for Alzheimer's disease targets TGF-beta type II receptor. *Brain Res*. 2010;1357:166–174.

86. Schonrock N, Humphreys DT, Preiss T, Gotz J. Target gene repression mediated by miRNAs miR-181c and miR-9, both of which are downregulated by amyloid-beta. *J Mol Neurosci*. 2012;46(2):324–335.

87. Zhu HC, Wang LM, Wang M, et al. MicroRNA-195 downregulates Alzheimer's disease amyloid-beta production by targeting BACE1. *Brain Res Bull*. 2012;88(6):596–601.

88. Liu W, Liu C, Zhu J, et al. MicroRNA-16 targets amyloid precursor protein to potentially modulate Alzheimer's-associated pathogenesis in SAMP8 mice. *Neurobiol Aging*. 2012;33(3):522–534.

89. Narasimhan M, Riar AK, Rathinam ML, Vedpathak D, Henderson G, Mahimainathan L. Hydrogen peroxide responsive miR153 targets Nrf2/ARE cytoprotection in paraquat induced dopaminergic neurotoxicity. *Toxicol Lett*. 2014;228(3):179–191.

90. Jiao G, Pan B, Zhou Z, Zhou L, Li Z, Zhang Z. MicroRNA-21 regulates cell proliferation and apoptosis in H(2)O(2)-stimulated rat spinal cord neurons. *Mol Med Rep*. 2015;12(5):7011–7016.

91. Zhang R, Zhang Q, Niu J, et al. Screening of microRNAs associated with Alzheimer's disease using oxidative stress cell model and different strains of senescence accelerated mice. *J Neurol Sci*. 2014;338(1–2):57–64.

92. Xu S, Zhang R, Niu J, et al. Oxidative stress mediated-alterations of the microRNA expression profile in mouse hippocampal neurons. *Int J Mol Sci*. 2012;13(12):16945–16960.

93. Bu H, Baraldo G, Lepperdinger G, Jansen-Durr P. mir-24 activity propagates stress-induced senescence by down regulating DNA topoisomerase 1. *Exp Gerontol*. 2016;75:48–52.

94. Li JJ, Dolios G, Wang R, Liao FF. Soluble beta-amyloid peptides, but not insoluble fibrils, have specific effect on neuronal microRNA expression. *PLoS One*. 2014;9(3):e90770.

95. Sun X, Wu Y, Gu M, Zhang Y. miR-342–5p decreases ankyrin G levels in Alzheimer's disease transgenic mouse models. *Cell Rep*. 2014;6(2):264–270.

96. Shi Q, Gibson GE. Up-regulation of the mitochondrial malate dehydrogenase by oxidative stress is mediated by miR-743a. *J Neurochem*. 2011;118(3):440–448.

97. Pogue AI, Percy ME, Cui JG, et al. Up-regulation of NF-kB-sensitive miRNA-125b and miRNA-146a in metal sulfate-stressed human astroglial (HAG) primary cell cultures. *J Inorg Biochem*. 2011;105(11):1434–1437.

98. Cui JG, Li YY, Zhao Y, Bhattacharjee S, Lukiw WJ. Differential regulation of interleukin-1 receptor-associated kinase-1 (IRAK-1) and IRAK-2 by microRNA-146a and NF-kappaB in stressed human astroglial cells and in Alzheimer disease. *J Biol Chem*. 2010;285(50):38951–38960.

99. Zhao Y, Pogue AI, Lukiw WJ. MicroRNA (miRNA) signaling in the human CNS in sporadic Alzheimer's Disease (AD)-Novel and unique pathological features. *Int J Mol Sci*. 2015;16(12):30105–30116.

100. Lukiw WJ, Alexandrov PN, Zhao Y, Hill JM, Bhattacharjee S. Spreading of Alzheimer's disease inflammatory signaling through soluble micro-RNA. *Neuroreport.* 2012;23(10):621–626.
101. Lukiw WJ. NF-small ka, CyrillicB-regulated micro RNAs (miRNAs) in primary human brain cells. *Exp Neurol.* 2012;235(2):484–490.
102. Yang SF, Lee WJ, Tan P, et al. Upregulation of miR-328 and inhibition of CREB-DNA-binding activity are critical for resveratrol-mediated suppression of matrix metalloproteinase-2 and subsequent metastatic ability in human osteosarcomas. *Oncotarget.* 2015;6(5):2736–2753.
103. Ren X, Bai X, Zhang X, et al. Quantitative nuclear proteomics identifies that miR-137-mediated EZH2 reduction regulates resveratrol-induced apoptosis of neuroblastoma cells. *Mol Cell Proteomics.* 2015;14(2):316–328.
104. Tili E, Michaille JJ, Alder H, et al. Resveratrol modulates the levels of microRNAs targeting genes encoding tumor-suppressors and effectors of TGFbeta signaling pathway in SW480 cells. *Biochem Pharmacol.* 2010;80(12):2057–2065.
105. Han Z, Yang Q, Liu B, et al. MicroRNA-622 functions as a tumor suppressor by targeting K-Ras and enhancing the anticarcinogenic effect of resveratrol. *Carcinogenesis.* 2012;33(1):131–139.
106. Zhao YN, Li WF, Li F, et al. Resveratrol improves learning and memory in normally aged mice through microRNA-CREB pathway. *Biochem Biophys Res Commun.* 2013;435(4):597–602.
107. Zhou C, Ding J, Wu Y. Resveratrol induces apoptosis of bladder cancer cells via miR21 regulation of the Akt/Bcl2 signaling pathway. *Mol Med Rep.* 2014;9(4):1467–1473.
108. Li H, Jia Z, Li A, et al. Resveratrol repressed viability of U251 cells by miR-21 inhibiting of NF-kappaB pathway. *Mol Cell Biochem.* 2013;382(1–2):137–143.
109. Liu P, Liang H, Xia Q, et al. Resveratrol induces apoptosis of pancreatic cancers cells by inhibiting miR-21 regulation of BCL-2 expression. *Clin Transl Oncol.* 2013;15(9):741–746.
110. Sheth S, Jajoo S, Kaur T, et al. Resveratrol reduces prostate cancer growth and metastasis by inhibiting the Akt/MicroRNA-21 pathway. *PLoS One.* 2012;7(12):e51655.
111. Baselga-Escudero L, Blade C, Ribas-Latre A, et al. Resveratrol and EGCG bind directly and distinctively to miR-33a and miR-122 and modulate divergently their levels in hepatic cells. *Nucleic Acids Res.* 2014;42(2):882–892.
112. Al-Amin MM, Rahman MM, Khan FR, Zaman F, Mahmud Reza H. Astaxanthin improves behavioral disorder and oxidative stress in prenatal valproic acid-induced mice model of autism. *Behav Brain Res.* 2015;286:112–121.
113. Li Y, VandenBoom TG, 2nd, Kong D, et al. Up-regulation of miR-200 and let-7 by natural agents leads to the reversal of epithelial-to-mesenchymal transition in gemcitabine-resistant pancreatic cancer cells. *Cancer Res.* 2009;69(16):6704–6712.
114. Hagiwara K, Gailhouste L, Yasukawa K, Kosaka N, Ochiya T. A robust screening method for dietary agents that activate tumour-suppressor microRNAs. *Sci Rep.* 2015;5:14697.
115. Ma J, Cheng L, Liu H, et al. Genistein down-regulates miR-223 expression in pancreatic cancer cells. *Curr Drug Targets.* 2013;14(10):1150–1156.
116. Xia J, Duan Q, Ahmad A, et al. Genistein inhibits cell growth and induces apoptosis through up-regulation of miR-34a in pancreatic cancer cells. *Curr Drug Targets.* 2012;13(14):1750–1756.
117. Tao SF, He HF, Chen Q. Quercetin inhibits proliferation and invasion acts by up-regulating miR-146a in human breast cancer cells. *Mol Cell Biochem.* 2015;402(1–2):93–100.
118. Boesch-Saadatmandi C, Wagner AE, Wolffram S, Rimbach G. Effect of quercetin on inflammatory gene expression in mice liver in vivo—role of redox factor 1, miRNA-122, and miRNA-125b. *Pharmacol Res.* 2012;65(5):523–530.
119. Li YY, Cui JG, Hill JM, Bhattacharjee S, Zhao Y, Lukiw WJ. Increased expression of miRNA-146a in Alzheimer's disease transgenic mouse models. *Neurosci Lett.* 2011;487(1):94–98.
120. Zhang W, Bai W, Zhang W. MiR-21 suppresses the anticancer activities of curcumin by targeting PTEN gene in human non-small-cell lung cancer A549 cells. *Clin Transl Oncol.* 2014;16(8):708–713.
121. Sun M, Estrov Z, Ji Y, Coombes KR, Harris DH, Kurzrock R. Curcumin (diferuloylmethane) alters the expression profiles of microRNAs in human pancreatic cancer cells. *Mol Cancer Ther.* 2008;7(3):464–473.
122. Saini S, Arora S, Majid S, et al. Curcumin modulates microRNA-203-mediated regulation of the Src-Akt axis in bladder cancer. *Cancer Prev Res (Phila).* 2011;4(10):1698–1709.
123. Kronski E, Fiori ME, Barbieri O, et al. miR181b is induced by the chemopreventive polyphenol curcumin and inhibits breast cancer metastasis via down-regulation of the inflammatory cytokines CXCL1 and -2. *Mol Oncol.* 2014;8(3):581–595.

124. Gao SM, Yang JJ, Chen CQ, et al. Pure curcumin decreases the expression of WT1 by upregulation of miR-15a and miR-16–1 in leukemic cells. *J Exp Clin Cancer Res.* 2012;31:27.

125. Olivieri F, Lazzarini R, Babini L, et al. Anti-inflammatory effect of ubiquinol-10 on young and senescent endothelial cells via miR-146a modulation. *Free Radic Biol Med.* 2013;63:410–420.

126. Pek SL, Tavintharan S, Woon K, Lin L, Ong CN, Lim SC, Sum CF. MicroRNAs as biomarkers of hepatotoxicity in a randomized placebo-controlled study of simvastatin and ubiquinol supplementation. *Exp Biol Med (Maywood).* 2016;241:317–330.

127. Giangreco AA, Vaishnav, A.,Wagner, D., Finelli, A., Fleshner, N., Van der Kwast, T., Vieth, R., Nonn, L. Tumor suppressor microRNAs, miR-100, and miR-125b, are regulated by 1,25-dihydroxyvitamin D in primary prostate cells and in patient tissue. *Cancer Prev Res (Phila).* 2013;6:483–494.

128. Lisse TS, Chun RF, Rieger S, Adams JS, Hewison M. Vitamin D activation of functionally distinct regulatory miRNAs in primary human osteoblasts. *J Bone Miner Res.* 2013;28(6):1478–1488.

129. Ting HJ, Messing J, Yasmin-Karim S, Lee YF. Identification of microRNA-98 as a therapeutic target inhibiting prostate cancer growth and a biomarker induced by vitamin D. *J Biol Chem.* 2013;288(1):1–9.

130. Kasiappan R, Shen Z, Tse AK, et al. 1,25-Dihydroxyvitamin D3 suppresses telomerase expression and human cancer growth through microRNA-498. *J Biol Chem.* 2012;287(49):41297–41309.

131. Alvarez-Diaz S, Valle N, Ferrer-Mayorga G, et al. MicroRNA-22 is induced by vitamin D and contributes to its antiproliferative, antimigratory, and gene regulatory effects in colon cancer cells. *Hum Mol Genet.* 2012;21(10):2157–2165.

132. Gocek E, Wang X, Liu X, Liu CG, Studzinski GP. MicroRNA-32 upregulation by 1,25-dihydroxyvitamin D3 in human myeloid leukemia cells leads to Bim targeting and inhibition of AraC-induced apoptosis. *Cancer Res.* 2011;71(19):6230–6239.

133. Choi SE, Fu T, Seok S, et al. Elevated microRNA-34a in obesity reduces NAD+ levels and SIRT1 activity by directly targeting NAMPT. *Aging Cell.* 2013;12(6):1062–1072.

134. Chen Z, Gu D, Zhou M, Shi H, Yan S, Cai Y. Regulatory role of miR-125a/b in the suppression by selenium of cadmium-induced apoptosis via the mitochondrial pathway in LLC-PK1 cells. *Chem Biol Interact.* 2016;243:35–44.

135. Gaedicke S, Zhang X, Schmelzer C, et al. Vitamin E dependent microRNA regulation in rat liver. *FEBS Lett.* 2008;582(23–24):3542–3546.

136. Ji X, Wang Z, Geamanu A, Goja A, Sarkar FH, Gupta SV. Delta-tocotrienol suppresses Notch-1 pathway by upregulating miR-34a in non-small-cell lung cancer cells. *Int J Cancer.* 2012;131(11):2668–2677.

137. Zhang J, Gao Y, Yu M, et al. Retinoic acid induces embryonic stem cell differentiation by altering both encoding RNA and microRNA expression. *PLoS One.* 2015;10(7):e0132566.

138. Khan S, Wall D, Curran C, Newell J, Kerin MJ, Dwyer RM. MicroRNA-10a is reduced in breast cancer and regulated in part through retinoic acid. *BMC Cancer.* 2015;15:345.

139. Jian P, Li ZW, Fang TY, et al. Retinoic acid induces HL-60 cell differentiation via the upregulation of miR-663. *J Hematol Oncol.* 2011;4:20.

140. Gao SM, Yang J, Chen C, et al. miR-15a/16-1 enhances retinoic acid-mediated differentiation of leukemic cells and is up-regulated by retinoic acid. *Leuk Lymphoma.* 2011;52(12):2365–2371.

141. Kim SM, Lim SM, Yoo JA, Woo MJ, Cho KH. Consumption of high-dose vitamin C (1250 mg per day) enhances functional and structural properties of serum lipoprotein to improve anti-oxidant, anti-atherosclerotic, and anti-aging effects via regulation of anti-inflammatory microRNA. *Food Funct.* 2015;6(11):3604–3612.

142. Ames BN, Shigenaga MK, Hagen TM. Oxidants, antioxidants, and the degenerative diseases of aging. *Proc Natl Acad Sci U S A.* 1993;90(17):7915–7922.

143. Boveris A, Chance B. The mitochondrial generation of hydrogen peroxide. General properties and effect of hyperbaric oxygen. *Biochem J.* 1973;134(3):707–716.

144. Coyle JT, Puttfarcken P. Oxidative stress, glutamate, and neurodegenerative disorders. *Science.* 1993;262(5134):689–695.

145. Graham DG. Oxidative pathways for catecholamines in the genesis of neuromelanin and cytotoxic quinones. *Mol Pharmacol.* 1978;14(4):633–643.

146. Chan PH, Fishman RA. Transient formation of superoxide radicals in polyunsaturated fatty acid-induced brain swelling. *J Neurochem.* 1980;35(4):1004–1007.

147. Lafon-Cazal M, Pietri S, Culcasi M, Bockaert J. NMDA-dependent superoxide production and neurotoxicity. *Nature.* 1993;364(6437):535–537.

148. Winterbourn CC. Toxicity of iron and hydrogen peroxide: The Fenton reaction. *Toxicol Lett.* 1995;82–83:969–974.

149. Prasad KN. Micronutrients in the prevention and improvement of the standard therapy for Alzheimer's disease. *Micronutrients in Health and Disease*. Boca Raton, FL: CRE Press; 2011.

150. Sompol P, Ittarat W, Tangpong J, et al. A neuronal model of Alzheimer's disease: An insight into the mechanisms of oxidative stress-mediated mitochondrial injury. *Neuroscience*. 2008;153(1):120–130.

151. Gu X, Sun J, Li S, Wu X, Li L. Oxidative stress induces DNA demethylation and histone acetylation in SH-SY5Y cells: Potential epigenetic mechanisms in gene transcription in Abeta production. *Neurobiol Aging*. 2013;34(4):1069–1079.

152. Hartl D, Schuldt V, Forler S, Zabel C, Klose J, Rohe M. Presymptomatic alterations in energy metabolism and oxidative stress in the APP23 mouse model of Alzheimer disease. *J Proteome Res*. 2012;11(6):3295–3304.

153. Clausen A, Xu X, Bi X, Baudry M. Effects of the superoxide dismutase/catalase mimetic EUK-207 in a mouse model of Alzheimer's disease: Protection against and interruption of progression of amyloid and tau pathology and cognitive decline. *J Alzheimers Dis*. 2012;30(1):183–208.

154. Conrad CC, Marshall PL, Talent JM, Malakowsky CA, Choi J, Gracy RW. Oxidized proteins in Alzheimer's plasma. *Biochem Biophys Res Commun*. 2000;275(2):678–681.

155. Ringman JM, Fithian AT, Gylys K, et al. Plasma methionine sulfoxide in persons with familial Alzheimer's disease mutations. *Dement Geriatr Cogn Disord*. 2012;33(4):219–225.

156. Barone E, Di Domenico F, Cenini G, et al. Oxidative and nitrosative modifications of biliverdin reductase-A in the brain of subjects with Alzheimer's disease and amnestic mild cognitive impairment. *J Alzheimers Dis*. 2011;25(4):623–633.

157. Cervellati C, Cremonini E, Bosi C, et al. Systemic oxidative stress in older patients with mild cognitive impairment or late onset Alzheimer's disease. *Curr Alzheimer Res*. 2013;10(4):365–372.

158. Torres LL, Quaglio NB, de Souza GT, et al. Peripheral oxidative stress biomarkers in mild cognitive impairment and Alzheimer's disease. *J Alzheimers Dis*. 2011;26(1):59–68.

159. Leuner K, Schulz K, Schutt T, et al. Peripheral mitochondrial dysfunction in Alzheimer's disease: Focus on lymphocytes. *Mol Neurobiol*. 2012;46(1):194–204.

160. de la Monte SM, Wands JR. Molecular indices of oxidative stress and mitochondrial dysfunction occur early and often progress with severity of Alzheimer's disease. *J Alzheimers Dis*. 2006;9(2):167–181.

161. Schipper HM, Cisse S, Stopa EG. Expression of heme oxygenase-1 in the senescent and Alzheimer-diseased brain. *Ann Neurol*. 1995;37(6):758–768.

162. Sims NR, Bowen DM, Neary D, Davison AN. Metabolic processes in Alzheimer's disease: Adenine nucleotide content and production of 14CO2 from [U-14C] glucose in vitro in human neocortex. *J Neurochem*. 1983;41(5):1329–1334.

163. Saito K, Elce JS, Hamos JE, Nixon RA. Widespread activation of calcium-activated neutral proteinase (calpain) in the brain in Alzheimer disease: A potential molecular basis for neuronal degeneration. *Proc Natl Acad Sci U S A*. 1993;90(7):2628–2632.

164. Nixon RA, Cataldo AM. Free radicals, proteolysis, and the degeneration of neurons in Alzheimer disease: How essential is the beta-amyloid link? *Neurobiol Aging*. 1994;15(4):463–469; discussion 473.

165. Zhou Y, Richardson JS, Mombourquette MJ, Weil JA. Free radical formation in autopsy samples of Alzheimer and control cortex. *Neurosci Lett*. 1995;195(2):89–92.

166. Koppal T. Peroxynitrite-mediated damage to brain membrane alterations in Alzheimer's disease (AD). *Soc Neurosci*. 1998;24:1217a.

167. Simic G, Lucassen PJ, Krsnik Z, et al. nNOS expression in reactive astrocytes correlates with increased cell death related DNA damage in the hippocampus and entorhinal cortex in Alzheimer's disease. *Exp Neurol*. 2000;165(1):12–26.

168. Lovell MA, Xie C, Markesbery WR. Decreased glutathione transferase activity in brain and ventricular fluid in Alzheimer's disease. *Neurology*. 1998;51(6):1562–1566.

169. Ghosh T, Mustafa M, Kumar V, et al. A preliminary study on the influence of glutathione S transferase T1 (GSTT1) as a risk factor for late onset Alzheimer's disease in North Indian population. *Asian J Psychiatr*. 2012;5(2):160–163.

170. Tesco G, Latorraca S, Piersanti P, Piacentini S, Amaducci L, Sorbi S. Alzheimer skin fibroblasts show increased susceptibility to free radicals. *Mech Ageing Dev*. 1992;66(2):117–120.

171. Ramamoorthy M, Sykora P, Scheibye-Knudsen M, et al. Sporadic Alzheimer disease fibroblasts display an oxidative stress phenotype. *Free Radic Biol Med*. 2012;53(6):1371–1380.

172. Zaman Z, Roche S, Fielden P, Frost PG, Niriella DC, Cayley AC. Plasma concentrations of vitamins A and E and carotenoids in Alzheimer's disease. *Age Ageing*. 1992;21(2):91–94.

173. Kosenko EA, Aliev G, Tikhonova LA, Li Y, Poghosyan AC, Kaminsky YG. Antioxidant status and energy state of erythrocytes in Alzheimer dementia: Probing for markers. *CNS Neurol Disord Drug Targets*. 2012;11(7):926–932.

174. Kish SJ, Bergeron C, Rajput A, et al. Brain cytochrome oxidase in Alzheimer's disease. *J Neurochem*. 1992;59(2):776–779.

175. Mutisya EM, Bowling AC, Beal MF. Cortical cytochrome oxidase activity is reduced in Alzheimer's disease. *J Neurochem*. 1994;63(6):2179–2184.

176. Mattson MP. Calcium and neuronal injury in Alzheimer's disease. Contributions of beta-amyloid precursor protein mismetabolism, free radicals, and metabolic compromise. *Ann N Y Acad Sci*. 1994;747:50–76.

177. Gabuzda D, Busciglio J, Chen LB, Matsudaira P, Yankner BA. Inhibition of energy metabolism alters the processing of amyloid precursor protein and induces a potentially amyloidogenic derivative. *J Biol Chem*. 1994;269(18):13623–13628.

178. Sultana R, Butterfield DA. Oxidatively modified, mitochondria-relevant brain proteins in subjects with Alzheimer disease and mild cognitive impairment. *J Bioenerg Biomembr*. 2009;41(5):441–446.

179. Piaceri I, Rinnoci V, Bagnoli S, Failli Y, Sorbi S. Mitochondria and Alzheimer's disease. *J Neurol Sci*. 2012;322(1–2):31–34.

180. Joachim CL, Selkoe DJ. The seminal role of beta-amyloid in the pathogenesis of Alzheimer disease. *Alzheimer Dis Assoc Disord*. 1992;6(1):7–34.

181. Postina R. A closer look at alpha-secretase. *Curr Alzheimer Res*. 2008;5(2):179–186.

182. Simmons LK, May PC, Tomaselli KJ, et al. Secondary structure of amyloid beta peptide correlates with neurotoxic activity in vitro. *Mol Pharmacol*. 1994;45(3):373–379.

183. Lorenzo A, Yankner BA. Beta-amyloid neurotoxicity requires fibril formation and is inhibited by congo red. *Proc Natl Acad Sci U S A*. 1994;91(25):12243–12247.

184. Loo G. Redox-sensitive mechanisms of phytochemical-mediated inhibition of cancer cell proliferation (review). *J Nutr Biochem*. 2003;14(2):64–73.

185. Koh JY, Suh SW, Gwag BJ, He YY, Hsu CY, Choi DW. The role of zinc in selective neuronal death after transient global cerebral ischemia. *Science*. 1996;272(5264):1013–1016.

186. Bondy SC, Truong A. Potentiation of beta-folding of beta-amyloid peptide 25–35 by aluminum salts. *Neurosci Lett*. 1999;267(1):25–28.

187. Eikelenboom P, Stam FC. Immunoglobulins and complement factors in senile plaques. An immunoperoxidase study. *Acta Neuropathol (Berl)*. 1982;57(2–3):239–242.

188. Misonou H, Morishima-Kawashima M, Ihara Y. Oxidative stress induces intracellular accumulation of amyloid beta-protein (Abeta) in human neuroblastoma cells. *Biochemistry*. 2000;39(23):6951–6959.

189. Koppaka V, Axelsen PH. Accelerated accumulation of amyloid beta proteins on oxidatively damaged lipid membranes. *Biochemistry*. 2000;39(32):10011–10016.

190. Murakami K, Murata N, Noda Y, Irie K, Shirasawa T, Shimizu T. Stimulation of the amyloidogenic pathway by cytoplasmic superoxide radicals in an Alzheimer's disease mouse model. *Biosci Biotechnol Biochem*. 2012;76(6):1098–1103.

191. Gwon AR, Park JS, Arumugam TV, et al. Oxidative lipid modification of nicastrin enhances amyloidogenic gamma-secretase activity in Alzheimer's disease. *Aging Cell*. 2012;11(4):559–568.

192. Nakagawa K, Kiko T, Miyazawa T, Sookwong P, Tsuduki T, Satoh A. Amyloid beta-induced erythrocytic damage and its attenuation by carotenoids. *FEBS Lett*. 2011;585(8):1249–1254.

193. Varadarajan S, Yatin S, Kanski J, Jahanshahi F, Butterfield DA. Methionine residue 35 is important in amyloid beta-peptide-associated free radical oxidative stress. *Brain Res Bull*. 1999;50(2):133–141.

194. Tabaton M, Tamagno E. The molecular link between beta- and gamma-secretase activity on the amyloid beta precursor protein. *Cell Mol Life Sci*. 2007;64(17):2211–2218.

195. Placanica L, Tarassishin L, Yang G, et al. Pen2 and presenilin-1 modulate the dynamic equilibrium of presenilin-1 and presenilin-2 gamma-secretase complexes. *J Biol Chem*. 2009;284(5):2967–2977.

196. Naslund J, Haroutunian V, Mohs R, et al. Correlation between elevated levels of amyloid beta-peptide in the brain and cognitive decline. *JAMA*. 2000;283(12):1571–1577.

197. Irwin DJ, Cohen TJ, Grossman M, et al. Acetylated tau, a novel pathological signature in Alzheimer's disease and other tauopathies. *Brain*. 2012;135(Pt 3):807–818.

198. Gregori L, Hainfeld JF, Simon MN, Goldgaber D. Binding of amyloid beta protein to the 20 S proteasome. *J Biol Chem*. 1997;272(1):58–62.

199. Nahreini P, Andreatta C, Prasad KN. Proteasome activity is critical for the cAMP-induced differentiation of neuroblastoma cells. *Cell Mol Neurobiol*. 2001;21(5):509–521.

200. Rockwell P, Yuan H, Magnusson R, Figueiredo-Pereira ME. Proteasome inhibition in neuronal cells induces a proinflammatory response manifested by upregulation of cyclooxygenase-2, its accumulation as ubiquitin conjugates, and production of the prostaglandin PGE(2). *Arch Biochem Biophys.* 2000;374(2):325–333.

201. Jenkinson ML, Bliss MR, Brain AT, Scott DL. Rheumatoid arthritis and senile dementia of the Alzheimer's type. *Br J Rheumatol.* 1989;28(1):86–88.

202. Breitner JC, Gau BA, Welsh KA, et al. Inverse association of anti-inflammatory treatments and Alzheimer's disease: Initial results of a co-twin control study. *Neurology.* 1994;44(2):227–232.

203. McGeer PL, Schulzer M, McGeer EG. Arthritis and anti-inflammatory agents as possible protective factors for Alzheimer's disease: A review of 17 epidemiologic studies. *Neurology.* 1996;47(2):425–432.

204. McGeer EG, McGeer PL. The importance of inflammatory mechanisms in Alzheimer disease. *Exp Gerontol.* 1998;33(5):371–378.

205. Shalit F, Sredni B, Stern L, Kott E, Huberman M. Elevated interleukin-6 secretion levels by mononuclear cells of Alzheimer's patients. *Neurosci Lett.* 1994;174(2):130–132.

206. Sharif SF, Hariri RJ, Chang VA, Barie PS, Wang RS, Ghajar JB. Human astrocyte production of tumour necrosis factor-alpha, interleukin-1 beta, and interleukin-6 following exposure to lipopolysaccharide endotoxin. *Neurol Res.* 1993;15(2):109–112.

207. Rogers J, Cooper NR, Webster S, et al. Complement activation by beta-amyloid in Alzheimer disease. *Proc Natl Acad Sci U S A.* 1992;89(21):10016–10020.

208. Rogers J, Lue L-F, Brachova L, Webster S, Schultz J. Inflammation as a response and a cause of Alzheimer's pathophysiology. *Dementia.* 1995;9:133–138.

209. Webster S, O'Barr S, Rogers J. Enhanced aggregation and beta structure of amyloid beta peptide after coincubation with C1q. *J Neurosci Res.* 1994;39(4):448–456.

210. Chen L, Richardson JS, Caldwell JE, Ang LC. Regional brain activity of free radical defense enzymes in autopsy samples from patients with Alzheimer's disease and from nondemented controls. *Int J Neurosci.* 1994;75(1–2):83–90.

211. Richardson JS, Subbarao KV, Ang LC. On the possible role of iron-induced free radical peroxidation in neural degeneration in Alzheimer's disease. *Ann N Y Acad Sci.* 1992;648:326–327.

212. Smith MA, Sayre LM, Monnier VM, Perry G. Radical ageing in Alzheimer's disease. *Trends Neurosci.* 1995;18(4):172–176.

213. Harman D. A hypothesis on the pathogenesis of Alzheimer's disease. *Ann N Y Acad Sci.* 1996;786:152–168.

214. Frohman EM, Frohman TC, Gupta S, de Fougerolles A, van den Noort S. Expression of intercellular adhesion molecule 1 (ICAM-1) in Alzheimer's disease. *J Neurol Sci.* 1991;106(1):105–111.

215. Verbeek MM, Otte-Holler I, Westphal JR, Wesseling P, Ruiter DJ, de Waal RM. Accumulation of intercellular adhesion molecule-1 in senile plaques in brain tissue of patients with Alzheimer's disease. *Am J Pathol.* 1994;144(1):104–116.

216. Rozemuller JM, Eikelenboom P, Pals ST, Stam FC. Microglial cells around amyloid plaques in Alzheimer's disease express leucocyte adhesion molecules of the LFA-1 family. *Neurosci Lett.* 1989;101(3):288–292.

217. Prasad KN, Hovland AR, La Rosa FG, Hovland PG. Prostaglandins as putative neurotoxins in Alzheimer's disease. *Proc Soc Exp Biol Med.* 1998;219(2):120–125.

218. Prasad KN, La Rosa FG, Prasad JE. Prostaglandins act as neurotoxin for differentiated neuroblastoma cells in culture and increase levels of ubiquitin and beta-amyloid. *In Vitro Cell Dev Biol Anim.* 1998;34(3):265–274.

219. Blasko I, Marx F, Steiner E, Hartmann T, Grubeck-Loebenstein B. TNFalpha plus IFNgamma induce the production of Alzheimer beta-amyloid peptides and decrease the secretion of APPs. *FASEB J.* 1999;13(1):63–68.

220. Patel JR, Brewer GJ. Age-related changes to tumor necrosis factor receptors affect neuron survival in the presence of beta-amyloid. *J Neurosci Res.* 2008;86(10):2303–2313.

221. Liao YF, Wang BJ, Cheng HT, Kuo LH, Wolfe MS. Tumor necrosis factor-alpha, interleukin-1beta, and interferon-gamma stimulate gamma-secretase-mediated cleavage of amyloid precursor protein through a JNK-dependent MAPK pathway. *J Biol Chem.* 2004;279(47):49523–49532.

222. Qiu Z, Gruol DL. Interleukin-6, beta-amyloid peptide and NMDA interactions in rat cortical neurons. *J Neuroimmunol.* 2003;139(1–2):51–57.

223. Shelat PB, Chalimoniuk M, Wang JH, et al. Amyloid beta peptide and NMDA induce ROS from NADPH oxidase and AA release from cytosolic phospholipase A2 in cortical neurons. *J Neurochem.* 2008;106(1):45–55.

224. Rich JB, Rasmusson DX, Folstein MF, Carson KA, Kawas C, Brandt J. Nonsteroidal anti-inflammatory drugs in Alzheimer's disease. *Neurology*. 1995;45(1):51–55.

225. McGeer PL, McGeer E, Rogers J, Sibley J. Anti-inflammatory drugs and Alzheimer disease. *Lancet*. 1990;335(8696):1037.

226. Lucca U, Tettamanti M, Forloni G, Spagnoli A. Nonsteroidal antiinflammatory drug use in Alzheimer's disease. *Biol Psychiatry*. 1994;36(12):854–856.

227. Rogers J, Kirby LC, Hempelman SR, et al. Clinical trial of indomethacin in Alzheimer's disease. *Neurology*. 1993;43(8):1609–1611.

228. Martin BK, Szekely C, Brandt J, et al. Cognitive function over time in the Alzheimer's Disease Anti-inflammatory Prevention Trial (ADAPT): Results of a randomized, controlled trial of naproxen and celecoxib. *Arch Neurol*. 2008;65(7):896–905.

229. Babiloni C, Frisoni GB, Del Percio C, et al. Ibuprofen treatment modifies cortical sources of EEG rhythms in mild Alzheimer's disease. *Clin Neurophysiol*. 2009;120(4):709–718.

230. Hirohata M, Ono K, Naiki H, Yamada M. Non-steroidal anti-inflammatory drugs have anti-amyloidogenic effects for Alzheimer's beta-amyloid fibrils in vitro. *Neuropharmacology*. 2005;49(7):1088–1099.

231. McKee AC, Carreras I, Hossain L, et al. Ibuprofen reduces Abeta, hyperphosphorylated tau and memory deficits in Alzheimer mice. *Brain Res*. 2008;1207:225–236.

232. Busciglio J, Hartmann H, Lorenzo A, et al. Neuronal localization of presenilin-1 and association with amyloid plaques and neurofibrillary tangles in Alzheimer's disease. *J Neurosci*. 1997;17(13):5101–5107.

233. Mohmmad Abdul H, Wenk GL, Gramling M, Hauss-Wegrzyniak B, Butterfield DA. APP and PS-1 mutations induce brain oxidative stress independent of dietary cholesterol: Implications for Alzheimer's disease. *Neurosci Lett*. 2004;368(2):148–150.

234. Refolo LM, Malester B, LaFrancois J, et al. Hypercholesterolemia accelerates the Alzheimer's amyloid pathology in a transgenic mouse model. *Neurobiol Dis*. 2000;7(4):321–331.

235. Simons M, Keller P, De Strooper B, Beyreuther K, Dotti CG, Simons K. Cholesterol depletion inhibits the generation of beta-amyloid in hippocampal neurons. *Proc Natl Acad Sci U S A*. 1998;95(11):6460–6464.

236. Jick H, Zornberg GL, Jick SS, Seshadri S, Drachman DA. Statins and the risk of dementia. *Lancet*. 2000;356(9242):1627–1631.

237. Haag MD, Hofman A, Koudstaal PJ, Stricker BH, Breteler MM. Statins are associated with a reduced risk of Alzheimer disease regardless of lipophilicity. The Rotterdam Study. *J Neurol Neurosurg Psychiatry*. 2009;80(1):13–17.

238. Rao S, Porter DC, Chen X, Herliczek T, Lowe M, Keyomarsi K. Lovastatin-mediated G1 arrest is through inhibition of the proteasome, independent of hydroxymethyl glutaryl-CoA reductase. *Proc Natl Acad Sci U S A*. 1999;96(14):7797–7802.

239. Kumar B, Andreatta C, Koustas WT, Cole WC, Edwards-Prasad J, Prasad KN. Mevastatin induces degeneration and decreases viability of cAMP-induced differentiated neuroblastoma cells in culture by inhibiting proteasome activity, and mevalonic acid lactone prevents these effects. *J Neurosci Res*. 2002;68(5):627–635.

240. Farrer LA, Cupples LA, Haines JL, et al. Effects of age, sex, and ethnicity on the association between apolipoprotein E genotype and Alzheimer disease. A meta-analysis. APOE and Alzheimer disease meta analysis consortium. *JAMA*. 1997;278(16):1349–1356.

241. Marx J. New gene tied to common form of Alzheimer's. *Science*. 1998;281(5376):507, 509.

242. McConnell LM, Koenig BA, Greely HT, Raffin TA. Genetic testing and Alzheimer disease: Has the time come? Alzheimer disease working group of the Stanford program in genomics, ethics & society. *Nat Med*. 1998;4(7):757–759.

243. Blacker D, Wilcox MA, Laird NM, et al. Alpha-2 macroglobulin is genetically associated with Alzheimer disease. *Nat Genet*. 1998;19(4):357–360.

244. Kehoe P, Wavrant-De Vrieze F, Crook R, et al. A full genome scan for late onset Alzheimer's disease. *Hum Mol Genet*. 1999;8(2):237–245.

245. McMillan PJ, Leverenz JB, Dorsa DM. Specific downregulation of presenilin 2 gene expression is prominent during early stages of sporadic late-onset Alzheimer's disease. *Brain Res Mol Brain Res*. 2000;78(1–2):138–145.

246. Cruts M, Van Broeckhoven C. Molecular genetics of Alzheimer's disease. *Ann Med*. 1998;30(6):560–565.

247. Hanson AJ, Prasad JE, Nahreini P, et al. Overexpression of amyloid precursor protein is associated with degeneration, decreased viability, and increased damage caused by neurotoxins (prostaglandins A1 and E2, hydrogen peroxide, and nitric oxide) in differentiated neuroblastoma cells. *J Neurosci Res*. 2003;74(1):148–159.

248. Candore G, Balistreri CR, Grimaldi MP, et al. Age-related inflammatory diseases: Role of genetics and gender in the pathophysiology of Alzheimer's disease. *Ann N Y Acad Sci.* 2006;1089:472–486.

249. Candore G, Balistreri CR, Grimaldi MP, et al. Polymorphisms of pro-inflammatory genes and Alzheimer's disease risk: A pharmacogenomic approach. *Mech Ageing Dev.* 2007;128(1):67–75.

250. Zhao J, Fu Y, Yasvoina M, et al. Beta-site amyloid precursor protein cleaving enzyme 1 levels become elevated in neurons around amyloid plaques: Implications for Alzheimer's disease pathogenesis. *J Neurosci.* 2007;27(14):3639–3649.

251. Velliquette RA, O'Connor T, Vassar R. Energy inhibition elevates beta-secretase levels and activity and is potentially amyloidogenic in APP transgenic mice: Possible early events in Alzheimer's disease pathogenesis. *J Neurosci.* 2005;25(47):10874–10883.

252. Lesne S, Docagne F, Gabriel C, et al. Transforming growth factor-beta 1 potentiates amyloid-beta generation in astrocytes and in transgenic mice. *J Biol Chem.* 2003;278(20):18408–18418.

253. Song W, Nadeau P, Yuan M, Yang X, Shen J, Yankner BA. Proteolytic release and nuclear translocation of Notch-1 are induced by presenilin-1 and impaired by pathogenic presenilin-1 mutations. *Proc Natl Acad Sci U S A.* 1999;96(12):6959–6963.

254. Wakasugi K, Kitatsuji C, Morishima I. Possible neuroprotective mechanism of human neuroglobin. *Ann N Y Acad Sci.* 2005;1053:220–230.

255. Liu J, Yu Z, Guo S, et al. Effects of neuroglobin overexpression on mitochondrial function and oxidative stress following hypoxia/reoxygenation in cultured neurons. *J Neurosci Res.* 2009;87(1):164–170.

256. Yu Z, Liu J, Guo S, et al. Neuroglobin-overexpression alters hypoxic response gene expression in primary neuron culture following oxygen glucose deprivation. *Neuroscience.* 2009.

257. Sun Y, Jin K, Peel A, Mao XO, Xie L, Greenberg DA. Neuroglobin protects the brain from experimental stroke in vivo. *Proc Natl Acad Sci U S A.* 2003;100(6):3497–3500.

258. Sun Y, Jin K, Mao XO, et al. Effect of aging on neuroglobin expression in rodent brain. *Neurobiol Aging.* 2005;26(2):275–278.

259. Greenberg DA, Jin K, Khan AA. Neuroglobin: An endogenous neuroprotectant. *Curr Opin Pharmacol.* 2008;8(1):20–24.

260. Li RC, Morris MW, Lee SK, Pouranfar F, Wang Y, Gozal D. Neuroglobin protects PC12 cells against oxidative stress. *Brain Res.* 2008;1190:159–166.

261. Li RC, Pouranfar F, Lee SK, Morris MW, Wang Y, Gozal D. Neuroglobin protects PC12 cells against beta-amyloid-induced cell injury. *Neurobiol Aging.* 2008;29(12):1815–1822.

262. Khan AA, Mao XO, Banwait S, Jin K, Greenberg DA. Neuroglobin attenuates beta-amyloid neurotoxicity in vitro and transgenic Alzheimer phenotype in vivo. *Proc Natl Acad Sci U S A.* 2007;104(48):19114–19119.

263. Szymanski M, Wang R, Fallin MD, Bassett SS, Avramopoulos D. Neuroglobin and Alzheimer's dementia: Genetic association and gene expression changes. *Neurobiol Aging.* 2008.

264. Hager K, Kenklies M, McAfoose J, Engel J, Munch G. Alpha-lipoic acid as a new treatment option for Alzheimer's disease—A 48-month follow-up analysis. *J Neural Transm Suppl.* 2007(72):189–193.

265. Moreira PI, Harris PL, Zhu X, et al. Lipoic acid and N-acetylcysteine decrease mitochondrial-related oxidative stress in Alzheimer disease patient fibroblasts. *J Alzheimers Dis.* 2007;12(2):195–206.

266. Zhang L, Xing GQ, Barker JL, et al. Alpha-lipoic acid protects rat cortical neurons against cell death induced by amyloid and hydrogen peroxide through the Akt signalling pathway. *Neurosci Lett.* 2001;312(3):125–128.

267. Carlson DA, Smith AR, Fischer SJ, Young KL, Packer L. The plasma pharmacokinetics of R-(+)-lipoic acid administered as sodium R-(+)-lipoate to healthy human subjects. *Altern Med Rev.* 2007;12(4):343–351.

268. Chng HT, New LS, Neo AH, Goh CW, Browne ER, Chan EC. Distribution study of orally administered lipoic acid in rat brain tissues. *Brain Res.* 2009;1251:80–86.

269. Siedlak SL, Casadesus G, Webber KM, et al. Chronic antioxidant therapy reduces oxidative stress in a mouse model of Alzheimer's disease. *Free Radic Res.* 2009;43(2):156–164.

270. Quinn JF, Bussiere JR, Hammond RS, et al. Chronic dietary alpha-lipoic acid reduces deficits in hippocampal memory of aged Tg2576 mice. *Neurobiol Aging.* 2007;28(2):213–225.

271. Suchy J, Chan A, Shea TB. Dietary supplementation with a combination of alpha-lipoic acid, acetyl-L-carnitine, glycerophosphocholine, docosahexaenoic acid, and phosphatidylserine reduces oxidative damage to murine brain and improves cognitive performance. *Nutr Res.* 2009;29(1):70–74.

272. Yang X, Yang Y, Li G, Wang J, Yang ES. Coenzyme Q10 attenuates beta-amyloid pathology in the aged transgenic mice with Alzheimer presenilin 1 mutation. *J Mol Neurosci.* 2008;34(2):165–171.

273. Ono K, Hasegawa K, Naiki H, Yamada M. Preformed beta-amyloid fibrils are destabilized by coenzyme Q10 in vitro. *Biochem Biophys Res Commun.* 2005;330(1):111–116.

274. Moreira PI, Santos MS, Sena C, Nunes E, Seica R, Oliveira CR. CoQ10 therapy attenuates amyloid beta-peptide toxicity in brain mitochondria isolated from aged diabetic rats. *Exp Neurol*. 2005;196(1):112–119.

275. de Bustos F, Molina JA, Jimenez-Jimenez FJ, et al. Serum levels of coenzyme Q10 in patients with Alzheimer's disease. *J Neural Transm*. 2000;107(2):233–239.

276. McDonald SR, Sohal RS, Forster MJ. Concurrent administration of coenzyme Q10 and alpha-tocopherol improves learning in aged mice. *Free Radic Biol Med*. 2005;38(6):729–736.

277. Feng Z, Qin C, Chang Y, Zhang JT. Early melatonin supplementation alleviates oxidative stress in a transgenic mouse model of Alzheimer's disease. *Free Radic Biol Med*. 2006;40(1):101–109.

278. Olcese JM, Cao C, Mori T, et al. Protection against cognitive deficits and markers of neurodegeneration by long-term oral administration of melatonin in a transgenic model of Alzheimer disease. *J Pineal Res*. 2009;47(1):82–96.

279. Gehrman PR, Connor DJ, Martin JL, Shochat T, Corey-Bloom J, Ancoli-Israel S. Melatonin fails to improve sleep or agitation in double-blind randomized placebo-controlled trial of institutionalized patients with Alzheimer disease. *Am J Geriatr Psychiatry*. 2009;17(2):166–169.

280. Furio AM, Brusco LI, Cardinali DP. Possible therapeutic value of melatonin in mild cognitive impairment: A retrospective study. *J Pineal Res*. 2007;43(4):404–409.

281. Green KN, Steffan JS, Martinez-Coria H, et al. Nicotinamide restores cognition in Alzheimer's disease transgenic mice via a mechanism involving sirtuin inhibition and selective reduction of Thr231-phosphotau. *J Neurosci*. 2008;28(45):11500–11510.

282. Liu D, Pitta M, Mattson MP. Preventing NAD(+) depletion protects neurons against excitotoxicity: Bioenergetic effects of mild mitochondrial uncoupling and caloric restriction. *Ann N Y Acad Sci*. 2008;1147:275–282.

283. Qin W, Yang T, Ho L, et al. Neuronal SIRT1 activation as a novel mechanism underlying the prevention of Alzheimer disease amyloid neuropathology by calorie restriction. *J Biol Chem*. 2006;281(31):21745–21754.

284. Qin W, Chachich M, Lane M, et al. Calorie restriction attenuates Alzheimer's disease type brain amyloidosis in Squirrel monkeys (Saimiri sciureus). *J Alzheimers Dis*. 2006;10(4):417–422.

285. Ono K, Yoshiike Y, Takashima A, Hasegawa K, Naiki H, Yamada M. Vitamin A exhibits potent anti-amyloidogenic and fibril-destabilizing effects in vitro. *Exp Neurol*. 2004;189(2):380–392.

286. Ding Y, Qiao A, Wang Z, et al. Retinoic acid attenuates beta-amyloid deposition and rescues memory deficits in an Alzheimer's disease transgenic mouse model. *J Neurosci*. 2008;28(45):11622–11634.

287. Peng QL, Buz'Zard AR, Lau BH. Pycnogenol protects neurons from amyloid-beta peptide-induced apoptosis. *Brain Res Mol Brain Res*. 2002;104(1):55–65.

288. Isaac MG, Quinn R, Tabet N. Vitamin E for Alzheimer's disease and mild cognitive impairment. *Cochrane Database Syst Rev*. 2008;(3):CD002854.

289. Sano M, Ernesto C, Thomas RG, et al. A controlled trial of selegiline, alpha-tocopherol, or both as treatment for Alzheimer's disease. The Alzheimer's Disease Cooperative Study. *N Engl J Med*. 1997;336(17):1216–1222.

290. Fillenbaum GG, Kuchibhatla MN, Hanlon JT, et al. Dementia and Alzheimer's disease in community-dwelling elders taking vitamin C and/or vitamin E. *Ann Pharmacother*. 2005;39(12):2009–2014.

291. Gray SL, Anderson ML, Crane PK, et al. Antioxidant vitamin supplement use and risk of dementia or Alzheimer's disease in older adults. *J Am Geriatr Soc*. 2008;56(2):291–295.

292. Zandi PP, Anthony JC, Khachaturian AS, et al. Reduced risk of Alzheimer disease in users of antioxidant vitamin supplements: The Cache County Study. *Arch Neurol*. 2004;61(1):82–88.

293. Sung S, Yao Y, Uryu K, et al. Early vitamin E supplementation in young but not aged mice reduces Abeta levels and amyloid deposition in a transgenic model of Alzheimer's disease. *FASEB J*. 2004;18(2):323–325.

294. Lockrow J, Prakasam A, Huang P, Bimonte-Nelson H, Sambamurti K, Granholm AC. Cholinergic degeneration and memory loss delayed by vitamin E in a Down syndrome mouse model. *Exp Neurol*. 2009;216(2):278–289.

295. Jimenez-Jimenez FJ, Molina JA, de Bustos F, et al. Serum levels of beta-carotene, alpha-carotene and vitamin A in patients with Alzheimer's disease. *Eur J Neurol*. 1999;6(4):495–497.

296. Jimenez-Jimenez FJ, de Bustos F, Molina JA, et al. Cerebrospinal fluid levels of alpha-tocopherol (vitamin E) in Alzheimer's disease. *J Neural Transm*. 1997;104(6–7):703–710.

297. Rinaldi P, Polidori MC, Metastasio A, et al. Plasma antioxidants are similarly depleted in mild cognitive impairment and in Alzheimer's disease. *Neurobiol Aging*. 2003;24(7):915–919.

298. Charlton KE, Rabinowitz TL, Geffen LN, Dhansay MA. Lowered plasma vitamin C, but not vitamin E, concentrations in dementia patients. *J Nutr Health Aging*. 2004;8(2):99–107.

299. Cole MG, Prchal JF. Low serum vitamin B12 in Alzheimer-type dementia. *Age Ageing.* 1984;13(2):101–105.

300. Regland B, Gottfries CG, Oreland L. Vitamin B12-induced reduction of platelet monoamine oxidase activity in patients with dementia and pernicious anaemia. *Eur Arch Psychiatry Clin Neurosci.* 1991;240(4–5):288–291.

301. Nadeau A, Roberge AG. Effects of vitamin B12 supplementation on choline acetyltransferase activity in cat brain. *Int J Vitam Nutr Res. Internationale Zeitschrift fur Vitamin und Ernahrungsforschung. Journal international de vitaminologie et de nutrition.* 1988;58(4):402–406.

302. Ikeda T, Yamamoto K, Takahashi K, et al. Treatment of Alzheimer-type dementia with intravenous mecobalamin. *Clin Ther.* 1992;14(3):426–437.

303. Malouf R, Grimley Evans J. Folic acid with or without vitamin B12 for the prevention and treatment of healthy elderly and demented people. *Cochrane Database Syst Rev.* 2008(4):CD004514.

304. Aisen PS, Schneider LS, Sano M, et al. High-dose B vitamin supplementation and cognitive decline in Alzheimer disease: A randomized controlled trial. *JAMA.* 2008;300(15):1774–1783.

305. van Dyck CH, Lyness JM, Rohrbaugh RM, Siegal AP. Cognitive and psychiatric effects of vitamin B12 replacement in dementia with low serum B12 levels: A nursing home study. *Int Psychogeriatr.* 2009;21(1):138–147.

306. Vingtdeux V, Dreses-Werringloer U, Zhao H, Davies P, Marambaud P. Therapeutic potential of resveratrol in Alzheimer's disease. *BMC Neurosci.* 2008;9 Suppl 2:S6.

307. Wang J, Ho L, Zhao Z, et al. Moderate consumption of Cabernet Sauvignon attenuates Abeta neuropathology in a mouse model of Alzheimer's disease. *FASEB J.* 2006;20(13):2313–2320.

308. Luchsinger JA, Tang MX, Siddiqui M, Shea S, Mayeux R. Alcohol intake and risk of dementia. *J Am Geriatr Soc.* 2004;52(4):540–546.

309. Savaskan E, Olivieri G, Meier F, Seifritz E, Wirz-Justice A, Muller-Spahn F. Red wine ingredient resveratrol protects from beta-amyloid neurotoxicity. *Gerontology.* 2003;49(6):380–383.

310. Marambaud P, Zhao H, Davies P. Resveratrol promotes clearance of Alzheimer's disease amyloid-beta peptides. *J Biol Chem.* 2005;280(45):37377–37382.

311. Anekonda TS. Resveratrol--a boon for treating Alzheimer's disease? *Brain Res Rev.* 2006;52(2):316–326.

312. Tang BL, Chua CE. SIRT1 and neuronal diseases. *Mol Aspects Med.* 2008;29(3):187–200.

313. DeKosky ST, Williamson JD, Fitzpatrick AL, et al. Ginkgo biloba for prevention of dementia: A randomized controlled trial. *JAMA.* 2008;300(19):2253–2262.

314. Augustin S, Rimbach G, Augustin K, Schliebs R, Wolffram S, Cermak R. Effect of a short- and long-term treatment with Ginkgo biloba extract on amyloid precursor protein levels in a transgenic mouse model relevant to Alzheimer's disease. *Arch Biochem Biophys.* 2009;481(2):177–182.

315. Freund-Levi Y, Eriksdotter-Jonhagen M, Cederholm T, et al. Omega-3 fatty acid treatment in 174 patients with mild to moderate Alzheimer disease: OmegAD study: A randomized double-blind trial. *Arch Neurol.* 2006;63(10):1402–1408.

316. Fotuhi M, Mohassel P, Yaffe K. Fish consumption, long-chain omega-3 fatty acids and risk of cognitive decline or Alzheimer disease: A complex association. *Nat Clin Pract Neurol.* 2009;5(3):140–152.

317. Kroger E, Verreault R, Carmichael PH, et al. Omega-3 fatty acids and risk of dementia: The canadian study of health and aging. *Am J Clin Nutr.* 2009;90(1):184–192.

318. Chiu CC, Su KP, Cheng TC, et al. The effects of omega-3 fatty acids monotherapy in Alzheimer's disease and mild cognitive impairment: A preliminary randomized double-blind placebo-controlled study. *Prog Neuropsychopharmacol Biol Psychiatry.* 2008;32(6):1538–1544.

319. Rezai-Zadeh K, Arendash GW, Hou H, et al. Green tea epigallocatechin-3-gallate (EGCG) reduces beta-amyloid mediated cognitive impairment and modulates tau pathology in Alzheimer transgenic mice. *Brain Res.* 2008;1214:177–187.

320. Arendash GW, Schleif W, Rezai-Zadeh K, et al. Caffeine protects Alzheimer's mice against cognitive impairment and reduces brain beta-amyloid production. *Neuroscience.* 2006;142(4):941–952.

321. Myllykangas-Luosujarvi R, Isomaki H. Alzheimer's disease and rheumatoid arthritis. *Br J Rheumatol.* 1994;33(5):501–502.

322. Breitner JC, Welsh KA, Helms MJ, et al. Delayed onset of Alzheimer's disease with nonsteroidal anti-inflammatory and histamine H2 blocking drugs. *Neurobiol Aging.* 1995;16(4):523–530.

323. Andersen K, Launer LJ, Ott A, Hoes AW, Breteler MM, Hofman A. Do nonsteroidal anti-inflammatory drugs decrease the risk for Alzheimer's disease? The Rotterdam Study. *Neurology.* 1995;45(8):1441–1445.

324. Brown AM, Kristal BS, Effron MS, et al. Zn2+ inhibits alpha-ketoglutarate-stimulated mitochondrial respiration and the isolated alpha-ketoglutarate dehydrogenase complex. *J Biol Chem.* 2000;275(18):13441–13447.

325. Aisen PS, Davis KL, Berg JD, et al. A randomized controlled trial of prednisone in Alzheimer's disease. Alzheimer's Disease Cooperative Study. *Neurology*. 2000;54(3):588–593.
326. Scharf S, Mander A, Ugoni A, Vajda F, Christophidis N. A double-blind placebo-controlled trial of diclofenac/misoprostol in Alzheimer's disease. *Neurology*. 1999;53(1):197–201.
327. Sainati S, Ingram D, Talwalker S. Results of a double-blind, placebo-controlled study of celecoxib in the treatment of progression of Alzheimer's disease. *Paper presented at: Sixth International Stockholm-Spingfield Symposium of Advances in Alzheimer's Therapy*. Stockholm, Sweden; 2000:5–8.
328. Vile GF, Winterbourn CC. Inhibition of adriamycin-promoted microsomal lipid peroxidation by beta-carotene, alpha-tocopherol and retinol at high and low oxygen partial pressures. *FEBS Lett*. 1988;238(2):353–356.
329. Niki E. Interaction of ascorbate and alpha-tocopherol. *Ann N Y Acad Sci*. 1987;498:186–199.
330. Wu H, Kong L, Tan Y, et al. C66 ameliorates diabetic nephropathy in mice by both upregulating NRF2 function via increase in miR-200a and inhibiting miR-21. *Diabetologia*. 2016;59:1558–1568.
331. Jaramillo MC, Zhang DD. The emerging role of the Nrf2-Keap1 signaling pathway in cancer. *Genes Dev*. 2013;27(20):2179–2191.
332. Williamson TP, Johnson DA, Johnson JA. Activation of the Nrf2-ARE pathway by siRNA knockdown of Keap1 reduces oxidative stress and provides partial protection from MPTP-mediated neurotoxicity. *Neurotoxicology*. 2012;33(3):272–279.
333. Itoh K, Chiba T, Takahashi S, et al. An Nrf2/small Maf heterodimer mediates the induction of phase II detoxifying enzyme genes through antioxidant response elements. *Biochemi Biophys Res Commun*. 1997;236(2):313–322.
334. Hayes JD, Chanas SA, Henderson CJ, et al. The Nrf2 transcription factor contributes both to the basal expression of glutathione S-transferases in mouse liver and to their induction by the chemo-preventive synthetic antioxidants, butylated hydroxyanisole, and ethoxyquin. *Biochem Soc Trans*. 2000;28(2):33–41.
335. Chan K, Han XD, Kan YW. An important function of Nrf2 in combating oxidative stress: Detoxification of acetaminophen. *Proc Natl Acad Sci U S A*. 2001;98(8):4611–4616.
336. Ramsey CP, Glass CA, Montgomery MB, et al. Expression of Nrf2 in neurodegenerative diseases. *J Neuropathol Exp Neurol*. 2007;66(1):75–85.
337. Chen PC, Vargas MR, Pani AK, et al. Nrf2-mediated neuroprotection in the MPTP mouse model of Parkinson's disease: Critical role for the astrocyte. *Proc Natl Acad Sci U S A*. 2009;106(8):2933–2938.
338. Lastres-Becker I, Ulusoy A, Innamorato NG, et al. alpha-synuclein expression and Nrf2 deficiency cooperate to aggravate protein aggregation, neuronal death, and inflammation in early-stage Parkinson's disease. *Hum Mol Genet*. 2012;21(14):3173–3192.
339. Xi YD, Yu HL, Ding J, et al. Flavonoids protect cerebrovascular endothelial cells through Nrf2 and PI3K from beta-amyloid peptide-induced oxidative damage. *Curr Neurovasc Res*. 2012;9(1):32–41.
340. Suh JH, Shenvi SV, Dixon BM, et al. Decline in transcriptional activity of Nrf2 causes age-related loss of glutathione synthesis, which is reversible with lipoic acid. *Proc Natl Acad Sci U S A*. 2004;101(10):3381–3386.
341. Trujillo J, Chirino YI, Molina-Jijon E, Anderica-Romero AC, Tapia E, Pedraza-Chaverri J. Renoprotective effect of the antioxidant curcumin: Recent findings. *Redox Biol*. 2013;1(1):448–456.
342. Steele ML, Fuller S, Patel M, Kersaitis C, Ooi L, Munch G. Effect of Nrf2 activators on release of glutathione, cysteinylglycine and homocysteine by human U373 astroglial cells. *Redox Biol*. 2013;1(1):441–445.
343. Kode A, Rajendrasozhan S, Caito S, Yang SR, Megson IL, Rahman I. Resveratrol induces glutathione synthesis by activation of Nrf2 and protects against cigarette smoke-mediated oxidative stress in human lung epithelial cells. *Am J Physiol Lung Cell Mol Physiol*. 2008;294(3):L478–488.
344. Gao L, Wang J, Sekhar KR, et al. Novel n-3 fatty acid oxidation products activate Nrf2 by destabilizing the association between Keap1 and Cullin3. *J Biol Chem*. 2007;282(4):2529–2537.
345. Saw CL, Yang AY, Guo Y, Kong AN. Astaxanthin and omega-3 fatty acids individually and in combination protect against oxidative stress via the Nrf2-ARE pathway. *Food Chem Toxicol*. 2013;62:869–875.
346. Song J, Kang SM, Lee WT, Park KA, Lee KM, Lee JE. Glutathione protects brain endothelial cells from hydrogen peroxide-induced oxidative stress by increasing nrf2 expression. *Exp Neurobiol*. 2014;23(1):93–103.
347. Ji L, Liu R, Zhang XD, et al. N-acetylcysteine attenuates phosgene-induced acute lung injury via up-regulation of Nrf2 expression. *Inhal Toxicol*. 2010;22(7):535–542.
348. Choi HK, Pokharel YR, Lim SC, et al. Inhibition of liver fibrosis by solubilized coenzyme Q10: Role of Nrf2 activation in inhibiting transforming growth factor-beta1 expression. *Toxicol Appl Pharmacol*. 2009;240(3):377–384.

349. Bai H, Liu R, Chen HL, et al. Enhanced antioxidant effect of caffeic acid phenethyl ester and Trolox in combination against radiation induced-oxidative stress. *Chem Biol Interact.* 2014;207:7–15.

350. Cui L, Jeong H, Borovecki F, Parkhurst CN, Tanese N, Krainc D. Transcriptional repression of PGC-1alpha by mutant huntingtin leads to mitochondrial dysfunction and neurodegeneration. *Cell.* 2006;127(1):59–69.

351. Li XH, Li CY, Lu JM, Tian RB, Wei J. Allicin ameliorates cognitive deficits ageing-induced learning and memory deficits through enhancing of Nrf2 antioxidant signaling pathways. *Neurosci Lett.* 2012;514(1):46–50.

352. Bergstrom P, Andersson HC, Gao Y, et al. Repeated transient sulforaphane stimulation in astrocytes leads to prolonged Nrf2-mediated gene expression and protection from superoxide-induced damage. *Neuropharmacology.* 2011;60(2–3):343–353.

353. Wruck CJ, Gotz ME, Herdegen T, Varoga D, Brandenburg LO, Pufe T. Kavalactones protect neural cells against amyloid beta peptide-induced neurotoxicity via extracellular signal-regulated kinase 1/2-dependent nuclear factor erythroid 2-related factor 2 activation. *Mol Pharmacol.* 2008;73(6):1785–1795.

354. Li W, Khor TO, Xu C, et al. Activation of Nrf2-antioxidant signaling attenuates NFkappaB-inflammatory response and elicits apoptosis. *Biochem Pharmacol.* 2008;76(11):1485–1489.

355. Kim J, Cha YN, Surh YJ. A protective role of nuclear factor-erythroid 2-related factor-2 (Nrf2) in inflammatory disorders. *Mutat Res.* 2010;690(1–2):12–23.

356. Abate A, Yang G, Dennery PA, Oberle S, Schroder H. Synergistic inhibition of cyclooxygenase-2 expression by vitamin E and aspirin. *Free Radic Biol Med.* 2000;29(11):1135–1142.

357. Devaraj S, Tang R, Adams-Huet B, et al. Effect of high-dose alpha-tocopherol supplementation on biomarkers of oxidative stress and inflammation and carotid atherosclerosis in patients with coronary artery disease. *Am J Clin Nutr.* 2007;86(5):1392–1398.

358. Fu Y, Zheng S, Lin J, Ryerse J, Chen A. Curcumin protects the rat liver from CCl4-caused injury and fibrogenesis by attenuating oxidative stress and suppressing inflammation. *Mol Pharmacol.* 2008;73(2):399–409.

359. Lee HS, Jung KK, Cho JY, et al. Neuroprotective effect of curcumin is mainly mediated by blockade of microglial cell activation. *Pharmazie.* 2007;62(12):937–942.

360. Peairs AT, Rankin JW. Inflammatory response to a high-fat, low-carbohydrate weight loss diet: Effect of antioxidants. *Obesity (Silver Spring).* 2008;16(7):1573–1578.

361. Rahman S, Bhatia K, Khan AQ, et al. Topically applied vitamin E prevents massive cutaneous inflammatory and oxidative stress responses induced by double application of 12-O-tetradecanoylphorbol-13-acetate (TPA) in mice. *Chem Biol Interact.* 2008;172(3):195–205.

362. Reznick AZ, Cross CE, Hu ML, et al. Modification of plasma proteins by cigarette smoke as measured by protein carbonyl formation. *Biochem J.* 1992;286 (Pt 2):607–611.

363. Zhu J, Yong W, Wu X, et al. Anti-inflammatory effect of resveratrol on TNF-alpha-induced MCP-1 expression in adipocytes. *Biochem Biophys Res Commun.* 2008;369(2):471–477.

364. Kanninen K, Malm TM, Jyrkkanen HK, et al. Nuclear factor erythroid 2-related factor 2 protects against beta amyloid. *Mol Cell Neurosci.* 2008;39(3):302–313.

365. Albanes D, Till C, Klein EA, et al. Plasma tocopherols and risk of prostate cancer in the Selenium and Vitamin E Cancer Prevention Trial (SELECT). *Cancer Prev Res (Phila).* 2014;7(9):886–895.

366. Lee DS, Ko W, Kim DC, Kim YC, Jeong GS. Cudarflavone B provides neuroprotection against glutamate-induced mouse hippocampal HT22 cell damage through the Nrf2 and PI3K/Akt signaling pathways. *Molecules.* 2014;19(8):10818–10831.

367. Song J, Hur BE, Bokara KK, et al. Agmatine improves cognitive dysfunction and prevents cell death in a streptozotocin-induced Alzheimer rat model. *Yonsei Med J.* 2014;55(3):689–699.

368. Zou Y, Hong B, Fan L, et al. Protective effect of puerarin against beta-amyloid-induced oxidative stress in neuronal cultures from rat hippocampus: Involvement of the GSK-3beta/Nrf2 signaling pathway. *Free Radic Res.* 2013;47(1):55–63.

369. Joshi G, Gan KA, Johnson DA, Johnson JA. Increased Alzheimer's disease-like pathology in the APP/PS1DeltaE9 mouse model lacking Nrf2 through modulation of autophagy. *Neurobiol Aging.* 2014;36(2):664–679.

370. Karkkainen V, Pomeshchik Y, Savchenko E, et al. Nrf2 regulates neurogenesis and protects neural progenitor cells against Abeta toxicity. *Stem Cells.* 2014;32(7):1904–1916.

371. Jo C, Gundemir S, Pritchard S, Jin YN, Rahman I, Johnson GV. Nrf2 reduces levels of phosphorylated tau protein by inducing autophagy adaptor protein NDP52. *Nat Commun.* 2014;5:3496.

10 Micronutrients for the Prevention and Improvement of the Standard Therapy for Parkinson's Disease

INTRODUCTION

Parkinson's disease (PD) is a slow, progressive, neurological disorder of the central nervous system.[1] In 1917, Dr. James Parkinson, a British physician, published an article on "The Shaky Palsy" describing the major symptoms of the disease that would later bear his name. Since then, pathologists and neurologists have repeatedly reported that loss of dopamine (DA) neurons from the substantia nigra region of the brains is primarily responsible for the most motor control abnormalities observed in PD patients, although other cells are also affected in this disease. It is estimated that in normal individuals, about 3%–5% of DA neurons are lost every decade; however, in PD patients, the rate of loss is greater than that found in normal individuals.[2] The analysis of autopsied samples of PD brain revealed that about 70%–75% of DA neurons are lost by the time the disease becomes detectable.[2] This suggests that DA neurons possess a high degree of functional plasticity.

The major environmental-, dietary-, or lifestyle-related factors that initiate or promote the progression of degeneration of DA neurons in PD are not known. However, the research of the past several decades has identified several cellular defects that may be contributing factors. Among them, increased oxidative stress, inflammation, and mitochondrial defects are the most important in sporadic PD. Even in familial PD, in which some genetic defects have been identified, these biological mechanisms play a central role in the initiation and progression of PD. Thus, they could serve as a biological basis for developing preventive treatments and improving current treatment strategies for both sporadic and familial PD. At present, there is no effective strategy for reducing the incidence or progression of PD in high-risk populations (familial cases, early stage PD and individuals over the age of 65 years). The current drug and surgical treatments are very effective at improving the major symptoms of PD; but the efficacy of these treatments only lasts for as long as DA neurons remain viable. Additionally, the severe side effects of levodopa, a gold standard therapy, are observed after some time, possibly mediated via increased oxidative stress and chronic inflammation. It is known that auto-oxidation of L-dopa and dopamine generates excessive amounts of free radicals that could damage not only DA neurons but neurons in other regions of the brain. The toxic side effects become a limiting factor for the continuation of levodopa therapy. None of the current treatments with drugs or surgical procedures affect the levels of oxidative stress and inflammation that are major contributors to the degeneration of DA neurons. Antioxidants that have potentials to reduce the rate of degeneration of DA neurons by reducing oxidative stress and inflammation have not been utilized on the basis of a scientific rationale in all clinical studies published thus far. The clinical trials to evaluate the role of antioxidants in the progression of PD have utilized only one dietary antioxidant, primarily vitamin E, which may not be adequate to reduce both oxidative stress and chronic inflammation in the brain. Therefore, additional clinical studies should be initiated, using an appropriate mixture of micronutrients at appropriate dose and dose-schedule for reducing the risk and progression of PD and improving the efficacy of standard therapy in PD Patients.

Increased oxidative stress and chronic inflammation are also involved in impaired nonmotor functions of PD, such as dementia,[3–6] psychiatry disorders,[7–10] impaired olfaction,[11–13] and autonomic failure.[14,15]

MicroRNAs that are evolutionarily conserved small noncoding single-stranded RNAs that play an important role in the pathogenesis of neurodegenerative disease such as AD (Chapter 9 of this book). Therefore, they play a similar role in the pathogenesis of PD. Enhanced oxidative stress and pro-inflammatory cytokines associated with PD also alter the expressions of microRNAs. A review has discussed the role of antioxidant compounds in protecting dopaminergic neurons by reducing oxidative stress in preclinical studies.[16] It is possible that one of the neuroprotective actions of antioxidants is mediated by altering the levels of specific RNAs.

This chapter describes the incidence, prevalence, cost, etiology, neuropathology, genetic defects, and evidence for the involvement of oxidative stress, chronic inflammation, mitochondrial dysfunction, and glutamate release in the initiation and progression of PD. This chapter also discusses the role of microRNAs in the pathogenesis of PD. It proposes a novel hypothesis that simultaneous elevation of the levels of antioxidant enzymes and dietary and endogenous antioxidants may be necessary for optimally reducing oxidative stress, chronic inflammation, and glutamate release in human PD. The levels of antioxidants can be enhanced, while glutamate release and toxicity can be decreased by an oral supplementation. However, elevation of the levels of antioxidant enzymes is complex requiring activation of the Nrf2/ARE (nuclear transcriptional factor-2/antioxidant response element) pathway. This review briefly discusses the activation of Nrf2, and proposes a mixture of micronutrients that can simultaneously activate Nrf2 and enhance the levels of antioxidants for testing in the prevention, and in combination with standard therapy, in the improved management of PD.

INCIDENCE, PREVALENCE, AND COST OF PD

Incidence: Parkinson Foundation estimates about 60,000 new cases each year in the United States, and approximately 4% of the people are diagnosed with PD before the age of 50 years. The risk of this disease increases after the age of 50 years. The incidence of PD is 1.5 times more in men than in women.

Prevalence: Approximately 500,000 people have this disease in the United States. Prevalence increases with age and affects 1% of the population over the age of 60.[17]

Incidence per 100,000 in ethnic groups in the US population

Non-Hispanic white	3.6
Hispanic	6.6
Black	10.2
Asian	11.3

Cost: The total direct and indirect cost of PD increased from $6 billion per year in 1992[18] to $25 billion now (Parkinson's Foundation, 2017). This cost is likely to increase in the future, because the disease occurs primarily in older people over the age of 50, and because the average age of Americans will increase, and the number of this group of people will also continue to increase.

ETIOLOGY OF PD

Age is a risk factor for most idiopathic (sporadic) neurological diseases including PD. In addition, a sustained adverse interaction between environmental toxins and internal toxins increases oxidative stress, chronic inflammation, and gene mutations, leading to degeneration and eventually death of DA neurons. An exposure to excessive amounts of manganese such as observed among manganese miners increased the incidence of PD-like disease.[19] This is because increased brain levels of free manganese can enhance production of free radicals, which then gradually cause damage to DA neurons. In 1980, increased incidence of PD-like disease was seen among users of the designer drug, meperidene, which contains 1-methyl-4-phenyl-1,2,3,6-tetrahydropyridine (MPTP), a neurotoxic byproduct formed during the synthesis of this drug.[20] At least one of the mechanisms of action of MPTP-induced degeneration of DA neurons is mediated by free radicals.[20]

In an effort to identify other external agents as risk factors, several epidemiologic identified some potential risk factors, such as rural living, well water consumption, exposure to herbicides and pesticides (e.g., dieldrin and dithiocarbamates).[21–24] Although no particular dietary risk factors for PD were identified, the consumption of nuts and salad oil (pressed from seeds) appeared to be of protective value.[22] Vitamin E consumption was found to be lower among patients with PD than among normal control.[24]

NEUROPATHOLOGY AND SYMPTOMS OF PD

The degeneration of DA neurons of the substantia nigra is a characteristic feature of PD. Surviving neurons contains Lewy bodies, a pathological hallmark of PD. The Lewy bodies are present in other area of the brain, particularly brain stems area like the locus coeruleus that sends out processes throughout the brain. Thus, PD is not just a disease of substantia nigra DA neurons alone. The incidence of Lewy bodies in 139 autopsied brain samples of elderly individuals with normal cognitive function and without any type of movement disorders was evaluated. The results showed that about 23% of the samples contained Lewy bodies in various regions of the brains. The most common regions involved were medulla (26%), amygdale (24%), pons (20%), and midbrain (20%).[25] Lewy bodies contain predominantly neurofilaments that are important components of the neuronal cytoskeleton and ubiquitin that degrades abnormal proteins. Lewy bodies also contain high levels of alpha-synuclein. The presence of another protein FOXO3 (a transcriptional activator that can trigger neuronal death upon oxidative stress) was demonstrated in Lewy bodies in the autopsied brain samples of PD as well as in the Lewy body dementia.[26] Lewy bodies are considered consequences of neuronal damage. They can be transferred from one neuron to another by endocytosis. This was demonstrated by the fact that Lewy bodies were present in the neurons grafted in patients with PD and in a transgenic animal model of PD.[27]

The major symptoms of PD include tremor, muscle rigidity, postural problems, gait disorders, speaking difficulties, cognitive dysfunction, and immobility that ultimately lead to total disability and death.

GENETIC OF PD

Mutations in six genes have been identified in familial PD, and their actions in degeneration of DA neurons have been elucidated. Mutations in alpha-synuclein (SNCA), PARKIN, PTEN-induced kinase 1 (PINK1), DJ-1, and leucin-rich repeat kinase 2 (LRRK2) are associated with familial PD,[28–31] and account for about 2%–3% of all cases of PD. In addition, the levels of ATP13A2 gene that encodes a lysosomal ATPase increased in the brains of patients with sporadic or idiopathic PD.[32] The transgenic animal models confirm the role of these mutations in the pathology of PD.[33,34] Among familial PD, mutations in PARKIN gene account for about 50%, PINK1 8-15%, and DJ-1 about 1% of cases.[35] The mutation in LRRK2 gene is involved not only in familial PD but also in some sporadic PD. Several variants in LRRK2 and SNCA have been associated with an increased risk of sporadic PD.[36] There appears to be interaction between PARKIN, PINK1, and DJ-1genes. It was demonstrated that these genes formed a complex referred to as PPD complex to promote ubiquitination and degradation of PARKIN substrates, including PRKIN itself in neuroblastoma cells in culture and human brain lysates.[37] Genetic ablation of either PINK1 or DJ-1 reduced ubiquitination of endogenous PARKIN and decreased degradation of aberrantly expressed PRKIN substrates. Expression of PINK1 increased PARKIN-mediated degradation of heat shock-induced misfolded protein. However, mutations in PARKIN and PINK1 reduced degradation of PARKIN substrates by impairing ubiquitin E3 ligase activity.[37]

PD GENES AND OXIDATIVE STRESS

DJ-1 Gene

DJ-1 was originally identified as an oncogene. Overexpression of the wild-type DJ-1 protects DA neurons against oxidative damage induced by H_2O_2[38] and dopamine- and 6-hydroxydopamine (6-OHDA)-induced toxicity.[39,40] It acts as a stress sensor and increases its level in response to elevated oxidative stress.[41] However, DJ-1 is easily damaged by free radicals. As matter of fact, increased levels of oxidized DJ-1 have been found in the autopsied brain tissues of sporadic as well as in familial PD.[42] Therefore, it can be considered as a biomarker for sporadic PD.[43] In contrast to the wild-type DJ-1, mutated DJ-1 makes DA neurons more vulnerable to oxidative stress-induced apoptosis.[44] Mutated DJ-1 also promotes aggregation of alpha-synuclein that impairs mitochondrial function causing DA neurons to degenerate slowly.[45]

Alpha-Synuclein Gene

A family of homologous proteins, alpha- and beta-synuclein, is located primarily in the presynaptic regions of brain neurons, whereas gamma-synuclein is present in the peripheral nervous system and retina.[46] Lewy bodies, hallmark of PD, contain predominantly alpha-synuclein in aggregated form, which has been implicated in the pathogenesis of PD. The overexpression of wild-type alpha-synuclein caused degenerative changes in human DA neurons in culture,[47] and in transgenic rat DA neurons.[48,49]

The overexpression of human wild-type alpha-synuclein in differentiated neuroblastoma cells decreased their viability and increased their sensitivity to oxidative stress and neurotoxins, such as H_2O_2, nitric oxide, and prostaglandin E2.[50] Increased oxidative stress, proteasome inhibition, and endoplasmic reticulum stress upregulated wild-type alpha-synuclein expression in fibroblasts obtained from patients with PD compared to those obtained from normal subjects.[51] Overexpression of wild-type alpha-synuclein is associated with degeneration of DA neurons. Increased oxidative stress also causes aggregation of alpha-synuclein that is toxic to DA neurons. The mechanisms of action of alpha-synuclein are not well understood; however, it has been suggested that alpha-synuclein-induced neurotoxicity is related to increased oxidative stress[52,53] that is caused by impaired mitochondria. Alpha-synuclein enters mitochondria through an import receptors located in both the outer and inner mitochondrial membranes,[54] and excessive accumulation of alpha-synuclein causes mitochondrial dysfunction. This is due to the fact that overexpression of alpha-synuclein caused nitration of mitochondrial proteins and the release of cytochrome c from the mitochondria.[55] These biological events that are related to increased oxidative stress may initiate degeneration of DA neurons. The overexpression of human wild-type or mutant (A53T or A30P) alpha-synuclein in human neuroblastoma cells in culture enhanced aggregation of alpha-synuclein.[56] Mutant alpha-synuclein (A53T) transfected mice developed intraneuronal Lewy bodies-like inclusions, mitochondrial dysfunction, and apoptotic death in neocortical, brain stem, and motor neurons.[57] The role of dysfunctional mitochondria in the pathogenesis of PD is further substantiated by the fact that chronic inhibition of complex I activity by rotenone induced neurodegeneration characteristics of PD in rats.

This effect of rotenone caused accumulation and aggregation of alpha-synuclein and ubiquitin, progressive oxidative damage, and caspase-dependent death in human neuroblastoma cells in culture.[58]

Dopamine metabolite, 3,4-dihydroxyphenylacetaldehyde, interacts with alpha-synuclein protein causing them to aggregate.[49]

The aggregated form of alpha-synuclein plays an important role in the pathogenesis of PD.[59] Mitochondrial dysfunction can also induce alpha-synuclein oligomerization through increased protein oxidation and microtubule depolymerization.[60] Alpha-synuclein-knockout mice developed without gross abnormality but are resistant to MPTP-induced degeneration of DA neurons. In addition, genetic ablation of alpha-synuclein protected neuronal cells in culture against oxidative stress,[59] increased the resistance of human DA neuron-like cells to 1-methy-4-phenylpyridine (MPP+).[61,62] Conversely, overexpression of wild-type alpha-synuclein or mutant alpha-synuclein (A53T) increased the sensitivity of neurons to MPP+, which induced mitochondrial dysfunction, and 6-hydroxydopamine, which increased oxidative stress in human neuroblastoma cells in culture.[63] Antioxidants such as Edaravone protected only against MPP+-induced toxicity, and epigallo-catechin-3-o-gallate protected only against 6-hydroxydopamine–induced neurodegeneration.[63] This study suggests that one type of antioxidant is not sufficient to affect neurodegeneration induced by diverse groups of toxins. Mutant alpha-synuclein (A53T), but not other variants such as A30P, induced adult-onset of PD in transgenic mice, and this effect was associated with abnormal accumulation of detergent insoluble alpha-synuclein protein.[64]

Overexpression of wild-type alpha-synuclein or mutated alpha-synuclein had no effect on proteasome activity in neuronal cells in culture or in transgenic mice,[65,66] although alpha-synuclein directly and reversibly inhibited the activity of purified 20S subunits of proteasome in vitro.[66] The inhibition of proteasome activity in human neuroblastoma cells in culture failed to induce alpha-synuclein aggregation.[66] These results suggest that proteasome inhibition and overexpression of alpha-synuclein that are associated with PD are not related. It is likely that increased oxidative stress that up-regulates alpha-synuclein and inhibits proteasome activity is a primary event in the pathogenesis of PD. Since alpha-synuclein is degraded by proteasome and by autophagic pathways,[67,68] any defects in one or both pathways can lead to an accumulation of alpha synuclein in neurons. Whether or not a protein forms aggregation depends upon the cellular concentration of the protein and thermodynamics properties inherent to each protein. Therefore, an increase in cellular concentration of alpha-synuclein can lead to aggregation. Oxidation of alpha-synuclein can also cause aggregation. Tyrosinase, a rate-limiting enzyme in the synthesis of melanin, in combination with alpha-synuclein, allows aggregation of alpha-synuclein.[69] The abnormal aggregation of alpha-synuclein plays a central role in the degeneration of DA neurons.[67] The interaction between alpha-synuclein and PARKIN resulted in decreased PARKIN and alpha-tubulin ubiquitation, accumulation of insoluble PARKIN, and cytoskeletal alterations, with reduced neurite outgrowth.[70]

PTEN-Induced Putative Kinase 1 (PINK1)

PINK1, a mitochondrial Ser/Thr kinase, is a ubiquitous protein expressed throughout the human brain and is primarily located to the mitochondrial membrane and the cytosol. One of the functions of wild-type PINK1 is to protect mitochondria against a variety of stress-signaling pathways. Genetic ablation of wild-type PINK1caused loss of mitochondrial membrane potential, decrease in ATP synthesis, complex IV activity, and mitochondrial electron transport chain function.[71] Impairment of mitochondrial electron transport chain and an increased frequency of deletions of mitochondrial DNA which codes some of the subunits of mitochondrial electron transport chain have been found in the autopsied samples of the substantia nigra of PD brains. PINK1 is also present in the Lewy bodies.[72] Like mutated alpha-synuclein, mutated PINK1 also impairs mitochondrial function. Mutant PINK1 (W437X) enhanced the levels of mutant synuclein (A53T)-induced mitochondrial dysfunction. This effect was associated with increased intracellular calcium levels.[73]

Coexpression of mutated PINK1 and alpha-synuclein altered mitochondrial structure and neurite growth that were totally blocked by the inhibitor of mitochondrial calcium flux.[73] Mutant PINK1 or PNK1 knockdown reduced mitochondrial respiration and ATP synthesis, inhibited proteasome activity and increased alpha-synuclein aggregation in neuronal cells in culture.[74]

The wild-type PARKIN is considered one of the most important factors that improve mitochondrial dysfunction.[75] PINK1 and PARKIN play a central role in the regulation of mitochondrial dynamics and function (fission, fusion and migration, and energy generation); therefore, mutations in these genes can impair mitochondrial function and dynamics.[37] Mitochondrial dysfunction interferes with the generation of energy and produces more free radicals that initiate degeneration of DA neurons and eventually causing neuronal death. Mutated PINK1 increased oxidative damage in the fibroblasts obtained from PD patients as well as upregulated wild-type alpha-synuclein expression in fibroblasts obtained from normal subjects.[51]

PARKIN GENE

The wild-type PARKIN improves mitochondrial function.[75] Mutations in this gene can impair mitochondrial function and dynamics.[37] Nitric oxide and oxidative stress inhibit PARKIN function, which can lead to degeneration of DA neurons. Loss of PARKIN gene in human midbrain DA neurons increases the transcription of monoamine oxidases, and oxidative stress reduces DA uptake and enhances spontaneous release of DA. Insertion of a wild-type PARKIN gene into these DA neurons prevents the above changes.[76]

The above studies suggest mutations in alpha-synuclein, DJ-1, PINK-1, and PARKIN genes cause damage to mitochondria that can increase oxidative stress. Reducing oxidative stress may block the deleterious effects of these mutated genes on the survival of DA neurons.

MicroRNAs IN THE PATHOGENESIS OF PD

MICRORNAS

MicroRNAs (miRs) are evolutionarily conserved small noncoding single-stranded RNAs of approximately 22 nucleotides in length, and are present in all living organisms including humans.[77–80] The biogenesis of miRs is very complex and involves multiple biochemical steps. The majority of miRs are transcribed by RNA polymerase II (Pol II), while some are transcribed by RNA polymerase III (Pol III) from the noncoding region of the DNA to produce primary miRs (pri-miRs). Pri-miRs undergo a nuclear cleavage by ribonuclease III Drosa to generate precursor-miRs (pre-miRs) that migrate to the cytoplasm where they are further cleaved by ribonuclease III Dicer to ultimately form mature single-stranded miRs with the help of another protein argonaute (Ago).[79,81–83] Each microRNA binds to its complementary sequences in the 3′-untranslated region (3′-UTR) of the mRNA, promotes degradation of the m RNA transcript, and prevents translation of the message of protein. In this manner, miRs regulate the translation of proapoptotic or antiapoptotic proteins from their respective mRNAs, depending upon whether the DNA receives damaging or protective signal. The binding site of the mRNA for a microRNA is only about 6–8 base pairs; therefore, one miRNA may target as many as 100 different mRNAs,[79,84] altering the levels of these proteins to regulate cellular functions. On the other hand, individual mRNA contains multiple binding sites for different microRNAs.

CHANGES IN THE EXPRESSIONS OF MicroRNAs IN NEURONAL CELL CULTURE MODELS OF PD

1-METHYL-4-PHENYLPYRIDINIUM (MPP+) TREATMENT

Treatment of dopaminergic neurons (SH-SY5Y) in culture with MPP+ decreased the expression of miR-7 and enhanced the levels of its target protein Keap1 (Kelch-like ECH-associated protein 1), an inhibitor of Nrf2, leading to increased oxidative stress and neurodegeneration.[85] Upregulation of the expression of miR-7 protected dopaminergic neurons against MPP+-induced toxicity by reducing oxidative stress.[85]

Elevation of miR-7 reduced the levels of alpha-synuclein by binding to its 3'-UTR mRNA, and protected neurons against oxidative stress.[59] Upregulation of miR-7 protected dopaminergic neurons against MPP+-induced toxicity by reducing the levels of alpha-synuclein. Upregulation of miR-152 also reduced the levels of alpha-synuclein by: binding to its 3'-UTR mRNA.[86] Overexpressions of miR-7 and miR-153 protected neurons against MPP+-induced cell death by elevating the levels of rapamycin signaling pathway that plays a role in cell survival.[87]

Upregulation of miR-34b and miR-34c protected neurons by decreasing the levels of alpha-synuclein in human dopaminergic neurons.[88] These results suggest that multiple microRNAs may target alpha synuclein. In contrast, upregulation of miR-320a and miR-16-1 enhanced the accumulation and aggregation of alpha-synuclein indirectly by decreasing the levels of Hsc70 (heat shock protein 70) that prevented the degradation of alpha-synuclein in dopaminergic neurons overexpressing alpha-synuclein (SH-SY5Y-syn+).[89,90] Thus, the levels of alpha-synuclein can be increased or decreased depending upon the types and expressions levels of microRNAs.

MiR-7 also targets RelA (v-rel-avian reticuloendotheliosis viral oncogene homolog A) protein involved in the regulation of activation of NF-kB.[91] Overexpression of miR-7 protected neurons against MPP+-induced cell death by decreasing the levels of RelA. Downregulation of miR-7 increased the levels of RelA that eventually led to neuronal death via activation of NF-kB pathway.

6-Hydroxydopamine (6-OHDA) Treatment

Treatment of dopaminergic neurons in culture with 6-OHDA enhanced the expression of miR-126 and reduced the levels of its target protein insulin growth factor-1 (IGF-1) causing neurodegeneration.[92] Downregulation of miR-126 expression increased the levels of IGF-1 that provided neuroprotection against 6-OHDA-induced toxicity.

Rotenone Treatment

Treatment of DA neurons with rotenone, a mitochondrial toxin, upregulated the expression of miR-384-5p and reduced the levels of its target protein glucose regulated protein 78 (GRP78), a major ER chaperone protein, leading to decreased cell viability.[93] Therefore, inhibition of the expression of miR-384-5p protected neurons against rotenone-induced toxicity by increasing the levels of GRP78 protein.

CHANGES IN THE EXPRESSIONS OF MicroRNAs IN ANIMAL MODELS OF PD

Downregulation of the expression of miR-124 was reduced the levels of its target protein Bim, a proapoptotic protein of Bcl2 family, and induced neurodegeneration in the MPTP mouse model of PD.[94] The treatment with miR-124 agomir (a synthetic miR-124) protected DA neurons against MPTP-induced toxicity by decreasing the level of Bim. Another protein target for miR-124 was calpain 1, a calcium-dependent non-lysosomal cysteine proteases. MPTP treatment caused death of dopaminergic neurons by decreasing the expression of miR-124 and increasing the levels of calpain1.[95] Overexpression of miR-124 decreased the levels of calpain1 and improved the survival of neurons. Silencing miR-124 increased production of reactive oxygen species (ROS) and hydrogen peroxide (H_2O_2). The results suggest that one microRNA targets more than one mRNAs.

MPTP treatment enhanced the expression of miR-494 and decreased the levels of its target protein DJ-1, leading to increased oxidative stress and degeneration of DA neurons.[96] This suggested that decreasing the expression of miR-494 might be of neuroprotective value.

CHANGES IN THE EXPRESSIONS OF MicroRNAs IN HUMAN PD

Decreased expression of miR-205 and elevated levels of its target protein LRRK2 were found in the autopsied frontal cortex tissues of patients with sporadic PD.[97] Reduced expression of miR-34b and increased levels of its target protein adenosine A2A receptor (A2AR) were found in the autopsied brain tissue of PD patients as well as in the putamen of incidental PD cases (Braak stages 1-2).[87] In early-stage PD, decreased expression levels of miR-34b and elevated levels of pathogenic protein A2AR were found in the brain.[98] Deletion of these microRNAs reduced the viability of differentiated dopaminergic neurons (SH-SY5Y cell line). Downregulation of the expression of miR-34b and miR-34c increased the levels of alpha-synuclein causing neurodegeneration.[99] These findings suggest that miR-34b and miR-34c may target more than one protein. Alterations in the levels of microRNAs in PD could be due to changes in their transcription, processing by Dorsa and Dicer in the nucleus and cytoplasm, respectively or their stability.

Table 10.1 summarizes the changes in the expression levels of microRNAs and their target proteins in experimental and human PD.

TABLE 10.1

Changes in Expression Levels of MicroRNAs and Their Target Proteins, and Their Consequences on Neurodegeneration in PD

PD Model	Upregulation	Downregulation	Target Proteins	Results
In vitro models		miR-7	[a]Keap1	Degeneration
MPP+		miR-7	[a]α-synuclein	" " " " "
" " " " " "		miR-7, miR-153	[a]α-synuclein	" " " " "
" " " " "		miR-7, miR-153	[b]mTOR	" " " " "
" " " " "		miR-34b, miR-34c	[a]α-synuclein	" " " " "
" " " " "	miR-320, miR-16-1		[b]Hsc70	" " " " "
" " " " "		miR-7	[a]RelA	" " " " "
6-OHDA	miR-126		IGF-1	" " " " "
Rotenone	miR-384-5p		[b]GRP78	" " " " "
MPTP		miR-124	[a]Bim, calpain-1	" " " " "
" " " " "	miR-494		[b]DJ-1	" " " " "
Human PD	miR-494		[b]DJ-1	" " " " "
" " " " "		miR-34b	[a]A2AR	" " " " "
" " " " "		miR-34b, miR-34c	[b]DJ-1,Parkin	" " " " "
" " " " "		miR-205	[a]LRRK2	" " " " "

Note: a = increased; b = decreased.

1-Methyl-4-phenylpyridinium (MPP+) 6-Hydroxydopamine (6-OHDA); 1-Methyl-4-phenyl-1, 2, 3, 6-tetrahydropyridine (MPTP); Mammalian target of rapamycin (mTOR); Heat shock protein 70 (Hsc70); v-Rel-avian reticuloendotheliosis viral oncogene homolog A (RelA); Insulin growth factor-1 (IGF-1); Glucose regulated protein 78 (GRP78); Adenosine A2A receptor (A2AR); Leucine-rich repeat kinase 2 (LRRK2).

CHANGES IN THE EXPRESSIONS OF MicroRNAs IN IMPAIRED NON-MOTOR SYMPTOMS IN PD

Some studies suggest that the expression levels of microRNAs are also altered in impaired nonmotor symptoms associated with PD, such as dementia, psychiatry disorders, and impaired olfaction.[100] A few studies on this issue are described here.

Fragile-X-associated tremor and ataxia syndrome (FXTAS) is a neurodegenerative disease that appears in primarily in men of over 50 years carrying permutation (55–200 repeats of CGG) in FMIR (Fragile-X-mental retardation-1) gene. Individuals with this heritable disorder exhibit mental retardation, intentional tremor, gait ataxia, autonomic dysfunction, and peripheral neuropathy.[101,102] Three microRNAs, miR-10, miR-129-5p, and miR-221, bind with 3′-UTR FMRI mRNA. The expression of miR-221 was downregulated in synaptosomal preparation of young FXTAS mice that would increase the levels of FMRI protein in synaptosomes.[103] Thus, decreased expression levels of these microRNAs may be involved in cognitive dysfunction and autistic behavior.

Downregulation of three microRNAs miR-132, miR-124, and miR-34 were associated with dementia in PD.[104] The expression levels of four microRNAs, miR-146a, miR-221, miR-654-5p, miR-656, were downregulated in olfactory mucosal stem cells obtained from patients with Autism spectrum disorders.[105] Increased expression of miR-137 caused downregulation of presynaptic target genescomplexin-1, N-ethylmaleimide-sensitive factor, and synaptotagmin-1 that resulted in changes in synaptic vesicle pool distribution, impaired induction of mossy fiber long-term potentiation, and deficits in hippocampal-dependent learning and memory. Silencing the expression of miR-137 abolished the above changes.[106] The expression levels of miR-19b were downregulated in patients with idiopathic rapid eye movement sleep behavior disorder.[107]

REACTIVE OXYGEN SPECIES (ROS) REGULATES THE EXPRESSIONS OF MicroRNAs IN NEURONAL CELLS

Increased oxidative stress is one of the earliest biochemical defects that initiate and participate in the progression of PD.[108] Therefore, it may act as one of the signals to alter the expression levels of certain specific microRNAs. The evidence for this has been presented in a recent review[16] and in Chapter 9 of this edition.

PRO-INFLAMMATORY CYTOKINES UPREGULATE THE EXPRESSIONS OF MicroRNAs

Since chronic inflammation plays an important role in the pathogenesis of PD, it is likely that pro-inflammatory cytokines may alter the expression of microRNAs in PD. This issue has been discussed in detail in a previous review[16] and discussed in Chapter 9 of this edition.

ANTIOXIDANTS REGULATE THE EXPRESSIONS OF MicroRNAs

Since antioxidants protect neurons against oxidative damage and chronic inflammation, it is likely that antioxidant may provide neuroprotection by altering the expressions of microRNAs in PD.[16] The evidence for this has been described in Chapter 9 of this edition.

EVIDENCE FOR INCREASED OXIDATIVE STRESS IN PD

Several studies have demonstrated the presence of high levels of oxidative stress in autopsied brain samples of PD patients. The normal brain has the highest concentration of unsaturated fatty acids of all organs, and these fatty acids are very susceptible to lipid peroxidation. Indeed, high levels of oxidative damage have been observed in the autopsied samples of substantia nigra of PD brains.[109–112] Autopsied samples of substantia nigra of PD brain contained reduced levels of antioxidant enzymes[113,114] and antioxidants.[115–117]

The levels of markers of oxidative damage and vitamin E were measured in 211 patients with PD and 135 healthy controls. The results showed that leukocyte 8-hydroxyguanosine and plasma malondialdehyde (MDA) were elevated, whereas erythrocyte glutathione peroxidase and plasma vitamin E levels were reduced in PD patients compared to the control subjects.[118,119] Reduced glutathione levels were observed in the substantia nigra of the autopsied brain samples of PD patients indicating the presence of high oxidative stress.[120–122] Reduced glutathione can impair mitochondrial function. Isofurans are products of lipid peroxidation and their formation is favored in the presence of high oxygen tension. The levels of Isofurans but not F2-isoprostane are elevated in the autopsied samples of the substantia nigra of PD patients.[123] Heme oxygenase-1 (HO-1) is a cellular stress protein expressed in brain and other tissues, and becomes elevated in response to increased oxidative stress. The expression of HO-1 is upregulated in the autopsied samples of the substantia nigra of PD brain.[124] The antioxidant capacity in the autopsied substantia nigra of PD brain was lower than control subjects.[125] It has been reported that the NADH dehydrogenase activity in the platelets of PD patients were lowered compared to healthy age- and gender-matched controls, whereas the activity of succinate dehydrogenase was similar in both groups.[126]

The serum levels of vitamin A, vitamin E, or vitamin C in PD patients did not differ from controls[127–130]; however, plasma levels of vitamin C and vitamin E were decreased in patients with vascular PD.[130] These data suggest that serum or plasma levels of vitamin A, vitamin C, or vitamin E do not play any significant role in the pathogenesis of PD, because they did not reflect the brain levels of antioxidants. Thus, brain tissue levels of antioxidants rather than the blood levels of antioxidants may play significant role in the initiation and progression of both sporadic and familial PD.

Several studies have confirmed that PD is associated with a significant increase in free iron in the degenerating substantia nigra.[131–133] The effects of iron on degeneration of DA neurons are via increased oxidative stress. The mechanisms of accumulation of iron in the substantia nigra are unknown; however, an isoforms of the divalent metal transporter-1 (DMT1) is elevated in the substantia nigra of PD brain.[134]

Using a MPTP model of rat PD, it was demonstrated that the expression of DMT1and the levels of iron increased in treated animals. These two biological events were associated with increased oxidative stress and neuronal death.[134] The mutation in DMT1 protected rats against toxicity produced by MPTP or 6-hydroxydopamine. Manganese-enhanced DA-induced apoptosis in mesencephalic neurons.[135] The effect of manganese is mediated by induction of NF-kappaB and activation of nitric oxide synthase that generates increased amounts of free radicals.

It has been reported that the neuromelanin granules accumulate in the substantia nigra of PD patients. Neuromelanins are formed from auto-oxidation of catecholamines in the substantia nigra of PD brain, and contain significant amounts of iron.[136,137] Neuromelanin can cause degeneration in DA neurons by generating H_2O_2 when it is intact, or by releasing redox active metals such as iron if it is impaired. In addition, dying DA neurons can release melanin that can initiate chronic inflammatory responses by activating microglia cells. Excessive production NO by the treatment with MPTP plays a significant role in degeneration of DA neurons, because nitric oxide can be oxidized to form peroxynitrite, a form of nitrogen-derived free radicals that is highly neurotoxic. Therefore, the involvement of NO in the pathophysiology of PD has been proposed.[138]

MITOCHONDRIAL DYSFUNCTION IN PD

Mitochondrial dysfunction plays a central role in most neurodegenerative diseases including PD,[139,140] but can be considered as a secondary event in the initiation and progression of PD, because mitochondrial dysfunctions can be induced by diverse groups of external and internal agents. External agents include MPTP, insecticides and pesticides, whereas internal agents include increased oxidative stress and chronic inflammation, and mutated or aggregated alpha-synuclein, mutated PINK1, DJ-1, and PARKIN genes.[31,141,142] The mitochondrial dysfunctions include impaired electron transport chain, mitochondrial DNA defects, impaired calcium buffering, reduced ATP synthesis, and anomalies of morphology and dynamics of mitochondria.[143,144] The consequences of mitochondrial dysfunction include increased oxidative stress, release of cytochrome c, activation of caspase, release of calcium, upregulation of Bax expression and its translocation to mitochondria, and proteasome inhibition all of which contribute to degeneration of DA neurons and eventually their death.[139,145,146] Thus, reducing oxidative stress by antioxidants should protect mitochondria, thereby decrease the risk of PD.

EVIDENCE FOR INCREASED CHRONIC INFLAMMATION IN PD

Oxidative damage, if not repaired, leads to chronic inflammation. Microglia initiated chronic inflammation responses also play an important role in the mechanism of degeneration of DA neurons in PD.[147,148] Aggregated or nitrated alpha-synuclein activates microglia that contributes to the degeneration of DA neurons by releasing pro-inflammatory cytokines and other neurotoxic factors.[149–151] It has been reported that nitric oxide and superoxide released by activated microglia may promote inflammation as well as abnormal alpha-synuclein (excessive amount or mutated form) to cause degeneration of DA neurons in transgenic mice model of PD.[152] In autopsied brain samples of PD brains, the number of activated microglia cells increased in the substantia nigra during the progression of PD. The levels of pro-inflammatory cytokines IL-6 and TNF-alpha increased in both PD and Lewy body disease.[153] The analysis of neuronal loss in autopsied samples of substantia nigra suggests that neurons containing melanin are primarily lost.[154] Indeed, pathologists have consistently observed depigmentation of the substantia nigra in the autopsied samples of PD brains. The addition of human neuromelanin to microglia cell cultures induced chemotactic effects and activated the pro-inflammatory transcription factor NF-kappaB.[154] This treatment of microglia cells also upregulated TNF-alpha, IL-6, and nitric oxide. These results suggest that the presence of extracellular neuromelanin serves as a chronic source of inflammation that aggravates the rate of degeneration of DA neurons. Although inflammatory response is considered a protective response, but chronic activation of microglia cells may produce excessive amounts of pro-inflammatory cytokines, complement proteins, adhesion molecules, and reactive oxygen species, all of which are neurotoxic. It has been reported that cyclooxygenase (COX) is the rate-limiting enzyme in the synthesis of prostaglandins that are neurotoxic in excessive amounts.[155] The inducible isoforms COX-2 is upregulated in the DA neurons in autopsied brain samples of PD patients, and in neurotoxin-induced animal PD models. The overexpression of COX-2 in human neuroblastoma cells facilitated oxidation of DA, and proteins including alpha-synuclein.[156] The studies presented in this section clearly show that chronic inflammation plays an important role in degeneration and apoptosis of DA neurons in PD. Therefore, agents such as high-dose antioxidants and a low-dose non-steroidal anti-inflammatory drug (NSAID) as such aspirin that can inhibit chronic inflammation may help in reducing the incidence of PD in high risk populations, and when used as an adjunctive therapy, they may improve the efficacy of standard therapy in the treatment of PD.

EVIDENCE FOR INCREASED GLUTAMATE IN PD

Glutamate is a major excitatory transmitter in the mammalian central nervous system, and is neurotoxic when present in excess at the synapses. With the depletion of nigrostriatal DA neurons, the glutamatergic projections from subthalamic nucleus to the basal ganglia output nuclei become overactive.[157] The glutamatergic activity also increased in the striatal region of the PD brain. One of the neurotoxic effects of glutamate is mediated via free radicals.[158,159]

Increased glutamate signaling in the substantia nigra played an important role in the mechanisms of neuronal death induced by chronic treatment of mice with MPTP.[160] This is substantiated by the fact that inhibitors of glutamate receptors ameliorated abnormality in motor movements in the animal model of PD.[161,162] Antioxidants also block the toxic effects of glutamate,[158,159] confirming that neurotoxic effect of glutamate is mediated via free radicals.

LABORATORY AND HUMAN STUDIES IN PD AFTER TREATMENT WITH MICRONUTRIENTS

Several in vitro and animal studies suggest that supplementation with individual micronutrients should be useful in reducing the risk and progression of PD; however, clinical studies with individual antioxidants have produced inconsistent results varying from no effect to minimal beneficial effects.

IN VITRO STUDIES WITH MICRONUTRIENTS

Alpha-synuclein fibrils are considered toxic to DA neurons. It has been reported that certain antioxidants such as vitamin A, beta-carotene, and coenzyme Q10 inhibited formation of alpha-synuclein fibrils in a dose-dependent manner, whereas vitamin B2, vitamin B6, vitamin C, and vitamin E were ineffective in vitro.[163] In addition, vitamin A, beta-carotene, and coenzyme Q10 destabilized preformed alpha-synuclein fibrils in a dose-dependent manner. The results of these studies cannot be extrapolated to human PD, but they would suggest that supplementation with these antioxidants may help to reduce the risk of PD by preventing the aggregation of alpha-synuclein and by destabilizing the preformed alpha-synuclein fibrils.

CELL CULTURE STUDIES WITH MICRONUTRIENTS

Dopamine is known to induce apoptosis in several lines of neuronal cells in culture by increasing oxidative stress. The viability of DA-treated human melanocytes significantly decreased in a dose-dependent manner, whereas keratinocytes exhibited less sensitivity to DA treatment. N-acetylcysteine (NAC) or glutathione protected against DA-induced toxicity in normal human melanocytes, whereas other antioxidants such as vitamin C, vitamin E, trolox, and quercetin were ineffective.[164] Melatonin, deprenyl, and vitamin E inhibited autooxidation of DA in a dose-dependent manner, whereas vitamin C was ineffective.[165] These studies further confirmed that only certain antioxidants could protect DA neuron against free radicals generated by auto-oxidation of DA. Treatment with ascorbate completely prevented the neurotoxin-induced degeneration in both normal and glutamate-depleted neurons in culture.[166] Glutamate, an excitatory neurotransmitter, in excessive amounts is toxic to DA neurons by causing increase in oxidative stress. This effect of glutamate can be blocked by an analog of NAC (N-acetylcysteine amide),[167] vitamin E,[158] and coenzyme Q10.[159]

ANTIOXIDANT STUDIES IN ANIMAL MODELS OF PD

Treatment with 6-OHDA, MPTP, quinolinic acid, 3-nitropropionic acid and rotenone induce oxidative damage to DA neurons and behavior alterations in animals resembling those observed in PD patients. Pre-treatment of rats with d-alpha-tocopherol or dl-alpha-tocopherol significantly reduced 6-OHDA-induced behavior and biochemical abnormalities.[168,169] Intramuscular administration of d-alpha-tocopheryl succinate, the most effective form of vitamin E,[170] protected 6-OHDA-induced death of locus coeruleus neurons as well as behavioral and biochemical defects in rats.[171,172] Administration of L-carnitine, coenzyme Q10, vitamin E, alpha-lipoic acid, or resveratrol reduced oxidative damage and behavior abnormalities in animal model of PD induced by diverse groups of neurotoxins.[173,174] Supplementation with NAC decreased the levels of alpha-synuclein in mice overexpressing wild-type human alpha-synuclein in the brain, and partially prevented the loss of dopaminergic terminals in these mice.[175]

Resveratrol is also an activator of SIRT1, and thus, stimulated mitochondrial biogenesis in mice and reduces production of reactive oxygen species.[176] Pretreatment of fibroblasts obtained from patients with early-onset PD carrying mutated Park2 gene with resveratrol enhanced mitochondrial oxidative function by activating Peroxisome proliferator-activated receptor-gamma coactivator-1α (PGC-1α).[177] Both curcumin and a mixture of dietary and endogenous antioxidants (a gift from Premier Micronutrient Corporation, Nashville, TN) reduced the incidence of death and hypokinesia induced by MPTP treatment in mice. Although both curcumin and an antioxidant mixture markedly blocked MPTP-induced depletion of tyrosine hydroxylase (TH) activity, only the antioxidant mixture enhanced the TH activity.[178] This suggested that an antioxidant mixture treatment was more effective than the curcumin treatment in preventing MPTP-induced depletion of TH in mice. Treatment of neuroblastoma cells (PC-12 derived from the rat and SH-SY5Y derived from the human) with curcumin prevented mutated alpha-synuclein (A53T)-induced cell death by inhibiting oxidative stress, mitochondrial depolarization, cytochrome c release, and caspase-9 and caspase-3 activation[179,180] Pretreatment of rats with a flavonoid quercetin reduced 6-OHDA-induced increase in the levels of protein carbonyl, glutathione, dopamine, and SOD in the striatum.[181]

Treatment with some phytochemicals such as methanol extract of Garcinia Indica fruits,[182] silymarin, derived from the seeds of the plant Silyburn marianum,[183] and silibinin, a major constituent of silymarin 184 reduced MPTP- and 6-OHDA-induced toxicity on dopaminergic neurons in the substantia nigra of rats. These agents exhibit antioxidant and anti-inflammation activities.

Nicotinamide, an inhibitor of histone deacetylase, preserves the activity of silent information regulator-1 (SIRT-1), a regulator of mitochondrial biogenesis.[185] This vitamin inhibits oxidative damage and improves mitochondrial function and thus can protect neurodegeneration and improve motor functions. In addition, in Drosophila melanogaster model of PD (an alpha-synuclein transgenic fly), nicotinamide treatment significantly improved the motor function (climbing ability).[186]

Pre-treatment treatment of mice with fish oil, melatonin, or vitamin E decreased the levels of MPTP-induced elevation of the activity of COX-2 and lipid peroxides in the homogenates of midbrain. Treatment with fish oil was more effective in reducing MPTP-induced rise in COX-2 activity than vitamin E or melatonin, whereas melatonin was more effective in reducing MPTP-induced rise in lipid peroxides than fish oil or vitamin E.[187] These results suggest that different antioxidants affect markers of increased oxidative stress and chronic inflammation differently. Omega-3-fatty acids restricted diet increased the levels of NO in the striatum of young and adult rats but not in the substantia nigra; however, increased lipoperoxidation and decreased catalase activity were found in both regions of the brain, while total SOD activity was lowered in the striatum. In addition, fewer tyrosine hydroxylase- and brain-derived nerve growth factor-positive cells were present in the substantia nigra compared to the controls.

ANTIOXIDANT STUDIES IN HUMAN PD

Several epidemiologic studies suggested that diet rich in vitamin E might reduce the risk of PD.[188,189] In addition, animal studies revealed that supplementation with a single antioxidant compound may be also useful in reducing oxidative stress and delaying or improving the symptoms of PD. To test this possibility, most clinical trials utilized a single antioxidant, primarily vitamin E, that may have contributed to the inconsistent results. Deprenyl and Tocopherol Antioxidative Therapy of Parkinsonism (DATATOP), a randomized, double-blind, placebo-controlled, multicenter clinical trial was initiated in 1989 in order to evaluate the efficacy of deprenyl (10 mg per day) and dl-tocopherol (2,000 IU per day) individually and in combination in patients with early-stage PD when no therapy was required. The primary outcome was prolongation of the time needed for levodopa therapy. After a follow-up period of 8.2 years, deprenyl significantly delay the time when levodopa therapy was needed, but alpha tocopherol was ineffective.[190,191] The use of a single dietary antioxidant vitamin E was a major flaw in this study design. There was another flaw in the DATATOP study design. A multiple vitamin preparation (One a Day™) was allowed for all individuals who wished to take it. It was argued that the effect of 30 IU of vitamin E in the multiple vitamin preparation would not significantly contribute to the effect of 2,000 IU of vitamin E. This argument may not be valid, since it has been shown that antioxidants when used individually had no effect of growth of mammalian cancer cells in culture, but when they are combined at the same doses produced pronounced effect on growth inhibition, suggesting they may interact with each other in a synergistic manner.[192,193] Therefore, the impact of 30 IU of vitamin E in a multiple vitamin preparation would be more pronounced than that produced by 30 IU of vitamin E alone. Hence, the consumption of a multiple vitamin preparation containing a low dose of vitamin E by control subjects is likely to create an unacceptable variable while evaluating the efficacy of high dose of vitamin E alone in early PD patients, especially when both experimental and placebo group were allowed to have a multiple vitamin preparation in an uncontrolled fashion. Patients with PD have a high oxidative environment in the brain. It is known that individual antioxidants when oxidized act as prooxidants. Therefore, the conclusion of the DATATOP study that antioxidants are not useful in reducing the progression of PD is not valid.

In an open-labeled clinical trial, the efficacy of high doses of alpha-tocopherol and ascorbate was tested in early PD patients. Patients were allowed to receive amantadine and anticholinergics, but not levodopa or a DA agonist. The primary outcome was delay of the time when levodopa therapy is needed. The results showed that these antioxidants delayed the time when levodopa therapy was needed by 2.5 years.[194] This study shows that a mixture of antioxidants may be a better approach for delaying the time when levodopa therapy is needed than a single antioxidant in patients with an early-stage PD.

In a multi-center, randomized, double-blind, placebo-controlled trial involving 80 early-stage PD patients who did not require any therapy, the efficacy of coenzyme Q10 at doses of 300, 600, or 1200 mg per day was evaluated. The primary outcome was Unified Parkinson Disease Rating Score (UPDRS), and the patients were followed up for 16 months or until disability requiring levodopa therapy is needed. The results showed that coenzyme Q10 at the highest dose of 1200 mg per day was safe and well-tolerated by patients. The results also revealed that less disability developed in patients receiving coenzyme Q10 compared to placebo controls; the benefit was greater in patients receiving the highest dosage.[195] Reviews of several open and controlled clinical studies revealed that daily supplementation with coenzyme Q10 either has no effect or has minimal benefit in early stage PD patients.[196,197]

In a randomized, double-blind, placebo-controlled trial involving 35 patients with tardive dyskinesia (17 patients received vitamin E and 18 patients received placebo), the efficacy of vitamin E alone at a dose of 800 IU per day was evaluated. Twenty-nine of these patients had a diagnosis of schizophrenia and 6 of mood disorder. They were followed up for two months. Patients were assessed using modified Abnormal Involuntary Movement Scale (mAIMS), Simpson-Angus Scale for extrapyramidal side effects, brief Psychiatric Rating Scale, and dyskinesia. The results showed that vitamin E supplementation reduced the severity of tardive dyskinesia in patients who had this disease for 5 years or less.[198]

The efficacy of reduced nicotinamide adenine dinucleotide (NADH) in the treatment of PD patients has become controversial. A review on the clinical efficacy of NADH has concluded that it is premature to recommend NADH alone for the treatment of PD.[199]

POTENTIAL REASONS FOR INCONSISTENT RESULTS WITH INDIVIDUAL MICRONUTRIENTS IN AD PREVENTION STUDIES

The reasons for individual micronutrients or aspirin producing no effects or some transient beneficial effects on PD are not known; however, some potentials causes are described here: (a) antioxidants show differential subcellular distribution and different mechanisms of action; therefore, a single antioxidant cannot protect all parts of the cell; (b) a single antioxidant in a high internal oxidative environment in high-risk patients is oxidized and can then itself act as a prooxidant rather than as an antioxidant; (c) the body protects against oxidative damage by elevating antioxidant enzymes, and dietary and endogenous antioxidants; (d) antioxidants neutralize free radicals by donating electrons to those molecules with unpaired electron, whereas antioxidant enzymes destroy free radicals by catalysis, converting them to harmless molecules such as water and oxygen. Therefore, both of these agents should be enhanced to achieve substantial protection against oxidative damage; (e) the affinity of different antioxidants for free radicals differs, depending upon their lipophilicity; (f) both the aqueous and lipid compartments of the cell need to be protected together. Water-soluble antioxidants such as vitamin C and glutathione protect molecules in the aqueous environment of the cells, whereas lipid soluble antioxidants such as vitamin A and vitamin E protect molecules in the lipid compartment; (g) vitamin E is more effective in quenching free radicals in a reduced oxygenated cellular environment, whereas vitamin C and alpha-tocopherol are more effective in a higher oxygenated environment of the cells[200]; (h) vitamin C is important for recycling the oxidized form of alpha-tocopherol to the antioxidant form at the lipid/aqueous interface[201]; (i) antioxidants produce cell protective proteins by altering the expression of different microRNAs.[202] For example, some antioxidants can activate Nrf2 by upregulating miR-200a that inhibits its target protein Keap1, whereas others activate Nrf2 by downregulating miR-21 that binds with 3'-UTR Nrf2 mRNA.[203]

The use of a single micronutrient is not expected to yield any beneficial effects on PD prevention. For this reason, a mixture of micronutrients that can simultaneously reduce oxidative stress and inflammation by enhancing the levels of antioxidant enzymes through the activation of Nrf2 pathway together with dietary and endogenous antioxidants for Alzheimer's disease and Parkinson's disease has been suggested.[16,202] Oral supplementation can increase the levels of dietary and endogenous antioxidants; however, elevation of the levels of antioxidant enzymes requires an activation of Nrf2. Therefore it is essential to understand the regulation of activation of Nrf2.

ACTIVATION OF Nrf2 (NUCLEAR FACTOR-ERYTHROID-2-RELATED FACTOR 2)

Nrf2

The nuclear transcriptional factor, Nrf2 (nuclear factor-erythroid-2-related factor 2) belongs to the Cap 'n' Collar (CNC) family that contains a conserved basic leucine zipper (bZIP) transcriptional factor.[204] Under physiological condition, Nrf2 is associated with Kelch-like ECH associated protein 1 (Keap1), which acts as an inhibitor of Nrf2.[205] Keap1 protein serves as an adaptor to link Nrf2 to the ubiquitin ligase CuI-Rbx1 complex for degradation by proteasomes and maintains the steady levels of Nrf2 in the cytoplasm. Nrf2-keap1 complex is primarily located in the cytoplasm; Keap1 acts as a sensor for ROS/electrophilic stress.

ROS ACTIVATES Nrf2

During acute oxidative stress, ROS is needed to activate Nrf2, which then dissociates itself from Keap1-CuI-Rbx1 complex and translocates in the nucleus where it heterodimerizes with a small Maf protein, and binds with ARE, leading to increased expression of target genes coding for several cytoprotective enzymes, including antioxidant enzymes.[206–208]

ROS-Resistant Nrf2: During chronic oxidative stress, Nrf2 becomes resistant to ROS,[209–211] suggesting that activation of Nrf2 by a ROS-independent mechanism exists. This is evidenced by the fact that increased chronic oxidative stress occurs in PD despite the presence of Nrf2. The question arises as to how to activate ROS-resistant Nrf2 in PD.

Antioxidants Activate ROS-Resistant Nrf2: Some examples are vitamin E and genistein,[212] alpha-lipoic acid,[213] curcumin,[214] resveratrol,[215,216] omega-3-fatty acids,[217,218] glutathione,[219] NAC,[220] and coenzyme Q10.[221] Several plant-derived phytochemicals, such as epigallocatechin-3-gallate, carestol, kahweol, cinnamonyl-based compounds, zerumbone, lycopene and carnosol,[204,222,223] genistein,[212] allicin, a major organosulfur compound found in garlic,[224] sulforaphane, a organosulfur compound, found in cruciferous vegetables,[225] and kavalactones (methysticin, kavain, and yangonin).[226] The reasons for the activation of Nrf2 without ROS by antioxidant compounds are not known.

Binding of Nrf2 with ARE in the Nucleus: An activation of Nrf2 alone is not sufficient to increase the levels of antioxidant enzymes. Activated Nrf2 must bind with ARE in the nucleus for increasing the expression of target genes coding for antioxidant enzymes. This binding ability of Nrf2 with ARE was impaired in aged rats and this defect was restored by supplementation with alpha-lipoic acid.[213] It is unknown whether the binding ability of Nrf2 with ARE is impaired in PD.

Nrf2 IN PD

6-hydroxydopamine (6-OHDA) and 1-methyl-4-phenyl-1,2,3,6-tetrahydropyridine (MPT) are neurotoxins commonly used for inducing Parkinson disease-like symptoms in animals and degeneration and death of dopaminergic neurons in cell culture models. These neurotoxins produced above effects by increasing the levels of chronic oxidative stress and inflammation. Pretreatment of human neuroblastoma cells in culture and mice with naringenin, a natural flavonoid, protected neurons against 6-OHDA-induced toxicity. The protective effect of naringenin was dependent upon the presence of Nrf2, because deletion of Nrf2 blocked its protective effect.[227] Puerarin treatment reduced neurodegeneration in the substantia nigra of rats following injection with 6-OHDA by activating the Nrf2/ARE pathway and elevating the levels of brain-derived neurotrophic factor (BDNF).[228] Licochalcone E (Lico-E), a glycyrrhiza inflate-derived chaocone, reduced inflammation in microglia cells and protected human neuroblastoma cells against 6-OHDA- and MPTP-induced neurotoxicity by activating the Nrf2/ARE pathway.[229] Resveratrol reduced paraquat-induced ROS and inflammation by activating the Nrf2/ARE pathway.[230] Several other phytochemicals, such as gastrodin, a main constituent of Chinese herbal medicine *Gastrodia elata*,[231] tetramethylpyrazine, an extract of Ligusticum wallichii Franchat (ChuanXiong),[232] Mangiferin, a polyphenolic compound[233] protected against MPTP-induced oxidative stress, neurodegenerative changes, and motor deficits by activating the Nrf2/ARE pathway.

Importance of Nrf2 in neuroprotection is demonstrated by the fact that deficiency of Nrf2 enhanced alpha-synuclein aggregation and chronic inflammation that contribute to the degeneration of DA neurons in PD.[211] Nrf2 deficiency also increased the sensitivity of mice to MPTP-induced behavior and biochemical changes. Overexpression of Nrf2 in astrocyte was sufficient to provide neuroprotection in MPTP mouse model of PD.[210]

The above studies suggest that activation Nrf2 is essential for neuroprotection in laboratory experiments; however, in human PD, activation of Nrf2 alone may not be sufficient for prevention or improved management, because the levels of dietary and endogenous antioxidants decrease in a high oxidative environment; therefore, they must also be elevated simultaneously.

REDUCING GLUTAMATE RELEASE AND TOXICITY

Release of glutamate was blocked by antioxidants, such as vitamin E,[234] tempol, a superoxide dismutase mimetic, and edaravone, a synthetic antioxidant,[235] quercetin,[236] glutathione and vitamin E,[237] alpha-lipoic acid,[238] and coenzyme Q10.[239] In addition to antioxidants, vitamin B6,[240] vitamin B12,[241] and vitamin B2 (riboflavin)[242] also reduce release of glutamate. Antioxidants such as alpha-tocopherol[243] and coenzyme Q10[159] also protected neurons against glutamate-induced degeneration and death.

PROPOSED MICRONUTRIENT MIXTURE FOR PREVENTION AND IMPROVED MANAGEMENT OF PD

I propose a micronutrient mixture containing multiple dietary (vitamin A, vitamin C, vitamin E succinate, vitamin E acetate, natural carotenoids, curcumin, resveratrol, and selenomethionine,) and endogenous (alpha-lipoic acid, L-carnitine, and coenzyme Q10), a synthetic antioxidant

N-acetylcysteine (NAC), omega-3-fatty acids, vitamin D3, zinc, and all B-vitamins. This mixture may optimally reduce oxidative stress, chronic inflammation, and glutamate release and toxicity by simultaneously enhancing the levels of antioxidant enzymes through activation of the Nrf2/ARE pathway and antioxidants. These micronutrients can cross blood-brain-barrier at varying amounts. This is supported by the fact that administration of many of these micronutrients improved some PD symptoms in animals and humans.

PRIMARY PREVENTION

The major objective of primary prevention is to protect healthy individuals from developing PD. Individuals 50 years or older, and individuals with a family history of PD who have not developed any clinical symptoms of PD are suitable for the primary prevention study. The proposed mixture of micronutrients is recommended for the study of primary prevention. At present, there are not strategies to prevent or delay the onset of PD in individuals carrying mutated PD genes. The proposed mixture may be effective at least in delaying the onset of PD in these individuals. Following experimental evidence supports this possibility.

The gene HOP (TUM-1) is essential for the development of *Drosophila melanogaster* (fruit fly). A mutation in this gene markedly increases the risk of developing a leukemia-like tumor in female flies. In collaboration with Dr. Bhattacharya of NASA Moffat Field, CA, we observed that whole-body irradiation of these flies with proton radiation dramatically increased the incidence of cancer compared to that in unirradiated flies. Treatment with a mixture of antioxidants before and after irradiation blocked the proton radiation-induced cancer in fruit flies.[244] This finding is of particular interest, because it suggests that heritable genetic basis of the disease can be prevented by antioxidant treatment.

SECONDARY PREVENTION

The purpose of secondary prevention is to stop or slow the progression of PD. Individuals who exhibit early sign of PD, but are not taking any medication, can be included in the secondary prevention study. The mixture of micronutrients recommended for the primary prevention study can also be used for the secondary prevention study.

CURRENT TREATMENTS OF PD

The current treatment strategies involve increasing the function of surviving DA neurons by maintaining adequate levels of DA. To accomplish this, L-dopa, a precursor of DA and DA receptor agonists are used. Deprenyl and catechol-o-methyl transferase (COMT) inhibitor are used to prevent degradation of DA. In addition, in some cases acetylcholinesterase inhibitor is utilized in order to balance between two neurotransmitters, DA and acetylcholine, by reducing the levels of acetylcholine. In cases where drug therapy becomes ineffective, highly effective surgical methods to relieve some of the symptoms of PD such as tremor are available. None of these treatments prevents DA neurons from dying due to increased oxidative stress and chronic inflammation.

PROPOSED MICRONUTRIENT MIXTURE IN COMBINATION WITH STANDARD THERAPY

Standard therapy includes primarily drugs that elevate dopamine in the surviving DA neurons. These drugs do not address oxidative stress, chronic inflammation, or glutamate release; therefore, DA neurons continue to die despite drug treatment. The effectiveness of Levodopa therapy that is considered a gold standard lasts only for about 5 years, after which serious side effects of this therapy are manifested.

In some cases, surgery may be appropriate, if the disease doesn't respond to a standard drug therapy. Deep brain stimulation (DBS), an FDA-approved therapy improves major symptoms of PD for a short period of time, but does not reduce oxidative stress or chronic inflammation. The proposed mixture of micronutrients recommended for the primary prevention studies can also be used in combination with standard drug therapy or after DBS. This strategy may reduce the progression and prolong the beneficial effects of current drugs and surgery in patients with PD by protecting surviving DA neurons from damage produced by increased oxidative stress, chronic inflammation, and glutamate.

DIET AND LIFESTYLE RECOMMENDATIONS FOR PD

Even though, there is no direct link between the diet and lifestyle related factors and the initiation or progression of PD, it is always useful to include a balanced diet that contains low fat and plenty of fruits and vegetables. Among fruits, blueberries and raspberries are particularly important because of their protective role against oxidative injuries in the brain. Lifestyle recommendations include daily moderate exercise, reduced stress, and no tobacco smoking or drug use.

CONCLUSIONS

Parkinson's disease (PD) is a slow progressive neurological disorder of the central nervous system characterized by the loss of dopamine (DA) neurons from the substantia nigra region of the brains that is primarily responsible for the most motor control abnormalities, although cells from other regions of the brain are also affected in this disease. Increased oxidative stress and chronic inflammation play a central role in the initiation and progression of sporadic PD. Glutamate also participates in the progression of this disease. Even in familial PD, these biological events play a crucial role in the pathogenesis of this disease. Therefore, attenuation of these biological defects may reduce the risk of developing PD, and in combination of standard therapy, may improve the management of PD. Alterations in the expressions of microRNAs play an important role in the pathogenesis of PD. The expressions of microRNAs and their respective target proteins depend upon whether they receive damaging signals such as ROS and pro-inflammatory cytokines or protective signals such as antioxidants. Supplementation with a single micronutrient has yielded inconsistent results in varying from no effect to modest beneficial effect on PD prevention. Therefore, we have proposed that in order to simultaneously reduce oxidative stress and chronic inflammation, it is essential to enhance the levels of antioxidant enzymes and dietary and endogenous antioxidants at the same time. To accomplish this, a mixture of micronutrients that would enhance the levels of antioxidant enzymes through the activation of Nrf2 pathway together with dietary and endogenous antioxidants, is essential. Oral supplementation can increase the levels of dietary and endogenous antioxidants; however, elevation of the levels of antioxidant enzymes requires an activation of Nrf2 that becomes resistant to ROS in PD. Antioxidants activate ROS-resistant Nrf2. A mixture of micronutrients, which may increase the levels of antioxidant enzymes by activating the Nrf2/ARE pathway and dietary and endogenous antioxidants, is proposed. This micronutrient may also prevent the release and toxicity of glutamate. This mixture of micronutrients may reduce the risk of developing PD in high-risk populations, and in combination with the drug therapy, may improve the management of this disease by prolonging the efficacy of the drugs for a longer period of time, and by reducing long-term side effects.

REFERENCES

1. Olanow CW, Youdim MB. *Neurodegeneration and Neuroprotection in Parkinson's Disease*. New York: Academic Press; 1996.
2. Mandel S, Grunblatt E, Riederer P, Gerlach M, Levites Y, Youdim MB. Neuroprotective strategies in Parkinson's disease: An update on progress. *CNS Drugs*. 2003;17(10):729–762.

3. Fernandez-Viadero C, Jimenez-Sanz M, Fernandez-Perez A, Verduga Velez R, Crespo Santiago D. Inflammation and oxidation: Predictive and/or causative factors. *Rev Esp Geriatr Gerontol.* 2016;51 Suppl 1:27–33.

4. Desai A. Dietary Polyphenols as potential remedy for dementia. *Adv Neurobiol.* 2016;12:41–56.

5. Chi GC, Fitzpatrick AL, Sharma M, Jenny NS, Lopez OL, DeKosky ST. Inflammatory biomarkers predict domain-specific cognitive decline in older adults. *J Gerontol A Biol Sci Med Sci.* 2016;72(6):796–803.

6. Daulatzai MA. Fundamental role of pan-inflammation and oxidative-nitrosative pathways in neuropathogenesis of Alzheimer's disease in focal cerebral ischemic rats. *Am J Neurodegener Dis.* 2016;5(2):102–130.

7. Kim SY, Cohen BM, Chen X, et al. Redox dysregulation in Schizophrenia revealed by *in vivo* NAD+/NADH Measurement. *Schizophr Bull.* 2016;43(1):197–204.

8. Cudney LE, Sassi RB, Behr GA, et al. Alterations in circadian rhythms are associated with increased lipid peroxidation in females with bipolar disorder. *Int J Neuropsychopharmacol.* 2014;17(5):715–722.

9. de Sousa RT, Zarate CA, Jr., Zanetti MV, et al. Oxidative stress in early stage Bipolar Disorder and the association with response to lithium. *J Psychiatr Res.* 2014;50:36–41.

10. Morris G, Berk M, Klein H, Walder K, Galecki P, Maes M. Nitrosative stress, hypernitrosylation, and autoimmune responses to nitrosylated proteins: New pathways in neuroprogressive disorders including depression and chronic fatigue syndrome. *Mol Neurobiol.* 2016;54(6):4271–4291.

11. Garratt M, Pichaud N, Glaros EN, Kee AJ, Brooks RC. Superoxide dismutase deficiency impairs olfactory sexual signaling and alters bioenergetic function in mice. *Proc Natl Acad Sci U S A.* 2014;111(22):8119–8124.

12. Cabungcal JH, Preissmann D, Delseth C, Cuenod M, Do KQ, Schenk F. Transitory glutathione deficit during brain development induces cognitive impairment in juvenile and adult rats: Relevance to schizophrenia. *Neurobiol Dis.* 007;26(3):634–645.

13. Getchell ML, Shah DS, Buch SK, Davis DG, Getchell TV. 3-Nitrotyrosine immunoreactivity in olfactory receptor neurons of patients with Alzheimer's disease: Implications for impaired odor sensitivity. *Neurobiol Aging.* 2003;24(5):663–673.

14. Kasasbeh E, Chi DS, Krishnaswamy G. Inflammatory aspects of sleep apnea and their cardiovascular consequences. *South Med J.* 2006;99(1):58–67; quiz 68-59, 81.

15. Maes M, Mihaylova I, Kubera M, Uytterhoeven M, Vrydags N, Bosmans E. Coenzyme Q10 deficiency in myalgic encephalomyelitis/chronic fatigue syndrome (ME/CFS) is related to fatigue, autonomic and neurocognitive symptoms, and is another risk factor explaining the early mortality in ME/CFS due to cardiovascular disorder. *Neuro Endocrinol Lett.* 2009;30(4):470–476.

16. Prasad KN. Simultaneous activation of Nrf2 and elevation of antioxidant compounds for reducing oxidative stress and chronic inflammation in human Alzheimer's disease. *Mech Ageing Dev.* 2016;153:41–47.

17. Tysnes OB, Storstein A. Epidemiology of Parkinson's disease. *J Neural Transm (Vienna).* 2017;124(8):901–905.

18. NINDS. *Parkinson's Disease: A Research Planning Workshop.* Bethesda, MD: National Instutute of Health; 2008.

19. Mena I, Horiuchi K, Burke K, Cotzias GC. Chronic manganese poisoning: Individual susceptibility and absorption of iron. *Neurology.* 1969;19(10):1000–1006.

20. Ballard PA, Tetrud JW, Langston JW. Permanent human parkinsonism due to 1-methyl-4-phenyl-1,2,3,6-tetrahydropyridine (MPTP): Seven cases. *Neurology.* 1985;35(7):949–956.

21. Langston JW. Epidemiology versus genetics in Parkinson's disease: Progress in resolving an age-old debate. *Ann Neurol.* 1998;44(3 Suppl 1):S45–S52.

22. Golbe LI, Farrell TM, Davis PH. Case-control study of early life dietary factors in Parkinson's disease. *Arch Neurol.* 1988;45(12):1350–1353.

23. Seidler A, Hellenbrand W, Robra BP, et al. Possible environmental, occupational, and other etiologic factors for Parkinson's disease: A case-control study in Germany. *Neurology.* 1996;46(5):1275–1284.

24. de Rijk MC, Breteler MM, den Breeijen JH, et al. Dietary antioxidants and Parkinson disease. The Rotterdam Study. *Arch Neurol.* 1997;54(6):762–765.

25. Markesbery WR, Jicha GA, Liu H, Schmitt FA. Lewy body pathology in normal elderly subjects. *J Neuropathol Exp Neurol.* 2009;68(7):816–822.

26. Su B, Liu H, Wang X, et al. Ectopic localization of FOXO3a protein in Lewy bodies in Lewy body dementia and Parkinson's disease. *Mol Neurodegener.* 2009;4:32.

27. Desplats P, Lee HJ, Bae EJ, et al. Inclusion formation and neuronal cell death through neuron-to-neuron transmission of alpha-synuclein. *Proc Natl Acad Sci U S A.* 2009;106(31):13010–13015.

28. Gandhi PN, Chen SG, Wilson-Delfosse AL. Leucine-rich repeat kinase 2 (LRRK2): A key player in the pathogenesis of Parkinson's disease. *J Neurosci Res.* 2009;87(6):1283–1295.

29. Giaime E, Sunyach C, Druon C, et al. Loss of function of DJ-1 triggered by Parkinson's disease-associated mutation is due to proteolytic resistance to caspase-6. *Cell Death Differ.* 2009;17(1):158–169.

30. Fitzgerald JC, Plun-Favreau H. Emerging pathways in genetic Parkinson's disease: Autosomal-recessive genes in Parkinson's disease: A common pathway? *FEBS J.* 2008;275(23):5758–5766.

31. Dodson MW, Guo M. Pink1, Parkin, DJ-1 and mitochondrial dysfunction in Parkinson's disease. *Curr Opin Neurobiol.* 2007;17(3):331–337.

32. Klein C, Lohmann-Hedrich K. Impact of recent genetic findings in Parkinson's disease. *Curr Opin Neurol.* 2007;20(4):453–464.

33. Li Y, Liu W, Oo TF, et al. Mutant LRRK2(R1441G) BAC transgenic mice recapitulate cardinal features of Parkinson's disease. *Nat Neurosci.* 2009;12(7):826–828.

34. Giasson BI, Van Deerlin VM. Mutations in LRRK2 as a cause of Parkinson's disease. *Neurosignals.* 2008;16(1):99–105.

35. da Costa CA. DJ-1: A newcomer in Parkinson's disease pathology. *Curr Mol Med.* 2007;7(7):650–657.

36. Wider C, Wszolek ZK. Clinical genetics of Parkinson's disease and related disorders. *Parkinsonism Relat Disord.* 2007;13 Suppl 3:S229–232.

37. Bueler H. Impaired mitochondrial dynamics and function in the pathogenesis of Parkinson's disease. *Exp Neurol.* 2009;218(2):235–246.

38. Gu L, Cui T, Fan C, et al. Involvement of ERK1/2 signaling pathway in DJ-1-induced neuroprotection against oxidative stress. *Biochem Biophys Res Commun.* 2009;383(4):469–474.

39. Lev N, Ickowicz D, Barhum Y, Lev S, Melamed E, Offen D. DJ-1 protects against dopamine toxicity. *J Neural Transm.* 2009;116(2):151–160.

40. Lev N, Ickowicz D, Melamed E, Offen D. Oxidative insults induce DJ-1 upregulation and redistribution: Implications for neuroprotection. *Neurotoxicology.* 2008;29(3):397–405.

41. Ariga H, Takahashi-Niki K, Kato I, Maita H, Niki T, Iguchi-Ariga SM. Neuroprotective function of DJ-1 in Parkinson's disease. *Oxid Med Cell Longev.* 2013;2013:683920.

42. Kitamura Y, Watanabe S, Taguchi M, et al. Neuroprotective effect of a new DJ-1-binding compound against neurodegeneration in Parkinson's disease and stroke model rats. *Mol Neurodegener.* 2011;6(1):48.

43. Bandopadhyay R, Kingsbury AE, Cookson MR, et al. The expression of DJ-1 (PARK7) in normal human CNS and idiopathic Parkinson's disease. *Brain.* 2004;127(Pt 2):420–430.

44. Xu J, Zhong N, Wang H, et al. The Parkinson's disease-associated DJ-1 protein is a transcriptional co-activator that protects against neuronal apoptosis. *Hum Mol Genet.* 2005;14(9):1231–1241.

45. Batelli S, Albani D, Rametta R, et al. DJ-1 modulates alpha-synuclein aggregation state in a cellular model of oxidative stress: Relevance for Parkinson's disease and involvement of HSP70. *PLoS One.* 2008;3(4):e1884.

46. Duda JE, Shah U, Arnold SE, Lee VM, Trojanowski JQ. The expression of alpha-, beta-, and gamma-synucleins in olfactory mucosa from patients with and without neurodegenerative diseases. *Exp Neurol.* 1999;160(2):515–522.

47. Zhou W, Schaack J, Zawada WM, Freed CR. Overexpression of human alpha-synuclein causes dopamine neuron death in primary human mesencephalic culture. *Brain Res.* Feb 1 2002;926(1–2):42–50.

48. Lo Bianco C, Ridet JL, Schneider BL, Deglon N, Aebischer P. Alpha-synucleinopathy and selective dopaminergic neuron loss in a rat lentiviral-based model of Parkinson's disease. *Proc Natl Acad Sci U S A.* 2002;99(16):10813–10818.

49. Galvin JE. Interaction of alpha-synuclein and dopamine metabolites in the pathogenesis of Parkinson's disease: A case for the selective vulnerability of the substantia nigra. *Acta Neuropathol.* 2006;112(2):115–126.

50. Prasad JE, Kumar B, Andreatta C, et al. Overexpression of alpha-synuclein decreased viability and enhanced sensitivity to prostaglandin E(2), hydrogen peroxide, and a nitric oxide donor in differentiated neuroblastoma cells. *J Neurosci Res.* 2004;76(3):415–422.

51. Hoepken HH, Gispert S, Azizov M, et al. Parkinson patient fibroblasts show increased alpha-synuclein expression. *Exp Neurol.* 2008;212(2):307–313.

52. Lucking CB, Brice A. Alpha-synuclein and Parkinson's disease. *Cell Mol Life Sci.* 2000;57(13–14):1894–1908.

53. el-Agnaf OM, Irvine GB. Aggregation and neurotoxicity of alpha-synuclein and related peptides. *Biochem Soc Trans.* 2002;30(4):559–565.

54. Devi L, Anandatheerthavarada HK. Mitochondrial trafficking of APP and alpha synuclein: Relevance to mitochondrial dysfunction in Alzheimer's and Parkinson's diseases. *Biochim Biophys Acta.* 2009;1802(1):11–19.

55. Parihar MS, Parihar A, Fujita M, Hashimoto M, Ghafourifar P. Mitochondrial association of alpha-synuclein causes oxidative stress. *Cell Mol Life Sci.* 2008;65(7–8):1272–1284.

56. Parihar MS, Parihar A, Fujita M, Hashimoto M, Ghafourifar P. Alpha-synuclein overexpression and aggregation exacerbates impairment of mitochondrial functions by augmenting oxidative stress in human neuroblastoma cells. *Int J Biochem Cell Biol.* 2009;41(10):2015–2024.

57. Martin LJ, Pan Y, Price AC, et al. Parkinson's disease alpha-synuclein transgenic mice develop neuronal mitochondrial degeneration and cell death. *J Neurosci.* 2006;26(1):41–50.

58. Sherer TB, Betarbet R, Stout AK, et al. An in vitro model of Parkinson's disease: Linking mitochondrial impairment to altered alpha-synuclein metabolism and oxidative damage. *J Neurosci.* 2002;22(16):7006–7015.

59. Junn E, Lee KW, Jeong BS, Chan TW, Im JY, Mouradian MM. Repression of alpha-synuclein expression and toxicity by microRNA-7. *Proc Natl Acad Sci U S A.* 2009;106(31):13052–13057.

60. Esteves AR, Arduino DM, Swerdlow RH, Oliveira CR, Cardoso SM. Oxidative Stress involvement in alpha-synuclein oligomerization in Parkinsons disease cybrids. *Antioxid Redox Signal.* 2008;11(3):439–448.

61. Fountaine TM, Venda LL, Warrick N, et al. The effect of alpha-synuclein knockdown on MPP+ toxicity in models of human neurons. *Eur J Neurosci.* 2008;28(12):2459–2473.

62. Wu F, Poon WS, Lu G, et al. Alpha-synuclein knockdown attenuates MPP(+) induced mitochondrial dysfunction of SH-SY5Y cells. *Brain Res.* 2009;1292:173–179.

63. Ma L, Cao TT, Kandpal G, et al. Genome-wide microarray analysis of the differential neuroprotective effects of antioxidants in neuroblastoma cells overexpressing the familial Parkinson's Disease alpha-Synuclein A53T mutation. *Neurochem Res.* 2009;35:130–142.

64. Lee MK, Stirling W, Xu Y, et al. Human alpha-synuclein-harboring familial Parkinson's disease-linked Ala-53 --> Thr mutation causes neurodegenerative disease with alpha-synuclein aggregation in transgenic mice. *Proc Natl Acad Sci U S A.* 2002;99(13):8968–8973.

65. Martin-Clemente B, Alvarez-Castelao B, Mayo I, et al. Alpha-synuclein expression levels do not significantly affect proteasome function and expression in mice and stably transfected PC12 cell lines. *J Biol Chem.* 2004;279(51):52984–52990.

66. Dyllick-Brenzinger M, D'Souza CA, Dahlmann B, Kloetzel PM, Tandon A. Reciprocal effects of alpha-synuclein overexpression and proteasome inhibition in neuronal cells and tissue. *Neurotox Res.* 2010;17(3):215–227.

67. Kim C, Lee SJ. Controlling the mass action of alpha-synuclein in Parkinson's disease. *J Neurochem.* 2008;107(2):303–316.

68. Xilouri M, Vogiatzi T, Vekrellis K, Stefanis L. alpha-synuclein degradation by autophagic pathways: A potential key to Parkinson's disease pathogenesis. *Autophagy.* 2008;4(7):917–919.

69. Tessari I, Bisaglia M, Valle F, et al. The reaction of alpha-synuclein with tyrosinase: Possible implications for Parkinson disease. *J Biol Chem.* 2008;283(24):16808–16817.

70. Kawahara K, Hashimoto M, Bar-On P, et al. Alpha-synuclein aggregates interfere with Parkin solubility and distribution: Role in the pathogenesis of Parkinson disease. *J Biol Chem.* 2008;283(11):6979–6987.

71. Gegg ME, Cooper JM, Schapira AH, Taanman JW. Silencing of PINK1 expression affects mitochondrial DNA and oxidative phosphorylation in dopaminergic cells. *PLoS One.* 2009;4(3):e4756.

72. Gandhi S, Muqit MM, Stanyer L, et al. PINK1 protein in normal human brain and Parkinson's disease. *Brain.* 2006;129(Pt 7):1720–1731.

73. Marongiu R, Spencer B, Crews L, et al. Mutant Pink1 induces mitochondrial dysfunction in a neuronal cell model of Parkinson's disease by disturbing calcium flux. *J Neurochem.* 2009;108(6):1561–1574.

74. Liu W, Vives-Bauza C, Acin-Perez R, et al. PINK1 defect causes mitochondrial dysfunction, proteasomal deficit and alpha-synuclein aggregation in cell culture models of Parkinson's disease. *PLoS One.* 2009;4(2):e4597.

75. Mitsui T, Kuroda Y, Kaji R. Parkin and mitochondria. *Brain Nerve.* 2008;60(8):923–929.

76. Jiang H, Ren Y, Yuen EY, et al. Parkin controls dopamine utilization in human midbrain dopaminergic neurons derived from induced pluripotent stem cells. *Nat Commun.* 2012;3:668.

77. Lee RC, Feinbaum RL, Ambros V. The C. elegans heterochronic gene lin-4 encodes small RNAs with antisense complementarity to lin-14. *Cell.* 1993;75(5):843–854.

78. Wightman B, Ha I, Ruvkun G. Posttranscriptional regulation of the heterochronic gene lin-14 by lin-4 mediates temporal pattern formation in C. elegans. *Cell.* 1993;75(5):855–862.

79. Macfarlane LA, Murphy PR. MicroRNA: Biogenesis, function and role in cancer. *Curr Genomics.* 2010;11(7):537–561.

80. Londin E, Loher P, Telonis AG, et al. Analysis of 13 cell types reveals evidence for the expression of numerous novel primate- and tissue-specific microRNAs. *Proc Natl Acad Sci U S A.* 2015;112(10):E1106–E1115.

81. Denli AM, Tops BB, Plasterk RH, Ketting RF, Hannon GJ. Processing of primary microRNAs by the Microprocessor complex. *Nature.* 2004;432(7014):231–235.

82. Lee Y, Ahn C, Han J, et al. The nuclear RNase III Drosha initiates microRNA processing. *Nature.* 2003;425(6956):415–419.

83. Hutvagner G, McLachlan J, Pasquinelli AE, Balint E, Tuschl T, Zamore PD. A cellular function for the RNA-interference enzyme Dicer in the maturation of the let-7 small temporal RNA. *Science.* 2001;293(5531):834–838.

84. Bartel DP. MicroRNAs: Genomics, biogenesis, mechanism, and function. *Cell.* 2004;116(2):281–297.

85. Kabaria S, Choi DC, Chaudhuri AD, Jain MR, Li H, Junn E. MicroRNA-7 activates Nrf2 pathway by targeting Keap1 expression. *Free Radic Biol Medicine.* 2015;89:548–556.

86. Doxakis E. Post-transcriptional regulation of alpha-synuclein expression by mir-7 and mir-153. *J Biol Chem.* 2010;285(17):12726–12734.

87. Villar-Menendez I, Porta S, Buira SP, et al. Increased striatal adenosine A2A receptor levels is an early event in Parkinson's disease-related pathology and it is potentially regulated by miR-34b. *Neurobiol Dis.* 2014;69:206–214.

88. Fragkouli A, Doxakis E. miR-7 and miR-153 protect neurons against MPP(+)-induced cell death via upregulation of mTOR pathway. *Front Cell Neurosci.* 2014;8:182.

89. Li G, Yang H, Zhu D, Huang H, Liu G, Lun P. Targeted suppression of chaperone-mediated autophagy by miR-320a promotes alpha-synuclein aggregation. *Int J Mol Sci.* 2014;15(9):15845–15857.

90. Zhang Z, Cheng Y. miR-16-1 promotes the aberrant alpha-synuclein accumulation in parkinson disease via targeting heat shock protein 70. *ScientificWorldJournal.* 2014;2014:938348.

91. Choi DC, Chae YJ, Kabaria S, et al. MicroRNA-7 protects against 1-methyl-4-phenylpyridinium-induced cell death by targeting RelA. *J Neurosci: Off J Soc Neurosci.* 2014;34(38):12725–12737.

92. Kim W, Lee Y, McKenna ND, et al. miR-126 contributes to Parkinson's disease by dysregulating the insulin-like growth factor/phosphoinositide 3-kinase signaling. *Neurobiol Aging.* 2014;35(7):1712–1721.

93. Jiang M, Yun Q, Shi F, et al. Down-regulation of miR-384-5p attenuates rotenone-induced neurotoxicity in dopaminergic SH-SY5Y cells through inhibiting endoplasmic reticulum stress. *Am J Physiol Cell Physiol.* 2016. doi:10.1152/ajpcell.00226.2015.

94. Wang H, Ye Y, Zhu Z, et al. MiR-124 regulates apoptosis and autophagy process in MPTP model of Parkinson's disease by targeting to Bim. *Brain Pathol.* 2016;26(2):167–176.

95. Kanagaraj N, Beiping H, Dheen ST, Tay SS. Downregulation of miR-124 in MPTP-treated mouse model of Parkinson's disease and MPP iodide-treated MN9D cells modulates the expression of the calpain/cdk5 pathway proteins. *Neuroscience.* 2014;272:167–179.

96. Xiong R, Wang Z, Zhao Z, et al. MicroRNA-494 reduces DJ-1 expression and exacerbates neurodegeneration. *Neurobiol Aging.* 2014;35(3):705–714.

97. Cho HJ, Liu G, Jin SM, et al. MicroRNA-205 regulates the expression of Parkinson's disease-related leucine-rich repeat kinase 2 protein. *Hum Mol Genet.* 2013;22(3):608–620.

98. Minones-Moyano E, Porta S, Escaramis G, et al. MicroRNA profiling of Parkinson's disease brains identifies early downregulation of miR-34b/c which modulate mitochondrial function. *Hum Mol Genet.* 2011;20(15):3067–3078.

99. Kabaria S, Choi DC, Chaudhuri AD, Mouradian MM, Junn E. Inhibition of miR-34b and miR-34c enhances alpha-synuclein expression in Parkinson's disease. *FEBS Lett.* 2015;589(3):319–325.

100. Ha TY. MicroRNAs in human diseases: From autoimmune diseases to skin, psychiatric, and neurodegenerative diseases. *Immune Netw.* 2011;11(5):227–244.

101. Capelli LP, Goncalves MR, Leite CC, Barbosa ER, Nitrini R, Vianna-Morgante AM. The fragile X-associated tremor and ataxia syndrome (FXTAS). *Arq Neuropsiquiatr.* 2010;68(5):791–798.

102. Hagerman PJ, Hagerman RJ. Fragile X-associated tremor/ataxia syndrome (FXTAS). *Ment Retard Dev Disabil Res Rev.* 2004;10(1):25–30.

103. Zongaro S, Hukema R, D'Antoni S, et al. The 3' UTR of FMR1 mRNA is a target of miR-101, miR-129-5p and miR-221: Implications for the molecular pathology of FXTAS at the synapse. *Hum Mol Genet.* 2013;22(10):1971–1982.

104. Hernandez-Rapp J, Rainone S, Hebert SS. MicroRNAs underlying memory deficits in neurodegenerative disorders. *Prog Neuropsychopharmacol Biol Psychiatry.* 2016;73:79–86.

105. Nguyen LS, Lepleux M, Makhlouf M, et al. Profiling olfactory stem cells from living patients identifies miRNAs relevant for autism pathophysiology. *Mol Autism.* 2016;7:1.
106. Siegert S, Seo J, Kwon EJ, et al. The schizophrenia risk gene product miR-137 alters presynaptic plasticity. *Nat Neurosci.* 2015;18(7):1008–1016.
107. Fernandez-Santiago R, Iranzo A, Gaig C, et al. MicroRNA association with synucleinopathy conversion in rapid eye movement behavior disorder. *Ann Neurol.* 2015;77(5):895–901.
108. Prasad KN, Bondy SC. Inhibition of early upstream events in prodromal Alzheimer's disease by use of targeted antioxidants. *Curr Aging Sci.* 2014;7(2):77–90.
109. Dexter DT, Holley AE, Flitter WD, et al. Increased levels of lipid hydroperoxides in the parkinsonian substantia nigra: An HPLC and ESR study. *Mov Disord.* 1994;9(1):92–97.
110. Dexter DT, Carter CJ, Wells FR, et al. Basal lipid peroxidation in substantia nigra is increased in Parkinson's disease. *J Neurochem.* 1989;52(2):381–389.
111. Sanchez-Ramos J, Overvik E, Ames B. A marker of oxyradical-mediated DNA damage (8-hydroxy-2'-deoxyguanosine) is increased in nigro-striatum of Parkinson's disease brain. *Neurodegeneration.* 1994;3:197–204.
112. Ebadi M, Srinivasan SK, Baxi MD. Oxidative stress and antioxidant therapy in Parkinson's disease. *Prog Neurobiol.* 1996;48(1):1–19.
113. Ambani LM, Van Woert MH, Murphy S. Brain peroxidase and catalase in Parkinson disease. *Arch Neurol.* 1975;32(2):114–118.
114. Kish SJ, Morito C, Hornykiewicz O. Glutathione peroxidase activity in Parkinson's disease brain. *Neurosci Lett.* 1985;58(3):343–346.
115. Riederer P, Sofic E, Rausch WD, et al. Transition metals, ferritin, glutathione, and ascorbic acid in parkinsonian brains. *J Neurochem.* 1989;52(2):515–520.
116. Perry TL, Godin DV, Hansen S. Parkinson's disease: A disorder due to nigral glutathione deficiency? *Neurosci Lett.* 1982;33(3):305–310.
117. Sofic E, Lange KW, Jellinger K, Riederer P. Reduced and oxidized glutathione in the substantia nigra of patients with Parkinson's disease. *Neurosci Lett.* 1992;142(2):128–130.
118. Chen CM, Liu JL, Wu YR, et al. Increased oxidative damage in peripheral blood correlates with severity of Parkinson's disease. *Neurobiol Dis.* 2009;33(3):429–435.
119. Sanyal J, Bandyopadhyay SK, Banerjee TK, et al. Plasma levels of lipid peroxides in patients with Parkinson's disease. *Eur Rev Med Pharmacol Sci.* 2009;13(2):129–132.
120. Sian J, Dexter DT, Lees AJ, et al. Alterations in glutathione levels in Parkinson's disease and other neurodegenerative disorders affecting basal ganglia. *Ann Neurol.* 1994;36(3):348–355.
121. Jenner P. Oxidative mechanisms in nigral cell death in Parkinson's disease. *Mov Disord.* 1998;13 Suppl 1:24–34.
122. Fitzmaurice PS, Ang L, Guttman M, Rajput AH, Furukawa Y, Kish SJ. Nigral glutathione deficiency is not specific for idiopathic Parkinson's disease. *Mov Disord.* 2003;18(9):969–976.
123. Fessel JP, Hulette C, Powell S, Roberts LJ, 2nd, Zhang J. Isofurans, but not F2-isoprostanes, are increased in the substantia nigra of patients with Parkinson's disease and with dementia with Lewy body disease. *J Neurochem.* 2003;85(3):645–650.
124. Schipper HM, Liberman A, Stopa EG. Neural heme oxygenase-1 expression in idiopathic Parkinson's disease. *Exp Neurol.* 1998;150(1):60–68.
125. Sofic E, Sapcanin A, Tahirovic I, et al. Antioxidant capacity in postmortem brain tissues of Parkinson's and Alzheimer's diseases. *J Neural Transm Suppl.* 2006;(71):39–43.
126. Varghese M, Pandey M, Samanta A, Gangopadhyay PK, Mohanakumar KP. Reduced NADH coenzyme Q dehydrogenase activity in platelets of Parkinson's disease, but not Parkinson plus patients, from an Indian population. *J Neurol Sci.* 2009;279(1–2):39–42.
127. Fernandez-Calle P, Jimenez-Jimenez FJ, Molina JA, et al. Serum levels of ascorbic acid (vitamin C) in patients with Parkinson's disease. *J Neurol Sci.* ;118(1):25–28.
128. Fernandez-Calle P, Molina JA, Jimenez-Jimenez FJ, et al. Serum levels of alpha-tocopherol (vitamin E) in Parkinson's disease. *Neurology.* 1992;42(5):1064–1066.
129. King D, Playfer JR, Roberts NB. Concentrations of vitamins A, C and E in elderly patients with Parkinson's disease. *Postgrad Med J.* 1992;68(802):634–637.
130. Paraskevas GP, Kapaki E, Petropoulou O, Anagnostouli M, Vagenas V, Papageorgiou C. Plasma levels of antioxidant vitamins C and E are decreased in vascular parkinsonism. *J Neurol Sci.* 2003;215(1–2):51–55.
131. Double KL, Gerlach M, Youdim MB, Riederer P. Impaired iron homeostasis in Parkinson's disease. *J Neural Transm Suppl.* 2000;60:37–58.

132. Graham JM, Paley MN, Grunewald RA, Hoggard N, Griffiths PD. Brain iron deposition in Parkinson's disease imaged using the PRIME magnetic resonance sequence. *Brain*. 2000;123 Pt 12:2423–2431.
133. Andersen JK. Iron dysregulation and Parkinson's disease. *J Alzheimers Dis*. 2004;6(6 Suppl):S47–S52.
134. Salazar J, Mena N, Hunot S, et al. Divalent metal transporter 1 (DMT1) contributes to neurodegeneration in animal models of Parkinson's disease. *Proc Natl Acad Sci U S A*. 2008;105(47):18578–18583.
135. Prabhakaran K, Ghosh D, Chapman GD, Gunasekar PG. Molecular mechanism of manganese exposure-induced dopaminergic toxicity. *Brain Res Bull*. 2008;76(4):361–367.
136. Enochs WS, Sarna T, Zecca L, Riley PA, Swartz HM. The roles of neuromelanin, binding of metal ions, and oxidative cytotoxicity in the pathogenesis of Parkinson's disease: A hypothesis. *J Neural Transm Park Dis Dement Sect*. 1994;7(2):83–100.
137. Good PF, Olanow CW, Perl DP. Neuromelanin-containing neurons of the substantia nigra accumulate iron and aluminum in Parkinson's disease: A LAMMA study. *Brain Res*. 1992;593(2):343–346.
138. Ebadi M, Sharma SK. Peroxynitrite and mitochondrial dysfunction in the pathogenesis of Parkinson's disease. *Antioxid Redox Signal*. 2003;5(3):319–335.
139. Arduino DM, Esteves AR, Cardoso SM, Oliveira CR. Endoplasmic reticulum and mitochondria interplay mediates apoptotic cell death: Relevance to Parkinson's disease. *Neurochem Int*. 2009;55(5):341–348.
140. Gubellini P, Picconi B, Di Filippo M, Calabresi P. Downstream mechanisms triggered by mitochondrial dysfunction in the basal ganglia: From experimental models to neurodegenerative diseases. *Biochim Biophys Acta*. 2009;1802(1):151–161.
141. Gautier CA, Kitada T, Shen J. Loss of PINK1 causes mitochondrial functional defects and increased sensitivity to oxidative stress. *Proc Natl Acad Sci U S A*. 2008;105(32):11364–11369.
142. Lee SJ. Alpha-synuclein aggregation: A link between mitochondrial defects and Parkinson's disease? *Antioxid Redox Signal*. 2003;5(3):337–348.
143. Banerjee R, Starkov AA, Beal MF, Thomas B. Mitochondrial dysfunction in the limelight of Parkinson's disease pathogenesis. *Biochim Biophys Acta*. 2009;1792(7):651–663.
144. Yang JL, Weissman L, Bohr VA, Mattson MP. Mitochondrial DNA damage and repair in neurodegenerative disorders. *DNA Repair (Amst)*. 2008;7(7):1110–1120.
145. Perier C, Bove J, Wu DC, et al. Two molecular pathways initiate mitochondria-dependent dopaminergic neurodegeneration in experimental Parkinson's disease. *Proc Natl Acad Sci U S A*. 2007;104(19):8161–8166.
146. Domingues AF, Arduino DM, Esteves AR, Swerdlow RH, Oliveira CR, Cardoso SM. Mitochondria and ubiquitin-proteasomal system interplay: Relevance to Parkinson's disease. *Free Radic Biol Med*. 2008;45(6):820–825.
147. Whitton PS. Inflammation as a causative factor in the aetiology of Parkinson's disease. *Br J Pharmacol*. 2007;150(8):963–976.
148. McGeer PL, McGeer EG. Glial reactions in Parkinson's disease. *Mov Disord*. 2008;23(4):474–483.
149. Reynolds AD, Glanzer JG, Kadiu I, et al. Nitrated alpha-synuclein-activated microglial profiling for Parkinson's disease. *J Neurochem*. 2008;104(6):1504–1525.
150. Zhang W, Wang T, Pei Z, et al. Aggregated alpha-synuclein activates microglia: A process leading to disease progression in Parkinson's disease. *FASEB J*. 2005;19(6):533–542.
151. Roodveldt C, Christodoulou J, Dobson CM. Immunological features of alpha-synuclein in Parkinson's disease. *J Cell Mol Med*. 2008;12(5B):1820–1829.
152. Gao HM, Kotzbauer PT, Uryu K, Leight S, Trojanowski JQ, Lee VM. Neuroinflammation and oxidation/nitration of alpha-synuclein linked to dopaminergic neurodegeneration. *J Neurosci*. 2008;28(30):7687–7698.
153. Sawada M, Imamura K, Nagatsu T. Role of cytokines in inflammatory process in Parkinson's disease. *J Neural Transm Suppl*. 2006;(70):373–381.
154. Wilms H, Zecca L, Rosenstiel P, Sievers J, Deuschl G, Lucius R. Inflammation in Parkinson's diseases and other neurodegenerative diseases: Cause and therapeutic implications. *Curr Pharm Des*. 2007;13(18):1925–1928.
155. Prasad KN, Hovland AR, La Rosa FG, Hovland PG. Prostaglandins as putative neurotoxins in Alzheimer's disease. *Proc Soc Exp Biol Med*. 1998;219(2):120–125.
156. Chae SW, Kang BY, Hwang O, Choi HJ. Cyclooxygenase-2 is involved in oxidative damage and alpha-synuclein accumulation in dopaminergic cells. *Neurosci Lett*. 2008;436(2):205–209.
157. Blandini F, Porter RH, Greenamyre JT. Glutamate and Parkinson's disease. *Mol Neurobiol*. 1996;12(1):73–94.
158. Schubert D, Kimura H, Maher P. Growth factors and vitamin E modify neuronal glutamate toxicity. *Proc Natl Acad Sci U S A*. 1992;89(17):8264–8267.

159. Sandhu JK, Pandey S, Ribecco-Lutkiewicz M, et al. Molecular mechanisms of glutamate neurotoxicity in mixed cultures of NT2-derived neurons and astrocytes: Protective effects of coenzyme Q10. *J Neurosci Res*. 2003;72(6):691–703.

160. Meredith GE, Totterdell S, Beales M, Meshul CK. Impaired glutamate homeostasis and programmed cell death in a chronic MPTP mouse model of Parkinson's disease. *Exp Neurol*. 2009;219(1):334–340.

161. Bonsi P, Cuomo D, Picconi B, et al. Striatal metabotropic glutamate receptors as a target for pharmacotherapy in Parkinson's disease. *Amino Acids*. 2007;32(2):189–195.

162. Ossowska K, Konieczny J, Wardas J, et al. An influence of ligands of metabotropic glutamate receptor subtypes on parkinsonian-like symptoms and the striatopallidal pathway in rats. *Amino Acids*. 2007;32(2):179–188.

163. Ono K, Yamada M. Vitamin A potently destabilizes preformed alpha-synuclein fibrils in vitro: Implications for Lewy body diseases. *Neurobiol Dis*. 2007;25(2):446–454.

164. Park ES, Kim SY, Na JI, et al. Glutathione prevented dopamine-induced apoptosis of melanocytes and its signaling. *J Dermatol Sci*. 2007;47(2):141–149.

165. Khaldy H, Escames G, Leon J, Vives F, Luna JD, Acuna-Castroviejo D. Comparative effects of melatonin, L-deprenyl, Trolox, and ascorbate in the suppression of hydroxyl radical formation during dopamine autoxidation *in vitro*. *J Pineal Res*. 2000;29(2):100–107.

166. Ehrhart J, Zeevalk GD. Cooperative interaction between ascorbate and glutathione during mitochondrial impairment in mesencephalic cultures. *J Neurochem*. 2003;86(6):1487–1497.

167. Penugonda S, Mare S, Goldstein G, Banks WA, Ercal N. Effects of N-acetylcysteine amide (NACA), a novel thiol antioxidant against glutamate-induced cytotoxicity in neuronal cell line PC12. *Brain Res*. 2005;1056(2):132–138.

168. Cadet JL, Katz M, Jackson-Lewis V, Fahn S. Vitamin E attenuates the toxic effects of intrastriatal injection of 6-hydroxydopamine (6-OHDA) in rats: Behavioral and biochemical evidence. *Brain Res*. 1989;476(1):10–15.

169. Heim C, Kolasiewicz W, Kurz T, Sontag KH. Behavioral alterations after unilateral 6-hydroxydopamine lesions of the striatum. Effect of alpha-tocopherol. *Pol J Pharmacol*. 2001;53(5):435–448.

170. Hanson AJ, Prasad JE, Nahreini P, et al. Overexpression of amyloid precursor protein is associated with degeneration, decreased viability, and increased damage caused by neurotoxins (prostaglandins A1 and E2, hydrogen peroxide, and nitric oxide) in differentiated neuroblastoma cells. *J Neurosci Res*. 2003;74(1):148–159.

171. Pasbakhsh P, Omidi N, Mehrannia K, et al. The protective effect of vitamin E on locus coeruleus in early model of Parkinson's disease in rat: Immunoreactivity evidence. *Iran Biomed J*. 2008;12(4):217–222.

172. Roghani M, Behzadi G. Neuroprotective effect of vitamin E on the early model of Parkinson's disease in rat: Behavioral and histochemical evidence. *Brain Res*. 2001;892(1):211–217.

173. Silva-Adaya D, Perez-De La Cruz V, Herrera-Mundo MN, et al. Excitotoxic damage, disrupted energy metabolism, and oxidative stress in the rat brain: Antioxidant and neuroprotective effects of L-carnitine. *J Neurochem*. 2008;105(3):677–689.

174. Virmani A, Gaetani F, Binienda Z. Effects of metabolic modifiers such as carnitines, coenzyme Q10, and PUFAs against different forms of neurotoxic insults: Metabolic inhibitors, MPTP, and methamphetamine. *Ann N Y Acad Sci*. 2005;1053:183–191.

175. Clark J, Clore EL, Zheng K, Adame A, Masliah E, Simon DK. Oral N-acetylcysteine attenuates loss of dopaminergic terminals in alpha-synuclein overexpressing mice. *PLoS ONE*. 2010;5(8):e12333.

176. Guarente L. Sirtuins in aging and disease. *Cold Spring Harb Symp Quant Biol*. 2007;72:483–488.

177. Ferretta A, Gaballo A, Tanzarella P, et al. Effect of resveratrol on mitochondrial function: Implications in parkin-associated familiar Parkinson's disease. *Biochim Biophys Acta*. 2014;1842(7):902–915.

178. Muthian G, King, J, Mackey, V, Prasad, K, Charlton, CG. Blockage of the proposed precipitating stage for Parkinson's disease by antioxidants. A potential preventive measure for PD. *FASEB J*. 2008;Publication number 715.2.

179. Liu Z, Yu Y, Li X, Ross CA, Smith WW. Curcumin protects against A53T alpha-synuclein-induced toxicity in a PC12 inducible cell model for Parkinsonism. *Pharmacol Res*. 2011;63(5):439–444.

180. Jiang TF, Zhang YJ, Zhou HY, et al. Curcumin ameliorates the neurodegenerative pathology in A53T alpha-synuclein cell model of Parkinson's disease through the downregulation of mTOR/p70S6K signaling and the recovery of macroautophagy. *J Neuroimmune Pharmacol*. 2013;8(1):356–369.

181. Haleagrahara N, Siew CJ, Ponnusamy K. Effect of quercetin and desferrioxamine on 6-hydroxydopamine (6-OHDA) induced neurotoxicity in striatum of rats. *J Toxicol Sci*. 2013;38(1):25–33.

182. Antala BV, Patel MS, Bhuva SV, Gupta S, Rabadiya S, Lahkar M. Protective effect of methanolic extract of Garcinia indica fruits in 6-OHDA rat model of Parkinson's disease. *Indian J Pharmacol.* 2012;44(6):683–687.

183. Perez HJ, Carrillo SC, Garcia E, Ruiz-Mar G, Perez-Tamayo R, Chavarria A. Neuroprotective effect of silymarin in a MPTP mouse model of Parkinson's disease. *Toxicology.* 2014;319:38–43.

184. Geed M, Garabadu D, Ahmad A, Krishnamurthy S. Silibinin pretreatment attenuates biochemical and behavioral changes induced by intrastriatal MPP+ injection in rats. *Pharmacol Biochem Behav.* 2014;117:92–103.

185. Liu D, Pitta M, Mattson MP. Preventing NAD(+) depletion protects neurons against excitotoxicity: Bioenergetic effects of mild mitochondrial uncoupling and caloric restriction. *Ann N Y Acad Sci.* 2008;1147:275–282.

186. Jia H, Li X, Gao H, et al. High doses of nicotinamide prevent oxidative mitochondrial dysfunction in a cellular model and improve motor deficit in a Drosophila model of Parkinson's disease. *J Neurosci Res.* 2008;86(9):2083–2090.

187. Ortiz GG, Pacheco-Moises, FP., Gomez-Rodriguez, VM., Gonzalez-Renovato, ED, Torres-Sanchez, ED, Ramirez-Anguiano, AC. Fish oil, Melatonin and vitamin E attenuates midbrain cyclooxygenase-2 activity and oxidative stress after administration of 1-methyl-4-phenyl-1,2,3,6-tetrahydropyridine. *Matab Brain Dis.* 2013, (Epub ahead of publication).

188. Zhang SM, Hernan MA, Chen H, Spiegelman D, Willett WC, Ascherio A. Intakes of vitamins E and C, carotenoids, vitamin supplements, and PD risk. *Neurology.* 2002;59(8):1161–1169.

189. Etminan M, Gill SS, Samii A. Intake of vitamin E, vitamin C, and carotenoids and the risk of Parkinson's disease: A meta-analysis. *Lancet Neurol.* 2005;4(6):362–365.

190. Shoulson I. DATATOP: A decade of neuroprotective inquiry. Parkinson study group. Deprenyl and tocopherol antioxidative therapy of parkinsonism. *Ann Neurol.* 1998;44(3 Suppl 1):S160–S166.

191. Group TPS. Effects of tocopherol and deprenyl on the progression of disability in early parkinson's disease. *N Engl J Med.* 1993;328(3):176–183.

192. Prasad KN, Hernandez C, Edwards-Prasad J, Nelson J, Borus T, Robinson WA. Modification of the effect of tamoxifen, cis-platin, DTIC, and interferon-alpha 2b on human melanoma cells in culture by a mixture of vitamins. *Nutr Cancer.* 1994;22(3):233–245.

193. Prasad KN, Kumar R. Effect of individual and multiple antioxidant vitamins on growth and morphology of human nontumorigenic and tumorigenic parotid acinar cells in culture. *Nutr Cancer.* 1996;26(1):11–19.

194. Fahn S. A pilot trial of high-dose alpha-tocopherol and ascorbate in early Parkinson's disease. *Ann Neurol.* 1992;32 Suppl:S128–S132.

195. Shults CW, Oakes D, Kieburtz K, et al. Effects of coenzyme Q10 in early Parkinson disease: Evidence of slowing of the functional decline. *Arch Neurol.* 2002;59(10):1541–1550.

196. Weber CA, Ernst ME. Antioxidants, supplements, and Parkinson's disease. *Ann Pharmacother.* 2006;40(5):935–938.

197. Storch A, Jost WH, Vieregge P, et al. Randomized, double-blind, placebo-controlled trial on symptomatic effects of coenzyme Q(10) in Parkinson disease. *Arch Neurol.* 2007;64(7):938–944.

198. Lohr JB, Caligiuri MP. A double-blind placebo-controlled study of vitamin E treatment of tardive dyskinesia. *J Clin Psychiatry.* 1996;57(4):167–173.

199. Swerdlow RH. Is NADH effective in the treatment of Parkinson's disease? *Drugs Aging.* 1998;13(4):263–268.

200. Vile GF, Winterbourn CC. Inhibition of adriamycin-promoted microsomal lipid peroxidation by beta-carotene, alpha-tocopherol, and retinol at high and low oxygen partial pressures. *FEBS Lett.* 1988;238(2):353–356.

201. Niki E. Interaction of ascorbate and alpha-tocopherol. *Ann N Y Acad Sci.* 1987;498:186–199.

202. Prasad KN. Oxidative stress and pro-inflammatory cytokines may act as one of signals for regulating MicroRNAs expression in Alzheimer's disease. *Mech Ageing Dev.* 2017;162:63–71.

203. Wu H, Kong L, Tan Y, et al. C66 ameliorates diabetic nephropathy in mice by both upregulating NRF2 function via increase in miR-200a and inhibiting miR-21. *Diabetologia.* 2016;59:1558–1568.

204. Jaramillo MC, Zhang DD. The emerging role of the Nrf2-Keap1 signaling pathway in cancer. *Genes Dev.* 2013;27(20):2179–2191.

205. Williamson TP, Johnson DA, Johnson JA. Activation of the Nrf2-ARE pathway by siRNA knockdown of Keap1 reduces oxidative stress and provides partial protection from MPTP-mediated neurotoxicity. *Neurotoxicology.* 2012;33(3):272–279.

206. Itoh K, Chiba T, Takahashi S, et al. An Nrf2/small Maf heterodimer mediates the induction of phase II detoxifying enzyme genes through antioxidant response elements. *Biochem Biophys Res Commun.* 1997;236(2):313–322.

207. Hayes JD, Chanas SA, Henderson CJ, et al. The Nrf2 transcription factor contributes both to the basal expression of glutathione S-transferases in mouse liver and to their induction by the chemopreventive synthetic antioxidants, butylated hydroxyanisole, and ethoxyquin. *Biochem Soc Trans.* 2000;28(2):33–41.

208. Chan K, Han XD, Kan YW. An important function of Nrf2 in combating oxidative stress: Detoxification of acetaminophen. *Proc Natl Acad Sci USA.* 2001;98(8):4611–4616.

209. Ramsey CP, Glass CA, Montgomery MB, et al. Expression of Nrf2 in neurodegenerative diseases. *J Neuropathol Exp Neurol.* 2007;66(1):75–85.

210. Chen PC, Vargas MR, Pani AK, et al. Nrf2-mediated neuroprotection in the MPTP mouse model of Parkinson's disease: Critical role for the astrocyte. *Proc Natl Acad Sci U S A.* 2009;106(8):2933–2938.

211. Lastres-Becker I, Ulusoy A, Innamorato NG, et al. Alpha-synuclein expression and Nrf2 deficiency cooperate to aggravate protein aggregation, neuronal death, and inflammation in early-stage Parkinson's disease. *Hum Mol Genet.* 2012;21(14):3173–3192.

212. Xi YD, Yu HL, Ding J, et al. Flavonoids protect cerebrovascular endothelial cells through Nrf2 and PI3K from beta-amyloid peptide-induced oxidative damage. *Curr Neurovasc Res.* 2012;9(1):32–41.

213. Suh JH, Shenvi SV, Dixon BM, et al. Decline in transcriptional activity of Nrf2 causes age-related loss of glutathione synthesis, which is reversible with lipoic acid. *Proc Natl Acad Sci U S A.* 2004;101(10):3381–3386.

214. Trujillo J, Chirino YI, Molina-Jijon E, Anderica-Romero AC, Tapia E, Pedraza-Chaverri J. Renoprotective effect of the antioxidant curcumin: Recent findings. *Redox Biol.* 2013;1(1):448–456.

215. Steele ML, Fuller S, Patel M, Kersaitis C, Ooi L, Munch G. Effect of Nrf2 activators on release of glutathione, cysteinylglycine, and homocysteine by human U373 astroglial cells. *Redox Biol.* 2013;1(1):441–445.

216. Kode A, Rajendrasozhan S, Caito S, Yang SR, Megson IL, Rahman I. Resveratrol induces glutathione synthesis by activation of Nrf2 and protects against cigarette smoke-mediated oxidative stress in human lung epithelial cells. *Am J Physiol. Lung Cell Mol Physiol.* 2008;294(3):L478–L488.

217. Gao L, Wang J, Sekhar KR, et al. Novel n-3 fatty acid oxidation products activate Nrf2 by destabilizing the association between Keap1 and Cullin3. *J Biol Chem.* 2007;282(4):2529–2537.

218. Saw CL, Yang AY, Guo Y, Kong AN. Astaxanthin and omega-3 fatty acids individually and in combination protect against oxidative stress via the Nrf2-ARE pathway. *Food Chem Toxicol.* 2013;62:869–875.

219. Song J, Kang SM, Lee WT, Park KA, Lee KM, Lee JE. Glutathione protects brain endothelial cells from hydrogen peroxide-induced oxidative stress by increasing nrf2 expression. *Exp Neurobiol.* 2014;23(1):93–103.

220. Ji L, Liu R, Zhang XD, et al. N-acetylcysteine attenuates phosgene-induced acute lung injury via up-regulation of Nrf2 expression. *Inhal Toxicol.* 2010;22(7):535–542.

221. Choi HK, Pokharel YR, Lim SC, et al. Inhibition of liver fibrosis by solubilized coenzyme Q10: Role of Nrf2 activation in inhibiting transforming growth factor-beta1 expression. *Toxicol Appl Pharmacol.* 2009;240(3):377–384.

222. Bai H, Liu R, Chen HL, et al. Enhanced antioxidant effect of caffeic acid phenethyl ester and Trolox in combination against radiation induced-oxidative stress. *Chem Biol Interact.* 2014;207:7–15.

223. Cui L, Jeong H, Borovecki F, Parkhurst CN, Tanese N, Krainc D. Transcriptional repression of PGC-1alpha by mutant huntingtin leads to mitochondrial dysfunction and neurodegeneration. *Cell.* 2006;127(1):59–69.

224. Li XH, Li CY, Lu JM, Tian RB, Wei J. Allicin ameliorates cognitive deficits ageing-induced learning and memory deficits through enhancing of Nrf2 antioxidant signaling pathways. *Neurosci Lett.* 2012;514(1):46–50.

225. Bergstrom P, Andersson HC, Gao Y, et al. Repeated transient sulforaphane stimulation in astrocytes leads to prolonged Nrf2-mediated gene expression and protection from superoxide-induced damage. *Neuropharmacology.* 2011;60(2–3):343–353.

226. Wruck CJ, Gotz ME, Herdegen T, Varoga D, Brandenburg LO, Pufe T. Kavalactones protect neural cells against amyloid beta peptide-induced neurotoxicity via extracellular signal-regulated kinase 1/2-dependent nuclear factor erythroid 2-related factor 2 activation. *Mol Pharmacol.* 2008;73(6):1785–1795.

227. Lou H, Jing X, Wei X, Shi H, Ren D, Zhang X. Naringenin protects against 6-OHDA-induced neurotoxicity via activation of the Nrf2/ARE signaling pathway. *Neuropharmacology.* 2013;79:380–388.

228. Li R, Liang T, Xu L, Zheng N, Zhang K, Duan X. Puerarin attenuates neuronal degeneration in the substantia nigra of 6-OHDA-lesioned rats through regulating BDNF expression and activating the Nrf2/ARE signaling pathway. *Brain Res.* 2013;1523:1–9.

229. Kim SS, Lim J, Bang Y, et al. Licochalcone E activates Nrf2/antioxidant response element signaling pathway in both neuronal and microglial cells: Therapeutic relevance to neurodegenerative disease. *J Nutr Biochem.* 2012;23(10):1314–1323.

230. He X, Wang L, Szklarz G, Bi Y, Ma Q. Resveratrol inhibits paraquat-induced oxidative stress and fibrogenic response by activating the nuclear factor erythroid 2-related factor 2 pathway. *J Pharmacol Exp Ther.* 2012;342(1):81–90.

231. Wang XL, Xing GH, Hong B, et al. Gastrodin prevents motor deficits and oxidative stress in the MPTP mouse model of Parkinson's disease: Involvement of ERK1/2-Nrf2 signaling pathway. *Life Sci.* 2014;114(2):77–85.

232. Lu C, Zhang J, Shi X, et al. Neuroprotective effects of tetramethylpyrazine against dopaminergic neuron injury in a rat model of Parkinson's disease induced by MPTP. *Int J Biol Sci.* 2014;10(4):350–357.

233. Kavitha M, Nataraj J, Essa MM, Memon MA, Manivasagam T. Mangiferin attenuates MPTP induced dopaminergic neurodegeneration and improves motor impairment, redox balance, and Bcl-2/Bax expression in experimental Parkinson's disease mice. *Chem Biol Interact.* 2013;206(2):239–247.

234. Barger SW, Goodwin ME, Porter MM, Beggs ML. Glutamate release from activated microglia requires the oxidative burst and lipid peroxidation. *J Neurochem.* 2007;101(5):1205–1213.

235. Dohare P, Hyzinski-Garcia MC, Vipani A, et al. The neuroprotective properties of the superoxide dismutase mimetic tempol correlate with its ability to reduce pathological glutamate release in a rodent model of stroke. *Free Radic Biol Med.* 2014;77:168–182.

236. Lu CW, Lin TY, Wang SJ. Quercetin inhibits depolarization-evoked glutamate release in nerve terminals from rat cerebral cortex. *Neurotoxicology.* 2013;39:1–9.

237. Hurtado O, De Cristobal J, Sanchez V, et al. Inhibition of glutamate release by delaying ATP fall accounts for neuroprotective effects of antioxidants in experimental stroke. *FASEB J.* 2003;17(14):2082–2084.

238. Santos PS, Campelo LM, Freitas RL, Feitosa CM, Saldanha GB, Freitas RM. Lipoic acid effects on glutamate and taurine concentrations in rat hippocampus after pilocarpine-induced seizures. *Arquivos de Neuro-psiquiatria.* 2011;69(2B):360–364.

239. Chang Y, Huang SK, Wang SJ. Coenzyme Q10 inhibits the release of glutamate in rat cerebrocortical nerve terminals by suppression of voltage-dependent calcium influx and mitogen-activated protein kinase signaling pathway. *J Agric Food Chem.* 2012;60(48):11909–11918.

240. Yang TT, Wang SJ. Pyridoxine inhibits depolarization-evoked glutamate release in nerve terminals from rat cerebral cortex: A possible neuroprotective mechanism? *J Pharmacol Exper Ther.* 2009;331(1):244–254.

241. Hung KL, Wang CC, Huang CY, Wang SJ. Cyanocobalamin, vitamin B12, depresses glutamate release through inhibition of voltage-dependent Ca2+ influx in rat cerebrocortical nerve terminals (synaptosomes). *Eur J Pharmacol.* 2009;602(2–3):230–237.

242. Wang SJ, Wu WM, Yang FL, Hsu GS, Huang CY. Vitamin B2 inhibits glutamate release from rat cerebrocortical nerve terminals. *Neuroreport.* 2008;19(13):1335–1338.

243. Behl C, Davis J, Cole GM, Schubert D. Vitamin E protects nerve cells from amyloid beta protein toxicity. *Biochem Biophys Res Commun.* 1992;186(2):944–950.

244. Prasad KN. Micronutrients in the prevention and improvement of the standard therapy for Alzheimer's disease. *Micronutrients in Health and Disease.* Boca Raton, FL: CRE Press; 2011.

11 Micronutrients in Prevention and Improvement of the Standard Therapy in Hearing Disorders

INTRODUCTION

Hearing disorders are a complex disease of the ear and include a partial or full loss of hearing, tinnitus, and Meniere's disease (MD). They are caused by advanced age, diverse groups of ototoxic agents, such as chronic and intense noise, vibrations, gentamicin, ionizing radiation, cisplatin, large doses of aspirin, bacterial and viral infection, and gene mutations. In addition, health conditions, such as ear canal obstruction, and mechanical damage to the tympanic membrane and ossicles of the middle ear and inner ear also contribute to the hearing loss.

Congenital hearing defects could be primarily due to cytomegalovirus infection during pregnancy or gene mutation. Troops in combat zones, musicians, or industrial workers are likely to develop varying degrees of hearing loss despite the use of earplugs. Thus, hearing problems represent a major health concern both for civilians and the military in the USA.

Except for ear protective devices, there are no preventive strategies for reducing the risk of noise-induced hearing loss (NIHL). However, despite the use of earplugs, the energy generated from the noise can penetrate the inner ear, damaging the hair cells. In order to develop an effective preventive strategy, the major cellular defects that initiate and promote hearing loss should be identified.

Several studies indicate that increased oxidative stress,[1–6] inflammation,[7–13] and glutamate level[14–16] play a central role in the initiation and progression of hearing defects. Therefore, reducing these biochemical defects simultaneously may be one of the rational strategies for the prevention of hearing disorders.

Since reactive oxygen species (ROS) and pro-inflammatory cytokines are involved in the development and progression of hearing disorders, and since these cellular events regulate the expressions of microRNAs in other neurodegenerative diseases, it is likely that alterations in the expressions of microRNAs and their target proteins might be involved in the pathogenesis of hearing loss.

Animal studies showed that the use of primarily one antioxidant reduced the risk of developing hearing loss.[17–24] However, a few human studies, using one or a mixture of a few arbitrarily selected antioxidants or steroids produced variable degrees of reduction in hearing loss with or without standard therapy.[25–31] The potential reasons for this discrepancy are discussed later in this chapter.

Since antioxidants provide varying degree of protection against hearing loss, and since antioxidants regulate the expressions of microRNAs and the levels of their target proteins in other diseases, it is likely that one of the mechanisms of protection against hearing loss by antioxidants may involve alterations in the expressions of microRNAs and their target proteins.

The treatment of hearing disorders includes steroids,[32,33] glutamate antagonist,[34,35] various types of hearing aids,[36–38] and cochlear transplants.[39,40] Although these treatments produce varying degrees of improvements, they are considered unsatisfactory. One of the reasons could be that none of these treatment modalities simultaneously reduce oxidative stress, chronic inflammation, and glutamate level. Therefore, the disease continue to progress. The central question remains how to attenuate these cellular defects at the same time.

A previous review has proposed that simultaneous elevation of the levels of antioxidant enzymes, and dietary and endogenous antioxidants may be necessary for optimally reducing oxidative stress, inflammation, and glutamate levels in human neurodegenerative diseases.[41] A similar strategy may be needed for reducing the risk and progression of hearing loss. Supplementation with micronutrients can increase the levels of antioxidants and reduce the release and toxicity of glutamate; however, elevating the levels of antioxidant enzymes requires an activation of a nuclear transcriptional factor-2 (Nrf2).

This chapter briefly describes incidence and cost, types of hearing loss, agents and conditions causing hearing disorders, linkage between increased oxidative stress, inflammation, and glutamate level, and presents evidence to show that increased oxidative stress, inflammation, and glutamate levels are involved in the pathogenesis of hearing disorders. This review also discusses the role of microRNAs in the development of hearing loss. It briefly discusses the regulation of activation of Nrf2 and proposes a mixture of micronutrients that can simultaneously activate Nrf2, enhance the levels of antioxidants, and reduce the release and toxicity of glutamate for the prevention, and in combination with standard care, for the improvement of the management of hearing defects.

PREVALENCE AND COST

PREVALENCE

The prevalence of hearing disorders in adults has increased from 28.6 million in 2000 to about 40 million in 2014.[42] Two to three per 1000 children born in the United States have detectable level of hearing loss.[43] About 50 million Americans experience symptoms of tinnitus. Approximately 20 million struggle with burdensome chronic tinnitus, while 2 million have an extreme and debilitating condition.[44]

In sudden sensorineural hearing loss (SSHL), also referred to as sudden deafness, a rapid hearing loss occurs within a few hours or over a period of 3 days.[45] The incidence of SSHL is estimated to be 5–20 cases per 100,000 persons.[46]

It has been estimated that about 0.2%–2% of the US population suffer from MD. The majority of the people with MD are over the age of 40 years. This disease equally affects men and women.

COST

It has been estimated that 1st year treatment cost of hearing disorders is expected to rise from $8.2 billion in 2002 to $51.4 billion in 2030. If 20% of noise-induced hearing loss is prevented, projected savings would be about $123 billion.[42]

TYPES OF HEARING DISORDERS

CONDUCTIVE HEARING LOSS

Conductive hearing loss may occur when sound is not transmitted properly through the outer or middle ear or both. This form of hearing loss is generally mild to moderate, because sound still can be detected by the inner ear. Conductive hearing loss occurs due to ear canal obstruction, damage to tympanic membrane and ossicles of the middle ear, injury to inner ear, and otosclerosis.

SENSORINEURAL HEARING LOSS

Sensorineural hearing loss is due to insensitivity of the inner ear, the cochlea, or to impaired function of the auditory nervous system. This form of hearing loss could be moderate to severe and can lead to complete deafness. The sensorineural hearing loss is caused due to damage to hair cells of the cochlea. It also can be caused by the damage to the VIII cranial nerve and the vestibulocochlear nerve.

TINNITUS

Injury to the hair cells can cause hearing loss, tinnitus, or balance problems. When hair cells are damaged, glutamate, an excitatory neurotransmitter responsible for converting vibration sound into electrical signal, is produced in excessive amounts. Excessive amounts of glutamate are very toxic to neurons. Damage to peripheral auditory and somatosensory systems causes imbalance between excitatory and inhibitory neurotransmitters in the mid brain auditory cortex and brain stem. This imbalance causes hyperactivity in the auditory cortex leading to the perception of phantom sounds (tinnitus).

MENIERE'S DISEASE (MD)

Meniere's disease (MD) is a disorder of the inner ear that can cause episodes of vertigo (the abnormal sensation of movement), dizziness, ringing in the ears (tinnitus), fluctuating and progressive hearing loss, balance problem, and a feeling of fullness or pressure. In addition to hearing loss, sounds may appear distorted in some patients experiencing unusual sensitivity to noises (hyperacusis). These changes can occur in one or both ears. This disease is named after a French physician, Prosper Meniere, who first described this inner ear disorder in 1861.

MD usually starts in one ear, and over time (usually within 5 years) both ears are affected with this disease. In most cases, progressive hearing loss occurs in the affected ears. MD causes death of cochlear (hearing) hair cells, and it also gradually damages vestibular (motion-sensing) hair cells.

The fluid-filled hearing and balance membranous structures of the inner ear normally function independent of other fluid systems in the body, and the volume of the fluid (known as endolymph) remains constant. However, this changes with the injury or degeneration of the inner ear structures. One of the established pathological features includes fluctuating pressure of the fluid within the inner ear, referred to as endolymphatic hydrops or excess fluid in the inner ear. The membranous structure in the inner ear called labyrinth contains endolymph. This structure can become dilated like a balloon when pressure increases due to either blockage of the drainage system or entry of excess amounts of fluid. It is believed that endolymphatic fluid bursts from its normal channel in the ear and flows into other areas, causing damage to the auditory and vestibular systems.

AGENTS OR HEALTH CONDITIONS CAUSING HEARING DISORDERS

Prolonged exposure to intense noise is known to be a risk factor for hearing loss.[47] It is estimated that more than 30 million Americans are exposed to hazardous levels of sound intensity on a regular basis.[48] In addition, industrial workers, and troops in training and in combat are exposed to high intensity and vibration. Additional agents that can cause hearing loss include cancer chemotherapeutic agents such as cisplatin, and antibiotics such as gentamicin, diseases such as ear infection (otitis media) and meningitis, MD, trauma, aging, and heredity. Cytomegalovirus (CMV) is the leading cause of infectious-related congenital sensorineural hearing loss worldwide. The CMV inflammatory genes play a significant role in causing hearing loss.[49] Age-related hearing loss referred to as Presbycusis is caused by cochlear degeneration that is induced by increased oxidative stress and mutations in mitochondria. Hearing loss progresses very slowly as a function of aging. Causes of tinnitus include blows to the head, large doses of certain drugs, such as aspirin, anemia, hypertension, noise exposure, stress, earwax blockage, and certain types of tumor. Both dominant and recessive genes exist, which can cause mild to severe hearing loss.

MEASUREMENTS OF HEARING LOSS

The severity of hearing loss is measured by the degree of loudness, as measured in decibels (dB). The levels of dB ranges as function of severity of hearing loss are described below.

Normal hearing	0–25 dB
Mild hearing loss	26–40 dB
Moderate hearing loss	41–55 dB
Moderate-severe hearing loss	56–70 dB
Severe hearing loss	71–90 dB
Profound hearing loss	greater than 90 dB

EVIDENCE FOR INCREASED OXIDATIVE STRESS IN HEARING DISORDERS

Noise-Induced Oxidative Stress (NIHL)

Exposure to high-intensity noise decreased the levels of serum total antioxidant capacity and increased the levels of nitric oxide in guinea pigs.[50] Increased nitric oxide levels can form peroxynitrite that damages the hair cells. Impulse noise exposure also enhanced oxidative stress in some animal studies. The levels of nitric oxide, peroxynitrite, oxidative stress, nuclear factor-kappa-beta (NF-kB), glutamate receptor (N-methyl-D-aspartate), and calcium are elevated in patients with tinnitus.[1–3,51–54] Noise exposure induced approximately 21%–42% of tinnitus in humans.[4,55,56] About 34% of tinnitus patients had posttraumatic stress disorders (PTSDs).[57] These studies suggested that some common biochemical defects that cause both tinnitus and PTSD might exist in these diseases. Indeed, a recent review has shown that increased oxidative stress occurs in patients with PTSD and tinnitus.[58]

NADPH (nicotinamide adenine dinucleotide) oxidases (NOXs) transport electron across the plasma membrane and produce superoxide radicals from oxygen. Exposure to moderate or intense noise increased NOXs activities in the cochlea of rats. Treatment of rats with diphenyleneiodonium, an inhibitor of NOX, after noise exposure, prevented hearing loss.[5] Pravastatin treatment also decreased NIHL by inhibiting NOX activity in mice.[59] Figure 11.1 shows a diagrammatic presentation of noise-induced hearing loss.

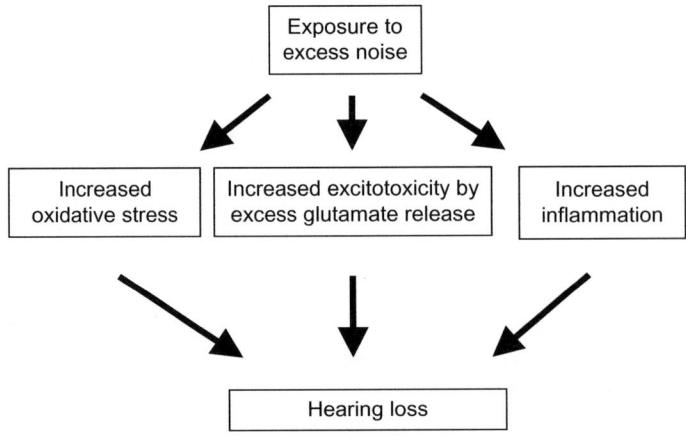

FIGURE 11.1 Diagrammatic representation of noise-induced hearing loss pathways.

Noise and/or Vibration-Induced Oxidative Stress

Frequent exposure to vibration also produces hearing disorders. The older guinea pigs were 2-fold more sensitive to vibration than younger animals.[57] The combination of noise and vibration during the use of handheld vibrating tools increased the risk of hearing loss in industrial workers.[6,60]

Cisplatin-Induced Oxidative Stress

Cisplatin caused hearing loss by generating free radicals. Treatment with this drug significantly depressed the levels of antioxidant enzymes, superoxide dismutase (SOD), glutathione peroxidase, glutathione reductase, glutathione transferase, and catalase, and enhanced the levels of lipid peroxidation.[61] Carboplatin also depleted the level of glutathione.[62] Cisplatin treatment also reduced the intracellular levels of nicotinamide adenine dinucleotide (NAD+); thereby, interfered with energy metabolism. Activation of NAD (P) H: quinone oxidoreductase 1 (NQO1) by beta-lapachone that exhibits antioxidant and anti-inflammation activities, protected against cisplatin-induced ototoxicity by increasing the levels NAD+ and sirtuin-1 protein.[63]

Advanced Age-Induced Oxidative Stress

Age-related progressive hearing disorder is the result of the effects of environment and genetic predisposition[64,65] and is characterized by the loss hair cells, stria vascularis atrophy, and loss of spiral ganglion neurons as well as alterations in central auditory pathways.[66] Increased oxidative stress and chronic inflammation are also associated with ageing,[67] and age-related cochlear structural alterations and degeneration of sensory and neural cells.[68] Hearing loss occurred due to increased oxidative stress in a model of aging rats. In addition, accumulation of mutated mitochondrial DNA was found in the peripheral and central auditory cells.[69–71] Furthermore, increased oxidative stress and mitochondrial DNA deletion play an important role in the pathogenesis of age-related hearing defects.[66]

In Mn-SOD heterozygous knockout mice, reduction in oxidative stress was not sufficient to accelerate age-related hearing loss (ARHL)[72]; however, in Cu/Zn homozygous and heterozygous knockout mice, increased rate of hearing loss was associated with greater cochlear pathology and loss of spiral ganglion neurons compared to wild-type mice.[73]

Oxidative Stress in the Meniere's Disease (MD)

The role for oxidative stress in MD is supported by the fact that free radical scavengers such as rebamipide, vitamin C, and glutathione, when administered orally for 8 weeks to patients with poorly controlled MD, improved tinnitus, hearing loss, and disability.[74]

EVIDENCE FOR INFLAMMATION IN HEARING DISORDERS

Noise-Induced Inflammation

Inflammation also plays an important role in hearing disorders induced by noise, drugs, and advancing age. Noise exposure can damage cochlear function by inducing inflammation in animal models.[7,75] This is supported by the fact that exposure to noise increased the levels of intracellular adhesion molecules and migration of leukocytes. Intense noise exposure can also activate the nuclear transcription factor-kappaB (NF-kB) in the cochlea of mice that causes over-expression of pro-inflammatory products including intracellular adhesion molecule-1 (ICAM-1) and vascular cell adhesion molecule-1 (VCAM-1), and inducible nitric oxide synthase (iNOS) in the inner ear that contribute to hearing loss.[8] Polymorphism of interleukin-6 (IL-6) increased the sensitivity of noise-induced hearing disorders in individuals over the age of 60 years.[76]

GENTAMICIN- AND CISPLATIN-INDUCED INFLAMMATION

Aspirin and other anti-inflammatory drugs prevented gentamicin-induced hearing loss and improved hearing ability.[25,77] Pro-inflammatory cytokines and activation of NF-kB contribute to the cisplatin-induced ototoxicity in mice and immortalized cochlear cells in culture.[9,78]

BACTERIAL INFECTION-INDUCED INFLAMMATION

Tumor necrosis factor-alpha (TNF-α) also induced cochlear degeneration after bacterial meningitis. Administration of TNF-α antibody reduced meningitis-induced hearing loss in Mongolian gerbils.[10]

HEALTH CONDITIONS-INDUCED INFLAMMATION

Increased levels of TNF-α were also associated with trauma-induced hearing loss. Treatment with dexamethasone reduced TNF-α-induced damage to the organ of Corti explants cultures.[79] A study has reported that otosclerosis-induced sensorineural hearing loss is due to the chronic release of TNF-α from the foci of otic capsule.[80,81] Chronic inflammatory reactions produce sac dysfunction leading to MD.[82]

ADVANCED AGE-INDUCED INFLAMMATION

Increased inflammation in the elder individuals was associated with (ARHL)[12] and sensorineural hearing loss.[13] Mouse strain SAMP8 exhibits premature aging associated with hearing loss and cochlear degeneration that resemble human ARHL. Increased oxidative damage and chronic inflammation, and decreased in the activities of mitochondrial complexes were associated with ARHL in SAMP8 mice.[83] An epidemiologic study suggested that prolonged elevation of serum C-reactive protein was associated with increased the risk of developing hearing impairment in individuals under the age of 60 years; however, this association was not observed in persons over the age of 60 years.[84]

EVIDENCE FOR INCREASED GLUTAMATE LEVEL IN HEARING DISORDERS

NOISE RELEASES GLUTAMATE

Afferent transmission between inner hair cells and auditory neurons is mediated by the glutamate receptors in the cochlea. Intense noise causes release of excessive amounts of glutamate that damage the inner hair cells and auditory synapses.[85] Kynurenate, a glutamate antagonist, protected guinea pigs against NIHL.[14] The glutamate-aspartate transporter (GLAST) that plays an important role in maintaining the normal level of glutamate was decreased in the cochlea after exposure to noise leading to increased accumulation of glutamate in the perilymphs. The resulting increased level of glutamate was associated with an enhanced rate of progression of hearing loss.[15] Inhibitors of GLAST protected the synapse from exposure to excessive extracellular glutamate and reduced noise-induced hearing defects.[86] Treatment with riluzole, an inhibitor of glutamatergic neurotransmission, protected guinea pigs against NIHL.[87] Treatment with D (-)-2-amino-5-phosphonopentanoic acid (D-AP5), a selective inhibitor of glutamate receptor N-methyl D-aspartate

(NMDA), attenuated noise-induced tinnitus.[16] Exposure to high-intensity noise enhanced the levels of glutamate and aspartate in the cochlea and caused degeneration of afferent dendrites under the inner hair cells, and loss of outer hair cells. Treatment with a NMDA antagonist (MK801) before noise exposure prevented release of glutamate and aspartate and reduced hearing loss in guinea pigs.[88] Diagrammatic representation of noise-induced biochemical events leading to hearing loss is represented in Figure 11.1.

SALICYLATE ACTIVATES GLUTAMATE RECEPTOR

Salicylate induced tinnitus by activating cochlear glutamate receptors NMDAs in rats.[34] This effect of salicylate was related to the inhibition of cyclooxygenase activity. Treatment of rats with antagonist of NMDA receptors blocked salicylate-induced tinnitus.

AMINOGLYCOSIDE, COCHLEA ISCHEMIA, OR TRAUMA-INDUCED RELEASE OF GLUTAMATE

Exposure to noise, aminoglycoside antibiotics, cochlea ischemia, or trauma caused excessive release of glutamate from the inner hair cells into the synaptic cleft. The high levels of glutamate caused swelling and degeneration of the dendrites of spiral ganglion neurons as well as loss of neurons.[89]

MicroRNAs IN THE PATHOGENESIS OF HEARING DISORDERS

MicroRNAs

MicroRNAs (miRs) are evolutionarily conserved small noncoding single-stranded RNAs of approximately 22 nucleotides in length, and are present in all living organisms including humans.[90–93] The biogenesis of miRs is very complex and involves multiple biochemical steps. The majority of miRs are transcribed by RNA polymerase II (Pol II), while some are transcribed by RNA polymerase III (Pol III) from the noncoding region of the DNA to produce primary miRs (pri-miRs). Pri-miRs undergo a nuclear cleavage by ribonuclease III Drosa to generate precursor-miRs (pre-miRs) that migrate to the cytoplasm where they are further cleaved by ribonuclease III Dicer to ultimately form mature single-stranded miRs with the help of another protein argonaute (Ago).[92,94–96] Each miR binds to its complementary sequences in the 3′-untranslated region (3′-UTR) of the mRNA, promotes degradation of the mRNA transcript, and prevents translation of the message of protein. In this manner, miRs regulate the translation of proapoptotic or antiapoptotic proteins from their respective mRNAs, depending upon whether they receive damaging or protective signal.

EXPRESSION OF MicroRNAs IN THE NORMAL EARS

MicroRNAs are expressed in the normal inner ear cells, and play an essential role in their development, differentiation, and survival.[97,98] In mouse embryonic inner ears, increased expressions of miR-376a-3p, miR-376-b-3p, and miR-376-c-3p that regulate the levels of phosphoribosyl pyrophosphate synthetase 1 (PRPS 1) were found.[99] The PRPS 1 protein is important for preserving hair cell function. Mutations in the gene coding for this protein are associated with a spectrum of non-syndromic and syndromic forms of hearing loss. MiR-96 and miR-183 was found to regulate the levels of chloride intracellular channel 5 (CLIC5) protein in inner hair cell line (HE1-OC1 cells), Overexpression of these microRNAs reduced the levels of CLIC5.[100] Expression of 157 microRNAs in the inner ear sensory epithelial cells and 53 microRNAs in the cochlear and vestibular cells were differently expressed.[101] Among these, miR-135b regulates the levels of PSIP1-p75 that had multiple cellular functions including DNA repair[102] and attenuates oxidative stress.[103] Using embryonic inner ear cell line (UB/OC-1), it was shown that overexpression of miR-210 supports differentiation from epithelial cells to sensory hair cells.[104] There were 455 microRNAs common to both the cochlear and vestibular sensory epithelial cells, with 30 microRNAs unique to the cochlea, and 44 microRNAs unique to the vestibule. Among these, miR-675-5p with its target protein Arhgap12, a GTPase activating protein has been identified.[105] MiR-194 is expressed in the spiral ganglia neurons of mouse inner ear where it may play a role in differentiation of neurons.[106] The family of miR-183 consisting of miR-96, miR-182, and miR-183 was strongly expressed in the inner ear hair cells where they play a role in differentiation of primary sensory cells.[107,108] MiR-124 regulates the fate of cells in the developing organ of Corti that contains sensory hair cells and supporting cells.[109]

Since microRNAs are prominently expressed in the inner ear, it is likely that they may be involved in hearing disorders induced by diverse groups of ototoxic agents. Indeed, changes in the expression of microRNAs occur in hearing disorders, but it is not known what signal causes these changes in the expression of microRNAs that play a role in the pathogenesis of hearing loss. In neurodegenerative disease such as Alzheimer's disease (AD), ROS and pro-inflammatory cytokines act as one of the signals that mediate the damaging effects of these biochemical events by changing the expressions of microRNAs and their target proteins in the nonauditory neurons.[110] Since increased oxidative stress[1–6] and inflammation[7–13] play a central role in the pathogenesis of hearing defects induced by the ototoxic agents, it is likely that ROS and pro-inflammatory cytokines may mediate their damaging effects on the hair cells by altering the expression of microRNAs.

In the nonauditory neuronal cells, antioxidants mediate their protective effects against oxidative damage by altering the expression of miRs.[110] Since antioxidants reduced the risk of developing hearing defects by decreasing oxidative stress,[17–24,26–31] it is likely that protective mechanisms of antioxidants in the auditory cells may be mediated via altering the expression of miRs and their target proteins.

ALTERATIONS IN MicroRNAs EXPRESSION IN HEARING DISORDERS

CHANGES IN THE EXPRESSIONS OF MicroRNAs IN AGE-RELATED HEARING DISORDERS

Age-related hearing loss is caused by the cochlear degeneration. Overexpression of miR-29b induced degeneration of cochlear hair cells by decreasing the levels of its target proteins. These key proteins are (a) silent mating type information regulation 2 homolog 1 (SIRT1), a NAD+ dependent protein deacetylase, which downregulates inflammatory processes, and (b) proliferator-activated receptor-gamma coactivator 1α (PGC-1α). PGC-1alpha is a stimulator of mitochondrial biogenesis and a regulator of energy metabolism, whose inhibition can lead to impaired mitochondrial function and cochlear hair cell apoptosis in mice.[111] This study was confirmed by the opposite experiment in which inhibition of miR-29b increased the levels of SIRT1 and PGC-1aα, and deceased apoptosis of cochlear hair cells (HEI-OC1 inner ear cell line).

The expression of Dicer, a ribonuclease III that cleaves pre-miR to form mature miR in the cytoplasm was downregulated in the whole blood of patients with idiopathic sudden sensorineural hearing loss (SSNHL).[112] Thus, the expression of miRs may also be reduced in this form of hearing loss. However, the expression of Drosha was not altered in the whole blood of these patients suggesting that the processing of miRs at the nuclear level was not affected. This suggests that in SSNHL, alterations in the expression of miRs are controlled at the level of cytoplasm and not at the level of nucleus.

The expression of miR-34a, which causes apoptosis increased in the cochlea of mice as function of aging, whereas the levels of SIRT1 decreased in these animals. Overexpression of miR-34a also inhibited SIRT1in the inner hair cell line (HE1-OCI). Resveratrol, an activator of SIRT1, decreased miR-34a overexpression, protected hair cells, and reduced hearing loss in mice.[113]

Degeneration of the organ of Corti, the auditory hair cells, which transduces mechanical stimuli to electrical signal in the inner ear, is the major cause of ARHL. The expression of miR-29 family and miR-34 family that regulate pro-apoptotic pathways was upregulated with aging. However, members of miR-181 and miR-183 responsible for proliferation and differentiation were downregulated during ARHL.[114]

MiR-431, which targets the protein Eya4, is highly expressed in the spinal ganglion neurons (SGNs) of the cochlea of newborn mice, and decreases during further development. Inhibition of the cochlear Eya4 protein in miR-431 overexpressing mice led to apoptosis of SGNs and caused hearing loss.[115]

Mutation in MicroRNA Induces Nonsyndromic Hearing Loss (NSHL)

Point mutation in miR-96 has been associated with the progressive hearing loss in hereditary NSHL both in humans and mice.[116,117] Treatment of mice with N-ethyl-N-nitrosurea (ENU) resulted in mutation in miR-96 that caused hearing loss associated with the damage to the hair cell function and differentiation.[118] The mouse model carrying mutated miR-96 is referred to as diminuendo and is considered a good model to study mechanisms of hearing loss. Mutation in miR-96 was also found in 2 Spanish families with autosomal dominant NSH.[119]

Changes in the Expressions of MicroRNAs in Noise-Induced Hearing Loss

Exposure to intense noise that caused damage to the cochlear hair cells, led to simultaneous decrease of miR-183 levels and corresponding enhancement of its target protein Taok1 (Tao kinase 1, a serine/threonine-protein kinase 1). This observation was confirmed in the cochlear organotypic culture where inhibition of miR-183 expression resulted in enhanced levels of Taok1 together with apoptosis of hair cells.[120] Exposure to noise downregulated the expression of miR-176 leading to increased Taok1 levels and apoptosis of the cochlear sensory epithelial cells.[120]

The expressions of three microRNAs miR-183, miR-96, and miR-182 were decreased 28 days after exposure to noise. This was associated with reduced number of outer hair cells many of which were damaged.[121]

In male textile workers with noise-induced hearing loss, the plasma levels of miR-16-5p, miR-24-3p, miR-185-5p, and miR-451a were upregulated in comparison to those who were exposed to noise exposure but had not developed hearing loss, whereas the plasma levels of miR-24-3p and miR-185-5p and miR-451a were downregulated in individuals exposed to noise compared to those not exposed to noise.[122] The protein targets for these miRs were not identified. Plasma levels of these miRs could be of diagnostic value of noise exposure-induced hearing disorders as well as to noise exposure. Further studies are needed to confirm these results.

Changes in the Expressions of MicroRNAs in Kanamycin-Induced Hearing Disorders

Treatment of mice with kanamycin increased the expression of miR-34a and miR-34c, and induced apoptosis in the cochlear hair cells, including stria vascularis cells, supporting cells, and spiral ganglion neurons.[123] These effects of kanamycin were associated with increased levels of calpain.

Changes in the Expressions of MicroRNAs in Damaged Auditory Nervous System

Progressive degeneration of spiral ganglion neurons (SGNs) caused sensorineural hearing loss (SNHL). Overexpression of miR-204 suppressed the viability of SGNs by reducing the levels of its target transmembrane protease, serine-3 (TMPRSS3).[124] Therefore, reducing the expression of miR-204 may prevent the development of SNHL. Mutation in the TMPRSS3 gene also caused non-syndromic autosomal recessive deafness with bilateral hearing loss in utero or in immature mice. This disease is characterized by degeneration of the organ of Corti and cochlear hair cell loss. Reducing the expression of miR-204 may also help to decrease the development of SNHL and may constitute a therapeutic approach to non-syndromic autosomal recessive deafness.

It is not established, whether changes in the expression of specific microRNAs are due to alterations in the rate of their transcription, processing by Drosha in the nucleus and Dicer in the cytoplasm or their stability.

Additional studies are needed to explore the effects of different ototoxic agents on the expression of microRNAs and their respective target proteins in the hair cells and spiral ganglion neurons in culture as well as in animals. In addition, the blood levels of microRNAs in patients with established hearing loss, and those who have been exposed to an ototoxic agent, but have not developed hearing defects, would also be useful and could readily be investigated.

Table 11.1 summarizes the alterations in expression of miRs in hearing loss induced by diverse agents and adverse health conditions.

TABLE 11.1
Upregulated and Downregulated MicroRNAs in Induced-Hearing Loss

Inducing Agents	Upregulated MicroRNAs	Target Proteins
Age	miR-29b, miR-34a	SIRT1, PGC-1α
	miR-29 and miR-34 families	Eya4
	miR-431	
Noise	[a]miR-16-5p, miR-24-3p, miR-185p5	Not identified
	miR-451a	
SNHL	miR-204	TMPRSS3
Downregulated MicroRNAs		
NSHL	Mutated miR-96	Not identified
SSNHL	Dicer	
Noise	miR-181, miR-176	Toak1
	[b]miR-96, miR-182, miR-183	Not identified
	miR-24-3p, miR-185-5p, miR-451a	

Note: SIRT1, Silent mating type information regulation 2 homolog 1; PGC-1α, Proliferator-activated receptor-gamma coactivator1α; Eya4, Eye absent homolog protein4; TMPRSS3, Transmembrane protease, serine-3; Taok1, Tao kinase1 (serine/theorine-protein kinase1); SNHL, Sensorineural hearing loss; SSNHL, Sudden sensorineural hearing loss; NSHL, Nonsyndromic hearing loss.

[a] Levels of noise exposure leading to hearing loss.

[b] Levels of noise exposure not causing hearing loss.

OXIDATIVE STRESS REGULATES THE EXPRESSION OF MicroRNAs IN HEARING DISORDERS

As mentioned earlier in this manuscript, increased oxidative stress is important in the development of hearing defects and alterations in the expressions of miRs occur in this disease. Therefore, it is likely that damaging effects of oxidative stress may be mediated by such alterations in hearing disorders. This is substantiated by the studies on auditory and nonauditory cells. These studies are briefly described here.

AUDITORY CELLS

Although increased oxidative stress is involved in the pathogenesis of hearing disorders, only a few studies are available on the effects of this biochemical event on changes in the expression of miRs in the cochlear hair cells.

1. Increased oxidative stress induced by t-BHP (tert-butylhydroperoxide) enhanced the expression of 24 microRNAs. Among these, 6 microRNAs: miR-1934, miR-411, miR-717, miR-503, miR-467e, and miR-699o that regulate apoptosis and proliferation of the cochlear hair cells were strongly expressed.[125] ROS generated by the treatment with t-BHO increased the expression of 35 microRNAs and decreased the expression of 40 microRNAs, and inhibited the proliferation of hair cells (HE1-C1).[126]
2. Reactive oxygen species (ROS) generated by exposure to ionizing radiation enhanced the expression of miR-207 in the hair cell line (HE1-OC1). This microRNA increased radiation-induced apoptosis and DNA damage by inhibiting its target protein AKt3. This was further supported by the fact that inhibiting the levels of AKt3 mimicked the effects of miR-207.[127]
3. In diabetic mice with a high level of internal oxidative stress, the expression of miR-34a was elevated and the level of SIRT1 was inhibited and promoted apoptosis in the hair cells (HE1-OC1). This finding indicated that downregulation of miR-34a may help in diabetic-related hearing loss.[128]

NON-AUDITORY CELLS (NEURONS AND NON-NEURONAL CELLS)

In the nonauditory cells oxidative stress mediates its damaging effects by altering the expression of microRNAs and their target proteins.[110] The details have been presented in Chapter 9.

PRO-INFLAMMATORY CYTOKINES COULD UPREGULATE THE EXPRESSIONS OF MicroRNAs IN HEARING DISORDERS

Since inflammation is involved in the pathogenesis of hearing defects, and since pro-inflammatory cytokines regulate the expressions of microRNAs and the levels of their target proteins in non-auditory neurons,[110] it is likely that damaging effects of inflammation on the hair cells may be mediated by alterations in the expressions of microRNAs. No such studies have been performed on the hair cells. The investigations on nonauditory cells (neurons and astroglia) showing that pro-inflammatory cytokines bring about their damaging effects in part, by altering the expression of miRs are discussed in Chapter 9.

ANTIOXIDANTS COULD REGULATE THE EXPRESSIONS OF MicroRNAs IN HEARING DISORDERS

Since antioxidants protect hearing defects, and since antioxidants regulate the expressions of microRNAs and the levels of their target proteins in non-auditory neurons,[110] it is likely that protective effects of antioxidants on the hair cells may be mediated by alterations in the expressions of microRNAs.

No such studies have been performed on the hair cells. The investigations showing that antioxidants protect mammalian cells, in part, by altering the expression of miRs are discussed in Chapter 9.

STUDIES ON ANTIOXIDANTS IN HEARING DISORDERS

ANIMAL STUDIES

Vitamin E, when administered intraperitoneally 3 days before and 3 days after noise exposure, reduced noise-induced cochlear damage and hearing loss in guinea pigs.[129,130] Vitamin E protected against noise-induced damage to the inner ear in cyprinid fish.[131] Alpha-lipoic acid protects against NIHL in guinea pigs.[50] An intraperitoneal injection of N-acetylcysteine (NAC) or glutathione significantly reduced hair cell loss in the cochlear cells of rats and guinea pigs.[132,133] NAC treatment attenuated NIHL in guinea pigs.[134] Acetyl-L-carnitine and NAC administered twice a day for 2 days and 1 hour before and 1 hour after noise exposure for an additional 2 days provided protection against hearing loss in Chinchilla model.[135] The role of NAC in reducing NIHL has been reviewed.[20] Coenzyme Q10 helped in recovery from hypoxia-induced sudden deafness by protecting damage to auditory hair cells as well as preventing respiratory metabolic impairment of hair cells.[21] Idebenone, a synthetic analog of coenzyme Q10 with antioxidant properties, protected guinea pigs against NIHL.[136] The soluble form of coenzyme Q10 was effective in reducing NIHL by promoting the survival of hair cells in guinea pigs.[137] The combination of vitamin E and idebenone did not produce additive protective effect against NIHL, suggesting that these two antioxidants may be acting by similar mechanisms.[138] Vitamin C also protected against NIHL in albino guinea pigs.[23] D-methionine, an antioxidant, attenuated NIHL and functional loss of cochlea in mice.[139]

Vitamin E protected against cisplatin-induced damage to cochlear hair cells in rats.[18] Trolox, a water-soluble analog of vitamin E, when applied locally, reduced cisplatin-induced ototoxicity in guinea pigs.[140] Vitamin E reduced gentamicin-induced hearing loss and vestibular dysfunction.[141] Cisplatin-induced cochlear damage is reduced by vitamin E in an animal model.[141] NAC treatment protected against cisplatin-induced damage to inner ear auditory sensory cells in culture.[142] Antioxidants attenuate aminoglycoside-induced hearing loss and vestibular dysfunction in an animal model (chinchilla).[143] Alpha-lipoic acid protected against carboplatin-induced toxicity in hair cells of rats.[19]

In mice and dogs, a diet rich in antioxidants reduced age-related cochlear degeneration.[67] Age-related hearing loss is characterized by progressive decline in sensitivity to sound; however, caloric restriction and treatment with individual antioxidants such as vitamin E, vitamin C, acetyl-L-carnitine, alpha-lipoic acid, and melatonin improved auditory sensitivity to sound and reduced mitochondrial DNA deletion and loss of hair cells in aging rats.[144–146] In a mice model of premature age-related hearing loss, treatment with N-acetyl-L-carnitine failed to protect against hearing loss.[147]

HUMAN STUDIES

In a prospective, double-blind study design, supplementation with vitamin E alone provided better recovery than the standard therapy in patients with idiopathic sudden hearing loss.[148] In a prospective, double-blind study, vitamin E alone administered orally improved the efficacy of standard therapy.[130] In a prospective randomized study, intravenous administration of magnesium sulfate improved hearing recovery in patients with idiopathic SSH.[149] Coenzyme Q10 delayed the progression of hearing loss in patients with a genetic defect, 7445A→G mitochondrial mutation.[26] The use of glutamate antagonists, steroids, and antioxidants may be useful in the management of hearing loss and tinnitus.[150] An oral supplementation with antioxidants (vitamin E, vitamin C, beta-carotene, and phospholipids) reduced the subjective discomfort and tinnitus intensity in patients with idiopathic tinnitus.[27] NAC protected against aminoglycoside-induced ototoxicity in hemodialysis patients.[151] An antioxidant mixture containing reduced glutathione, alpha-lipoic acid, cysteine, and other antioxidants improved the symptoms of MD.[152] Figure 11.2 shows diagrammatic presentation of pathways of antioxidant protection.

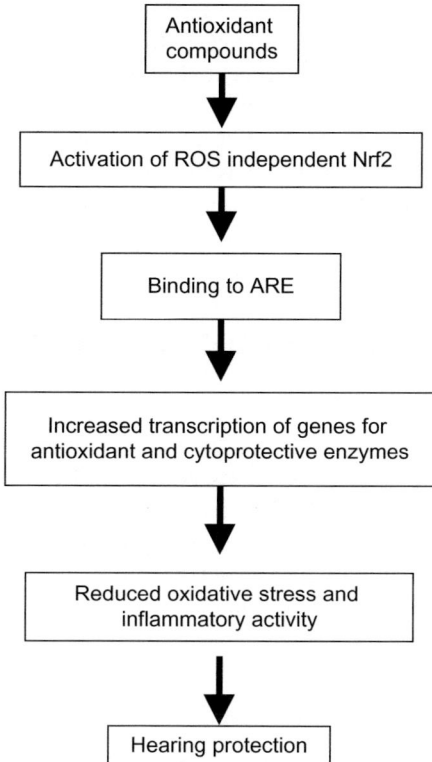

FIGURE 11.2 Proposed pathway of protection against hearing loss by antioxidant micronutrients.

POTENTIAL REASONS FOR SUBOPTIMAL BENEFICIAL EFFECTS WITH INDIVIDUAL MICRONUTRIENTS IN HEARING DISORDERS

The reasons for individual or multiple micronutrients in producing suboptimal protection of hearing disorders in humans are not known; however, some potentials causes are described here: (a) antioxidants show differential subcellular distribution and different mechanisms of action; therefore, a single antioxidant cannot protect all parts of the cell; (b) a single antioxidant in a high internal oxidative environment in high-risk patients is oxidized and can then itself act as a pro-oxidant rather than as an antioxidant; (c) the body protects against oxidative damage by elevating antioxidant enzymes, and dietary and endogenous antioxidants; (d) antioxidants neutralize free radicals by donating electrons to those molecules with unpaired electron, whereas antioxidant enzymes destroy free radicals by catalysis, converting them to harmless molecules such as water and oxygen. Therefore, both of these agents should be enhanced to achieve substantial protection against oxidative damage; (e) the affinity of different antioxidants for free radicals differs, depending upon their solubility; (f) both the aqueous and lipid compartments of the cell need to be protected together. Water-soluble antioxidants such as vitamin C and glutathione protect molecules in the aqueous environment of the cells, whereas lipid soluble antioxidants such as vitamin A and vitamin E protect molecules in the lipid compartment; (g) vitamin E is more effective in quenching free radicals in a reduced oxygenated cellular environment, whereas vitamin C and alpha-tocopherol are more effective in a higher oxygenated environment of the cells[153]; (h) vitamin C is important for recycling the oxidized form of alpha-tocopherol to the antioxidant form[154]; (i) antioxidants produce cell protective proteins by altering the expression of different microRNAs.[110] For example, some antioxidants can activate Nrf2 by upregulating miR-200a that inhibits its target protein Keap1, whereas others activate Nrf2 by downregulating miR-21 that binds with 3′-UTR Nrf2 mRNA.[155]

The use of a single micronutrient is not expected to produce optimal protection against oxidative and inflammatory events, which contribute to hearing disorders. For this reason, it is proposed that an elevation of the levels of antioxidant enzymes and dietary and endogenous antioxidants may be essential for simultaneously reducing oxidative stress and inflammation. Oral supplementation can increase the levels of dietary and endogenous antioxidants; however, elevation of the levels of antioxidant enzymes requires an activation of Nrf2. Therefore it is essential to understand the regulation of activation of Nrf2.

ACTIVATION OF Nrf2 (NUCLEAR FACTOR-ERYTHROID-2-RELATED FACTOR 2)

Nrf2

The nuclear transcriptional factor, Nrf2 (nuclear factor-erythroid-2-related factor 2) belongs to the Cap 'n' Collar (CNC) family that contains a conserved basic leucine zipper (bZIP) transcriptional factor.[156] Under physiological condition, Nrf2 is associated with Kelch-like ECH associated protein 1 (Keap1), which acts as an inhibitor of Nrf2.[157] Keap1 protein serves as an adaptor to link Nrf2 to the ubiquitin ligase CuI-Rbx1 complex for degradation by proteasomes and maintains the steady levels of Nrf2 in the cytoplasm. Nrf2-keap1 complex is primarily located in the cytoplasm; Keap1 acts as a sensor for ROS/electrophilic stress.

ACTIVATION OF Nrf2 DURING ACUTE OXIDATIVE STRESS

During acute oxidative stress, ROS is needed to activate Nrf2 which then dissociates itself from Keap1-CuI-Rbx1 complex and translocates in the nucleus where it heterodimerizes with a small Maf protein, binds with ARE leading to increased expression of target genes coding for several cytoprotective enzymes including antioxidant enzymes.[158–160]

FAILURE TO ACTIVATE Nrf2 DURING CHRONIC OXIDATIVE STRESS

During chronic oxidative stress, Nrf2 becomes resistant to ROS,[161–163] suggesting that activation of Nrf2 by a ROS-independent mechanism exists. This is evidenced by the fact that increased chronic oxidative stress occurs despite the presence of Nrf2 in hearing disorders. The question arises as to how to activate ROS-resistant Nrf2 in hearing disorders.

ANTIOXIDANTS ACTIVATE ROS-RESISTANT Nrf2

Some examples are vitamin E and genistein,[164] alpha-lipoic acid,[165] curcumin,[166] resveratrol,[167,168] omega-3-fatty acids,[169,170] glutathione,[171] NAC,[172] and coenzyme Q10.[173] Several plant-derived phytochemicals, such as epigallocatechin-3-gallate, carestol, kahweol, cinnamonyl-based compounds, zerumbone, lycopene and carnosol,[156,174,175] genistein,[164] allicin, a major organosulfur compound found in garlic,[176] sulforaphane, a organosulfur compound, found in cruciferous vegetables,[177] and kavalactones (methysticin, kavain, and yangonin).[178] The reasons for the activation of Nrf2 without ROS by antioxidant compounds are not known.

BINDING OF Nrf2 WITH ARE IN THE NUCLEUS

An activation of Nrf2 alone is not sufficient to increase the levels of antioxidant enzymes. Activated Nrf2 must bind with ARE in the nucleus for increasing the expression of target genes coding for antioxidant enzymes. This binding ability of Nrf2 with ARE was impaired in aged rats and this defect was restored by supplementation with alpha-lipoic acid.[165] It is unknown whether the binding ability of Nrf2 with ARE is impaired in hearing disorders.

IMPORTANCE OF ACTIVATION OF Nrf2 IN AUDITORY CELLS

In Nrf2 deleted mice (–/–), hair cells become more sensitive to noise-induced oxidative damage in comparison to wild-type mice. Pre-treatment with an activator of Nrf2 preserved integrity of hair cells and improved hearing levels in wild-type mice but not in Nrf2 deleted mice (–/–). These results suggest that high level of Nrf2 in the cochlear protects against noise-induced hearing loss.[179]

Cisplatin can cause hearing loss by increasing levels of oxidative damage and pro-inflammatory cytokines in hair cells. Pretreatment with an activator of Nrf2, such as Erdosteine,[180] flunarizine,[181] Ebselen,[182] Ginkgolide B, a major component of *Ginkgo biloba*,[183] and phloretin[184] protected hair cells (HE1-OC1) by reducing oxidative damage, pro-inflammatory cytokines, inhibiting pro-apoptotic expression, and enhancing the levels of cytoprotective enzymes, including antioxidant enzymes,

Increased oxidative stress contributes to cochlear damage, including AEHL, and gentamicin-induced ototoxicity. The Nrf2-knockout mice maintained normal auditory thresholds at their age of 3 months; however, their hearing ability was significantly impaired as they grow older (6 and 11 months) in comparison to age-matched wild-type mice.[185] In addition, the number of hair cells and spiral ganglion cells was markedly decreased in Nrf2-knockout mice. In the explants culture of Corte, treatment with gentamicin enhanced the loss of hair cells in Nrf2-deficient tissue more than that found in wild-type mice. Activation of Nrf2 occurred only in the wild-type mice, but not in Nrf2-knockout mice. These results further suggest importance of Nrf2 in the auditory for protection of hearing disorders.

CURRENT PREVENTION AND TREATMENTS STRATEGIES

Although physical ear protection devices can reduce the impact of noise and vibration somewhat, the energy generated from high levels of noise intensity and vibration can penetrate the inner ear to cause damage to hair cells. Physical protection of the ear plays no role in chemical-induced or ARHL. Some individuals, such as troops in combat, musicians, or industrial workers do develop varying degree of hearing loss despite physical ear protection. There is no biological protection strategy to reduce the risk of hearing loss. The development of such a strategy may compliment the physical ear protection devices in the prevention of hearing disorders.

Except for hearing aids of various types and cochlear transplant, there are no effective biological treatment strategies to improve the efficacy of physical ear devices. The hearing loss progresses in spite of hearing aids. Therefore, the development of a biological treatment strategy may compliment the ear devices in improving the management of hearing disorders.

Glucocorticoids are widely used to treat SSHL, possibly because of involvement of inflammation. Treatment of mice with dexamethasone improves the synthesis of glutathione in the cochlear spiral ganglion by increasing the expression of gamma-glutamylcysteine synthetase, a rate-limiting enzyme in the biosynthesis of glutathione.[186] Thus, the mechanisms of protection by dexamethasone involve both reduction in inflammation and oxidative stress.

The current treatment of MD includes medication, surgery and diet. Medications commonly used for acute episodes are Meclizine (Antivert), Lorazepam (Ativan), Phenergan, Compazine, Dexamethasone (Decadron), and calcium channel blockers. Medications used between attacks include diuretics, dyazide (Triamterine/HCTZ). Steroids and immune suppressants are rarely used. Surgical treatment is the last resort in severe cases of MD. Dietary recommendations include food and adequate fluid intake evenly throughout the day, reduced intake of salt and sugar, avoidance of caffeine and foods containing monosodium glutamate, and limited alcohol consumption.

These treatment methodologies have been useful to manage the symptoms of the disease but have failed to prevent the progressive damage to cochlear and vestibular hair cells. To address this problem, it is essential to understand the mechanisms that are involved in the death of these cells.

In order to develop an effective biological strategy for prevention or treatment of hearing disorders, it is important to identify some major biochemical events that contribute to the initiation and progression of hearing disorders. From the analysis of published data on laboratory and clinical studies, it appears that increased oxidative stress and chronic inflammation play a central role in the pathogenesis of hearing disorders.

REDUCING OXIDATIVE STRESS LEVEL

Activation of Nrf2 may not be sufficient to optimally reduce oxidative stress, because antioxidants compounds are also decreased during chronic oxidative stress[187–189]; therefore, their levels must also be simultaneously elevated.

REDUCING INFLAMMATION LEVEL

Activation of Nrf2[190,191] and some individual antioxidant compounds reduced chronic inflammation.[192–198]

REDUCING GLUTAMATE LEVEL

Some antioxidants decrease the release of glutamate as well as its neurotoxicity.[199–201] In addition, certain B-vitamins can also decrease the release of glutamate.[202,203]

PROPOSED MICRONUTRIENTS FOR SIMULTANEOUSLY REDUCING OXIDATIVE STRESS, INFLAMMATION, AND GLUTAMATE LEVELS IN HEARING DISORDERS

Because of failure to produce optimal benefits in improving the symptoms of hearing disorders with one or two micronutrients, a comprehensive micronutrient mixture is proposed. This mixture contains multiple dietary antioxidant compounds (vitamin A, natural mixed carotenoids, vitamin C, vitamin E succinate, vitamin E acetate, selenomethionine, curcumin, and resveratrol), endogenous antioxidants (alpha-lipoic acid, L-carnitine, and coenzyme Q10), a synthetic antioxidant N-acetylcysteine (NAC), omega-3-fatty acids, vitamin D3, zinc, and all B-vitamins. This mixture of micronutrients may optimally reduce oxidative stress and chronic inflammation by simultaneously enhancing the levels of antioxidant enzymes through activation of the Nrf2/ARE pathway, and elevating the levels of antioxidants. The same micronutrient mixture may also reduce the release and toxicity of glutamate at the same time.

PREVENTION OF HEARING DISORDERS

PRIMARY PREVENTION

The purpose of primary prevention is to protect healthy individuals from developing hearing disorders. Older individuals, musicians, industrial workers, troops who are likely to be employed in the war zones, individuals who are likely to receive certain antibiotics and cisplatin for their health conditions, and individuals carrying mutations in genes responsible for hearing loss are suitable subjects for the primary prevention studies.

At present, there are no strategies to prevent or delay the onset of hearing loss in individuals with mutated genes. The proposed mixture of micronutrients may be effective in preventing or delaying the onset of symptoms of hearing disorders in these individuals. This possibility is indirectly supported by the experiments on the fruit flies described here.

The gene HOP (TUM-1) is essential for the development of *Drosophila melanogaster* (fruit fly). A mutation in this gene markedly increases the risk of developing a leukemia-like tumor in female flies. In collaboration with Dr. Bhattacharya of NASA Moffat Field, CA, we observed that whole-body irradiation of these flies with proton radiation dramatically increased the incidence of cancer compared to that observed in unirradiated female flies. Treatment with a mixture of multiple antioxidants before and after irradiation blocked the development of proton radiation-induced cancer in female fruit flies.[204]

SECONDARY PREVENTION

The purpose of secondary prevention is to stop or slow the progression of hearing disorders after exposure to ototoxic agents. Individuals who have been exposed to such agents, but have not developed any hearing problems, and are not taking any medication, are suitable subjects for the secondary prevention studies. The micronutrient mixture suggested for the primary prevention studies is also proposed for the secondary prevention studies.

IMPROVED MANAGEMENT

The patients with hearing disorders who are receiving standard care are suitable for this study. The micronutrient mixture suggested for the primary prevention studies is also proposed in combination with standard care for the improved management of hearing disorders studies.

CONCLUSIONS

The hearing disorders include a partial or full loss of hearing, tinnitus, and Meniere's disease (MD). Advanced age, chronic and intense noise, vibrations, gentamicin, ionizing radiation, cisplatin, large doses of aspirin, bacterial and viral infections, ear canal obstruction, mechanical damage to the tympanic membrane and ossicles of the middle ear and inner ear, and gene mutations cause them. Congenital hearing defects could be primarily due to cytomegalovirus infection during pregnancy or gene mutation. Troops in combat zones, musicians, or industrial workers are likely to develop varying degrees of hearing loss despite the use of earplugs. Except for physical ear protection, there are no effective biological strategies for the prevention of hearing loss. Analysis of published studies suggests that increased oxidative stress, chronic inflammation, and glutamate play a key role in the initiation and progression of hearing disorders. Therefore, attenuation of these cellular defects may prevent, and in combination of standard therapy, may improve the management of hearing loss. Changes in the expressions of microRNAs are involved in the pathogenesis and that alterations in their expressions depend upon whether they receive damaging signals from ROS and pro-inflammatory cytokines or protective signals from antioxidants. Previous results with antioxidants produced suboptimal benefit in reducing hearing loss. In order to reduce oxidative stress, chronic inflammation, and glutamate levels, it is essential to enhance the levels of antioxidant enzymes and dietary and endogenous antioxidants. The levels of antioxidants can easily be increased by supplementation, but increasing the levels of antioxidant enzymes requires activation of Nrf2. A mixture of micronutrients that would optimally reduce oxidative stress, chronic inflammation by simultaneously enhancing the levels of antioxidant enzymes through activating the Nrf2/ARE pathway, and dietary and endogenous antioxidants by supplementation. Such a micronutrient mixture may also reduce the release and toxicity of glutamate. The efficacy of this mixture of micronutrients should be tested in the primary prevention, secondary prevention, as well as in combination with standard care, in the improved management of hearing disorders.

REFERENCES

1. Clerici WJ, DiMartino DL, Prasad MR. Direct effects of reactive oxygen species on cochlear outer hair cell shape in vitro. *Hear Res.* 1995;84(1–2):30–40.
2. Henderson D, Bielefeld EC, Harris KC, Hu BH. The role of oxidative stress in noise-induced hearing loss. *Ear Hear.* 2006;27(1):1–19.
3. Van Campen LE, Murphy WJ, Franks JR, Mathias PI, Toraason MA. Oxidative DNA damage is associated with intense noise exposure in the rat. *Hear Res.* 2002;164(1–2):29–38.
4. Neri S, Signorelli S, Pulvirenti D, et al. Oxidative stress, nitric oxide, endothelial dysfunction, and tinnitus. *Free Radic Res.* 2006;40(6):615–618.
5. Vlajkovic SM, Lin SC, Wong AC, Wackrow B, Thorne PR. Noise-induced changes in expression levels of NADPH oxidases in the cochlea. *Hear Res.* 2013;304:145–152.
6. Turcot A, Girard SA, Courteau M, Baril J, Larocque R. Noise-induced hearing loss and combined noise and vibration exposure. *Occup Med (Lond).* 2015;65(3):238–244.
7. Yamamoto H, Omelchenko I, Shi X, Nuttall AL. The influence of NF-kappaB signal-transduction pathways on the murine inner ear by acoustic overstimulation. *J Neurosci Res.* 2009;87(8):1832–1840.
8. Masuda M, Nagashima R, Kanzaki S, Fujioka M, Ogita K, Ogawa K. Nuclear factor-kappa B nuclear translocation in the cochlea of mice following acoustic overstimulation. *Brain Res.* 2006;1068(1):237–247.
9. Kim HJ, So HS, Lee JH, et al. Role of proinflammatory cytokines in cisplatin-induced vestibular hair cell damage. *Head Neck.* 2008;30(11):1445–1456.
10. Aminpour S, Tinling SP, Brodie HA. Role of tumor necrosis factor-alpha in sensorineural hearing loss after bacterial meningitis. *Otol Neurotol.* 2005;26(4):602–609.
11. Sziklai I, Batta TJ, Karosi T. Otosclerosis: An organ-specific inflammatory disease with sensorineural hearing loss. *Eur Arch Otorhinolaryngol.* 2009;266(11):1711–1718.
12. Verschuur C, Agyemang-Prempeh A, Newman TA. Inflammation is associated with a worsening of presbycusis: Evidence from the MRC national study of hearing. *Int J Audiol.* 2014;53(7):469–475.
13. Masuda M, Kanzaki S, Minami S, et al. Correlations of inflammatory biomarkers with the onset and prognosis of idiopathic sudden sensorineural hearing loss. *Otol Neurotol.* 2012;33(7):1142–1150.
14. Puel JL, Ruel J, Gervais d'Aldin C, Pujol R. Excitotoxicity and repair of cochlear synapses after noise-trauma induced hearing loss. *Neuroreport.* 1998;9(9):2109–2114.
15. Hakuba N, Koga K, Gyo K, Usami SI, Tanaka K. Exacerbation of noise-induced hearing loss in mice lacking the glutamate transporter GLAST. *J Neurosci.* 2000;20(23):8750–8753.
16. Brozoski TJ, Wisner KW, Odintsov B, Bauer CA. Local NMDA receptor blockade attenuates chronic tinnitus and associated brain activity in an animal model. *PLoS One.* 2013;8(10):e77674.
17. Hou F, Wang S, Zhai S, Hu Y, Yang W, He L. Effects of alpha-tocopherol on noise-induced hearing loss in guinea pigs. *Hear Res.* 2003;179(1–2):1–8.
18. Kalkanis JG, Whitworth C, Rybak LP. Vitamin E reduces cisplatin ototoxicity. *Laryngoscope.* 2004;114(3):538–542.
19. Husain K, Whitworth C, Somani SM, Rybak LP. Partial protection by lipoic acid against carboplantin-induced ototoxicity in rats. *Biomed Environ Sci.* 2005;18(3):198–206.
20. Kopke RD, Jackson RL, Coleman JK, Liu J, Bielefeld EC, Balough BJ. NAC for noise: From the bench top to the clinic. *Hear Res.* 2007;226(1–2):114–125.
21. Sato K. Pharmacokinetics of coenzyme Q10 in recovery of acute sensorineural hearing loss due to hypoxia. *Acta Otolaryngol Suppl.* 1988;458:95–102.
22. Ojano-Dirain CP, Antonelli PJ, Le Prell CG. Mitochondria-targeted antioxidant MitoQ reduces gentamicin-induced ototoxicity. *Otol Neurotol.* 2014;35(3):533–539.
23. McFadden SL, Woo JM, Michalak N, Ding D. Dietary vitamin C supplementation reduces noise-induced hearing loss in guinea pigs. *Hear Res.* 2005;202(1–2):200–208.
24. Seidman MD, Tang W, Bai VU, et al. Resveratrol decreases noise-induced cyclooxygenase-2 expression in the rat cochlea. *Otolaryngol Head Neck Surg.* 2013;148(5):827–833.
25. Wang X, Truong T, Billings PB, Harris JP, Keithley EM. Blockage of immune-mediated inner ear damage by etanercept. *Otol Neurotol.* 2003;24(1):52–57.
26. Angeli SI, Liu XZ, Yan D, Balkany T, Telischi F. Coenzyme Q-10 treatment of patients with a 7445A→G mitochondrial DNA mutation stops the progression of hearing loss. *Acta Otolaryngol.* 2005;125(5):510–512.
27. Savastano M, Brescia G, Marioni G. Antioxidant therapy in idiopathic tinnitus: Preliminary outcomes. *Arch Med Res.* 2007;38(4):456–459.

28. Kaya H, Koc AK, Sayin I, et al. Vitamins A, C, and E and selenium in the treatment of idiopathic sudden sensorineural hearing loss. *Eur Arch Otorhinolaryngol.* 2015;272(5):1119–1125.
29. Kang HS, Park JJ, Ahn SK, Hur DG, Kim HY. Effect of high dose intravenous vitamin C on idiopathic sudden sensorineural hearing loss: A prospective single-blind randomized controlled trial. *Eur Arch Otorhinolaryngol.* 2013;270(10):2631–2636.
30. Kapoor N, Mani KV, Shyam R, Sharma RK, Singh AP, Selvamurthy W. Effect of vitamin E supplementation on carbogen-induced amelioration of noise induced hearing loss in man. *Noise Health.* 2011;13(55):452–458.
31. Haase GM, Prasad KN, Cole WC, Baggett-Strelau JM, Wyatt SE. Antioxidant micronutrient impact on hearing disorders: Concept, rationale, and evidence. *Am J Otolaryngol-Head Neck Med Surg.* 2011;32:55–61.
32. Chen P, Wang S, Zhang Y, Huang H, Zhang C, Xiao Z. Intratympanic versus systemic steroid initial treatment for idiopathic sudden hearing loss: A Meta-analysis. *Lin Chung Er Bi Yan Hou Tou Jing Wai Ke Za Zhi.* 2015;29(22):1970–1977.
33. Langguth B, Elgoyhen AB. Current pharmacological treatments for tinnitus. *Expert Opin Pharmacother.* 2012;13(17):2495–2509.
34. Guitton MJ, Dudai Y. Blockade of cochlear NMDA receptors prevents long-term tinnitus during a brief consolidation window after acoustic trauma. *Neural Plast.* 2007;2007:80904.
35. Bing D, Lee SC, Campanelli D, et al. Cochlear NMDA receptors as a therapeutic target of noise-induced tinnitus. *Cell Physiol Biochem.* 2015;35(5):1905–1923.
36. Kirkby-Strachan G, Que-Hee C. Implantable hearing devices: An update. *Aust Fam Physician.* 2016;45(6):370–373.
37. Rezaei M, Rashedi V, Morasae EK. Reading skills in Persian deaf children with cochlear implants and hearing aids. *Int J Pediatr Otorhinolaryngol.* 2016;89:1–5.
38. Walravens E, Keidser G, Hickson L. Provision, perception, and use of trainable hearing aids in Australia: A survey of clinicians and hearing impaired adults. *Int J Audiol.* 2016:1–9.
39. de Carvalho GM, Guimaraes AC, Duarte AS, et al. Hearing preservation after cochlear implantation: UNICAMP outcomes. *Int J Otolaryngol.* 2013;2013:107186.
40. Colletti V, Fiorino FG, Saccetto L, Giarbini N, Carner M. Improved auditory performance of cochlear implant patients using the middle fossa approach. *Audiology.* 1999;38(4):225–234.
41. Prasad KN. Simultaneous activation of Nrf2 and elevation of antioxidant compounds for reducing oxidative stress and chronic inflammation in human Alzheimer's disease. *Mech Ageing Dev.* 2016;153:41–47.
42. Federal Trade Commission. Adult hearing loss: Recent data from CDC. In: CDC, ed. *Now Hear This: Competition, Innovation, and Consumer Protection Issues in Hearing Health Care,* Washington, DC, 2017.
43. National Institute of Deafness and Other Communication Disorders (NIDOCD). Quick statistics about hearing. 2017.
44. American Tinnitus Association (ATA). Understanding the facts. 2017.
45. National Institute of Deafness and Other Communication Disorders (NIDOCD). Sudden deafness (NIH pub. No. 00-4757). Bethesda, MD. 2003.
46. Byl FM, Jr. Sudden hearing loss: Eight years' experience and suggested prognostic table. *Laryngoscope.* 1984;94(5 Pt 1):647–661.
47. Dalton DS, Cruickshanks KJ, Wiley TL, Klein BE, Klein R, Tweed TS. Association of leisure-time noise exposure and hearing loss. *Audiology.* 2001;40(1):1–9.
48. National Institute of Deafness and Other Communication Disorders (NIDOCD). Noise-induced hearing loss (NIH Pub. No. 97-4233, Bethesda, MD. 2002).
49. Schraff SA, Brown DK, Schleiss MR, Meinzen-Derr J, Greinwald JH, Choo DI. The role of CMV inflammatory genes in hearing loss. *Otol Neurotol.* 2007;28(7):964–969.
50. Diao MF, Liu HY, Zhang YM, Gao WY. Changes in antioxidant capacity of the guinea pig exposed to noise and the protective effect of alpha-lipoic acid against acoustic trauma. *Sheng Li Xue Bao.* 25 2003;55(6):672–676.
51. Henderson D, McFadden SL, Liu CC, Hight N, Zheng XY. The role of antioxidants in protection from impulse noise. *Ann N Y Acad Sci.* 28 1999;884:368–380.
52. Ohlemiller KK, McFadden SL, Ding DL, et al. Targeted deletion of the cytosolic Cu/Zn-superoxide dismutase gene (Sod1) increases susceptibility to noise-induced hearing loss. *Audiol Neurootol.* 1999;4(5):237–246.
53. Yamane H, Nakai Y, Takayama M, et al. The emergence of free radicals after acoustic trauma and strial blood flow. *Acta Otolaryngol Suppl.* 1995;519:87–92.
54. Minami SB, Yamashita D, Schacht J, Miller JM. Calcineurin activation contributes to noise-induced hearing loss. *J Neurosci Res.* 2004;78(3):383–392.

55. Ossowska K, Konieczny J, Wardas J, et al. An influence of ligands of metabotropic glutamate receptor subtypes on parkinsonian-like symptoms and the striatopallidal pathway in rats. *Amino Acids*. 2007;32(2):179–188.

56. Kowalska S, Sulkowski W. Tinnitus in noise-induced hearing impairment. *Med Pr*. 2001;52(5):305–313.

57. Fagelson MA. The association between tinnitus and posttraumatic stress disorder. *Am J Audiol*. 2007;16(2):107–117.

58. Prasad KN. Simultaneous activation of Nrf2 and elevation of antioxidant chemicals in management of posttraumatic stress disorders and traumatic brain injury. *BMMR*. 2015;18:116–127.

59. Park JS, Kim SW, Park K, Choung YH, Jou I, Park SM. Pravastatin attenuates noise-induced cochlear injury in mice. *Neuroscience*. 2012;208:123–132.

60. Pettersson H, Burstrom L, Hagberg M, Lundstrom R, Nilsson T. Risk of hearing loss among workers with vibration-induced white fingers. *Am J Ind Med*. 2014;57(12):1311–1318.

61. Minami SB, Sha SH, Schacht J. Antioxidant protection in a new animal model of cisplatin-induced ototoxicity. *Hear Res*. 2004;198(1–2):137–143.

62. Husain K, Scott RB, Whitworth C, Somani SM, Rybak LP. Dose response of carboplatin-induced hearing loss in rats: Antioxidant defense system. *Hear Res*. 2001;151(1–2):71–78.

63. Kim HJ, Oh GS, Shen A, et al. Augmentation of NAD(+) by NQO1 attenuates cisplatin-mediated hearing impairment. *Cell Death Dis*. 2014;5:e1292.

64. Barashkov NA, Teryutin FM, Pshennikova VG, et al. Age-Related Hearing Impairment (ARHI) associated with GJB2 single mutation IVS1 + 1G>A in the Yakut population isolate in Eastern Siberia. *PLoS One*. 2014;9(6):e100848.

65. Momi SK, Wolber LE, Fabiane SM, MacGregor AJ, Williams FM. Genetic and environmental factors in age-related hearing impairment. *Twin Res Hum Genet*. 2015;18(4):383–392.

66. Tavanai E, Mohammadkhani G. Role of antioxidants in prevention of age-related hearing loss: A review of literature. *Eur Arch Otorhinolaryngol*. 2017;274(4):1821–1834.

67. Le T, Keithley EM. Effects of antioxidants on the aging inner ear. *Hear Res*. 2007;226(1–2):194–202.

68. Zou J, Bretlau P, Pyykko I, Starck J, Toppila E. Sensorineural hearing loss after vibration: An animal model for evaluating prevention and treatment of inner ear hearing loss. *Acta Otolaryngol*. 2001;121(2):143–148.

69. Du Z, Yang Q, Liu L, et al. NADPH oxidase 2-dependent oxidative stress, mitochondrial damage and apoptosis in the ventral cochlear nucleus of D-galactose-induced aging rats. *Neuroscience*. 12 2015;286:281–292.

70. Chen B, Zhong Y, Peng W, Sun Y, Kong WJ. Age-related changes in the central auditory system: Comparison of D-galactose-induced aging rats and naturally aging rats. *Brain Res*. 16 2010;1344:43–53.

71. Zhong Y, Hu YJ, Chen B, et al. Mitochondrial transcription factor A overexpression and base excision repair deficiency in the inner ear of rats with D-galactose-induced aging. *FEBS J*. 2011;278(14):2500–2510.

72. Kinoshita M, Sakamoto T, Kashio A, Shimizu T, Yamasoba T. Age-related hearing loss in Mn-SOD heterozygous knockout mice. *Oxid Med Cell Longev*. 2013;2013:325702.

73. McFadden SL, Ding D, Burkard RF, et al. Cu/Zn SOD deficiency potentiates hearing loss and cochlear pathology in aged 129,CD-1 mice. *J Comp Neurol*. 1999;413(1):101–112.

74. Takumida M, Anniko M, Ohtani M. Radical scavengers for Meniere's disease after failure of conventional therapy: A pilot study. *Acta Otolaryngol*. 2003;123(6):697–703.

75. Shi X, Nuttall AL. Expression of adhesion molecular proteins in the cochlear lateral wall of normal and PARP-1 mutant mice. *Hear Res*. 2007;224(1–2):1–14.

76. Braga MP, Maciel SM, Marchiori LL, Poli-Frederico RC. Association between interleukin-6 polymorphism in the-174 G/C region and hearing loss in the elderly with a history of occupational noise exposure. *Braz J Otorhinolaryngol*. 2014;80(5):373–378.

77. Chen Y, Huang WG, Zha DJ, et al. Aspirin attenuates gentamicin ototoxicity: From the laboratory to the clinic. *Hear Res*. 2007;226(1–2):178–182.

78. So H, Kim H, Lee JH, et al. Cisplatin cytotoxicity of auditory cells requires secretions of proinflammatory cytokines via activation of ERK and NF-kappaB. *J Assoc Res Otolaryngol*. 2007;8(3):338–355.

79. Haake SM, Dinh CT, Chen S, Eshraghi AA, Van De Water TR. Dexamethasone protects auditory hair cells against TNFalpha-initiated apoptosis via activation of PI3K/Akt and NFkappaB signaling. *Hear Res*. 2009;255(1–2):22–32.

80. Van De Water TR, Dinh CT, Vivero R, Hoosien G, Eshraghi AA, Balkany TJ. Mechanisms of hearing loss from trauma and inflammation: Otoprotective therapies from the laboratory to the clinic. *Acta Otolaryngol*. 2009:1–4.

81. Sziklai I, Batta TJ, Karosi T. Otosclerosis: An organ-specific inflammatory disease with sensorineural hearing loss. *Eur Arch Otorhinolaryngol.* 2009:266(11):1711–1718.

82. Derebery MJ. Allergic and immunologic aspects of Meniere's disease. *Otolaryngol Head Neck Surg.* 1996;114(3):360–365.

83. Menardo J, Tang Y, Ladrech S, et al. Oxidative stress, inflammation, and autophagic stress as the key mechanisms of premature age-related hearing loss in SAMP8 mouse Cochlea. *Antioxid Redox Signal.* 2012;16(3):263–274.

84. Nash SD, Cruickshanks KJ, Zhan W, et al. Long-term assessment of systemic inflammation and the cumulative incidence of age-related hearing impairment in the epidemiology of hearing loss study. *J Gerontol A Biol Sci Med Sci.* 2014;69(2):207–214.

85. Zhang YM, Ma B, Gao WY, Wen W, Liu HY. Role of glutamate receptors in the spiral ganglion neuron damage induced by acoustic noise. *Sheng Li Xue Bao.* 2007;59(1):103–110.

86. Bai XY, Ma Y, Ding R, Fu B, Shi S, Chen XM. MiR-335 and miR-34a promote renal senescence by suppressing mitochondrial antioxidative enzymes. *J Am Soc Nephrol.* 2011;22(7):1252–1261.

87. Ruel J, Wang J, Pujol R, Hameg A, Dib M, Puel JL. Neuroprotective effect of riluzole in acute noise-induced hearing loss. *Neuroreport.* 2005;16(10):1087–1090.

88. Jager W, Goiny M, Herrera-Marschitz M, Brundin L, Fransson A, Canlon B. Noise-induced aspartate and glutamate efflux in the guinea pig cochlea and hearing loss. *Exp Brain Res.* 2000;134(4):426–434.

89. Steinbach S, Lutz J. Glutamate induces apoptosis in cultured spiral ganglion explants. *Biochem Biophys Res Commun.* 2007;357(1):14–19.

90. Lee RC, Feinbaum RL, Ambros V. The C. elegans heterochronic gene lin-4 encodes small RNAs with antisense complementarity to lin-14. *Cell.* 1993;75(5):843–854.

91. Wightman B, Ha I, Ruvkun G. Posttranscriptional regulation of the heterochronic gene lin-14 by lin-4 mediates temporal pattern formation in C. elegans. *Cell.* 1993;75(5):855–862.

92. Macfarlane LA, Murphy PR. MicroRNA: Biogenesis, function, and role in cancer. *Curr Genomics.* 2010;11(7):537–561.

93. Londin E, Loher P, Telonis AG, et al. Analysis of 13 cell types reveals evidence for the expression of numerous novel primate- and tissue-specific microRNAs. *Proc Natl Acad Sci USA.* 2015;112(10):E1106–E1115.

94. Denli AM, Tops BB, Plasterk RH, Ketting RF, Hannon GJ. Processing of primary microRNAs by the Microprocessor complex. *Nature.* 2004;432(7014):231–235.

95. Lee Y, Ahn C, Han J, et al. The nuclear RNase III Drosha initiates microRNA processing. *Nature.* 2003;425(6956):415–419.

96. Hutvagner G, McLachlan J, Pasquinelli AE, Balint E, Tuschl T, Zamore PD. A cellular function for the RNA-interference enzyme Dicer in the maturation of the let-7 small temporal RNA. *Science.* 2001;293(5531):834–838.

97. Ushakov K, Rudnicki A, Avraham KB. MicroRNAs in sensorineural diseases of the ear. *Front Mol Neurosci.* 2013;6:52.

98. Friedman LM, Dror AA, Mor E, et al. MicroRNAs are essential for development and function of inner ear hair cells in vertebrates. *Proc Natl Acad Sci USA.* 2009;106(19):7915–7920.

99. Yan D, Xing Y, Ouyang X, et al. Analysis of miR-376 RNA cluster members in the mouse inner ear. *Int J Exp Pathol.* 2012;93(6):450–457.

100. Gu C, Li X, Tan Q, Wang Z, Chen L, Liu Y. MiR-183 family regulates chloride intracellular channel 5 expression in inner ear hair cells. *Toxicol In Vitro.* 2013;27(1):486–491.

101. Elkan-Miller T, Ulitsky I, Hertzano R, et al. Integration of transcriptomics, proteomics, and microRNA analyses reveals novel microRNA regulation of targets in the mammalian inner ear. *PloS One.* 2011;6(4):e18195.

102. Pradeepa MM, Grimes GR, Taylor GC, Sutherland HG, Bickmore WA. Psip1/Ledgf p75 restrains Hox gene expression by recruiting both trithorax and polycomb group proteins. *Nucleic Acids Res.* 2014;42(14):9021–9032.

103. Basu A, Drame A, Munoz R, et al. Pathway specific gene expression profiling reveals oxidative stress genes potentially regulated by transcription co-activator LEDGF/p75 in prostate cancer cells. *Prostate.* 2012;72(6):597–611.

104. Riccardi S, Bergling S, Sigoillot F, et al. MiR-210 promotes sensory hair cell formation in the organ of corti. *BMC Genomics.* 27 2016;17:309.

105. Rudnicki A, Isakov O, Ushakov K, et al. Next-generation sequencing of small RNAs from inner ear sensory epithelium identifies microRNAs and defines regulatory pathways. *BMC Genomics.* 2014;15:484.

106. Wang XR, Zhang XM, Zhen J, Zhang PX, Xu G, Jiang H. MicroRNA expression in the embryonic mouse inner ear. *Neuroreport*. 2010;21(9):611–617.

107. Li H, Kloosterman W, Fekete DM. MicroRNA-183 family members regulate sensorineural fates in the inner ear. *J Neurosci*. 2010;30(9):3254–3263.

108. Zhang KD, Stoller ML, Fekete DM. Expression and misexpression of the miR-183 family in the developing hearing organ of the chicken. *PLoS One*. 2015;10(7):e0132796.

109. Huyghe A, Van den Ackerveken P, Sacheli R, et al. MicroRNA-124 regulates cell specification in the cochlea through modulation of Sfrp4/5. *Cell Rep*. 2015;13(1):31–42.

110. Prasad KN. Oxidative stress and pro-inflammatory cytokines may act as one of signals for regulating microRNAs expression in Alzheimer's disease. *Mech Ageing Dev*. 2017;162:63–71.

111. Xue T, Wei L, Zha DJ, et al. MiR-29b overexpression induces cochlear hair cell apoptosis through the regulation of SIRT1/PGC-1alpha signaling: Implications for age-related hearing loss. *Int J Mol Med*. 2016;38(5):1387–1394.

112. Kim S, Lee JH, Nam SI. Dicer is downregulated and correlated with Drosha in idiopathic sudden sensorineural hearing loss. *J Korean Med Sci*. 2015;30(8):1183–1188.

113. Xiong H, Pang J, Yang H, et al. Activation of miR-34a/SIRT1/p53 signaling contributes to cochlear hair cell apoptosis: Implications for age-related hearing loss. *Neurobiol Aging*. 2015;36(4):1692–1701.

114. Zhang Q, Liu H, McGee J, Walsh EJ, Soukup GA, He DZ. Identifying microRNAs involved in degeneration of the organ of corti during age-related hearing loss. *PLoS One*. 2013;8(4):e62786.

115. Fan Y, Zhang Y, Wu R, et al. miR-431 is involved in regulating cochlear function by targeting Eya4. *Biochim Biophys Acta*. 2016;1862(11):2119–2126.

116. Kuhn S, Johnson SL, Furness DN, et al. MiR-96 regulates the progression of differentiation in mammalian cochlear inner and outer hair cells. *Proc Natl Acad Sci USA*. 2011;108(6):2355–2360.

117. Friedman LM, Avraham KB. MicroRNAs and epigenetic regulation in the mammalian inner ear: Implications for deafness. *Mamm Genome*. 2009;20(9-10):581–603.

118. Lewis MA, Quint E, Glazier AM, et al. An ENU-induced mutation of miR-96 associated with progressive hearing loss in mice. *Nat Genet*. 2009;41(5):614–618.

119. Solda G, Robusto M, Primignani P, et al. A novel mutation within the MIR96 gene causes non-syndromic inherited hearing loss in an Italian family by altering pre-miRNA processing. *Hum Mol Genet*. 2012;21(3):577–585.

120. Patel M, Cai Q, Ding D, Salvi R, Hu Z, Hu BH. The miR-183/Taok1 target pair is implicated in cochlear responses to acoustic trauma. *PLoS One*. 2013;8(3):e58471.

121. Zhang Z, Liu K, Chen Y, Li Z, Yan N, Zhang J. The expression of miR-183 family in the pathogenesis and development of noise-induced deafness. *Lin Chung Er Bi Yan Hou Tou Jing Wai Ke Za Zhi*. 2014;28(7):468–472.

122. Ding L, Liu J, Shen HX, et al. Analysis of plasma microRNA expression profiles in male textile workers with noise-induced hearing loss. *Hear Res*. 2016;333:275–282.

123. Yu L, Tang H, Jiang XH, Tsang LL, Chung YW, Chan HC. Involvement of calpain-I and microRNA34 in kanamycin-induced apoptosis of inner ear cells. *Cell Biol Int*. 2010;34(12):1219–1225.

124. Li Y, Peng A, Ge S, Wang Q, Liu J. MiR-204 suppresses cochlear spiral ganglion neuron survival in vitro by targeting TMPRSS3. *Hear Res*. 2014;314:60–64.

125. Wang JY, Xia Y, Yang CC, Wang Z. Analysis of microRNA regulatory network in cochlear hair cells with oxidative stress injury. *Zhonghua Er Bi Yan Hou Tou Jing Wai Ke Za Zhi*. 2016;51(10):751–755.

126. Wang Z, Liu Y, Han N, et al. Profiles of oxidative stress-related microRNA and mRNA expression in auditory cells. *Brain Res*. 2010;1346:14–25.

127. Tan PX, Du SS, Ren C, et al. MicroRNA-207 enhances radiation-induced apoptosis by directly targeting Akt3 in cochlea hair cells. *Cell Death Dis*. 2014;5:e1433.

128. Lin Y, Shen J, Li D, et al. MiR-34a contributes to diabetes-related cochlear hair cell apoptosis via SIRT1/HIF-1alpha signaling. *Gen Comp Endocrinol*. 2017;246:63–70.

129. Farr SA, Poon HF, Dogrukol-Ak D, et al. The antioxidants alpha-lipoic acid and N-acetylcysteine reverse memory impairment and brain oxidative stress in aged SAMP8 mice. *J Neurochem*. 2003;84(5):1173–1183.

130. Joachims HZ, Segal J, Golz A, Netzer A, Goldenberg D. Antioxidants in treatment of idiopathic sudden hearing loss. *Otol Neurotol*. 2003;24(4):572–575.

131. Scholik AR, Lee US, Chow CK, Yan HY. Dietary vitamin E protects the fathead minnow, pimephales promelas, against noise exposure. *Comp Biochem Physiol C Toxicol Pharmacol*. 2004;137(4):313–323.

132. Duan M, Qiu J, Laurell G, Olofsson A, Counter SA, Borg E. Dose and time-dependent protection of the antioxidant N-L-acetylcysteine against impulse noise trauma. *Hear Res*. 2004;192(1–2):1–9.

133. Ohinata Y, Yamasoba T, Schacht J, Miller JM. Glutathione limits noise-induced hearing loss. *Hear Res.* 2000;146(1–2):28–34.

134. Ohinata Y, Miller JM, Schacht J. Protection from noise-induced lipid peroxidation and hair cell loss in the cochlea. *Brain Res.* 2003;966(2):265–273.

135. Kopke R, Bielefeld E, Liu J, et al. Prevention of impulse noise-induced hearing loss with antioxidants. *Acta Otolaryngol.* 2005;125(3):235–243.

136. Sergi B, Fetoni AR, Paludetti G, et al. Protective properties of idebenone in noise-induced hearing loss in the guinea pig. *Neuroreport.* 2006;17(9):857–861.

137. Fetoni AR, Piacentini R, Fiorita A, Paludetti G, Troiani D. Water-soluble coenzyme Q10 formulation (Q-ter) promotes outer hair cell survival in a guinea pig model of noise induced hearing loss (NIHL). *Brain Res.* 2009;1257:108–116.

138. Fetoni AR, Ferraresi A, Greca CL, et al. Antioxidant protection against acoustic trauma by coadministration of idebenone and vitamin E. *Neuroreport.* 2008;19(3):277–281.

139. Samson J, Wiktorek-Smagur A, Politanski P, et al. Noise-induced time-dependent changes in oxidative stress in the mouse cochlea and attenuation by D-methionine. *Neuroscience.* 2008;152(1):146–150.

140. Teranishi MA, Nakashima T. Effects of trolox, locally applied on round windows, on cisplatin-induced ototoxicity in guinea pigs. *Int J Pediatr Otorhinolaryngol.* 2003;67(2):133–139.

141. Fetoni AR, Sergi B, Ferraresi A, Paludetti G, Troiani D. alpha-Tocopherol protective effects on gentamicin ototoxicity: An experimental study. *Int J Audiol.* 2004;43(3):166–171.

142. Feghali JG, Liu W, Van De Water TR. L-n-acetyl-cysteine protection against cisplatin-induced auditory neuronal and hair cell toxicity. *Laryngoscope.* 2001;111(7):1147–1155.

143. Schacht J. Antioxidant therapy attenuates aminoglycoside-induced hearing loss. *Ann N Y Acad Sci.* 28 1999;884:125–130.

144. Seidman MD. Effects of dietary restriction and antioxidants on presbyacusis. *Laryngoscope.* 2000; 110(5 Pt 1):727–738.

145. Seidman MD, Ahmad N, Joshi D, Seidman J, Thawani S, Quirk WS. Age-related hearing loss and its association with reactive oxygen species and mitochondrial DNA damage. *Acta Otolaryngol Suppl.* 2004(552):16–24.

146. Derin A, Agirdir B, Derin N, et al. The effects of L-carnitine on presbyacusis in the rat model. *Clin Otolaryngol Allied Sci.* 2004;29(3):238–241.

147. Davis RR, Kuo MW, Stanton SG, Canlon B, Krieg E, Alagramam KN. N-Acetyl L-cysteine does not protect against premature age-related hearing loss in C57BL/6J mice: A pilot study. *Hear Res.* 2007;226(1–2):203–208.

148. Aabdallah DM, Eid NI. Possible neuroprotective effects of lecithin and alpha-tocopherol alone or in combination against ischemia/reperfusion insult in rat brain. *J Biochem Mol Toxicol.* 2004;18(5):273–278.

149. Gordin A, Goldenberg D, Golz A, Netzer A, Joachims HZ. Magnesium: A new therapy for idiopathic sudden sensorineural hearing loss. *Otol Neurotol.* 2002;23(4):447–451.

150. Seidman MD. Glutamate antagonists, steroids, and antioxidants as therapeutic options for hearing loss and tinnitus and the use of an inner ear drug delivery system. *Int Tinnitus J.* 1998;4(2):148–154.

151. Tepel M. N-Acetylcysteine in the prevention of ototoxicity. *Kidney Int.* 2007;72(3):231–232.

152. Raponi G, Alpini D, Volonte S, Capobianco S, Cesarani A. The role of free radicals and plasmatic antioxidant in Meniere's syndrome. *Int Tinnitus J.* 2003;9(2):104–108.

153. Vile GF, Winterbourn CC. Inhibition of adriamycin-promoted microsomal lipid peroxidation by beta-carotene, alpha-tocopherol and retinol at high and low oxygen partial pressures. *FEBS Lett.* 1988;238(2):353–356.

154. Niki E. Interaction of ascorbate and alpha-tocopherol. *Ann N Y Acad Sci.* 1987;498:186–199.

155. Wu H, Kong L, Tan Y, et al. C66 ameliorates diabetic nephropathy in mice by both upregulating NRF2 function via increase in miR-200a and inhibiting miR-21. *Diabetologia.* 2016;59:1558–1568.

156. Jaramillo MC, Zhang DD. The emerging role of the Nrf2-Keap1 signaling pathway in cancer. *Genes Dev.* 2013;27(20):2179–2191.

157. Williamson TP, Johnson DA, Johnson JA. Activation of the Nrf2-ARE pathway by siRNA knockdown of Keap1 reduces oxidative stress and provides partial protection from MPTP-mediated neurotoxicity. *Neurotoxicology.* 2012;33(3):272–279.

158. Itoh K, Chiba T, Takahashi S, et al. An Nrf2/small Maf heterodimer mediates the induction of phase II detoxifying enzyme genes through antioxidant response elements. *Biochem Biophys Res Commun.* 1997;236(2):313–322.

159. Hayes JD, Chanas SA, Henderson CJ, et al. The Nrf2 transcription factor contributes both to the basal expression of glutathione S-transferases in mouse liver and to their induction by the chemopreventive synthetic antioxidants, butylated hydroxyanisole, and ethoxyquin. *Biochem Soc Trans.* 2000;28(2):33–41.

160. Chan K, Han XD, Kan YW. An important function of Nrf2 in combating oxidative stress: Detoxification of acetaminophen. *Proc Natl Acad Sci USA.* 2001;98(8):4611–4616.

161. Ramsey CP, Glass CA, Montgomery MB, et al. Expression of Nrf2 in neurodegenerative diseases. *J Neuropathol Exp Neurol.* 2007;66(1):75–85.

162. Chen PC, Vargas MR, Pani AK, et al. Nrf2-mediated neuroprotection in the MPTP mouse model of Parkinson's disease: Critical role for the astrocyte. *Proc Natl Acad Sci USA.* 2009;106(8):2933–2938.

163. Lastres-Becker I, Ulusoy A, Innamorato NG, et al. Alpha-synuclein expression and Nrf2 deficiency cooperate to aggravate protein aggregation, neuronal death and inflammation in early-stage Parkinson's disease. *Hum Mol Genet.* 2012;21(14):3173–3192.

164. Xi YD, Yu HL, Ding J, et al. Flavonoids protect cerebrovascular endothelial cells through Nrf2 and PI3K from beta-amyloid peptide-induced oxidative damage. *Curr Neurovasc Res.* 2012;9(1):32–41.

165. Suh JH, Shenvi SV, Dixon BM, et al. Decline in transcriptional activity of Nrf2 causes age-related loss of glutathione synthesis, which is reversible with lipoic acid. *Proc Natl Acad Sci USA.* 2004;101(10):3381–3386.

166. Trujillo J, Chirino YI, Molina-Jijon E, Anderica-Romero AC, Tapia E, Pedraza-Chaverri J. Renoprotective effect of the antioxidant curcumin: Recent findings. *Redox Biol.* 2013;1(1):448–456.

167. Steele ML, Fuller S, Patel M, Kersaitis C, Ooi L, Munch G. Effect of Nrf2 activators on release of glutathione, cysteinylglycine, and homocysteine by human U373 astroglial cells. *Redox Biol.* 2013;1(1):441–445.

168. Kode A, Rajendrasozhan S, Caito S, Yang SR, Megson IL, Rahman I. Resveratrol induces glutathione synthesis by activation of Nrf2 and protects against cigarette smoke-mediated oxidative stress in human lung epithelial cells. *Am J Physiol Lung Cell Mol Physiol.* 2008;294(3):L478–L488.

169. Gao L, Wang J, Sekhar KR, et al. Novel n-3 fatty acid oxidation products activate Nrf2 by destabilizing the association between Keap1 and Cullin3. *J Biol Chem.* 2007;282(4):2529–2537.

170. Saw CL, Yang AY, Guo Y, Kong AN. Astaxanthin and omega-3 fatty acids individually and in combination protect against oxidative stress via the Nrf2-ARE pathway. *Food Chem Toxicol.* 2013;62:869–875.

171. Song J, Kang SM, Lee WT, Park KA, Lee KM, Lee JE. Glutathione protects brain endothelial cells from hydrogen peroxide-induced oxidative stress by increasing nrf2 expression. *Exp Neurobiol.* 2014;23(1):93–103.

172. Ji L, Liu R, Zhang XD, et al. N-acetylcysteine attenuates phosgene-induced acute lung injury via upregulation of Nrf2 expression. *Inhal Toxicol.* 2010;22(7):535–542.

173. Choi HK, Pokharel YR, Lim SC, et al. Inhibition of liver fibrosis by solubilized coenzyme Q10: Role of Nrf2 activation in inhibiting transforming growth factor-beta1 expression. *Toxicol Appl Pharmacol.* 2009;240(3):377–384.

174. Bai H, Liu R, Chen HL, et al. Enhanced antioxidant effect of caffeic acid phenethyl ester and Trolox in combination against radiation induced-oxidative stress. *Chem Biol Interact.* 2014;207:7–15.

175. Cui L, Jeong H, Borovecki F, Parkhurst CN, Tanese N, Krainc D. Transcriptional repression of PGC-1alpha by mutant huntingtin leads to mitochondrial dysfunction and neurodegeneration. *Cell.* 2006;127(1):59–69.

176. Li XH, Li CY, Lu JM, Tian RB, Wei J. Allicin ameliorates cognitive deficits ageing-induced learning and memory deficits through enhancing of Nrf2 antioxidant signaling pathways. *Neurosci Lett.* 2012;514(1):46–50.

177. Bergstrom P, Andersson HC, Gao Y, et al. Repeated transient sulforaphane stimulation in astrocytes leads to prolonged Nrf2-mediated gene expression and protection from superoxide-induced damage. *Neuropharmacology.* 2011;60(2–3):343–353.

178. Wruck CJ, Gotz ME, Herdegen T, Varoga D, Brandenburg LO, Pufe T. Kavalactones protect neural cells against amyloid beta peptide-induced neurotoxicity via extracellular signal-regulated kinase 1/2-dependent nuclear factor erythroid 2-related factor 2 activation. *Mol Pharmacol.* 2008;73(6):1785–1795.

179. Honkura Y, Matsuo H, Murakami S, et al. NRF2 is a key target for prevention of noise-induced hearing loss by reducing oxidative damage of cochlea. *Sci Rep.* 2016;6:19329.

180. Kim SJ, Park C, Lee JN, et al. Erdosteine protects HEI-OC1 auditory cells from cisplatin toxicity through suppression of inflammatory cytokines and induction of Nrf2 target proteins. *Toxicol Appl Pharmacol.* 2015;288(2):192–202.

181. So H, Kim H, Kim Y, et al. Evidence that cisplatin-induced auditory damage is attenuated by downregulation of pro-inflammatory cytokines via Nrf2/HO-1. *J Assoc Res Otolaryngol.* 2008;9(3):290–306.
182. Kim SJ, Park C, Han AL, et al. Ebselen attenuates cisplatin-induced ROS generation through Nrf2 activation in auditory cells. *Hear Res.* 2009;251(1–2):70–82.
183. Ma W, Hu J, Cheng Y, Wang J, Zhang X, Xu M. Ginkgolide B protects against cisplatin-induced ototoxicity: Enhancement of Akt-Nrf2-HO-1 signaling and reduction of NADPH oxidase. *Cancer Chemother Pharmacol.* 2015;75(5):949–959.
184. Choi BM, Chen XY, Gao SS, Zhu R, Kim BR. Anti-apoptotic effect of phloretin on cisplatin-induced apoptosis in HEI-OC1 auditory cells. *Pharmacol Rep.* 2011;63(3):708–716.
185. Hoshino T, Tabuchi K, Nishimura B, et al. Protective role of Nrf2 in age-related hearing loss and gentamicin ototoxicity. *Biochem Biophys Res Commun.* 2011;415(1):94–98.
186. Nagashima R, Ogita K. Enhanced biosynthesis of glutathione in the spiral ganglion of the cochlea after in vivo treatment with dexamethasone in mice. *Brain Res.* 2006;1117(1):101–108.
187. Song SM, Park YS, Lee A, et al. Concentrations of blood vitamin A, C, E, coenzyme Q10, and urine cotinine related to cigarette smoking exposure. *Korean J Lab Med.* 2009;29(1):10–16.
188. Galan P, Viteri FE, Bertrais S, et al. Serum concentrations of beta-carotene, vitamins C and E, zinc, and selenium are influenced by sex, age, diet, smoking status, alcohol consumption, and corpulence in a general French adult population. *Eur J Clin Nutr.* 2005;59(10):1181–1190.
189. Adhikari D, Baxi J, Risal S, Singh PP. Oxidative stress and antioxidant status in cancer patients and healthy subjects, a case-control study. *Nepal Med Coll J.* 2005;7(2):112–115.
190. Li W, Khor TO, Xu C, et al. Activation of Nrf2-antioxidant signaling attenuates NFkappaB-inflammatory response and elicits apoptosis. *Biochem Pharmacol.* 2008;76(11):1485–1489.
191. Kim J, Cha YN, Surh YJ. A protective role of nuclear factor-erythroid 2-related factor-2 (Nrf2) in inflammatory disorders. *Mutat Res.* 2010;690(1–2):12–23.
192. Abate A, Yang G, Dennery PA, Oberle S, Schroder H. Synergistic inhibition of cyclooxygenase-2 expression by vitamin E and aspirin. *Free Radic Biol Med.* 2000;29(11):1135–1142.
193. Devaraj S, Tang R, Adams-Huet B, et al. Effect of high-dose alpha-tocopherol supplementation on biomarkers of oxidative stress and inflammation and carotid atherosclerosis in patients with coronary artery disease. *Am J Clin Nutr.* 2007;86(5):1392–1398.
194. Fu Y, Zheng S, Lin J, Ryerse J, Chen A. Curcumin protects the rat liver from CCl4-caused injury and fibrogenesis by attenuating oxidative stress and suppressing inflammation. *Mol Pharmacol.* 2008;73(2):399–409.
195. Lee HS, Jung KK, Cho JY, et al. Neuroprotective effect of curcumin is mainly mediated by blockade of microglial cell activation. *Pharmazie.* 2007;62(12):937–942.
196. Rahman S, Bhatia K, Khan AQ, et al. Topically applied vitamin E prevents massive cutaneous inflammatory and oxidative stress responses induced by double application of 12-O-tetradecanoylphorbol-13-acetate (TPA) in mice. *Chem Biol Interact.* 2008;172(3):195–205.
197. Suzuki YJ, Aggarwal BB, Packer L. Alpha-lipoic acid is a potent inhibitor of NF-kappa B activation in human T cells. *Biochem Biophys Res Commun.* 1992;189(3):1709–1715.
198. Zhu J, Yong W, Wu X, et al. Anti-inflammatory effect of resveratrol on TNF-alpha-induced MCP-1 expression in adipocytes. *Biochem Biophys Res Commun.* 2008;369(2):471–477.
199. Chang Y, Huang SK, Wang SJ. Coenzyme Q10 inhibits the release of glutamate in rat cerebrocortical nerve terminals by suppression of voltage-dependent calcium influx and mitogen-activated protein kinase signaling pathway. *J Agric Food Chem.* 2012;60(48):11909–11918.
200. Schubert D, Kimura H, Maher P. Growth factors and vitamin E modify neuronal glutamate toxicity. *Proc Natl Acad Sci USA.* 1992;89(17):8264–8267.
201. Sandhu JK, Pandey S, Ribecco-Lutkiewicz M, et al. Molecular mechanisms of glutamate neurotoxicity in mixed cultures of NT2-derived neurons and astrocytes: Protective effects of coenzyme Q10. *J Neurosci Res.* 2003;72(6):691–703.
202. Yang TT, Wang SJ. Pyridoxine inhibits depolarization-evoked glutamate release in nerve terminals from rat cerebral cortex: A possible neuroprotective mechanism? *J Pharmacol Exp Ther.* 2009;331(1):244–254.
203. Hung KL, Wang CC, Huang CY, Wang SJ. Cyanocobalamin, vitamin B12, depresses glutamate release through inhibition of voltage-dependent Ca2+ influx in rat cerebrocortical nerve terminals (synaptosomes). *Eur J Pharmacol.* 2009;602(2–3):230–237.
204. Prasad KN. *Etiology of Alzheimer's Disease Prevention and Improved Management by Micronutrients.* Boca Raton, FL: CRC Press; 2015.

12 Micronutrients in Improvement of the Standard Therapy in Posttraumatic Stress Disorder (PTSD)

INTRODUCTION

Posttraumatic stress disorder (PTSD) is a complex mental disorder often resulting from exposure to sudden or repeatedly extreme traumatic events such as war, terrorism, natural- or human-caused disaster, as well as violent personal assault such as rape, mugging, domestic violence, and accidents. There is also a strong direct relationship between mild traumatic brain injury (TBI) and PTSD.[1,2] Approximately 17.6% of PTSD can develop mild to severe TBI over the first 4 years after injury.[3]

There are not effective prevention strategies for PTSD. The current gold standard management of PTSD involves antidepressant medications that rarely yield better than a 40% reduction in the Clinician Administered PTSD Scale (CAPS) scores, but most patients still exhibit PTSD symptoms at the end of any treatment trial.[4] Therefore, additional approaches that attenuate some cellular events that contribute to the initiation and progression of PTSD must be developed.

Analysis of studies shows that increased oxidative stress, chronic inflammation, and excessive release of glutamate are major cellular defects that increase the risk of developing PTSD and that promote the progression of PTSD.[5] Studies also show that increased oxidative stress precedes increased chronic inflammation glutamate level. Oxidative damage, if not repaired, leads to chronic inflammation. Enhanced glutamate level participates in the progression of PTSD. Therefore, attenuation of these cellular defects at the same time would help reduce the risk of developing PTSD, and in combination with standard care, may improve the management of this mental disease. In order to achieve this goal, it is essential to increase the levels of antioxidant enzymes and dietary and endogenous antioxidants.[6] The levels of antioxidants can be increased by supplementation, but enhancing the levels of antioxidant enzymes requires activation of a nuclear transcriptional factor Nrf2.

Despite the role of increased oxidative stress, chronic inflammation, and glutamate in initiation and promotion of PTSD, only limited studies on the effects of individual antioxidants in improving some symptoms in animal models of PTSD have been published.[5]

This chapter describes incidence, prevalence, and cost of PTSD, symptoms, and brain pathology, and presents evidence for increased oxidative stress, chronic inflammation, and glutamate level in the initiation and progression of PTSD. This review also discusses the role of microRNAs in the pathogenesis of PTSD. It briefly discusses the regulation of activation of Nrf2 and proposes a mixture of micronutrients that can simultaneously activate Nrf2, enhance the levels of antioxidants, and reduce the release and toxicity of glutamate for the prevention, and in combination with standard care, for the improvement in the management of PTSD.

PREVALENCE AND COST OF PTSD

PTSD affects about 7.7 million Americans over the ages of 18, or about 3.5% of people in this age group in a given year.[7] In the United States, lifetime prevalence of PTSD among ages 18 years and older is 6.8%. The prevalence of this disease among men is 5% and 10.4% among women.[8]

TABLE 12.1

Prevalence of Partial and Fully Established PTSD in US Military Personnel after Deployment

Source	Incidence (percent)
Veterans from Iraq, 2006	18–20
Veteran serving armed forced during Vietnam era	30.9 in men
	26.9 in women
Veterans of Vietnam theatre	15.2 in men
	8 in women
Gulf war veterans	12
OEF/OIF	13.8

Note: The incidence of PTSD in US troops before deployment was
5%. The incidence of PTSD appears to increase with time as
well as with repeated combat deployment.
OEF/OIF, Operation Enduring Freedom/Operation Iraqi Freedom.

Prevalence of PTSD among children and adolescent aged between 12–17 years is 3.7% in boys and 6.3% in girls.[9] The prevalence among veterans serving in US armed forces during Vietnam era, Vietnam theater, Gulf War, and Operation Educing Freedom/Operation Iraqi Freedom (OEF/OIF) was presented in Table 12.1.

In a large-scale study of military personnel in the current combat theatres, it was demonstrated that US Army and Marine Corps personnel returning from duty in Iraq exhibited PTSD rates of 18% and 20%, respectively.[10] Before deployment, only 5% of soldiers showed PTSD symptoms, but after a full year of deployment about 17% of soldiers exhibited PTSD symptoms. The rate of increase in PTSD was proportional to the length of their stay in Iraq[11] (Table 12.1). The number of soldiers with PTSD may further increase due to repeated combat deployments.[12]

An additional 22.5% of men and 21.2% of women have had partial PTSD. This constitutes about 1.7 million Vietnam veterans who have experienced clinically significant combat-related stress disorders.

The estimated societal cost of PTSD and depression among returning troops for 2 years after deployment varies from about $6,000 to more than $25,000 per case. The total cost including direct medical treatment and care, lost productivity, and suicide for 2 years ranges from $4 billion to $6.2 billion (Rand Corporation analysis, 2008).

SYMPTOMS OF PTSD

The symptoms of PTSD often appear within 3 months of the exposure to traumatic stressors, and they include unwanted re-experiencing of the trauma in memory (flashbacks, nightmares, triggered emotional responses), passive and active avoidance (emotional numbing, avoidance of discussions about the traumatic event), and hyperarousal.[13–15] In addition, PTSD is usually accompanied by other psychiatric and medical comorbidities, including depression, substance abuse, cognitive dysfunction, and other problems of physical and mental health.[16,17] These problems may lead to impairment of the ability to function in social or family life, including occupational instability, marital stress, and family problems. Some of the symptoms of PTSD overlap with other diseases including chronic fatigue syndrome, fibromyalgia, and multiple chemical sensitivities.[18,19] The severity in obstructive sleep apnea (OSA) was directly related to suicidal tendency in PTSD patients. Depression was considered a mediator of the association between respiratory disturbance index (RDI) and suicidal tendency.[20] PTSD patients with comorbid conditions and mild TBI exhibited increased self-reported pain intensity, whereas mild TBI patients did not.[21] The symptoms of hyperarousal in PTSD were associated with increased rate of DNA methylation.[22]

BRAIN PATHOLOGY OF PTSD

The neuropathology of PTSD patients is not well defined, possibly due to the lack of sufficient autopsied brain tissues. Most data on neuropathology have been obtained by examining the brain tissue by MRI (magnetic resonance imaging). The reduction in the volume of certain areas of the brain, particularly in the hippocampus, has been consistently observed. For example, reduction in the hippocampal volume was found in patients with PTSD.[23–25] Loss of hippocampal volume may account for cognitive dysfunction commonly observed in PTSD patients. In patients with PTSD, reduced cerebellar volume was associated with mood changes, depression, and anxiety.[26] MRI scanning of the brains of PTSD patients revealed that accelerated brain atrophy occurred throughout the brain, particularly in the brain stem, and frontal and temporal lobes. Accelerated brain atrophy was associated with increased severity of the PTSD symptoms.[27] In addition, it was observed that greater rates of brain atrophy were associated with greater rates of decline in verbal memory and delayed facial recognition. Another MRI study showed that the cortical gray matter abnormalities, particularly in the frontal and occipital lobes, decreased in patients with PTSD compared to that in healthy controls.[28] Using MRI technique, it was shown that reduction of gray matter volume in the left anterior cingulate cortex was associated with the development of PTSD, whereas reduction of gray matter volume in the right pulvinar and left pallidus was associated with severe trauma without PTSD.[29] In addition, the atrophy of the frontal and limbic cortices was associated with the severity of the PTSD symptoms. MRI study on the brains of twins with or without PTSD revealed that significant reduction in gray matter volume occurred in four brain regions: right hippocampus, pregenual anterior cingulate cortex, and left and right insulae in twins with PTSD compared to that in twins without PTSD.[30] Smaller ACC and insular cortex within the limbic-prefrontal circuit contribute to the development of PTSD.[31]

The cerebellum of the brain is involved in fear perception, anticipation, and recollection. Examination of the brain by the MRI technique showed that reduction in volume of the cerebellum was associated with mood change, anxiety, and PTSD symptoms, whereas reduction in volume of the vermis was associated with an early traumatic life experiences, and may be considered a risk factor for future development of PTSD.[26] Examination of the brain by MRI revealed that the volume of the left amygdala, right amygdala, and left hippocampus was reduced in PTSD patients compared to trauma-exposed individuals without PTSD; however, the right hippocampus was not reduced in patients with PTSD.[32] Studies on the scanning of brain with MRI suggested that greater re-experiencing score predicted reduced volume of the middle temporal and inferior occipital cortices, whereas increased reports of flashback predicted reduced volume of the insula/parietal operculum and inferior temporal gyrus in patients with PTSD.[33] Alcohol consumption accelerates reduction in the hippocampus volume in PTSD patients.[34]

A review of 9 studies with 319 subjects revealed that reduction in gray matter in the anterior cingulate cortex, ventromedial prefrontal cortex, left temporal pole/middle temporal gyrus, and left hippocampus occurred in PTSD patients compared to individuals exposed to trauma without PTSD.[35]

Serotonin transporter (5-HTT) located in the amygdala regulates stress response. Therefore, deficient 5-HTT function and abnormal amygdala activity may contribute to the development of PTSD. This was shown by the fact that PTSD patients exhibited reduced amygdala expression of 5-HTT, as measured by PET (positron emission tomography) using a radioactive tracer of 5-HTT (^{11}C-AFM). It was observed that reduced amygdala 5-HTT binding was associated with higher anxiety and depression symptoms in PTSD patients.[36]

Using proton magnetic resonance spectroscopy, it was demonstrated that levels of GABA were lower in the insula of PTSD patients compared to control subjects. There was no difference in the levels of GABA in the dorsal anterior cingulated cortex (ACC). Although lower insula GABA level was not associated with the severity of PTSD symptoms, it was significantly associated with higher state and trait anxiety.[37] Using the same technique, it was found that lower GABA and higher glutamate levels in parieto-occipital cortex were correlated with poor sleep quality that is consistent with the hyperarousal theory of both PTSD and primary insomnia.[38]

Both TBI and PTSD exhibit common neuropsychiatry disorders, such as anxiety, irritability, insomnia, personality changes, and memory deficits, and both disrupt neural connections, such as asymmetrical white matter tract abnormalities and gray matter changes in the basolateral amygdala, hippocampus, and prefrontal cortex. The neural disruptions are also shared comorbid conditions shared by PTSD and TBI. These disturbances in neural connections cause behavior changes that include impairments in executive function and memory, fear retention, fear extinction deficiencies, and other abnormalities.[39]

MicroRNAs IN PTSD

Expression of DROSA1, a cytoplasmic enzyme that generates mature microRNAs was reduced in the blood of patients with PTSD with comorbid depression compared to control subjects.[40] The expression of miR-125a was downregulated and the levels of its target protein INF-γ in PTSD patients.[41] Downregulation of several microRNAs including has-miR-193a-5p was associated with the increased levels of IFN-γ and IL-12 in the peripheral blood mononuclear cells of PTSD patients.[42] In serum and amygdala of animal model of PTSD, a panel of 9 stress-responsive microRNAs: miR-142-5p, miR-19b, miR-1928, miR-223-3p, miR-322, miR-324, miR-421-5p, miR-463, and miR-674 were identified.[43] It was suggested that these microRNAs could serve as biomarkers for PTSD. Among 9 microRNAs, 5 of them, miR-142-5p, miR-19b, miR-1928, miR-223-3p, and miR-421-5p, play a role in regulation of genes associated with delayed and exaggerated fear.

EVIDENCE FOR INCREASED OXIDATIVE STRESS IN PTSD

There are some studies that show that increased oxidative stress may be involved in the initiation and progression of some human chronic neurological disorders, including psychiatric disorders and PTSD.[44] Stress evokes a sustained increase in nitric oxide synthase (NOS) activity that can generate excessive amounts of nitric oxide.[45,46] Oxidation of nitric oxide produces peroxynitrite, which is very toxic to nerve cells.[19] It has been proposed that deficiency of tetrahydrobioptrin causes NOS to produce superoxide,[47] which can oxidize nitric oxide to produce peroxynitrite. Peroxynitrite can then damage vital molecules, thus repeating a vicious cycle of producing increased levels of peroxynitrite. The combination of high NOS activity and low levels of tetrahydrobioptrin can produce a sustained increase in peroxynitrite level. Indeed, elevated levels of peroxynitrite and its precursor nitric oxide have been observed in patients with PTSD.[48]

Platelet monoamine oxidase, which generates excessive amounts of free radicals while degrading catecholamines, is also elevated in patients with PTSD.[49] This is further confirmed by the fact that depletion of catecholamines has been observed in patients with PTSD.[50] Peroxynitrite and other free radicals increase the level of oxidative damage in the brain tissue of patients with PTSD, causing cognitive and other brain dysfunction. The above studies in humans support the view that increased levels of oxidative stress may contribute to the development of PTSD and associated cognitive dysfunctions. This was confirmed in animal models of PTSD.

Severe life stresses can induce PTSD-like symptoms. A review has described the impact of severe life stress in animals, which includes sleep deprivation and social isolation.[51] Rats exposed to single prolonged stress exhibit symptoms of PTSD. It has been demonstrated that rats exposed to single prolonged stress showed apoptosis in the hippocampus region of the brain and impaired spatial memory. These effects were mediated by Bcl2 (B-cell lymphoid-2) and Bax genes.[52] Rats exposed to foot shock and maternal separation (forms of stress) exhibited impaired spatial memory and increased number of DNA breaks in the hippocampus.[53] It is interesting to point out that increased oxidative stress has been also observed in other neurodegenerative diseases, such as Alzheimer's disease.[54] Thus, attenuation of oxidative stress appears to be one of the rational choices for reducing the risk of onset and progression of PTSD.

Platelet monoamine oxidase, which generates excessive amounts of free radicals while degrading catecholamines, is also elevated in patients with PTSD.[49] This is further confirmed by the fact that depletion of catecholamines has been observed in patients with PTSD.[50] Peroxynitrite and other free radicals increase the level of oxidative damage in brain tissue of patients with PTSD, causing cognitive and other brain dysfunction. Recently, the expression profiles of certain genes in mitochondria of autopsied samples of dorsolateral prefrontal cortex of patients with PTSD are altered in comparison to healthy control.[55] This study is important because the activity of dorsolateral prefrontal cortex region of the brain that regulates working memory and fear responses is decreased in PTSD patients.[55] The DNA microarray analysis of postmortem samples of prefrontal cortex from patients with major depression revealed that the gene expression profiles of some specific genes are altered in comparison to those from normal control.[56] The alterations in expression profile of certain genes are very interesting observations, but they have not been confirmed by real time PCR; therefore, additional studies would be needed to establish changes in the levels of specific genes that are associated with PTSD. Increased levels of oxidative stress may contribute to the cognitive dysfunctions commonly observed in patients with PTSD. It is interesting to point out that increased oxidative stress and chronic inflammation have been observed in other neurological diseases such as Alzheimer's disease.[54]

The levels of reactive oxygen species (ROS) and pro-inflammatory cytokines were increased in an animal model of PTSD. Treatment with valproic acid, an inhibitor of histone deacetylase, normalized these biochemical defects, decreased anxiety, and restored the levels of neurotransmitters such as catecholamines and serotonin.[57] In rat model of PTSD, the levels of oxidative stress and inflammatory cytokines were elevated in the brain (hippocampus, amygdala, and prefrontal cortex), adrenal glands, and whole blood, suggesting that damage to multiple organs were involved in the progression of PTSD.[58] Exposure to enriched environment reversed behavioral impairments (anxiety-like behavior, enhanced fear learning behavior, and spatial memory deficits) by reducing oxidative stress in the hippocampus and pre-frontal cortex.[59] Treatment with apocynin, a methoxy-substituted catechol, an inhibitor of NOX2 (nicotinamide adenosine dinucleotide phosphate NADPH-2) that produces free radicals, reduced the levels of markers of oxidative stress (malondialdehyde, NOX2, and 4-hydroxynonenal) and pro-inflammatory cytokine IL-6 in the hippocampus of rat model of PTSD.[60]

The levels of serum paraoxonase-1 (PON-1) enzyme activity were lower and those of malondialdehyde (MDA) were higher in PTSD patients who survived an earthquake compared to those earthquake survivors who did not develop this disease. This study suggests that increased oxidative stress is associated with the development of PTSD.[61] Thus, attenuation of oxidative stress appears to be one of the rational choices for reducing the risk of onset and progression of PTSD.

EVIDENCE FOR CHRONIC INFLAMMATION IN PTSD

In addition to increased oxidative stress, increased chronic inflammation due to activation of microglia may be associated with PTSD. For example, serum levels of interleukin-6 (IL-6) are elevated in patients with PTSD.[62] Increased levels of IL-6 and IL-6 receptors were found in patients with PTSD.[63] High levels of tumor necrosis factor-alpha (TNF-alpha) and IL-1beta were elevated in patients with PTSD in comparison to control subjects.[64] Psychological stress induces a chronic inflammatory process.[65] Chronic fear of terror in women, but not in men, is associated with elevated levels of C-reactive protein (CRP) that may contribute to increased risk of cardiovascular disease in PTSD patients.[66] The levels of CRP and receptor to IL-6 were elevated in patients with PTSD.[67] A study has reported that in men, but not in women, the episodes of depression is associated with increased levels of CRP[68]; however, others have reported no such association.[69] Increased levels of chronic inflammation may also contribute to the cognitive dysfunctions commonly observed in patients with PTSD. Increased chronic inflammation is also associated with certain neurological diseases such as Alzheimer's disease.[54] Elevated levels of neuroinflammation were repeatedly observed in patients with PTSD. A few reviews have been published on this issue.[70–74] Some recent studies on human PTSD are presented here. Inflammation markers C-reactive protein (CRP), white blood cells (WBC), and fibrinogen were elevated in patients with PTSD.[75] This study revealed that higher avoidance was associated with higher levels of fibrinogen. Among Gulf War veterans with PTSD, increased levels of inflammatory marker soluble receptor II for tumor necrosis factor (sTNF-RII), but not IL-6 was associated with reduced hippocampal volume and higher PTSD symptoms.[76] The levels of inflammatory markers IL-6, TNF-alpha, gamma-interferon, C-reactive protein (CRP) were elevated in war veterans with PTSD.[77] No significant correlations were found between the levels of inflammatory markers and severity of PTSD symptoms in this study.

One of the cellular abnormalities in PTSD involves reduced levels of nitric oxide (NO). A recently identified marker NO synthetic capacity in vivo Global Arginine Bioavailability ratio (GABR) was used to determine its dysfunction in combat-exposed male PTSD patients. The results showed that the value of GABR was lower in PTSD patients compared to combat-exposed males without PTSD, suggesting reduced production of NO in this disorder. Furthermore, the levels of GABR were inversely related to inflammation markers (IL-6 and TNF-alpha), and the severity of CAPS (Clinician Administered PTSD Scale).[78] In the Marine Resiliency Study, Plasma CRP levels were highly significant predictor of post-deployment CAPS scores.[79] Single-nucleotide polymorphisms (SNPs) in the CRP gene were associated with increased levels of plasma CRP, severity of PTSD symptoms, and enhanced fear-related startle to a safety signal.[80] In addition to inflammation, smoking and alcohol dependence contribute to the severity of PTSD symptoms.[81]

Activated glia that release pro-inflammatory cytokines are found in patients with PTSD.[62,63] The prevalence of chronic pain is high among patients with PTSD. Rat exposed to SPE (single prolonged exposure) enhanced the activation of glia cells (including microglia and astrocytes) and accumulation of pro-inflammatory cytokines in the spinal cord.[82] Administration of a novel anti-inflammatory agent, PHA-543613, a selective agonist of alpha-7 nicotinic acetylcholine receptor (alpha7nAChR) decreased SPS-induced chronic pain in a dose-dependent manner, and reduced glia activation and elevated levels of pro-inflammatory cytokines.[82] The studied discussed above suggest that chronic inflammation plays a role in the development and progression of this disease. Therefore, attenuation of chronic inflammation may be one of the rational strategies for reducing the risk of onset and progression of PTSD.

EVIDENCE FOR INCREASED RELEASE OF GLUTAMATE AND DECREASED LEVELS OF GABA IN PTSD

The glutamatergic systems appear to play an important role in the pathophysiology of PTSD.[83] Stress-induced glutamate release and glucocorticoids have been implicated to cause hippocampal atrophy in patients with PTSD. This observation is not unexpected because glutamate in high doses is known to be neurotoxic. Glutamate and nitric oxide (NO) released during stress play a central role in maintaining anxiety disorders.[45,83–85] Stress activates glutamate-NMDA receptors and decreases brain-derived neurotrophic factors, and excessive amounts of glutamate can cause death to cholinergic neurons that may account for the cognitive dysfunction associated with PTSD. Therefore, blocking the release of glutamate and reducing the toxicity of glutamate would be useful in reducing the risk and progression of PTSD symptoms. Indeed, anti-glutamatergic agents such as lamotrigine improve some of the symptoms of PTSD (re-experiencing hyperarousal, and avoidance).

Glutamate and GABA Levels in PTSD

Several studies suggest that the imbalances between activities of glutamatergic and GABAnergic neurons contribute to the severity of the symptoms of PTSD including fear and anxiety. They are briefly described here. The levels of glutamate in the serum of patients with established PTSD or partial PTSD were higher compared to those without PTSD. In addition, higher serum levels of glutamate were associated with the severity of PTSD and major depressive disorder.[86] This study also revealed that the glutamine/glutamate ratio was inversely associated with the severity of PTSD but not with the severity of major depressive disorder. Dysfunction of glutamate neurotransmission appears to be the main feature of stress-related psychiatric disorders including PTSD, anxiety, and mood changes.[87] Using in vivo proton magnetic resonance spectroscopy (1H MRS), it was found that the levels of GABA were lower and the levels of glutamate were higher in the parieto-occipital and temporal cortices of PTSD patients compared to those who were exposed to trauma but had not developed PTSD symptoms.[38] This study also demonstrated that increased anxiety symptoms scores and insomnia severity index (ISI) scores commonly found in PTSD were associated with the lower levels of GABA and higher levels of glutamate. Imbalances between glutamate and GABA contribute to the apoptosis in the hippocampus of animal model of PTSD.[88]

Glutamate action was mediated by enhancing the release of CRF (corticotropin-releasing factor) that activated the stress-response hormone cascade, which enhanced extracellular levels of glutamate and NMDA receptor expression.[83] This study suggested that increased levels of glutamate might cause atrophy to the hippocampus. The role CRF-mediated biochemical events in the pathogenesis of PTSD is further supported by the observation that patients with PTSD had increased levels of CRF.[89] Stress released excessive amounts of glutamate and nitric oxide and they play an important role in maintaining anxiety disorders.[46,84] Stress also activated glutamate-NMDA receptors and reduced the levels of BDNF (brain-derived neurotrophic factor) that contributed to the death of cholinergic neurons. This may account for the cognitive dysfunction in patients with PTSD.[46,83] Antagonists of two receptors of glutamate NMDA receptors and alpha-amino-3-hydroxy-5-methoxy-4-isoxazole-propionate (AMPA) receptors, a non-NMDA-type ionotropic transmembrane receptor for glutamate, reduced anxiety disorders.[90,91] From these studies, it appears rational to prevent the release of glutamate or block its action in order to improve some symptoms of PTSD. Indeed, antagonist agents such as aborigine improved some symptoms of PTSD, such as hyperarousal and avoidance.[83] In PTSD patients, the lower levels of GABA in the insular cortex were associated with higher state of anxiety.[92] Plasma levels of GABA were lower in PTSD patients than in control subjects.[93] Lower levels of GABA would allow increased glutamate transmission leading to anxiety and depression.

The studies discussed in the above paragraphs suggest that increased oxidative stress, chronic inflammation, and glutamatergic activities play an important role in the initiation and progression of PTSD symptoms; therefore, attenuation of these defects simultaneously may be beneficial in prevention, and in combination with standard care, in improving the management of this neurological disorders. The question arises how to simultaneously reduce these major biochemical defects associated with PTSD.

STUDIES ON ANTIOXIDANTS IN PTSD

The role of antioxidants in prevention or improved management of PTSD has not been evaluated in humans. A few studies on the effects antioxidants on PTSD disorders are described here.

Omega-3-Fatty Acids

It has been reported that daily supplementation with omega-3-fatty acids reduced some of the symptoms of PTSD in critically injured patients during the earthquake in Japan in 2011.[94] The question arose whether or not supplementation with omega-3-fatty acids during maturation of the brain can protect an adult brain against trauma that increased the risk of developing PTSD. To answer this, rats were fed diets enriched with or deficient in omega-3-fatty acids during the period of brain maturation. After attaining adulthood, rats were switched to a western diet and then subjected to mild traumatic brain injury (mTBI), which increases the risk of developing PTSD. The result showed the following: Animals fed omega-3-fatty acids-rich diet exhibited an increase in anxiety behavior and neuropeptide Y receptor type 1 (NPY1R), which are characteristics of PTSD.[95] These symptoms were aggravated in rats that were fed omega-3-fatty acids-deficient diet during brain maturation, suggesting that diet deficient in omega-3-fatty acids during development may lower the threshold for developing certain neurological disorders, such as PTSD, in response to trauma or accident. These preliminary animal and human studies suggest that omega-3-fatty acids may be some value in reducing the risk of developing PTSD; however, additional studies are needed to substantiate the role of omega-3-fatty acids in prevention of PTSD.

CURCUMIN

Administration of curcumin increased hippocampal neurogenesis in chronically stressed rats, similar to the effect of antidepressant imipramine treatment. New hippocampal cells mature and become neurons. In addition, curcumin treatment prevented stress-induced decline in serotonin receptor-1A (5-HT-1A) mRNA and brain-derived neurotrophic factor (BDNF) protein levels in the hippocampal regions.[96] Curcumin appears to be a promising agent for the treatment of varieties of neuropsychiatry disorders, such as depression, PTSD, obsessive-compulsive disorder, bipolar disorder, psychotic disorder, and autism.[97]

RESVERATROL

In rat model of PTSD, resveratrol treatment reduced anxiety-like behavior and fear and improved memory deficits by increasing phosphorylation of cAMP response element binding protein and brain-derived neurotrophic factor (BDNF) levels.[98]

PENTOXIFYLLINE AND TEMPOL

Pentoxifylline, a potent antioxidant, prevented memory deficits in single-prolonged stress-induced PTSD-like behavior in rats by improving antioxidant defense system and BDNF levels.[99] Another antioxidant tempol also prevented memory impairment by similar mechanisms as described above in rat model of PTSD.[100]

FLAVONOIDS

Xiaobuxin-Tang (XBXT), a traditional Chinese herbal product, has been used for the treatment of depressive disorders for centuries in China. Flavonoids (XBXT-2) isolated from the extract of XBXT increased neurogenesis in the hippocampus of chronically stressed rats. In addition, this treatment with flavonoids prevented stress-induced decrease in brain-derived neurotrophic factor (BDNF).[101]

VALPROIC ACID

Treatment of rat model of PTSD with valproic acid reduced oxidative stress and inflammation, enhance fear extinction, and restored neurotransmitter abnormalities.[57]

BLUEBERRY-RICH DIET

In rat model of PTSD, feeding blueberry-rich diet improved memory deficits, decreased anxiety, and increased the levels of 5-hydroxytryptophane (a precursor of serotonin) without affecting norepinephrine by attenuating oxidative stress and inflammation.[102]

EFFECT OF MULTIPLE MICRONUTRIENTS IN VETERANS

A commercial formulation of multiple micronutrients was tested in a clinical study in troops returning from Iraq and Afghanistan with mild to moderate TBI. Thirty-four patients with post-traumatic dizziness were admitted to the Naval Medical Center San Diego Clinic over a two-month period and agreed to participate in the study under the supervision of Dr. Michael Hoffer and his colleagues.[103] All patients had received their injury 3–20 weeks prior to admission, and they received identical treatment consisting of medical therapy (for any migraines), supportive care, steroids, and vestibular rehabilitation therapy. Fifteen of the 34 patients also received a dose of an antioxidant and micronutrient formula (two capsules by mouth twice a day). At the onset of therapy, all patients were evaluated in outcome measures, which included the Sensory Organization Test (SOT) by Computerized Dynamic Posturography (CDP), the Dynamic Gait Index (DGI), the Activities Balance Confidence (ABC) scale, the Dizziness Handicap Index (DHI), the Vestibular Disorders Activities of Daily Living (VADL) score, and the Balance Scoring System (BESS) test. The study was carried out for 12 weeks. The therapist who graded these outcomes and performed the testing was blinded as to whether the patient was receiving antioxidant therapy or not. The pre-trial test scores did not differ significantly between the two groups on any of the tests.

Both groups of patients showed trends toward significant improvement on all tests after the 12 weeks of therapy, but the combination treatment trend was stronger than that of the standard therapy alone group. After only 4 weeks, the SOT score by CDP was 78 for the antioxidant group as compared to 63 for the non-anti-oxidant group. This difference was statistically significant at the $P < 0.05$ levels. The improvement noted by the antioxidant group on the other tests was also greater than the non-antioxidant group, although these differences did not reach statistical significance because of the short trial period and small sample size. This study should be expanded using a randomized, double-blind, and placebo-control clinical study design in which the efficacy of the proposed multiple micronutrients preparation should be tested in soldiers returning from combat theaters exhibiting mild to moderate traumatic brain injury or any sign of mental disorders such as anxiety, fear, and depression.

Despite strong evidence for the involvement of increased oxidative stress, inflammation, and glutamate in the initiation and progression of PTSD, a few studies with individual antioxidants have been conducted in animal models of PTSD. Only one study with multiple micronutrients has been performed in veterans with concussive injury.

POTENTIAL REASONS FOR THE FAILURE OF INDIVIDUAL MICRONUTRIENTS IN PRODUCING CONSISTENT BENEFITS IN HUMAN

Although a few studies with individual antioxidants have been performed on animal models of PTSD, only one study with omega-3-fatty acids has been conducted in human PTSD with some improvements in symptoms. Investigations with individual antioxidants in other neurodegenerative diseases produced no effect or minimal beneficial effects, although animal studies showed consistent benefits.[6,104] It is likely that use of single antioxidants in human PTSD would produce similar inconsistent results. Some potentials causes are described here: (a) antioxidants show differential subcellular distribution and different mechanisms of action; therefore, a single antioxidant cannot protect all parts of the cell; (b) a single antioxidant in a high internal oxidative environment in high-risk patients is oxidized and can then itself act as a prooxidant rather than as an antioxidant; (c) the body protects against oxidative damage by elevating antioxidant enzymes, and dietary and endogenous antioxidants; (d) antioxidants neutralize free radicals by donating electrons to those molecules with unpaired electron, whereas antioxidant enzymes destroy free radicals by catalysis, converting them to harmless molecules such as water and oxygen. Therefore, both of these agents should be enhanced to achieve substantial protection against oxidative damage; (e) the affinity of different antioxidants for free radicals differs, depending upon their solubility; (f) both the aqueous and lipid compartments of the cell need to be protected together. Water-soluble antioxidants such as vitamin C and glutathione protect molecules in the aqueous environment of the cells, whereas lipid soluble antioxidants such as vitamin A and vitamin E protect molecules in the lipid compartment; (g) vitamin E is more effective in quenching free radicals in a reduced oxygenated cellular environment, whereas vitamin C and alpha-tocopherol are more effective in a higher oxygenated environment of the cells[105]; (h) vitamin C is important for recycling the oxidized form of alpha-tocopherol to the antioxidant form[106]; (i) antioxidants produce cell protective proteins by altering the expression of different microRNAs.[107] For example, some antioxidants can activate Nrf2 by upregulating miR-200a that inhibits its target protein Keap1, whereas others activate Nrf2 by downregulating miR-21 that binds with 3′-UTR Nrf2 mRNA.[108]

In order to avoid the pitfalls of individual antioxidants in reducing oxidative stress and inflammation, it is proposed that an elevation of the levels of antioxidant enzymes and dietary and endogenous antioxidants may be essential for simultaneously reducing these cellular defects. Oral supplementation can increase the levels of dietary and endogenous antioxidants; however, elevation of the levels of antioxidant enzymes requires an activation of Nrf2. Therefore it is essential to understand the regulation of activation of Nrf2.

ACTIVATION OF Nrf2 (NUCLEAR FACTOR-ERYTHROID-2-RELATED FACTOR 2)

Nrf2

The nuclear transcriptional factor, Nrf2 (nuclear factor-erythroid-2-related factor 2) belongs to the Cap 'n' Collar (CNC) family that contains a conserved basic leucine zipper (bZIP) transcriptional factor.[109] Under physiological condition, Nrf2 is associated with Kelch-like ECH associated protein 1 (Keap1), which acts as an inhibitor of Nrf2.[110] Keap1 protein serves as an adaptor to link Nrf2 to the ubiquitin ligase CuI-Rbx1 complex for degradation by proteasomes and maintains the steady levels of Nrf2 in the cytoplasm. Nrf2-keap1 complex is primarily located in the cytoplasm; Keap1 acts as a sensor for ROS/electrophilic stress.

ACTIVATION OF Nrf2 DURING ACUTE OXIDATIVE STRESS

During acute oxidative stress, ROS is needed to activate Nrf2 which then dissociates itself from Keap1-CuI-Rbx1 complex and translocates in the nucleus where it heterodimerizes with a small Maf protein, binds with ARE leading to increased expression of target genes coding for several cytoprotective enzymes including antioxidant enzymes.[111–113]

FAILURE TO ACTIVATE Nrf2 DURING CHRONIC OXIDATIVE STRESS

During chronic oxidative stress, Nrf2 becomes resistant to ROS,[114–116] suggesting that activation of Nrf2 by a ROS-independent mechanism exists. This is evidenced by the fact that increased chronic oxidative stress occurs despite the presence of Nrf2 in PTSD. The question arises as to how to activate ROS-resistant Nrf2 in hearing disorders.

ANTIOXIDANTS ACTIVATE ROS-RESISTANT Nrf2

Some examples are vitamin E and genistein,[117] alpha-lipoic acid,[118] curcumin,[119] resveratrol,[120,121] omega-3-fatty acids,[122,123] glutathione,[124] NAC,[125] and coenzyme Q10.[126] Several plant-derived phytochemicals, such as epigallocatechin-3-gallate, carestol, kahweol, cinnamonyl-based compounds, zerumbone, lycopene and carnosol,[109,127,128] genistein,[117] allicin, a major organosulfur compound found in garlic,[129] sulforaphane, a organosulfur compound, found in cruciferous vegetables,[130] and kavalactones (methysticin, kavain, and yangonin).[131] The reasons for the activation of Nrf2 without ROS by antioxidant compounds are not known.

BINDING OF Nrf2 WITH ARE IN THE NUCLEUS

An activation of Nrf2 alone is not sufficient to increase the levels of antioxidant enzymes. Activated Nrf2 must bind with ARE in the nucleus for increasing the expression of target genes coding for antioxidant enzymes. This binding ability of Nrf2 with ARE was impaired in aged rats and this defect was restored by supplementation with alpha-lipoic acid.[118] It is unknown whether the binding ability of Nrf2 with ARE is impaired in hearing disorders.

PROPOSED MICRONUTRIENT MIXTURE FOR OPTIMALLY REDUCING OXIDATIVE STRESS, CHRONIC INFLAMMATION, AND GLUTAMATE LEVELS

REDUCING OXIDATIVE STRESS

Based on the differential mechanisms of action and subcellular distributions of various antioxidant compounds, a micronutrient mixture containing multiple dietary antioxidant compounds (vitamin A, natural mixed carotenoids, vitamin C, vitamin E succinate, vitamin E acetate, selenomethionine, curcumin, and resveratrol), endogenous antioxidants (alpha-lipoic acid, L-carnitine, and coenzyme Q10), a synthetic antioxidant N-acetylcysteine (NAC), vitamin D3, all B-vitamins, zinc, and omega-3-fatty acids is proposed. Supplementation with this mixture of micronutrients may maximally reduce oxidative stress by simultaneously enhancing the levels of antioxidant enzymes through activation of the Nrf2 pathway as well as intracellular levels of antioxidants.

REDUCING CHRONIC INFLAMMATION

Activation of Nrf2 also suppresses chronic inflammation.[132,133] Some individual antioxidant compounds also reduce chronic inflammation.[134–138] Therefore, the proposed micronutrient mixture may also maximally decrease chronic inflammation.

REDUCING GLUTAMATE RELEASE AND TOXICITY

Some antioxidants, such as vitamin E and coenzyme Q10, decreased the release of glutamate and its neurotoxicity.[139–141] In addition, certain B-vitamins such as vitamin B6 and vitamin B12 reduced the release of glutamate.[142,143] The proposed micronutrient mixture has these B-vitamins.

PREVENTION OF PTSD

PRIMARY PREVENTION OF PTSD

The purpose of primary prevention is to protect healthy individuals from developing PTSD symptoms. Individuals who are likely to be exposed to PTSD risk factors such as troops to be employed in war zone are suitable for the primary prevention. The proposed mixture of micronutrients may be effective in reducing the risk of developing PTSD symptoms by reducing chronic oxidative stress and inflammation in concert together.

SECONDARY PREVENTION OF PTSD

The purpose of secondary prevention is to stop or slow the progression of PTSD symptoms. Individuals who are exposed to PTSD risk factors, but have not developed symptoms of the disease are suitable for the secondary prevention. The proposed mixture of micronutrients may be effective in preventing or delaying the onset PTSD symptoms by reducing chronic oxidative stress, inflammation, and glutamate release at the same time.

STANDARD THERAPY IN PTSD

Standard therapy includes drugs and psychological/psychiatric treatment. Some examples of drug therapy that has produced limited success are described below.

In a 6-week randomized, double-blind, placebo-controlled trial using 22 chronic PTSD outpatients, it was found that d-serine, an endogenous agonist of NMDA receptor at the site of glycine may improve some of the symptoms of PTSD.[144] Anti-glutamatergic agents, such as lamotrigine were effective in reducing some of the symptoms of PTSD.[83] Selective serotonin reuptake inhibitors also were useful in improving the symptoms of PTSD.[145] The efficacy of other drugs in the treatment of PTSD, such as antidepressants, anti-adrenergic agents, anticonvulsants, benzodiazepines, and atypical antipsychotics yielding variable degrees of improvement has been reviewed.[146]

Extinction of conditioned fear appears to be defective in patients with PTSD. D-cycloserine, a partial agonist of NMDA receptor, was useful in enhancing extinction of learned fear in rats.[147] This was achieved when d-cycloserine was administered shortly before or after extinction training of rats.[148]

Persistent retrieval and maintenance of traumatic memories is a biological process that keeps these memories vivid and thereby maintains the symptoms of PTSD. It has been demonstrated that elevated glucocorticoid levels inhibit memory retrieval process in animals and humans.[149] In patients with PTSD, low-dose cortisol treatment for one month reduced symptoms of traumatic memories without causing adverse health effects, probably by preventing recall of traumatic memories.[149,150] Details can be found in the website of the United States Department of Veterans Affairs (National Center for PTSD, 2013).

None of the drugs that are currently used in the treatment of PTSD addressed the issue of increased oxidative stress and chronic inflammation that are associated with the initiation and progression of PTSD.

IMPROVED MANAGEMENT OF PTSD

Patients with established PTSD who are on one or more medications are suitable for this study. The proposed micronutrient mixture, in combination with standard care, might improve the management of PTSD symptoms by reducing oxidative stress, chronic inflammation, and glutamate release and its toxicity at the same time.

DIET AND LIFESTYLE RECOMMENDATIONS FOR PTSD

In addition to supplementation with micronutrient mixture, a balanced diet low in fat, high in fiber, and rich in fruits and vegetables is necessary for reducing the risk of developing PTSD, as well as for improving the efficacy of standard therapy in the management of PTSD. Lifestyle recommendations include daily moderate exercise, reduced stress, no tobacco smoking, and reduced intake of caffeine or alcoholic beverages.

CONCLUSIONS

Posttraumatic stress disorder (PTSD) is a complex mental disorder resulting from exposure to blasts, sudden or repeated extreme traumatic events, and possibly other stressful environmental stressors. At present, there are no strategies to reduce the risk of developing PTSD. The current standard therapy of PTSD that includes drug therapy and psychological counseling is considered unsatisfactory. In order to develop a rational strategy, it is essential to identify cellular defects that initiate and promote PTSD. The role of microRNAs in the pathogenesis of PTSD has not been adequately studied. Several studies show that increased levels of oxidative stress, chronic inflammation, and glutamate initiate and promote PTSD. Therefore, simultaneous attenuation of these cellular defects may be useful in prevention, and in combination with standard therapy, in improved management of this disease. The use of individual antioxidants has improved some symptoms of PTSD in animal models. Only one study with omega-3-fatty acids has produced limited benefits in PTSD patients. The potential reasons of individual antioxidants for producing limited benefits are discussed. To avoid the pitfalls of using single antioxidants, a mixture of micronutrients that would enhance the levels of cytoprotective enzymes including antioxidant enzymes by activating the Nrf2/ARE pathway, and dietary and endogenous antioxidants is proposed. The same mixture would also prevent the release and toxicity of glutamate. The proposed mixture of micronutrients in combination with standard therapy might improve the management of human PTSD. Preclinical and clinical studies using proposed micronutrient mixture in primary prevention, secondary prevention, and in combination with standard therapy, for improved management of PTSD, are suggested.

REFERENCES

1. Hoge CW, McGurk D, Thomas JL, Cox AL, Engel CC, Castro CA. Mild traumatic brain injury in US soldiers returning from Iraq. *N Engl J Med.* 2008;358(5):453–463.
2. Schneiderman AI, Braver ER, Kang HK. Understanding sequelae of injury mechanisms and mild traumatic brain injury incurred during the conflicts in Iraq and Afghanistan: Persistent postconcussive symptoms and posttraumatic stress disorder. *Am J Epidemiol.* 2008;167(12):1446–1452.
3. Alway Y, Gould KR, McKay A, Johnston L, Ponsford J. The evolution of posttraumatic stress disorder following moderate-to-severe traumatic brain injury. *J Neurotrauma.* 2016;33(9):825–831.
4. Hamner MB, Robert S, Frueh BC. Treatment-resistant posttraumatic stress disorder: Strategies for intervention. *CNS Spectr.* 2004;9(10):740–752.
5. Prasad KN. Micronutrients in improvement of the standard therapy in posttraumatic stress disorders. *Micronutrients in Health and Disease.* Boca Raton, FL: CRC Press; 2011:235–247.
6. Prasad KN. Simultaneous activation of Nrf2 and elevation of antioxidant compounds for reducing oxidative stress and chronic inflammation in human Alzheimer's disease. *Mech Ageing Dev.* 2016;153:41–47.
7. Kessler RC, Chiu WT, Demler O, Merikangas KR, Walters EE. Prevalence, severity, and comorbidity of 12-month DSM-IV disorders in the National Comorbidity Survey Replication. *Arch Gen Psychiatry.* 2005;62(6):617–627.
8. Gradus JL. Prevalence and prognosis of stress disorders: A review of the epidemiologic literature. *Clin Epidemiol.* 2017;9:251–260.
9. PTSD UDoVAPNCf. Epidemiology of PTSD2017.
10. Hoge CW, Castro CA, Messer SC, McGurk D, Cotting DI, Koffman RL. Combat duty in Iraq and Afghanistan, mental health problems, and barriers to care. *N Engl J Med.* 2004;351(1):13–22.
11. Castro C, Hoge, CW. Building psychological resiliency and mitigating the risks of combat and deplyment stressors faced by soldiers. *Presented at NATO Human Factors and Medicine Panel Symposium, Prague, Czech Republic,* 2005. 2005.
12. Friedman MJ. Veterans' mental health in the wake of war. *N Engl J Med.* 2005;352(13):1287–1290.
13. King DL, GA; Weathers, FW. Confirmatory factor analysis of the clinician-administered PTSD scale: Evidence for the dimensionality of postraumatic stress disorder. *Psychol Assess.* 1998;10:90–96.
14. Baskar R, Balajee AS, Geard CR, Hande MP. Isoform-specific activation of protein kinase c in irradiated human fibroblasts and their bystander cells. *Int J Biochem Cell Biol.* 2008;40(1):125–134.
15. Leskin GA, Kaloupek DG, Keane TM. Treatment for traumatic memories: Review and recommendations. *Clin Psychol Rev.* 1998;18(8):983–1001.
16. Brewin CR. A cognitive neuroscience account of posttraumatic stress disorder and its treatment. *Behav Res Ther.* 2001;39:373–393.
17. King LA, King DW, Fairbank JA, Keane TM, Adams GA. Resilience-recovery factors in posttraumatic stress disorder among female and male Vietnam veterans: Hardiness, postwar social support, and additional stressful life events. *J Pers Soc Psychol.* 1998;74(2):420–434.
18. Stander VA, Merrill LL, Thomsen CJ, Milner JS. Posttraumatic stress symptoms in Navy personnel: Prevalence rates among recruits in basic training. *J Anxiety Disord.* 2007;21(6):860–870.
19. Pall ML, Satterlee JD. Elevated nitric oxide/peroxynitrite mechanism for the common etiology of multiple chemical sensitivity, chronic fatigue syndrome, and posttraumatic stress disorder. *Ann N Y Acad Sci.* 2001;933:323–329.

20. Gupta MA, Jarosz P. Obstructive sleep apnea severity is directly related to suicidal ideation in posttraumatic stress disorder. *J Clin Sleep Med.* 2018;14(3):427–435.

21. Stojanovic MP, Fonda J, Fortier CB, et al. Influence of mild traumatic brain injury (TBI) and posttraumatic stress disorder (PTSD) on pain intensity levels in OEF/OIF/OND veterans. *Pain Med.* 2016;17(11):2017–2025.

22. Wolf EJ, Logue MW, Stoop TB, et al. Accelerated DNA methylation age: Associations with posttraumatic stress disorder and mortality. *Psychosom Med.* 2018;80(1):42–48.

23. Bremner JD, Scott TM, Delaney RC, et al. Deficits in short-term memory in posttraumatic stress disorder. *Am J Psychiatry.* 1993;150(7):1015–1019.

24. Tischler L, Brand SR, Stavitsky K, et al. The relationship between hippocampal volume and declarative memory in a population of combat veterans with and without PTSD. *Ann N Y Acad Sci.* 2006;1071:405–409.

25. Villarreal G, Hamilton DA, Petropoulos H, et al. Reduced hippocampal volume and total white matter volume in posttraumatic stress disorder. *Biol Psychiatry.* 2002;52(2):119–125.

26. Baldacara L, Jackowski AP, Schoedl A, et al. Reduced cerebellar left hemisphere and vermal volume in adults with PTSD from a community sample. *J Psychiatr Res.* 2011;45(12):1627–1633.

27. Cardenas VA, Samuelson K, Lenoci M, et al. Changes in brain anatomy during the course of posttraumatic stress disorder. *Psychiatry Res.* 2011;193(2):93–100.

28. Tavanti M, Battaglini M, Borgogni F, et al. Evidence of diffuse damage in frontal and occipital cortex in the brain of patients with posttraumatic stress disorder. *Neurol Sci.* 2012;33(1):59–68.

29. Chen Y, Fu K, Feng C, et al. Different regional gray matter loss in recent onset PTSD and nonPTSD after a single prolonged trauma exposure. *PLoS One.* 2012;7(11):e48298.

30. Kasai K, Yamasue H, Gilbertson MW, Shenton ME, Rauch SL, Pitman RK. Evidence for acquired pregenual anterior cingulate gray matter loss from a twin study of combat-related posttraumatic stress disorder. *Biol Psychiatry.* 2008;63(6):550–556.

31. Meng Y, Qiu C, Zhu H, et al. Anatomical deficits in adult posttraumatic stress disorder: A meta-analysis of voxel-based morphometry studies. *Behav Brain Res.* 2014;270:307–315.

32. Morey RA, Gold AL, LaBar KS, et al. Amygdala volume changes in posttraumatic stress disorder in a large case-controlled veterans group. *Arch Gen Psychiatry.* 2012;69(11):1169–1178.

33. Kroes MC, Whalley MG, Rugg MD, Brewin CR. Association between flashbacks and structural brain abnormalities in posttraumatic stress disorder. *Eur Psychiatry.* 2011;26(8):525–531.

34. Starcevic A, Dimitrijevic I, Aksic M, et al. Brain changes in patients with posttraumatic stress disorder and associated alcoholism: MRI based study. *Psychiatr Danub.* 2015;27(1):78–83.

35. Kuhn S, Gallinat J. Gray matter correlates of posttraumatic stress disorder: A quantitative meta-analysis. *Biol Psychiatry.* 2013;73(1):70–74.

36. Murrough JW, Huang Y, Hu J, et al. Reduced amygdala serotonin transporter binding in posttraumatic stress disorder. *Biol Psychiatry.* 2011;70(11):1033–1038.

37. Rosso IM, Weiner MR, Crowley DJ, Silveri MM, Rauch SL, Jensen JE. Insula and anterior cingulate GABA levels in posttraumatic stress disorder: Preliminary findings using magnetic resonance spectroscopy. *Depress Anxiety.* 2014;31(2):115–123.

38. Meyerhoff DJ, Mon A, Metzler T, Neylan TC. Cortical gamma-aminobutyric acid and glutamate in posttraumatic stress disorder and their relationships to self-reported sleep quality. *Sleep.* 2014;37(5):893–900.

39. Kaplan GB, Leite-Morris KA, Wang L, et al. Pathophysiological bases of comorbidity: Traumatic brain injury and posttraumatic stress disorder. *J Neurotrauma.* 2018;35(2):210–225.

40. Wingo AP, Almli LM, Stevens JS, et al. DICER1 and microRNA regulation in posttraumatic stress disorder with comorbid depression. *Nat Commun.* 2015;6:10106.

41. Zhou J, Nagarkatti P, Zhong Y, et al. Dysregulation in microRNA expression is associated with alterations in immune functions in combat veterans with posttraumatic stress disorder. *PLoS One.* 2014;9(4):e94075.

42. Bam M, Yang X, Zhou J, et al. Evidence for epigenetic regulation of pro-inflammatory cytokines, interleukin-12 and interferon gamma, in peripheral blood mononuclear cells from PTSD Patients. *J Neuroimmune Pharmacol.* 2016;11(1):168–181.

43. Balakathiresan NS, Chandran R, Bhomia M, Jia M, Li H, Maheshwari RK. Serum and amygdala microRNA signatures of posttraumatic stress: Fear correlation and biomarker potential. *J Psychiatr Res.* 2014;57:65–73.

44. Bremner JD. Stress and brain atrophy. *CNS Neurol Disord Drug Targets.* 2006;5(5):503–512.

45. Harvey BH, Bothma T, Nel A, Wegener G, Stein DJ. Involvement of the NMDA receptor, NO-cyclic GMP and nuclear factor K-beta in an animal model of repeated trauma. *Hum Psychopharmacol.* 2005;20(5):367–373.

46. Harvey BH, Oosthuizen F, Brand L, Wegener G, Stein DJ. Stress-restress evokes sustained iNOS activity and altered GABA levels and NMDA receptors in rat hippocampus. *Psychopharmacology (Berl).* 2004;175(4):494–502.

47. Pall ML. Nitric oxide synthase partial uncoupling as a key switching mechanism for the NO/ONOO- cycle. *Med Hypotheses.* 2007;69(4):821–825.

48. Tezcan E, Atmaca M, Kuloglu M, Ustundag B. Free radicals in patients with posttraumatic stress disorder. *Eur Arch Psychiatry Clin Neurosci.* 2003;253(2):89–91.

49. Richardson JS. On the functions of monoamine oxidase, the emotions, and adaptation to stress. *Int J Neurosci.* 1993;70(1–2):75–84.

50. Pivac N, Knezevic J, Kozaric-Kovacic D, et al. Monoamine oxidase (MAO) intron 13 polymorphism and platelet MAO-B activity in combat-related posttraumatic stress disorder. *J Affect Disord.* 2007;103(1–3):131–138.

51. Schiavone S, Jaquet V, Trabace L, Krause KH. Severe life stress and oxidative stress in the brain: From animal models to human pathology. *Antioxid Redox Signal.* 2013;18(12):1475–1490.

52. Li X, Han F, Liu D, Shi Y. Changes of Bax, Bcl-2 and apoptosis in hippocampus in the rat model of posttraumatic stress disorder. *Neurol Res.* 2010;32(6):579–586.

53. Diehl LA, Alvares LO, Noschang C, et al. Long-lasting effects of maternal separation on an animal model of posttraumatic stress disorder: Effects on memory and hippocampal oxidative stress. *Neurol Res.* 2012;37(4):700–707.

54. Prasad KN, Cole WC, Prasad KC. Risk factors for Alzheimer's disease: Role of multiple antioxidants, nonsteroidal, antiinflammatory, and cholinergic agents alone or in combination in prevention and treatment. *J Am Coll Nutr.* 2002;21(6):506–522.

55. Su YA, Wu J, Zhang L, et al. Dysregulated mitochondrial genes and networks with drug targets in postmortem brain of patients with posttraumatic stress disorder (PTSD) revealed by human mitochondria-focused cDNA microarrays. *Int J Biol Sci.* 2008;4(4):223–235.

56. Tochigi M, Iwamoto K, Bundo M, Sasaki T, Kato N, Kato T. Gene expression profiling of major depression and suicide in the prefrontal cortex of postmortem brains. *Neurosci Res.* 2008;60(2):184–191.

57. Wilson CB, McLaughlin LD, Ebenezer PJ, Nair AR, Francis J. Valproic acid effects in the hippocampus and prefrontal cortex in an animal model of posttraumatic stress disorder. *Behav Brain Res.* 2014;268:72–80.

58. Wilson CB, McLaughlin LD, Nair A, Ebenezer PJ, Dange R, Francis J. Inflammation and oxidative stress are elevated in the brain, blood, and adrenal glands during the progression of posttraumatic stress disorder in a predator exposure animal model. *PLoS One.* 2013;8(10):e76146.

59. Sun XR, Zhang H, Zhao HT, et al. Amelioration of oxidative stress-induced phenotype loss of parvalbumin interneurons might contribute to the beneficial effects of environmental enrichment in a rat model of posttraumatic stress disorder. *Behav Brain Res.* 2016;312:84–92.

60. Liu FF, Yang LD, Sun XR, et al. NOX2 mediated-parvalbumin interneuron loss might contribute to anxiety-like and enhanced fear learning behavior in a rat model of posttraumatic stress disorder. *Mol Neurobiol.* 2016;53(10):6680–6689.

61. Atli A, Bulut M, Bez Y, et al. Altered lipid peroxidation markers are related to posttraumatic stress disorder (PTSD) and not trauma itself in earthquake survivors. *Eur Arch Psychiatry Clin Neurosci.* 2016;266(4):329–336.

62. Yehuda R. Biology of posttraumatic stress disorder. *J Clin Psychiatry.* 2001;62 Suppl 17:41–46.

63. Maes M, Lin AH, Delmeire L, et al. Elevated serum interleukin-6 (IL-6) and IL-6 receptor concentrations in posttraumatic stress disorder following accidental manmade traumatic events. *Biol Psychiatry.* 1999;45(7):833–839.

64. von Kanel R, Hepp U, Kraemer B, et al. Evidence for low-grade systemic proinflammatory activity in patients with posttraumatic stress disorder. *J Psychiatr Res.* 2007;41(9):744–752.

65. Sutherland AG, Alexander DA, Hutchison JD. Disturbance of pro-inflammatory cytokines in posttraumatic psychopathology. *Cytokine.* 2003;24(5):219–225.

66. Melamed S, Shirom A, Toker S, Berliner S, Shapira I. Association of fear of terror with low-grade inflammation among apparently healthy employed adults. *Psychosom Med.* 2004;66(4):484–491.

67. Miller RJ, Sutherland AG, Hutchison JD, Alexander DA. C-reactive protein and interleukin 6 receptor in posttraumatic stress disorder: A pilot study. *Cytokine.* 2001;13(4):253–255.

68. Danner M, Kasl SV, Abramson JL, Vaccarino V. Association between depression and elevated C-reactive protein. *Psychosom Med.* 2003;65(3):347–356.

69. Douglas KM, Taylor AJ, O'Malley PG. Relationship between depression and C-reactive protein in a screening population. *Psychosom Med.* 2004;66(5):679–683.

70. Prasad KN, Bondy SC. Common biochemical defects linkage between posttraumatic stress disorders, mild traumatic brain injury (TBI), and penetrating TBI. *Brain Res.* 2014;1599: 103–114.

71. Bam M, Yang X, Zumbrun EE, et al. Dysregulated immune system networks in war veterans with PTSD is an outcome of altered miRNA expression and DNA methylation. *Sci Rep.* 2016;6:31209.

72. Michopoulos V, Powers A, Gillespie CF, Ressler KJ, Jovanovic T. Inflammation in fear- and anxiety-based disorders: PTSD, GAD, and beyond. *Neuropsychopharmacology.* 2017;42(1):254–270.

73. Wang Z, Young MR. PTSD, a Disorder with an immunological component. *Front Immunol.* 2016;7:219.

74. Singh K, Agrawal NK, Gupta SK, Sinha P, Singh K. Increased expression of TLR9 associated with pro-inflammatory S100A8 and IL-8 in diabetic wounds could lead to unresolved inflammation in type 2 diabetes mellitus (T2DM) cases with impaired wound healing. *J Diabetes Complications.* 2016;30(1):99–108.

75. O'Donovan A, Ahmadian AJ, Neylan TC, Pacult MA, Edmondson D, Cohen BE. Current posttraumatic stress disorder and exaggerated threat sensitivity associated with elevated inflammation in the Mind Your Heart Study. *Brain Behav Immun.* 2017;60:198–205.

76. O'Donovan A, Chao LL, Paulson J, et al. Altered inflammatory activity associated with reduced hippocampal volume and more severe posttraumatic stress symptoms in Gulf War veterans. *Psychoneuroendocrinology.* 2015;51:557–566.

77. Lindqvist D, Dhabhar FS, Mellon SH, et al. Increased pro-inflammatory milieu in combat related PTSD: A new cohort replication study. *Brain Behav Immun.* 2017;59:260–264.

78. Bersani FS, Wolkowitz OM, Lindqvist D, et al. Global arginine bioavailability, a marker of nitric oxide synthetic capacity, is decreased in PTSD and correlated with symptom severity and markers of inflammation. *Brain Behav Immun.* 2016;52:153–160.

79. Eraly SA, Nievergelt CM, Maihofer AX, et al. Assessment of plasma C-reactive protein as a biomarker of posttraumatic stress disorder risk. *JAMA Psychiatry.* 2014;71(4):423–431.

80. Michopoulos V, Rothbaum AO, Jovanovic T, et al. Association of CRP genetic variation and CRP level with elevated PTSD symptoms and physiological responses in a civilian population with high levels of trauma. *Am J Psychiatry.* 2015;172(4):353–362.

81. Dennis PA, Weinberg JB, Calhoun PS, et al. An investigation of vago-regulatory and health-behavior accounts for increased inflammation in posttraumatic stress disorder. *J Psychosom Res.* 2016;83:33–39.

82. Sun R, Zhang W, Bo J, et al. Spinal activation of alpha7-nicotinic acetylcholine receptor attenuates posttraumatic stress disorder-related chronic pain via suppression of glial activation. *Neuroscience.* 2016;344:243–254.

83. Nair J, Singh Ajit S. The role of the glutamatergic system in posttraumatic stress disorder. *CNS Spectr.* 2008;13(7):585–591.

84. Joca SR, Ferreira FR, Guimaraes FS. Modulation of stress consequences by hippocampal monoaminergic, glutamatergic and nitrergic neurotransmitter systems. *Stress.* 2007;10(3):227–249.

85. Trist DG. Excitatory amino acid agonists and antagonists: Pharmacology and therapeutic applications. *Pharm Acta Helv.* 2000;74(2–3):221–229.

86. Nishi D, Hashimoto K, Noguchi H, Hamazaki K, Hamazaki T, Matsuoka Y. Glutamatergic system abnormalities in posttraumatic stress disorder. *Psychopharmacology (Berl).* 2015;232(23):4261–4268.

87. Averill LA, Purohit P, Averill CL, Boesl MA, Krystal JH, Abdallah CG. Glutamate dysregulation and glutamatergic therapeutics for PTSD: Evidence from human studies. *Neurosci Lett.* 2016.

88. Gao J, Wang H, Liu Y, et al. Glutamate and GABA imbalance promotes neuronal apoptosis in hippocampus after stress. *Med Sci Monit.* 2014;20:499–512.

89. Bremner JD, Licinio J, Darnell A, et al. Elevated CSF corticotropin-releasing factor concentrations in posttraumatic stress disorder. *Am J Psychiatry.* 1997;154(5):624–629.

90. Riaza Bermudo-Soriano C, Perez-Rodriguez MM, Vaquero-Lorenzo C, Baca-Garcia E. New perspectives in glutamate and anxiety. *Pharmacol Biochem Behav* 2012;100(4):752–774.

91. Walker DL, Davis M. The role of amygdala glutamate receptors in fear learning, fear-potentiated startle, and extinction. *Pharmacol Biochem Behav.* 2002;71(3):379–392.

92. Rosso IM, Weiner MR, Crowley DJ, Silveri MM, Rauch SL, Jensen JE. Insula and anterior cingulate gaba levels in posttraumatic stress disorder: Preliminary findings using magnetic resonance spectroscopy. *Depress Anxiety.* 2013;31(2):115–123.

93. Vaiva G, Boss V, Ducrocq F, et al. Relationship between posttrauma GABA plasma levels and PTSD at 1-year follow-up. *Am J Psychiatry.* 2006;163(8):1446–1448.

94. Matsuoka Y, Nishi D, Nakaya N, et al. Attenuating posttraumatic distress with omega-3 polyunsaturated fatty acids among disaster medical assistance team members after the great east Japan earthquake: The APOP randomized controlled trial. *BMC psychiatry.* 2011;11:132.

95. Tyagi E, Agrawal R, Zhuang Y, Abad C, Waschek JA, Gomez-Pinilla F. Vulnerability imposed by diet and brain trauma for anxiety-like phenotype: Implications for posttraumatic stress disorders. *PLoS One.* 2013;8(3):e57945.

96. Xu Y, Ku B, Cui L, et al. Curcumin reverses impaired hippocampal neurogenesis and increases serotonin receptor 1A mRNA and brain-derived neurotrophic factor expression in chronically stressed rats. *Brain Res.* 2007;1162:9–18.

97. Lopresti AL. Curcumin for neuropsychiatric disorders: A review of in vitro, animal and human studies. *J Psychopharmacol.* 2017;31(3):287–302.

98. Li G, Wang G, Shi J, et al. Trans-resveratrol ameliorates anxiety-like behaviors and fear memory deficits in a rat model of posttraumatic stress disorder. *Neuropharmacology.* 2018;133:181–188.

99. Alzoubi KH, Khabour OF, Ahmed M. Pentoxifylline prevents posttraumatic stress disorder induced memory impairment. *Brain Res Bull.* 2018;139:263–268.

100. Alzoubi KH, Rababa'h AM, Al Yacoub ON. Tempol prevents posttraumatic stress disorder induced memory impairment. *Physiol Behav.* 2018;184:189–195.

101. Aarsland D, Rongve A, Nore SP, et al. Frequency and case identification of dementia with Lewy bodies using the revised consensus criteria. *Dement Geriatr Cogn Disord.* 2008;26(5):445–452.

102. Ebenezer PJ, Wilson CB, Wilson LD, Nair AR, J F. The anti-inflammatory effects of blueberries in an animal model of posttraumatic stress disorder (PTSD). *PLoS One.* 2016;11(9):e0160923.

103. Gottshall K, Hoffer, ME, Balough, BJ. Use of antioxidants micronutrient compounds in vestibular rehabilitation after operational head trauma or blast injury. *Paper Presented At: Barany International Balance Meeting,* 2006; Stockholm, Sweden.

104. Prasad KN. Simultaneous activation of Nrf2 and elevation of dietary and endogenous antioxidants for prevention and improved managment of Parkinson's disease. In: Bondy SCC, A., ed. *Inflammation, Aging and Oxidative Stress.* New York: Springer; 2016:277–301.

105. Vile GF, Winterbourn CC. Inhibition of adriamycin-promoted microsomal lipid peroxidation by beta-carotene, alpha-tocopherol, and retinol at high and low oxygen partial pressures. *FEBS Lett.* 1988;238(2):353–356.

106. Niki E. Interaction of ascorbate and alpha-tocopherol. *Ann N Y Acad Sci.* 1987;498:186–199.

107. Prasad KN. Oxidative stress and pro-inflammatory cytokines may act as one of signals for regulating MicroRNAs expression in Alzheimer's disease. *Mech Ageing Dev.* 2017;162:63–71.

108. Wu H, Kong L, Tan Y, et al. C66 ameliorates diabetic nephropathy in mice by both upregulating NRF2 function via increase in miR-200a and inhibiting miR-21. *Diabetologia.* 2016;59:1558–1568.

109. Jaramillo MC, Zhang DD. The emerging role of the Nrf2-Keap1 signaling pathway in cancer. *Genes Dev.* 2013;27(20):2179–2191.

110. Williamson TP, Johnson DA, Johnson JA. Activation of the Nrf2-ARE pathway by siRNA knockdown of Keap1 reduces oxidative stress and provides partial protection from MPTP-mediated neurotoxicity. *Neurotoxicology.* 2012;33(3):272–279.

111. Itoh K, Chiba T, Takahashi S, et al. An Nrf2/small Maf heterodimer mediates the induction of phase II detoxifying enzyme genes through antioxidant response elements. *Biochem Biophys Res Commun.* 1997;236(2):313–322.

112. Hayes JD, Chanas SA, Henderson CJ, et al. The Nrf2 transcription factor contributes both to the basal expression of glutathione S-transferases in mouse liver and to their induction by the chemopreventive synthetic antioxidants, butylated hydroxyanisole and ethoxyquin. *Biochem Soc Trans.* 2000;28(2):33–41.

113. Chan K, Han XD, Kan YW. An important function of Nrf2 in combating oxidative stress: Detoxification of acetaminophen. *Proc Natl Acad Sci USA.* 2001;98(8):4611–4616.

114. Ramsey CP, Glass CA, Montgomery MB, et al. Expression of Nrf2 in neurodegenerative diseases. *J Neuropathol Exp Neurol.* 2007;66(1):75–85.

115. Chen PC, Vargas MR, Pani AK, et al. Nrf2-mediated neuroprotection in the MPTP mouse model of Parkinson's disease: Critical role for the astrocyte. *Proc Natl Acad Sci USA.* 2009;106(8):2933–2938.

116. Lastres-Becker I, Ulusoy A, Innamorato NG, et al. Alpha-synuclein expression and Nrf2 deficiency cooperate to aggravate protein aggregation, neuronal death and inflammation in early-stage Parkinson's disease. *Hum Mol Genet.* 2012;21(14):3173–3192.

117. Xi YD, Yu HL, Ding J, et al. Flavonoids protect cerebrovascular endothelial cells through Nrf2 and PI3K from beta-amyloid peptide-induced oxidative damage. *Curr Neurovasc Res.* 2012;9(1):32–41.

118. Suh JH, Shenvi SV, Dixon BM, et al. Decline in transcriptional activity of Nrf2 causes age-related loss of glutathione synthesis, which is reversible with lipoic acid. *Proc Natl Acad Sci USA.* 2004;101(10):3381–3386.

119. Trujillo J, Chirino YI, Molina-Jijon E, Anderica-Romero AC, Tapia E, Pedraza-Chaverri J. Renoprotective effect of the antioxidant curcumin: Recent findings. *Redox Biol.* 2013;1(1):448–456.

120. Steele ML, Fuller S, Patel M, Kersaitis C, Ooi L, Munch G. Effect of Nrf2 activators on release of glutathione, cysteinylglycine, and homocysteine by human U373 astroglial cells. *Redox Biol.* 2013;1(1):441–445.

121. Kode A, Rajendrasozhan S, Caito S, Yang SR, Megson IL, Rahman I. Resveratrol induces glutathione synthesis by activation of Nrf2 and protects against cigarette smoke-mediated oxidative stress in human lung epithelial cells. *Am J Physiol Lung Cell Mol Physiol.* 2008;294(3):L478–488.

122. Gao L, Wang J, Sekhar KR, et al. Novel n-3 fatty acid oxidation products activate Nrf2 by destabilizing the association between Keap1 and Cullin3. *J Biol Chem.* 2007;282(4):2529–2537.

123. Saw CL, Yang AY, Guo Y, Kong AN. Astaxanthin and omega-3 fatty acids individually and in combination protect against oxidative stress via the Nrf2-ARE pathway. *Food Chem Toxicol.* 2013;62:869–875.

124. Song J, Kang SM, Lee WT, Park KA, Lee KM, Lee JE. Glutathione protects brain endothelial cells from hydrogen peroxide-induced oxidative stress by increasing nrf2 expression. *Exp Neurobiol.* 2014;23(1):93–103.

125. Ji L, Liu R, Zhang XD, et al. N-acetylcysteine attenuates phosgene-induced acute lung injury via upregulation of Nrf2 expression. *Inhal Toxicol.* 2010;22(7):535–542.

126. Choi HK, Pokharel YR, Lim SC, et al. Inhibition of liver fibrosis by solubilized coenzyme Q10: Role of Nrf2 activation in inhibiting transforming growth factor-beta1 expression. *Toxicol Appl Pharmacol.* 2009;240(3):377–384.

127. Bai H, Liu R, Chen HL, et al. Enhanced antioxidant effect of caffeic acid phenethyl ester and Trolox in combination against radiation induced-oxidative stress. *Chem Biol Interact.* 2014;207:7–15.

128. Cui L, Jeong H, Borovecki F, Parkhurst CN, Tanese N, Krainc D. Transcriptional repression of PGC-1alpha by mutant huntingtin leads to mitochondrial dysfunction and neurodegeneration. *Cell.* 2006;127(1):59–69.

129. Li XH, Li CY, Lu JM, Tian RB, Wei J. Allicin ameliorates cognitive deficits ageing-induced learning and memory deficits through enhancing of Nrf2 antioxidant signaling pathways. *Neurosci Lett.* 2012;514(1):46–50.

130. Bergstrom P, Andersson HC, Gao Y, et al. Repeated transient sulforaphane stimulation in astrocytes leads to prolonged Nrf2-mediated gene expression and protection from superoxide-induced damage. *Neuropharmacology.* 2011;60(2–3):343–353.

131. Wruck CJ, Gotz ME, Herdegen T, Varoga D, Brandenburg LO, Pufe T. Kavalactones protect neural cells against amyloid beta peptide-induced neurotoxicity via extracellular signal-regulated kinase 1/2-dependent nuclear factor erythroid 2-related factor 2 activation. *Mol Pharmacol.* 2008;73(6):1785–1795.

132. Li W, Khor TO, Xu C, et al. Activation of Nrf2-antioxidant signaling attenuates NFkappaB-inflammatory response and elicits apoptosis. *Biochem Pharmacol.* 2008;76(11):1485–1489.

133. Kim J, Cha YN, Surh YJ. A protective role of nuclear factor-erythroid 2-related factor-2 (Nrf2) in inflammatory disorders. *Mutat Res.* 2010;690(1–2):12–23.

134. Devaraj S, Tang R, Adams-Huet B, et al. Effect of high-dose alpha-tocopherol supplementation on biomarkers of oxidative stress and inflammation and carotid atherosclerosis in patients with coronary artery disease. *Am J Clin Nutr.* 2007;86(5):1392–1398.

135. Fu Y, Zheng S, Lin J, Ryerse J, Chen A. Curcumin protects the rat liver from CCl4-caused injury and fibrogenesis by attenuating oxidative stress and suppressing inflammation. *Mol Pharmacol.* 2008;73(2):399–409.

136. Lee HS, Jung KK, Cho JY, et al. Neuroprotective effect of curcumin is mainly mediated by blockade of microglial cell activation. *Pharmazie.* 2007;62(12):937–942.

137. Rahman S, Bhatia K, Khan AQ, et al. Topically applied vitamin E prevents massive cutaneous inflammatory and oxidative stress responses induced by double application of 12-O-tetradecanoylphorbol-13-acetate (TPA) in mice. *Chem Biol Interact.* 2008;172(3):195–205.

138. Zhu J, Yong W, Wu X, et al. Anti-inflammatory effect of resveratrol on TNF-alpha-induced MCP-1 expression in adipocytes. *Biochem Biophys Res Commun.* 2008;369(2):471–477.

139. Chang Y, Huang SK, Wang SJ. Coenzyme Q10 inhibits the release of glutamate in rat cerebrocortical nerve terminals by suppression of voltage-dependent calcium influx and mitogen-activated protein kinase signaling pathway. *J Agricul Food Chem.* 2012;60(48):11909–11918.

140. Schubert D, Kimura H, Maher P. Growth factors and vitamin E modify neuronal glutamate toxicity. *Proc Natl Acad Sci USA.* 1992;89(17):8264–8267.

141. Sandhu JK, Pandey S, Ribecco-Lutkiewicz M, et al. Molecular mechanisms of glutamate neurotoxicity in mixed cultures of NT2-derived neurons and astrocytes: Protective effects of coenzyme Q10. *J Neurosci Res.* 2003;72(6):691–703.

142. Yang TT, Wang SJ. Pyridoxine inhibits depolarization-evoked glutamate release in nerve terminals from rat cerebral cortex: A possible neuroprotective mechanism? *J Pharmacol Exp Ther.* 2009;331(1):244–254.

143. Hung KL, Wang CC, Huang CY, Wang SJ. Cyanocobalamin, vitamin B12, depresses glutamate release through inhibition of voltage-dependent Ca^{2+} influx in rat cerebrocortical nerve terminals (synaptosomes). *Eur J Pharmacol.* 2009;602(2–3):230–237.

144. Heresco-Levy U, Vass A, Bloch B, et al. Pilot controlled trial of d-serine for the treatment of posttraumatic stress disorder. *Int J Neuropsychopharmacol.* 2009:1–8.

145. Ipser J, Seedat S, Stein DJ. Pharmacotherapy for posttraumatic stress disorder: A systematic review and meta-analysis. *S Afr Med J.* 2006;96(10):1088–1096.

146. Ravindran LN, Stein MB. Pharmacotherapy of PTSD: Premises, principles, and priorities. *Brain Res.* 2009;1293:24–39.

147. Richardson R, Ledgerwood L, Cranney J. Facilitation of fear extinction by D-cycloserine: Theoretical and clinical implications. *Learn Mem.* 2004;11(5):510–516.

148. Vervliet B. Learning and memory in conditioned fear extinction: Effects of D-cycloserine. *Acta Psychol (Amst).* 2008;127(3):601–613.

149. de Quervain DJ, Margraf J. Glucocorticoids for the treatment of posttraumatic stress disorder and phobias: A novel therapeutic approach. *Eur J Pharmacol.* 2008;583(2–3):365–371.

150. Schelling G. Effects of stress hormones on traumatic memory formation and the development of posttraumatic stress disorder in critically ill patients. *Neurobiol Learn Mem.* 2002;78(3):596–609.

13 Micronutrients in Improvement of the Standard Therapy in Traumatic Brain Injury

INTRODUCTION

Traumatic brain injury (TBI) includes mild TBI (mTBI), also called concussion or concussive injury, and penetrating traumatic brain Injury (pTBI). TBI can be a mild, moderate, or severe form. Concussive injury occurs when the brain violently rocks back and forth within the skull following a blow to the head or neck, such as that observed in contact sports like football and soccer. Concussive injury can also occur during the rapid displacement and rotation of the cranium after peak head acceleration and momentum transfer after helmet impacts.[1] Among US combat troops, concussive injury occurs due to exposure to blast pressure waves following detonation of improvised explosive devices (IEDs). Current efforts on reducing the adverse impacts of concussion on brain function have focused on the development of physical protection for the head. Introduction of newer football helmets appears to lower the risk of concussion by about 10%–20%.[2] Despites newer head protective devices, concussive injuries remain a major health risk for professional football players,[3] as well as for US troops in combat zones. At present, there are no biological preventive or improved treatment strategies. The current management of TBI involving medications, psychotherapy, and physical therapy is considered not satisfactory.

pTBI occurs when an object penetrates the skull and damages the brain. This form of TBI is caused by vehicle crashes, gunshot wounds to the head, and exposure to explosions of IEDs and combat-related head injuries. pTBI can be a mild, moderate, or severe form. Although there has been significant improvement in the management of pTBI, treatment strategies for patients with pTBI remain unsatisfactory, and morbidity and mortality continue to be high. In addition, there is no effective strategy to reduce the risk of dementia and other forms of mental disorders among the survivors of pTBI.

In order to develop a rational strategy for prevention of concussion and improved management of both concussion and pTBI, it would be important to identify major cellular defects that play crucial role in the initiation and progression of TBI.

Animal and human studies suggest that increased levels of oxidative stress, inflammation, and glutamate in the brain are common cellular defects in the pathogenesis of both concussion and pTBI. Therefore, attenuation of these cellular defects may prevent concussion, and in combination of standard therapy, improve the management of concussion as well as pTBI. There has been no significant studies on the effectiveness of single or multiple micronutrients in TBI. In order to reduce the above cellular defects, previous studies using individual micronutrients have yielded inconsistent results in neurodegenerative diseases.

This chapter describes briefly the incidence, prevalence, cost, causes, and symptoms of concussion and pTBI, and discusses the role of microRNAs in the pathogenesis and diagnosis of TBI. This chapter also presents evidence for the involvement of increased levels of oxidative stress, inflammation, and glutamate in concussion and pTBI. In order to simultaneously reduce these cellular defects, increasing the levels of antioxidant enzymes and dietary and endogenous antioxidants are essential. The levels of antioxidants can be increased by supplementation; however, enhancing the levels of antioxidants enzymes requires activation of a nuclear transcriptional factor Nrf2. This chapter describes agents that activate the Nrf2/ARE pathway and proposes a mixture of micronutrients that would reduce oxidative stress and inflammation by activating the Nrf2/ARE pathway and enhancing the levels of antioxidants. This mixture may also prevent the release and toxicity of glutamate, and thus, reduce concussive injury, and in combination with standard care, improve the management of both concussion and pTBI,

INCIDENCE, PREVALENCE, AND COST OF TBI

CONCUSSION IN USA POPULATION

The Centers for Disease Control and Prevention (CDC, 2012) estimates that approximately 1.7 million people in the USA sustain a TBI annually from all causes, out of which about 75% represent concussive injury.

NATIONAL FOOTBALL LEAGUE (NFL)

Between 2002 and 2007, 152 players had repeat concussions.[4] The defensive secondary, kick unit, running back, and linebacker have the highest incidence of repeat concussions. About 7.6% of all repeat concussions occurred within 2 weeks of the prior concussion. More than half of players with repeat concussions were removed from play.

HIGH SCHOOL AND COLLEGE SPORTS

The number of students participating in high school and college sports is increasing. Between 2005 and 2006, more than 7 million high school students, and between 2004 and 2005, about 385,000 college students participated in various sports. According to the National Federation of State High School Associations, between 2008 and 2009, about 7.5 million high school students participated in sports. A prospective 11-year study revealed that annual increase in concussive injury was 14% among boys and 21% among girls.[5] Football accounted for more than half of all concussions. Among girls' sports, soccer accounted for the highest proportion of concussive injury. The concussive injury increased 4-fold between the years 1998–2008. Another study has estimated that about 300,000 sports-related TBI, primarily concussive injury, occurred among high school and college athletes. Concussive injury represented 8.9% of all high school athletic injuries and 5.8% of all collegiate athletic injuries.[6] The rates of concussions were highest among athletes playing football and soccer. The rate of concussive injury was higher among girls than among boys. For individuals ages 15–24 years, sports are second to motor vehicle crashes as the leading cause of TBI.

US VETERANS

Among US veterans returning from the military conflicts in Iraq and Afghanistan, TBI represents one of the major injuries. The prevalence of TBI ranges from 15% to 20%, and 85% of the TBI are mild concussions.[7] The majority of these concussions were due to exposure to blasts. Most of them experienced exposure to multiple blasts. About 20% of them were exposed to second blasts within 2 weeks of the first and 87% within 3 months.

US CIVILIAN

In civilians, falls, motor vehicle accident, struck by/against moving or stationary objects, and assaults involving the head contribute to mild to severe TBI (CDC, Traumatic Brain Injury and Causes, 2012). Falls contribute to 35.2% of TBI, motor vehicle accidents 17.3%, struck by/against moving or stationary objects 16.5%, assaults 10%, and other unknown factors 21%. Falls are the major causes of concussive injury among children ages up to 14 years and among adults ages 65 years or older.

PENETRATING TBI (pTBI)

US TROOPS

A total of 1,255 troops returning from Iraq and Afghanistan suffer TBI due to exposure to explosive devices. Among them, 774 had pTBI and 481 had concussion, representing about 62% of total TBI. The number of survivors after pTBI has increased due to an excellent trauma care facility in the war zone.

US CIVILIAN

The Centers for Disease Control and Prevention (CDC) estimates that about 1.7 million people sustain pTBI each year. pTBI accounts for about 30.5% of all injury-related deaths and for substantial cases of permanent disability. The CDC has estimated that at least 5.3 million Americans who suffered from pTBI have a long-term or lifelong need for help to perform activities of daily living.

COST

Direct medical costs and indirect costs such as lost productivity of TBI estimated to be $56 billion in the USA each year. The cost of mild TBI or concussive injury each year is estimated to be $17 billion (CDC, Traumatic Brain Injury and Causes, 2012).

CAUSES OF CONCUSSION

Concussive injury occurs when the brain violently rocks back and forth within the skull following a blow to the head or neck such as that observed in contact sports like football and soccer. In US combat troops, concussive injury also occurs when exposed to a blast pressure wave following detonation of an IED. Among civilians, falls, and crashes involving automobiles, motorcycles, and bicycles can cause concussive injury.

CAUSES OF PENETRATING TBI (pTBI)

pTBI occurs when an object penetrates the skull and damages the brain, which could be confined to small or larger area of the brain. Among US soldiers deployed to the wars in Iraq and Afghanistan, blasts, improvised explosive devices (IEDs), vehicle crashes, and other combat-related injuries are the main causes of the increased incidence of pTBI. Among civilians, transportation accidents involving automobiles, motorcycles, bicycles, and pedestrians, and gunshot wounds to the head are the major causes of pTBI. This is a serious and life-threatening injury and requires emergency medical care.

ACUTE SYMPTOMS OF CONCUSSION

The major acute physical symptoms include transient confusion, disorientation, and loss of consciousness, headache, dizziness, nausea, blurred vision, uneven gait, insomnia, blurred vision, and fatigue. The cognitive symptoms include memory loss, attention deficits, and lack of concentration. The behavioral changes include irritability, depression, fear and anxiety, loss of emotional control, and problems with relationship.

ACUTE SYMPTOMS OF pTBI

The symptoms depend upon the severity of brain damage and area of the brain affected. The acute symptoms of pTBI include (a) heavy bleeding from the head, (b) bleeding from the ears, (c) difficulty breathing, (d) seizure, (e) loss of bladder and bowel functions, (f) loss of movement and sensation in the limbs, and (g) loss of consciousness. If the damage to the brain is extensive, patients may die within a few days to a few weeks.

LONG-TERM HEALTH CONSEQUENCES OF TBI

CONCUSSION

Brain deformation may occur after the primary head acceleration.[1] Damage to the midbrain correlated with memory and cognitive problems after concussions. The major commonly symptoms observed after concussions include impairment of memory, processing speed, verbal memory, and executive function.[8,9] An early onset of dementia may be initiated by repetitive concussions in professional football players.[10,11] Balance disorders are also considered one of the major health problems with the concussive injury.[11]

A study on retired NFL retired players showed that 10.2% of participating players had depression, which increased with an increasing number of concussions compared to those retired players who reported no concussions.[12] An increase in concussion-induced depression was independent of depression induced by other physical conditions. Another study on retired professional football players showed that retired players with 3 or more concussions had a 5-fold prevalence of mild cognitive dysfunction and a 3-fold increase in significant memory loss compared to those retired players who did not suffer concussions.[10] There was no association between recurrent concussions and Alzheimer's disease; however, the onset of this disease in the retired players was earlier than in the general American population.

A study on college football players showed that about 85.2% of football players who sustained concussions reported headaches that lasted up to 82 hours. Previous concussions were associated with slower recovery.[13]

Increased risk of chronic traumatic encephalopathy (CTE) remains one of the measures of health concerns of repeated concussions. In a study with high school football players, it was found repetitive blows to the head are cumulative and that repeated mild concussions can cause CTE and neurophysiological abnormalities.[14]

Concussions can cause decline in motor and cognitive function and increased risk of Alzheimer's disease in young athletes. Animal models of TBI have shown that impaired learning ability was related to synaptic plasticity suppression. In humans, single or repeated concussions can cause lifelong or cumulative enhancement of gamma-aminobutyric acid (GABA)-mediated suppression of synaptic plasticity. It has been reported that repeated concussions induced persistent elevation of GABA-mediated inhibition in primary motor cortex, which was associated with suppressed synaptic plasticity.[15] These changes accounted for impaired learning ability.

A study on college athletes showed that concussed female athletes performed significantly worse than concussed male athletes on visual memory tasks.[16] Male athletes were more likely to report symptoms of vomiting and sadness than female athletes. The analysis of performance data further revealed that at 2 days after injury, 58% of concussed athletes exhibited decline in performance and increase in other symptoms, whereas at 8 days after concussions, 30% continue to show one or more changes in neuropsychological tests.

In a study on US Army soldiers, an anonymous mental health survey was performed at 4 to 6 months after returning from deployment to Iraq or Afghanistan.[17] The results showed that 17% of soldiers reported a mild TBI during their previous deployment, and 59% of these soldiers suffered more than one mild TBI. After adjusting for posttraumatic stress syndrome (PTSD), depression, and other factors, multiple mild TBI was associated with the loss of consciousness and increased risk of headache compare to those who had only one mild TBI. Mild TBI is also associated with an increased incidence of PTSD. The similarity in some of the symptoms makes it difficult to distinguish them while evaluating for the treatment of these brain dysfunctions. A review of 3 large studies, which evaluated the frequency of mild TBI and PTSD in veterans of Iraq and Afghanistan, showed that frequency of mild TBI/PTSD varied from 5% to 7%; however, among those with a mild TBI, frequency of PTSD varied from 33% to 39%.[18] Evidence from functional and metabolic imaging suggests that abnormalities in the electric responses, metabolic balance and oxygen consumption in neurons exist several months after concussions.[19]

pTBI

The long-term consequences also include impairment of cognitive function (attention and memory), motor (extreme weakness, poor coordination and balance), sensation (hearing, vision, impaired perception, and touch), and emotion (depression, anxiety, aggression, impulse control, and personality changes), and PTSD. The survivors of pTBI may face long-term serious disabilities that can cause very poor quality of life.

NEUROPATHOLOGY OF TBI

Concussion

Increased risk of chronic traumatic encephalopathy (CTE) remains one of the measure health concerns of repeated concussions. In study with high school football players, it was found repetitive blows to head are cumulative and that repeated subconcussive blows can cause CTE and neurophysiological abnormalities.[14]

pTBI

The neuropathology of pTBI is very complex, depending upon the type and velocity of inducing agents, area and the size of the affected brain tissue, and amounts of loss of brain tissue. Generally, swelling, edema, hematoma, hemorrhage, contusion, focal cerebral vasospasm, increased blood-brain-barrier (BBB) disruption, and diffuse axonal injury are observed immediately after injury.[20] It has been reported that penetrating ballistic-like injury and hemorrhagic shock can cause persistent damage of cerebral blood flow and brain tissue oxygen tension. These changes increase the probability of cortical spreading depolarization that may contribute to secondary neuropathology and compromise neurological recovery.[21] The damage to the brain after pTBI occurs into three phases. The first phase involves primary injury to the brain tissue that cannot be reversed. The second phase occurs soon after injury and continues for days to weeks and contributes to the development of secondary damage that eventually leads to neurological disorders and neuronal death. During this period, intervention with appropriate agents can slow down the progression of the damage. The third phase appears as late effects, which depend upon the initial areas of the brain damaged. The late effects may include cognitive dysfunction, PTSD, and other behavior abnormalities.

SCORING SYSTEM OF SEVERITY OF TBI

The Glasgow Coma Scale (GCS) is one of the most commonly used severity scoring systems. Individual with GCS scores of 3–8 are classified with a pTBI, those with scores of 9–12 classified with a moderate TBI, and those with scores of 13–15 are classified with a mild TBI. Other classification systems include the Abbreviated Injury Scale (AIS), the Trauma Score, and the Abbreviated Trauma Scores. These classifications are useful in clinical management of TBI, because the prognosis for concussion is better than for pTBI.

MicroRNAs IN PATHOGENESIS OF TBI

Changes in the expressions of microRNAs appear to be involved in the pathogenesis of TBI. The expressions of miR-144, miR-153, and miR-340-5p were enhanced, and the levels of their target proteins calcium/calmodulin-dependent serine kinase (CASK), nuclear factor erythroid 2-related factor 2 (Nrf2), and alpha-synuclein (SNCA) were reduced in the ipsilateral hippocampus after TBI injury in rats.[22] In the controlled cortical Impact (CCI) mice model of TBI, the expression of miR-21, miR-144, miR-184, miR-451, and 2137 were upregulated, while the expression of miR-107, miR-137, miR-190, and miR-541, were downregulated.[23] No target proteins were identified in this study. Expression of miR-711 increased and the levels of its target proteins pro-survival protein Akt decreased in the cortex CCI mice model of TBI.[24] Downregulation of Akt led to sequential activation of forkhead box O3 (FoxO3)a/glycogen synthase kinase 3 (GSK3)α/β, proapoptotic BH3-only molecules PUMA (Bcl2-binding component 3), and Bim (Bcl2-like 11 apoptotic facilitator), and mitochondrial release of cytochrome c and AUF. A miR-711 mimic enhanced neuronal death in these mice, while inhibitor of miR-711 protected TBI-induced neuronal death by increasing the levels of Akt.[24] In the CCI mice model of TBI, the expressions of miR-23a and miR-27a were elevated and the levels of their target proteins proapoptotic Bcl2 family members Noxa, Puma, and Bax in the cortex leading to neuronal apoptosis.[25] In the fluid percussion injury (FPI) rat model of TBI, upregulation of miR-21 level improved long-term neurological functions, alleviated brain edema, decreased lesion volume, prompted angiogenesis, and inhibited apoptosis by reducing its target protein PTEN leading to activation of Akt signaling pathway.[26] Increased expression of miR-21 also alleviated damage to the blood-brain barrier by activating angioprotein 1 (Ang-1) and Tie-2 in the FPI rat model.[27] In the CCI mouse model of TBI, upregulation of miR-let-7c-5p improved neurological function and brain edema by inhibiting neuroinflammation and activation of microglia/macrophages. In addition, this enhanced expression of this microRNA reduced its target protein caspase-3.[28] Overexpression of miR-23b improved neuronal functions including cognitive function, reduced lesion volume, brain edema, and apoptosis by decreasing the levels of its target autophagy-related genes (ATGs) leading to suppression of neuronal autophagy. Enhanced expression of ATGs abolished neuroprotective effects of miR-23b.[29] Overexpression of miR-144, miR-27a, and miR-155 provided neuroprotection in the hippocampus by reducing the levels of their respective target proteins ADAM10 (a disintegrin and metallopeptidase domain 10), FoxO3 (forkhead box P3), and interferons.[30–32] Table 13.1 summarizes the effect of upregulation of microRNAs in animal models of TBI. Additional studies are needed in autopsied brain tissues from patients with TBI.

TABLE 13.1

Effects of Upregulation of MicroRNAs on the Brain of Animal Models of TBI

TBI Models	Upregulation	Downregulation of Target Proteins	Results
Rat TBI[22]	miR-144, miR-153, miR-340-5p	CASK, Nrf2, SNCA	Apoptosis
CCI Mouse[23]	miR-21, miR-144, miR-184, miR-451, miR-2137	Not identified	Secondary brain damage
CCI Mouse[24]	miR-711	Akt	Apoptosis
CCI Mouse[25]	miR-23a, miR-27a	Bcl2-family	Survival
FPI Rat[26,27]	miR-21	PTEN, Ang1, Tie-2	Survival
CCI Mouse[28]	miR-let-7c-5p	Caspase-3	Survival
CCI Mouse[29]	miR-23b	ATG12	Survival
CCI Mouse[30–32]	miR-144, miR-27a, miR-155	ADAM10, FoxO3a	Survival

Note: CASK, calcium/calmodulin-dependent serine protein kinase; Nrf2, nuclear factor erythroid 2-related factor 2; SNCA, alpha-synuclein; CCI, controlled cortical impact; Akt, prosurvival, serine/threonine kinase, also called protein kinase B; Bcl2 family (PUMA-p53 upregulated modulator of apoptosis, Noxa-phorbol-12-myristate-13-acetate-incuced protein 1, also known as NOXA [Latin for damage]), and Bax-Bcl2-associated X-protein; PTEN, phosphatase and Tensin homolog; Ang-1, angioprotein-1; Tie-2, tyrosine kinase with immunoglobulin-like and EGF-like domain-2; ATG12, autophagy-related genes, IFN, interferon; ADAM10, a disintegrin and metallopeptidase domain 10; FoxO3a, forkhead box protein3.

Number in superscripts refers to the reference number.

MicroRNAs AS POTENTIAL BIOMARKERS FOR TBI

Increased in levels of miR-21, miR-93, miR-191, miR-425, and miR-499 in the serum/plasma, and imiR-328, miR-362-3p, miR-451, and miR-486a in the cerebrospinal fluid (CSF) in humans are indicators of severe TBI and poor prognosis (Table 13.2).[33] Enhanced expressions of miR-93, miR-191, and miR-499 in the serum indicate poor outcome in patients with TBI.[34] Plasma levels of miR-16, miR-92a, and miR-765 are indicator of severe TBI in humans.[35] Downregulation of miR-425-5p and miR-502 in the serum was indicator of mild TBI, whereas upregulation of miR-21 and miR-335 was indicator of severe TBI.[36]

TABLE 13.2

Expressions of MicroRNAs in the Serum/Plasma and Cerebro-Spinal Fluid (CSF) in Humans

Serum/Plasma	CSF	Diagnosis
miR-21, miR-93, miR-191, miR-425-p, miR-499	miR-328, miR-362-3p, miR-451, miR-486a	Severe TBI[33]
miR-93, miR-191, miR-499	Not done	Severe, moderate or mild TBI[34]
miR-16, miR-92a, miR-765	Not done	Severe TBI[35]
miR-425-5p, miR-502 (downregulated)	Not done	mild TBI[36]
miR-21, miR-335 (upregulated)	Not done	Severe TBI[36]

Note: Expressions of MicoRNAs are upregulated if not mentioned.
Number in superscripts refers to reference number.

EVIDENCE FOR INCREASED OXIDATIVE STRESS IN CONCUSSION

ANIMAL MODELS

Evidence for increased oxidative stress comes from the levels of markers of oxidative damage and from the use of antioxidants that reduce their levels in animal models of concussions. It has been reported that elevated levels of protein carbonyls (a marker of oxidative damage), and reduced levels of superoxide dismutase (SOS) and silent information regulator-2 (Sir2) in the rat hippocampus after a mild TBI were observed.[37] In addition, poor performance by the animals was associated with the reduced levels of brain-derived neurotrophic factor (BDNF). BDNF facilitates synaptic function and support learning by modulating the CaMKII system (Ca^{2+} -and calmodulin-dependent protein kinase II), synapsin1, and cAMP-response element-binding protein (CREB). Feeding diet supplemented with vitamin E for 4 weeks before a mild TBI prevented impairment in learning ability and above biochemical changes in these rats. These results suggest that increased oxidative stress may be involved in causing impaired learning ability in animals with a mild TBI.

In transgenic mouse model of Alzheimer amyloidosis (Tg2576 mice), repetitive concussive brain injury induced by a modified cortical impact model of closed head injury increased the levels of brain lipid peroxidation, accelerated beta amyloid deposition, and caused learning deficits. Feeding diet supplemented with vitamin E for 4 weeks before a mild TBI prevented lipid peroxidation, impairment in learning ability, and reduction in the levels of BDNF in these transgenic mice.[38] It has been reported that feeding a high-fat diet decreased hippocampal plasticity and cognitive function by reducing BDNF in rats with a mild TBI.[39] Feeding diet supplemented with curcumin, which exhibit antioxidant and anti-inflammation activities, prevented oxidative stress, restored BDNF, and improved synaptic plasticity and cognitive function in rats with a mild TBI.[40] Similar results were obtained by feeding diet supplemented with omega-3-fatty acid docosahexaenoic acid (DHA) prior to inducing a mild TBI in rats.[41] Repetitive concussive injuries increased the levels of markers of oxidative damage malondialdehyde (MDA), reduced/oxidized glutathione ratio, nitrite, and nitrate and decreased the levels of ascorbic acid and glutathione in rats. These biochemical changes were observed in rats in which a mild TBI was delivered 1, 2 or 3 days after the first one. However, if the time interval between first one and second one was 5 day, the levels of biochemical markers of oxidative damage and nitrosylative damage were nearly control levels.[42]

HUMANS

No human studies have been performed on changes in markers of oxidative damage or the levels of antioxidants before or after concussive injury in active or retired football players or in veterans of foreign wars. Other factors, such as excessive use of oxygen by football players during the game may aggravate the impact of concussions on brain injury. Normally, the brain uses about 25% of respired oxygen. Mitochondria utilize oxygen to generate energy and free radicals are produced during this process. About 2% of unused oxygen leaks out of mitochondria that makes about 20 billion molecules of superoxide anions and hydrogen peroxide per cell per day. Thus, it is likely that during the game, when excessive amounts of oxygen are used, the brain may be exposed to higher levels of oxidative stress that may overwhelm endogenous defense systems. Such an event may enhance the levels of acute- and long-term adverse consequences of concussions in the brain.

EVIDENCE FOR INCREASED INFLAMMATION IN CONCUSSION

ANIMAL MODELS

Rats exposed to repetitive concussions (1, 3, or 5 times) spaced 5 days apart displayed increased anxiety- and depression-like behaviors, short- and long-term cognitive dysfunction, neuroinflammation, and cortical damage.[43]

HUMANS

Time-dependent changes in inflammatory cellular response in human cortical contusion were investigated by immunohistochemistry during first 30 weeks after blunt head injury.[44] The results showed that CD-15 (3-fucosyl-N-acertyl-lactosamine)-labeled granulocytes were detected as early as 10 minutes after brain injury. In addition, increased numbers of mononuclear leukocytes labeled with LCA (leukocyte common antigen), CD-3 and UCHL-1, a clone of CD45RO that is an isoform of LCA, were detected at 1.1 days, 2 days and 3.7 days after injury in cortical contusions.

In another study, time-dependent alterations in inflammatory responses in 12 consecutive patients undergoing surgery for brain contusions 3 hours to 5 days after trauma were determined by immunohistochemistry.[45] If the inflammatory responses were determined in less than 24 after injury, they were limited to vascular margination of polymorphonuclear cells. In patients undergoing surgery 3–5 days after injury, an extensive inflammatory reaction consisting of monocyte/macrophages, reactive microglia, polymorphonuclear cells, and CD-4 and CD-8-labeld T lymphocytes was observed. Human lymphocyte antigen-DQ was expressed on reactive microglia and infiltrating leukocytes later on. These inflammatory reaction following contusions may produce several potentially harmful effects, including acute- and long-term degeneration of nerve cells. On the above brain tissues, the expression of pro- and anti-inflammatory cytokines was determined.[46] The results showed that in patients undergoing surgery in less than 24 hours after injury, strong expression of the pro-inflammatory cytokines interleukin-1 beta (IL-1 beta), IL-6, and interferon-gamma (INF-gamma) and the anti-inflammatory cytokine IL-4 was present. However, in patients undergoing surgery 3–5 days after injury, expression of IL-4 was lower compared to those who were operated earlier. However, expression of IL-1beta and IFN-gamma remained high compared to IL-6. The persistence of pro-inflammatory cytokines could cause neurodegeneration.

In a study involving brain tissue obtained at autopsy from 24 patients who had TBI and 5 control brains, changes in CD-14, a pattern recognition receptor of the immune system were investigated.[47] In control brains, CD-14 expressed constitutively in perivascular cells, but not in parenchymal cells. However, after TBI, expression of CD-14 in perivascular cells and parenchymal cells reached maximal levels within 4–8 days and remained elevated until weeks after injury. These results suggest that increased expression of CD-14 is one of the major responses of acute inflammatory reaction in the brain following TBI.

EVIDENCE FOR INCREASED GLUTAMATE LEVEL IN CONCUSSION

Mild traumatic injury (brain concussive injury) can cause cognitive and emotional dysfunction and increases the risk for the development of anxiety disorders, including posttraumatic disorder (PTSD) commonly observed in veterans of foreign wars. Glutamate receptor N-methyl-D-aspartate (NMDA) in the amygdala appears to regulate fear and anxiety. In a rat model of mild TBI, the levels of NMDA receptors in the amygdala increased. In addition, gamma-aminobutyric acid (GABA)-related inhibition decreased in amygdala and hippocampus.[48] These results suggest excitatory events created by an elevation of NMDA receptors levels and a decrease in GABA activity may increase the risk for developing fear and anxiety. It appears that following concussive brain injury, excessive amounts of glutamate are released that can cause a massive efflux of K^+ ions and increased accumulation of lactate. This was confirmed by the fact that administration of ouabain, an inhibitor of Na^+/K^+-ATPase, before injury reduced lactate accumulation.

MOLECULAR CHANGES IN THE BRAIN AFTER CONCUSSION

The expression of oncogene proteins, c-myc, and c-fos was elevated in rat brains after brain concussions.[49,50] In addition, cortical expression of nuclear factor kappaB (NF-kappaB) was elevated in human contused brain.[51] The fact that antioxidants reduced expression of c-myc oncogene[52] and activation of NF-KappaB[53] further suggested that supplementation with antioxidants may reduce acute and long-term term adverse health consequences of concussive injury in the brain. The levels of inducible nitric oxide synthase (iNOS) in human neurons, macrophages, neutrophils, astrocytes, and oligodendrocytes increased within 6 hours after trauma, and peaked at about 8–23 hours.[54] Increased levels of iNOS can generate excessive amounts of NO that can form peroxynitrite that is very toxic to nerve cells.

EVIDENCE FOR INCREASED OXIDATIVE STRESS AFTER pTBI

ANIMAL MODELS

Increased oxidative stress due to production of excessive amounts of free radicals derived from oxygen and nitrogen occur after TBI.[55–57] Increased production of superoxide radicals has been demonstrated in mice.[58] The extent of oxidative damage appeared to be directly proportion to the severity of TBI in a rat model of TBI.[59] The levels of antioxidant enzymes Mn-SOD (manganese-dependent superoxide dismutase) and glutathione reductase decreased more in older rats than the younger ones following TBI, whereas the levels of markers of oxidative damage such as products of lipid peroxidation (acrolein and 4-hydroxynonenal) increased more in the older rats than the younger rats.[57] In rats, there appears to be a close relationship between degree of oxidative stress and severity of brain damage following TBI as evidenced by the highest values of malondialdehyde (MDA) and lowest value of ascorbate.[60] The total antioxidant reserves of brain homogenates and water-soluble antioxidants reserves as well as tissue concentration of ascorbate, glutathione, and sulfhydryl proteins were reduced after TBI in rats.[61] Peroxynitrite-mediated oxidative damage to mitochondrial function after pTBI precedes neuronal loss in the brain. The oxidation of nitric oxide forms peroxynitrite. Animal studies have revealed that TBI increased nitric oxide (NO) production that impairs mitochondrial function by inhibiting cytochrome oxidase.[62] Cytochrome oxidase is a key enzyme needed to generate energy. Thus, the energy level in tissue decreased after TBI that may interfere with repair process. TBI also increased inducible nitric oxide synthase (iNOS) activity that contributes to neurological deficits but not to cerebral edema by generating excessive amounts of NO.[63] In a rat model of traumatic injury (unilateral moderate cortical contusion), increased oxidative damage occur as early as 3 hours following TBI that adversely affects synaptic function and plasticity of hippocampal neurons, and thereby, enhances cognitive dysfunction.[64] In another model of TBI (fluid percussion brain injury in rat), it was observed that protein carbonylation and thiobarbituric acid-reactive substances (TBARS) levels increased in parietal cortex 1 and 3 months following injury. These changes in markers of oxidative damage were associated with the progressive decrease in the activity of Na^+, K^+-ATPase.[65] These results suggest that increase in oxidative stress associated with decrease in Na^+, K^+-ATPase activity may account for cognitive dysfunction observed following TBI.

It has been found that Nrf2 pathway which activates antioxidant enzyme through ARE (antioxidant response element) is enhanced during early brain damage after inducing subarachnoid hemorrhage in rats.[66] Since transient increased in oxidative stress is required for the activation of Nrf2 pathway, it can be concluded that increased oxidative stress occurred as an early biochemical event, which may contribute to the progression of the lesion in the brain.

HUMANS

A few human studies also confirm the role of oxidative stress in the progression of brain damage after TBI. F2-isoprostane is a marker of lipid peroxidation, whereas neuron-specific enolase (NSE) is considered a marker of neuronal damage. The levels of F2-isoprostane and NSE increased in the cerebral spinal fluid samples following TBI in children and infants.[67] Both the levels of ascorbate and glutathione decreased in the CSF of children and infants following TBI.[68] Metabolic function of the brain in children with s pTBI is impaired. Although cerebral blood flow is variable after pTBI in children, low oxygen metabolic index and hypoperfusion were observed.[69] A clinical study showed that the level of 3-nitrotyrosine increased in the CSF of the patients with TBI.[70] Another clinical study reported that increased levels of cytochrome C and activated caspases-9 were detected in the CSF of the adult patients with severe TBI.[71] Increased levels of cytochrome C and activated caspase-9 play a significant role in causing neuronal death. It has been reported that the levels of beta-amyloid fragments (Aß1-42) increased in the cerebral spinal fluid of patients after severe TBI.[72] This peptide has been implicated in causing neuronal damage in patients with Alzheimer's disease, and one of the mechanisms of injury induced by amyloid beta fragments generated from splicing of amyloid precursor protein (APP) involves increased oxidative stress.[73–76]

The plasma levels of 8-iso-prostaglandin F2alpha, a marker of oxidative damage in vivo, were higher in patients with pTBI than in healthy subjects.[77] Another clinical study has shown a close relationship between oxidative stress and excitotoxicity following pTBI in humans.[78] Another study showed that the levels of erythrocyte thiobarbituric acid-reactive substances (TBARS) were significantly higher and the levels of glutathione lower in pTBI and mild TBI patients compared to those in healthy individuals[79] The plasma levels of TBARS and protein oxidation (carbonyl) increased significantly in the first 70 hours after pTBI.[80]

Copeptin, a stable glycopeptide, a product of vasopressin, is secreted from the posterior pituitary gland. It is also known as an antidiuretic hormone. Higher plasma levels of copeptin appear to be associated with poor clinical outcomes of severely ill patients. A study on children showed that the plasma levels of copeptin were elevated in patients with pTBI than in healthy children[81] Therefore, plasma levels of copeptin may be used as diagnostic marker for pTBI.

High levels of active Peroxiredoxin 6 (prdx6), a major antioxidant enzyme normally found in astrocytes, were detected in the CSF of healthy control subject; however, it was oxidized (inactive form) in patients with TBI.[82] Enhanced oxidative damage in the brain and higher levels of markers of oxidative damage F2-isoprostane and F4-neuroprostane in the CSF were present in patients with TBI.[83] Increased serum concentration of thioredoxin, a marker of oxidative damage, was associated with severe TBI symptoms including acute lung injury, acute traumatic coagulopathy, progressive hemorrhagic injury, and posttraumatic cerebral infarction.[84]

OXIDATIVE STRESS AND MITOCHONDRIAL DYSFUNCTION AFTER pTBI

ANIMAL MODELS

Increased oxidative stress contributes to mitochondrial dysfunction that plays a central role in causing cognitive impairment and eventually neuronal death following TBI.[85,86] Experimental TBI causes a significant loss of cortical tissue at the site of injury (primary damage) that is followed by a secondary injury involving mitochondria that enhances the primary injury leading to neurological dysfunction. In a rat model of TBI, several mitochondrial proteins involved in bioenergetics were oxidized following injury causing mitochondrial dysfunction that eventually leads to neuronal death.[87] In a rat model of TBI, it was found that the activity of mitochondrial enzyme pyruvate dehydrogenase decreased, acid-base balance disrupted and levels of oxidative stress increased in blood following injury. The decreased in blood levels of pyruvate dehydrogenase (PDH) was associated with increased gliosis and loss of subunit PDHE1-infinity of PDH in the brain tissue, and these effects can be prevented by pyruvate treatment.[88] These changes contribute to the severity of brain injury. Cytochrome c oxidase is important for oxidative phosphorylation in the mitochondria. The expression of cytochrome c oxidase I, II, and III mRNA in injured cortex was reduced following TBI in rats, whereas the expression of these mRNAs was slightly elevated in the contralateral cortex.[89] Generally, oxidative stress-induced mitochondrial dysfunction in a rat model of TBI is observed 1–3 h after TBI; suggesting the importance of an early intervention to reduce the oxidative stress.[90] In a mice model of TBI, it was observed that cortical mitochondrial damage include swelling, a disruption of cristae and rupture of outer membranes, a decrease in calcium-buffering capacity, and an increase in oxidation of protein and lipids. The levels of cortical 3-nitrotyrosine were elevated as early as 30 min after injury.[91]

N-methyl-4-isoleucine-cyclosporin (NIM811), a non-immunosuppressive cyclosporine analog, inhibits the mitochondrial permeability transition pore. Supplementation with NIM811 improved mitochondrial function, cognitive function, and reduced oxidative damage in a severe unilateral controlled cortical impact rat model of TBI.[92] Mitochondrial dysfunction can cause increased oxidative damage, loss of respiratory functions, and diminished ability to buffer cytosolic calcium, all of which can cause neuronal death. It was demonstrated that supplementation with U-83836E, a potent inhibitor of lipid peroxyl radicals, reduced both oxidative and nitrosylative damage in cortical homogenates and mitochondria after pTBI in mice model.[93]

HUMANS

It has been reported that mitochondrial DNA polymorphism was associated with mitochondrial dysfunction and neurobehavioral abnormalities after pTBI.[94] There is a direct link between energy metabolism and N-acetylaspartate. In a clinical study on 14 patients (6 patients with diffuse brain injury and 8 with focal brain lesions), it was observed that reduction in the brain levels of n-acetylaspartate in the absence of ischemic insult reflected mitochondrial dysfunction.[95] It has been proposed that reduction in extracellular levels of N-acetylaspartate can be used as a potential marker for mitochondrial function in humans after TBI.[96] The role of mitochondrial dysfunction in the progression of damage following TBI is further supported by the fact that treatment with mitochondrial uncouplers, 2,4-dinitrophenol (2,4-DNP), and p-trifluoromethoxyphenylhydrazone (FCCP) significantly reduced loss of cortical damage and improved behavioral deficits following TBI in rats.[97]

EVIDENCE FOR INCREASE LEVELS OF MARKERS OF INFLAMMATION AFTER pTBI

ANIMAL MODELS

The levels of inflammation markers such as iNOS and cyclooxygenase 2 (COX-2) activities, and markers of oxidative stress (loss of glutathione and oxidized: reduced glutathione ratio, 3-nitrotyrosine, and 4-hydroxynonenal) increased after TBI in an animal model, and treatment with fenofibrate reduced the levels of these markers.[98] The levels of pro-inflammatory cytokines, tumor necrosis factor-alpha (TNF-alpha), increased after TBI in rats. The delayed elevation of soluble tumor necrosis factor receptors p75 and p55 was observed in cerebral spinal fluid and plasma after TBI.[99] The levels of TNF-alpha and Fas are elevated after TBI. Using TNF-alpha and Fas deficient transgenic mice (TNFalpha/Fas-/-), it was demonstrated that the motor performance and spatial memory acquisition were improved in transgenic animal compared to wild-type mice after subjecting them with a controlled cortical impact (a model of TBI). The results suggested that TNF-alpha and FAS play an important role in TBI-induced neurological dysfunction. This was further supported by the fact that in immature mice model of TBI, genetic inhibition of TNF-alpha and Fas conferred beneficial effects on histology and spatial memory acquisition in adulthood.[100] In a rat model of TBI, animal received impact-acceleration head injury as a sustained mild head injury or a severe head injury. The levels of NO metabolites decreased in the cortex, cerebellum, hippocampus and brain stem in both groups after 5 min. The extent of decrease in NO levels depended upon the extent of injury being lowest in the brain regions where the direct trauma was most severe.[101]

The role of pro-inflammatory cytokines in the progression of damage after TBI is further supported by the fact that inhibitors of these cytokines improved neuronal loss and cognitive dysfunction in animal models of TBI. For example, IL-1 beta neutralizing antibody (IgG2a/k),[102] dexanabinol (HU-211), an inhibitor of TNF-alpha at a posttranscriptional stage,[103] antioxidants,[104]

Minozac (Mzc), an inhibitor of glial activation and pro-inflammatory cytokines,[105] a synthetic analogue of tripeptide glypromate (NNZ-2566),[106] simvastatin, an inhibitor of activation of astrocytes[107] provide neuroprotection by reducing neuronal loss and neurological deficits.

It has been reported that the levels of cerebral vascular permeability increased by 4-fold in TBI mice model compared to that in normal mice. In addition, the expression of aquaporin-4 (AQP-4), which causes blood-brain-barrier-mediated edema in brain was increased by 2-fold in TBI mice compared to that in normal mice. Vagal nerve stimulation after TBI decreased the levels of cerebral vascular permeability as well as expression of AQP-4.[108] It has been demonstrated that the levels of substance-P, a neuropeptide, increased after severe diffuse TBI in rats. These rats develop edema and functional neurological deficits. Neurokinin-1 (NK-1) antagonist acetyl-L-tryptophan inhibits action of substance P. Administration of NK-1 antagonist after TBI reduced edema and vascular permeability and improved both motor and cognitive functions. These data suggest that increased levels of substance P contribute to the development of brain edema and increased vascular permeability.[109]

HUMANS

A review on the role of inflammation in pTBI has revealed that a strong inflammatory response occurs immediately after injury. Inflammatory response activates resident glia cells, microglia, and astrocytes, which secrete pro-inflammatory cytokines (IL-1, IL-6, and tumor necrosis factor-alpha) and anti-inflammatory cytokines (IL-4, IL-10 and TGF-beta, and chemokines.[110] The levels of pro-inflammatory cytokines were elevated, whereas the levels of anti-inflammatory cytokines did not change in the autopsied brain samples from patients with pTBI.[111] This is in contrast to acute phase of TBI when both pro- and anti-inflammatory cytokines are released.[110] It has been demonstrated that activated microglia persists as long 17 years after injury.[112] This suggests that toxic products of inflammation continue to be released long after TBI.

Diffuse axonal injury is the leading cause of lasting vegetative state and death of the patients after pTBI. A clinical study on 159 patients with pTBI who survived acute phase showed that about 72% of the patients had diffuse axonal injury.[113] A review has shown that increased levels of pro-inflammatory cytokines play and important role in the development of diffuse axonal injury.[114]

Following pTBI, resident cells in the brain such as microglia generate excessive amounts of pro-inflammatory cytokines, prostaglandins, reactive oxygen species, complement proteins and adhesion molecules that are highly toxic to neurons.[115–119] The evidence of inflammation is also found by the infiltration and accumulation of polymorphonuclear leukocytes. Pro-inflammatory cytokines increased the expression of iNOS which can produce excessive amounts of NO that may in turn become oxidized to form peroxynitrite that contribute to the pathogenesis of TBI.[120–122] An inhibitor of iNOS provided neuroprotection against damage produced by peroxynitrite.[123] The pro-inflammatory cytokine interleukin-6 (IL-6) is elevated in patients with pTBI, and a significant relationship exists between the severity of TBI and the transcranial IL-6 gradient at admission.[124] In addition, activation of nuclear factor-kappa B (NF-kappaB) occurs after TBI in both animals and humans.[51,125] Treatment with beta-Aescin inhibited activation of NF-kappaB and expression of TNF-alpha in a rat model of TBI.[125]

A study on patients with moderate to pTBI showed that the levels of cytokines (IL-6 and IL-8) increased in all patients compared to healthy control subjects. In addition, the levels of two cytokines were higher and the levels of LDL were lower in non-survivors than in survivors of pTBI. These results suggested that the level of LDL alone or in combination with IL-6 and IL-8 could be a prognostic value for a 30-day survival outcome.[126]

pTBI in infant and children (N = 36) increased the levels of pro-inflammatory cytokines (IL-1beta, IL-6 and IL-12p70) and anti-inflammatory cytokines (IL-10) and chemokines (IL-8 and MIP-1alpha) compared to controls. Moderate hypothermia, which is frequently used in the management of TBI, did not decrease the levels of cytokines in children with pTBI.[127]

EVIDENCE FOR INCREASED GLUTAMATE LEVEL AFTER pTBI

ANIMAL MODELS

The levels of extracellular glutamate and aspartate increased in the brain regions following TBI in animals.[128] In a rat model of TBI, it was shown that the levels of two high-affinity sodium-dependent glial transporters, glutamate transporter 1(GLT-1) and glutamate-aspartame transporter (GLAST) decreased following TBI.[129,130] GLT-1 is primarily responsible for clearing extracellular glutamate; therefore, decreased levels of GLT-1 may contribute to the increased levels of extracellular glutamate. Thus, increased levels of GLT-1 appear to be of neuroprotective value by reducing the levels of glutamate. This is supported by the observation in which administration of ceftriaxone, which increases the expression of GLT-1, reversed TBI-induced elevation of glia fibrillary acid protein (GFAP) and seizures in a rat model of TBI.[131] It has been reported that disruption in calcium-dependent neuronal glutamate release and glia-regulated extracellular glutamate contribute to the progression of damage in the striatum of rats 2 days after diffuse brain injury.[132] It has been demonstrated that increases in the levels of extracellular levels of glutamate occur due to excessive release of glutamate from neurons.[133] Thus, both neurons and glia contribute to the increased levels of extracellular glutamate after pTBI.

In a rat model of TBI, hypothermia treatment reduced the levels of hydroxyl radicals and glutamate release.[134] Administration of N-methyl-D-aspartate, an (NMDA) antagonist, and significantly reduced glutamate release,[135,136] and improved motor function and cognitive dysfunction following TBI in animal models. It has been demonstrated that injection of Premarin, a conjugated estrogens commonly used as hormone replacement in postmenopausal women, decreased blood glutamate levels in a rat model of TBI.[137]

Activation of presynaptic group II metabotropic glutamate (mGlu II) receptor reduces synaptic glutamate release. Indeed, (-)-2-oxa-4-aminobicyclo (3.1.0) hexane-4,6-dicarboxylate (LY379268), a selective agonist of mGlu II, significantly reduced cell death following TBI in mice.[138] In another animal model of TBI (lateral fluid percussion-induced brain injury), administration of mGlu II agonist improved behavior deficits compared to control following injury.[139]

The extracellular levels of glutamate and adenosine increase rapidly after TBI; however, the relationship between them in the progression of injury is not well defined. Normally, adenosine A (2A) receptor (A2AR) exerts neuroprotective action, but it can contribute to neurodegeneration depending upon the levels of glutamate. It has been demonstrated that high concentration of glutamate switched the effect of activated A2AR from anti-inflammation to proinflammation in microglia cells in culture and in mice TBI model.[140]

HUMANS

The excitatory amino acids play a significant role in the progression of injury following pTBI. Excessive amounts of glutamate in the extracellular space may lead to uncontrolled shift of sodium, potassium, and calcium that may cause swelling, edema and eventually neuronal death. In addition, increased synaptic release of glutamate also occurs at the site of injury.[130,141] The levels of excitatory amino acids increased that may enhance neuronal damage in patients with pTBI.[142] In patients with focal and diffuse brain injury, the levels of glutamate were elevated in both cerebrospinal fluid and extracellular space following TBI.[143] In another clinical study, it was found that patients who died of their head injury had higher levels of dialysate glutamate and aspartame compared to those who recovered from injury. The highest levels of glutamate were present in patients with gunshot wounds, followed by those who had mass lesions. Patients with diffuse brain injury had the lowest levels of glutamate and aspartame.[128] Excessive amounts of glutamate and aspartame are released in 85 severely head injured patients, and the patients with contusions had the highest level of glutamate and aspartate.[144] The levels of glutamate and taurine in ventricular cerebrospinal fluid (CSF) were elevated in patients with subdural or epidural hematomas, contusions, and generalized brain edema. The simultaneous release of taurine, which has inhibitory and anti-excitotoxic functions with glutamate, suggests that the injured brain is attempting to counteract the action of glutamate.[145] Similar results were obtained in a rat model of TBI.[146] The increased levels of glutamate measured by microdialysis were correlated with higher mortality and poor functional outcomes in patients with pTBI.[147] The concentration of glutamate and glycerol in microdialysate from older patients with pTBI were higher compared to younger patients.[148] This suggested that increased concentrations of glycerol and glutamate would indicate more extensive damage in older patients. A study showed that higher concentrations of glutamate, glucose, lactate/pyruvate ratio, intracranial pressure, cerebrovascular pressure reactivity index, and age were predictors of increased mortality in patients with pTBI.[149]

The levels of adenosine and glutamate were elevated in the ventricular CSF following severe TBI in children. The release of adenosine following TBI may reflect an attempt by adenosine to provide neuroprotection against glutamate-induced toxicity.[150]

ROLE OF MATRIX METALLOPROTEINASES (MMPS) AFTER SEVERE TBI

Experimental data in animal models of severe TBI suggested that an increase in the levels of matrix metalloproteinases 3 and 9, which are considered responsible for inflammation in the blood-brain-barrier disruption, hemorrhage, and neuronal death occurred after TBI. Indeed, a clinical study on 6 patients with TBI showed that the CSF levels of MMP-9 were elevated; however, elevated levels of MMP-3 were observed in the plasma but not in the CSF.[151] These data suggest that MMPs play an important role in the progression of damage after TBI. Increased levels of MMP-8 and MMP-9 were associated with increased levels of pro-inflammatory cytokines (IL-1 alpha, IL-2, and TNF-alpha) in the microdialysis samples of 8 patients with severe TBI. In contrast, the levels of MMP-7 decreased with increases in the levels of IL-1beta, Il-2 and IL-6.[152]

STUDIES ON THE EFFECTS OF SINGLE ANTIOXIDANTS AFTER TBI

Despite great potential of antioxidants in the improved management of severe TBI, very little attention has been paid to test the efficacy of these micronutrients either for primary prevention or secondary prevention of severe TBI in humans. A few studies on the effect of antioxidants on severe TBI in animals and humans are described here.

ANIMAL MODELS

Resveratrol, a polyphenolic compound, which exhibit antioxidant and anti-inflammation activities, administered immediately after TBI reduced oxidative damage and lesion volume in rats.[153,154] Treatment with alpha-lipoic acid reduced markers of pro-inflammatory cytokines and oxidative stress, and improved histological changes in the brain, and preserved blood-brain-barrier (BBB) permeability and reduced edema following TBI in animals.[155] Administration of N-acetylcysteine provided neuroprotection (reduction in brain edema and BBB permeability) in animal models following TBI by reducing markers of pro-inflammatory cytokines and adhesion molecules.[156] The early rise in complex I and complex II proteins of mitochondria, which regulate excitatory neurotransmitter release after TBI, was blocked by N-acetylcysteine (NAC).[141] In addition, TBI-induced elevation of heme oxygenase-1 (HO-1) levels in glial cells as well as neurons, and loss of tissue volume was markedly reduced by N-acetylcysteine treatment in animal model of TBI (lateral fluid percussion injury).[157]

Melatonin, a pineal hormone exhibiting antioxidant activity, protected against TBI-induced damage by attenuation the activation of NF-kappaB and AP-1.[158] S-nitrosoglutathione (GSNO), a modulator of nitric oxide, plays an important role in maintaining redox balance. Administration of GSNO after severe TBI reduced blood-brain-barrier disruption, infiltration/activation of macrophages, and reduced expression of ICAM-1, MMPs, and iNOS. This treatment also reduced neuronal cell and myelin loss in TBI model rats.[159] Administration of an endogenous fatty acid palmitoylethanol-amide (PEA), which maintains redox balance, reduced edema, brain infarction, neuronal loss, and improved neurological functions in a mice model of severe TBI.[160]

In a rat model of TBI (mild fluid percussion injury), increased oxidation of proteins and reduced levels of SOD and Sir2 (silent information regulator), and poor performance associated with a decline in the levels of brain-derived neurotrophic factor (BDNF) and its downstream effectors on synaptic plasticity, synapsin I, and cAMP-response element-binding protein (CREB) were observed following injury. Dietary supplementation with vitamin E or curcumin protected brain against mild-TBI-induced damage by reducing above biochemical changes involved in synaptic plasticity and cognitive function.[40,161] Superoxide dismutase improved TBI-induced mitochondrial dysfunction in transgenic mice over-expressing CuZn SOD or Mn SOD.[162] In transgenic mice overexpressing glutathione peroxidase (GPxTg), it was observed that markers of oxidative stress including nitrotyrosine were reduced and spatial memory improved compared to wild-type animals following TBI.[163]

It has been reported that dietary supplementation of omega-3 fatty acids in animal model of TBI (mild fluid percussion injury) protected against TBI-induced reduced synaptic plasticity and cognitive impairment.[164] In contrast, supplementation with a saturated-fat diet[39] or caffeine[165] aggravated TBI-induced injury in animals.

Administration of curcumin reduced cortex injury, neutrophil infiltration, and microglia activation and improved neuronal survival by activation of Nrf2 pathway.[166] It also protected secondary brain injury induced by TBI by activating the Nrf2/ARE pathway.[167]

HUMANS

Edaravone, an FDA-approved drug, reduced oxidative damage by neutralizing free radicals after TBI in humans.[168] No significant studies on single or multiple antioxidants in human TBI have been performed.

A commercial preparation of micronutrients containing multiple dietary and endogenous antioxidants (military micronutrient formulation, now called microdaily) was tested in troops returning from Iraq with mild to moderate TBI at the Naval Medical Center San Diego Clinic.[169] All patients had received their injury 3–20 weeks prior to admission, and they received identical treatment consisting of medical therapy (for any migraines), supportive care, steroids, and vestibular rehabilitation therapy. Fifteen of the 34 patients also received micronutrients (2 capsules by mouth twice a day). At the onset of therapy, all patients were evaluated in outcome measures which included the Sensory Organization Test (SOT) by Computerized Dynamic Posturography (CDP), the Dynamic Gait Index (DGI), the Activities Balance Confidence (ABC) scale, the Dizziness Handicap Index (DHI), the Vestibular Disorders Activities of Daily Living (VADL) score, and the Balance Scoring System (BESS) test. The study was carried out for 12 weeks.

Both groups of patients showed trends toward significant improvement on all tests after the 12 weeks of therapy, but the combination treatment trend was stronger than that of the standard therapy alone group. After only 4 weeks, the SOT score by CDP was 78 for the antioxidant group as compared to 63 for the nonantioxidant group. This difference was statistically significant at the $P < 0.05$ levels The improvement noted by the antioxidant group on the other tests was also greater than the non-antioxidant group, although these differences did not reach statistical significance because of the short trial period and small sample size.

POTENTIAL REASONS FOR INCONSISTENT RESULTS WITH INDIVIDUAL MICRONUTRIENTS IN OTHER NEURODEGENERATIVE DISEASES

No significant studies with micronutrients have been performed in human TBI. Studies on other neurodegenerative diseases show that individual micronutrients produced no effect or minimal transient benefits in early phase of the disease.[170,171] Some potentials causes are described here: (a) antioxidants show differential subcellular distribution and different mechanisms of action; therefore, a single antioxidant cannot protect all parts of the cell; (b) a single antioxidant in a high internal oxidative environment in high-risk patients is oxidized and can then itself act as a prooxidant rather than as an antioxidant; (c) the body protects against oxidative damage by elevating antioxidant enzymes, and dietary and endogenous antioxidants; (d) antioxidants neutralize free radicals by donating electrons to those molecules with unpaired electron, whereas antioxidant enzymes destroy free radicals by catalysis, converting them to harmless molecules such as water and oxygen. Therefore, both of these agents should be enhanced to achieve substantial protection against oxidative damage; (e) the affinity of different antioxidants for free radicals differs, depending upon their solubility; (f) both the aqueous and lipid compartments of the cell need to be protected together. Water-soluble antioxidants such as vitamin C and glutathione protect molecules in the aqueous environment of the cells, whereas lipid soluble antioxidants such as vitamin A and vitamin E protect molecules in the lipid compartment; (g) vitamin E is more effective in quenching free radicals in a reduced oxygenated cellular environment, whereas vitamin C and alpha-tocopherol are more effective in a higher oxygenated environment of the cells[172]; (h) vitamin C is important for recycling the oxidized form of alpha-tocopherol to the antioxidant form[173]; (i) antioxidants produce cell protective proteins by altering the expression of different microRNAs.[171] For example, some antioxidants can activate Nrf2 by upregulating miR-200a that inhibits its target protein Keap1, whereas others activate Nrf2 by downregulating miR-21 that binds with 3′-UTR Nrf2 mRNA.[174]

The use of a single micronutrient is not expected to produce optimal protection against oxidative stress, inflammation, and glutamate, which contribute to concussion and pTBI. For this reason, it is proposed that an elevation of the levels of antioxidant enzymes and dietary and endogenous antioxidants may be essential for simultaneously reducing oxidative stress and inflammation. Oral supplementation can increase the levels of dietary and endogenous antioxidants; however, elevation of the levels of antioxidant enzymes requires an activation of Nrf2. Therefore it is essential to understand the regulation of activation of Nrf2.

ACTIVATION OF Nrf2 (NUCLEAR FACTOR-ERYTHROID-2-RELATED FACTOR 2)

Nrf2

The nuclear transcriptional factor, Nrf2 (nuclear factor-erythroid-2-related factor 2) belongs to the Cap 'n' Collar (CNC) family that contains a conserved basic leucine zipper (bZIP) transcriptional factor.[175] Under physiological condition, Nrf2 is associated with Kelch-like ECH associated protein 1 (Keap1), which acts as an inhibitor of Nrf2.[176] Keap1 protein serves as an adaptor to link Nrf2 to the ubiquitin ligase CuI-Rbx1 complex for degradation by proteasomes and maintains the steady levels of Nrf2 in the cytoplasm. Nrf2-keap1 complex is primarily located in the cytoplasm; Keap1 acts as a sensor for ROS/electrophilic stress.

ACTIVATION OF Nrf2 DURING ACUTE OXIDATIVE STRESS

During acute oxidative stress, ROS is needed to activate Nrf2 which then dissociates itself from Keap1-CuI-Rbx1 complex and translocates in the nucleus where it heterodimerizes with a small Maf protein, binds with ARE leading to increased expression of target genes coding for several cytoprotective enzymes including antioxidant enzymes.[177–179]

FAILURE TO ACTIVATE Nrf2 DURING CHRONIC OXIDATIVE STRESS

During chronic oxidative stress, Nrf2 becomes resistant to ROS,[180–182] suggesting that activation of Nrf2 by a ROS-independent mechanism exists. This is evidenced by the fact that increased chronic oxidative stress occurs despite the presence of Nrf2 in TBI. The question arises as to how to activate ROS-resistant Nrf2 in TBI.

Antioxidants Activate ROS-Resistant Nrf2

Some examples are vitamin E and genistein,[183] alpha-lipoic acid,[184] curcumin,[185] resveratrol,[186,187] omega-3-fatty acids,[188,189] glutathione,[190] NAC,[191] and coenzyme Q10.[192] Several plant-derived phytochemicals, such as epigallocatechin-3-gallate, carestol, kahweol, cinnamonyl-based compounds, zerumbone, lycopene and carnosol,[175,193,194] genistein,[183] allicin, a major organosulfur compound found in garlic,[195] sulforaphane, a organosulfur compound, found in cruciferous vegetables,[196] and kavalactones (methysticin, kavain, and yangonin).[197] The reasons for the activation of Nrf2 without ROS by antioxidant compounds are not known.

Binding of Nrf2 with ARE in the Nucleus

An activation of Nrf2 alone is not sufficient to increase the levels of antioxidant enzymes. Activated Nrf2 must bind with ARE in the nucleus for increasing the expression of target genes coding for antioxidant enzymes. This binding ability of Nrf2 with ARE was impaired in aged rats and this defect was restored by supplementation with alpha-lipoic acid.[184] It is unknown whether the binding ability of Nrf2 with ARE is impaired in TBI.

Nrf2 IN TBI

Using transgenic mice deficient in Nrf2 (−/−) it was demonstrated that activation of NF-kappaB, the levels of pro-inflammatory cytokines, TNF-alpha, IL-1beta, and IL-6, and expression of intracellular adhesion molecule 1 (ICAN-1) were higher in the brain compared to the wild-type Nrf2 (+/+) mice following TBI (moderate to severe weight-drop impact head injury).[198,199] The neurological deficits and brain edema were more advanced in mice with Nrf2 deficiency (−/−) compared to mice with Nrf2 sufficiency (+/+).[200] Studies on the presence of Nrf2 in autopsied brain tissue from patients with TBI should be performed.

REDUCING OXIDATIVE STRESS LEVEL

Activation of Nrf2 may not be sufficient to optimally reduce oxidative stress, because antioxidants compounds are also decreased during chronic oxidative stress[201–203]; therefore, their levels must also be simultaneously elevated.

REDUCING INFLAMMATION LEVEL

Activation of Nrf2[204,205] and some individual antioxidant compounds reduced chronic inflammation.[206–212]

REDUCING GLUTAMATE LEVEL

Some antioxidants decrease the release of glutamate as well as its neurotoxicity.[213–215] In addition, certain B-vitamins can also decrease the release of glutamate.[216,217]

PROPOSED MICRONUTRIENTS FOR REDUCING OXIDATIVE STRESS, INFLAMMATION, AND GLUTAMATE LEVELS IN TBI

Because of partial success in improving some symptoms of concussive injury with multiple micronutrients in veterans,[169] a comprehensive micronutrient mixture is proposed. This mixture contains multiple dietary antioxidant compounds (vitamin A, natural mixed carotenoids, vitamin C, vitamin E succinate, vitamin E acetate, selenomethionine, curcumin, and resveratrol), endogenous antioxidants (alpha-lipoic acid, L-carnitine, and coenzyme Q10), vitamin D3, a synthetic antioxidant N-acetylcysteine (NAC), omega-3-fatty acids, zinc, and all B-vitamins. This mixture of micronutrients may optimally reduce oxidative stress and chronic inflammation by simultaneously enhancing the levels of antioxidant enzymes through activation of the Nrf2/ARE pathway, and elevating the levels of antioxidants. The same micronutrient mixture may also reduce the release and toxicity of glutamate at the same time.

No iron, copper, or manganese is included in this micronutrient mixture, because these trace minerals are known to interact with vitamin C to produce free radicals. These trace minerals are absorbed from the intestinal tract more in the presence of antioxidants than in their absence that could results in increased body stores of free forms of these minerals. Increased iron stores have been linked to increased risk of some neurodegenerative diseases.[218] No heavy metals such as zirconium and molybdenum were added because of their potential neurotoxicity after long-term consumption.

The recommended micronutrient supplements should be taken daily orally divided into two doses, one-half in the morning and the other-half in the evening with meal. This is because the biological half-lives of micronutrients are highly variable, which can create high levels of fluctuations in the tissue levels of micronutrients. A 2-fold difference in the levels of certain micronutrients such as alpha-tocopherol succinate can cause a marked difference in the expression of gene profiles.[219] In order to maintain relatively steady levels of micronutrients in the brain, the proposed micronutrients should be taken twice a day.

TOXICITY OF INGREDIENTS IN PROPOSED MICRONUTRIENT PREPARATION

Only a few antioxidants at very high doses are considered toxic. Vitamin A at doses of 10,000 IU or more per day can cause birth defects in pregnant women, and beta-carotene at doses 50 mg or more can produce bronzing of the skin that is reversible on discontinuation. Vitamin C as ascorbic acid at high doses (10 grams or more per day) can cause diarrhea in some individuals. Vitamin E at high doses (2,000 IU or more per day) can induce clotting defects after long-term consumption. Vitamin B6 at high doses (50 mg or more per day) may produce peripheral neuropathy, and selenium at doses 400 mcg or more per day can cause skin and liver toxicity after long-term consumption. All ingredients present in the proposed micronutrient mixture are safe and come under the category of "food supplement" and therefore do not require FDA approval for their use.

PREVENTION STUDIES WITH PROPOSED MICRONUTRIENT MIXTURE IN TBI

PRIMARY PREVENTION

The purpose of primary prevention is to protect healthy individuals against TBI. The efficacy of proposed micronutrient mixture can be tested in Individuals involved in contact sports and US troops to be deployed in military conflicts. It is expected that the level of initial damage to the brain following TBI would be reduced.

SECONDARY PREVENTION

The purpose of secondary prevention is to reduce the progression of damage following TBI. The efficacy of proposed micronutrient mixture can be tested among individuals who have sustained concussion or who have survived pTBI, but are not any medication. It is expected that the progression of damage following TBI would be decreased.

STANDARD THERAPY OF TBI

The pTBI is extremely difficult to treat, because of the inherent complexity of the brain structures and functions as well as extreme variations in the pattern of injury. Approximately half of severely brain-injured patients will need surgery to remove or repair hematomas (rupture of blood vessels) or contusions (bruised brain tissue) (National Institute of Neurological Disorders and Stroke, 2009). Initial treatment focuses on preventing secondary injury following pTBI. This includes proper oxygen supply to the brain and the rest of the body, maintaining adequate blood flow, and controlling blood pressure.

Hypothermia (32°C–33°C) attenuated the levels of markers of oxidative stress in infants and children after severe TBI.[220] The effect of hypothermia was analyzed in 12 studies with 1,327 patients in which 8 studies cooled according to long-term or goal-directed strategy, and 4 studies cooled according to short-term strategy. The results revealed that when only short-term strategy cooling were performed, neither mortality nor neurological outcomes were improved; however, when long-term cooling was used, mortality was reduced and neurological outcomes were improved.[221] The optimal results were obtained when cooling was continued for at least 72 hours and/or until intracranial pressure is normalized for at least 24 hours.

The CSF levels of alpha-synuclein were elevated in children with severe TBI than in control subjects; however, the CSF levels of alpha-synuclein decreased after hypothermia treatment.[222]

Medications to reduce the secondary damage to the brain immediately after injury may include diuretics (to reduce pressure from the brain by eliminating fluid through urine), antiseizure drugs during first week (to avoid additional damage to the brain that might be caused by seizures, and coma-inducing drugs (brain at this state use less oxygen for survival and function; this procedure is particularly helpful if the blood vessels are unable to supply sufficient nutrient and oxygen supply to the brain). In addition, emergency surgery may be needed to remove blood clot, repair skull fractures, and open a window in the skull to relieve pressure inside the brain by draining accumulated fluid. Patients with severe TBI receive rehabilitation therapy that includes individually tailored treatment program in the area of physical therapy, occupational therapy, speech/language therapy, medications, psychology/psychiatry therapy, and social support. The standard therapy has markedly improved the management severe TBI and has improved the survival rate.

Based on the studies on animal models of TBI, several potential therapeutic agents have been identified. They include erythropoietin,[223,224] antibodies of serotonin receptors,[225] histone deacetylase inhibitor,[35,226] protease inhibitors,[227] fenofibrate, a peroxisomes proliferators-activated receptor alpha agonist,[98] meloxicam, a COX-2 inhibitor,[228] and interferon-gamma.[229] These drugs will require FDA approval.

PROPOSED MICRONUTRIENTS IN COMBINATION WITH STANDARD THERAPY

The efficacy of the proposed micronutrient mixture in combination with standard therapy can be tested in patients with concussion as well as with pTBI. Those individuals who have suffered concussion may start taking micronutrient mixture at any time after concussion; however, those who have sustained pTBI may start 24 h after the injury, and not immediately after injury. This is due to the fact that both anti- and pro-inflammatory cytokines are released immediately after injury. Anti-inflammatory cytokines help to repair cellular damage. Supplementation with the micronutrient mixture immediately after injury may reduce both pro-inflammatory and anti-inflammatory cytokines. Inhibition of anti-inflammatory cytokines release may interfere with the repair processes in the brain. Micronutrient mixture can be consumed daily for the entire lifespan in order to reduce late adverse health effects of TBI. It is expected that the micronutrient mixture, in combination with standard therapy, would improve the current management of pTBI during the acute and chronic phases of injury.

DIET AND LIFESTYLE RECOMMENDATIONS FOR TBI

A balanced diet rich in fruits, vegetables and fibers and low in fat is suggested, Lifestyle recommendations include daily moderate exercise, reduced stress, no tobacco smoking, and reduced intake of caffeine. A high saturated-fat diet[39] and caffeine[165] appear to increase the progression of damage following TBI in animal models.

CONCLUSIONS

Traumatic brain injury (TBI) includes mild TBI, also called concussive injury, and penetrating TBI (pTBI). Concussion occurs when the brain violently rocks back and forth within the skull following a blow to the head or neck such as that observed in contact sports like football and soccer. In US combat troops, concussion occurs due to exposure to blast pressure wave following detonation of improvised explosive devices (IEDs). Despite development of newer head protective devices, concussion remains a major health concern among professional football players as well as among US troops in the combat zone. There are no biological preventive strategies. The management of TBI involving medications, psychotherapy, and physical therapy are unsatisfactory. pTBI occurs when an object penetrates the skull and damages the brain. This form of TBI is caused by vehicle crashes, gunshot wound to the head, and exposure to explosion of the IED and combat-related head injuries. Despite significant improvement in the treatment of pTBI, morbidity and mortality continue to be high. The role of microRNAs in the pathogenesis and diagnosis of TBI is briefly discussed. Animal and human studies suggest that increased levels of oxidative stress, inflammation, and glutamate in the brain are common cellular abnormalities in the development of both concussion and pTBI. Therefore, attenuation of these cellular defects may prevent concussion, and in combination of standard therapy, improve the treatment of concussion and pTBI. Very little investigations have been performed with antioxidants in human TBI. We have proposed that in order to reduce oxidative stress and inflammation, elevation of the levels of antioxidant enzymes as well as dietary and endogenous antioxidants is essential. The levels of antioxidants can easily be increased by supplementation; however, increasing the levels of antioxidant enzymes requires an activation of the nuclear transcriptional factor Nrf2/ARE pathway. Agents that can activate the Nrf2/ARE pathway were identified. Certain antioxidants and B-vitamins can prevent release and toxicity of glutamate. A mixture of micronutrients that would activate the Nrf2/ARE pathway, enhance the levels of antioxidants, and reduce the release and toxicity of glutamate is proposed. This micronutrient mixture, when consumed before exposure to concussive injury, might reduce acute and long-term brain damage. The same mixture in combination of standard therapy may improve the management of TBI in humans.

REFERENCES

1. Viano DC, Casson IR, Pellman EJ, et al. Concussion in professional football: Comparison with boxing head impacts: Part 10. *Neurosurgery.* 2005;57(6):1154–1172; discussion 1154–1172.
2. Viano DC, Pellman EJ, Withnall C, Shewchenko N. Concussion in professional football: Performance of newer helmets in reconstructed game impacts—Part 13. *Neurosurgery.* 2006;59(3):591–606; discussion 591–606.
3. Levy ML, Ozgur BM, Berry C, Aryan HE, Apuzzo ML. Analysis and evolution of head injury in football. *Neurosurgery.* 2004;55(3):649–655.
4. Casson IR, Viano DC, Powell JW, Pellman EJ. Repeat concussions in the national football league. *Sports Health.* 2011;3(1):11–24.
5. Lincoln AE, Caswell SV, Almquist JL, Dunn RE, Norris JB, Hinton RY. Trends in concussion incidence in high school sports: A prospective 11-year study. *Am J Sports Med.* 2011;39(5):958–963.
6. Gessel LM, Fields SK, Collins CL, Dick RW, Comstock RD. Concussions among United States high school and collegiate athletes. *J Athl Train.* 2007;42(4):495–503.

7. MacGregor AJ, Dougherty AL, Morrison RH, Quinn KH, Galarneau MR. Repeated concussion among US military personnel during Operation Iraqi Freedom. *J Rehabil Res Dev*. 2011;48(10):1269–1278.

8. Rapoport MJ, McCullagh S, Shammi P, Feinstein A. Cognitive impairment associated with major depression following mild and moderate traumatic brain injury. *J Neuropsychiatry Clin Neurosci*. 2005;17(1):61–65.

9. van Donkelaar P, Langan J, Rodriguez E, et al. Attentional deficits in concussion. *Brain Inj*. 2005;19(12):1031–1039.

10. Guskiewicz KM, Marshall SW, Bailes J, et al. Association between recurrent concussion and late-life cognitive impairment in retired professional football players. *Neurosurgery*. 2005;57(4):719–726; discussion 719–726.

11. Gottshall K, Drake A, Gray N, McDonald E, Hoffer ME. Objective vestibular tests as outcome measures in head injury patients. *Laryngoscope*. 2003;113(10):1746–1750.

12. Kerr ZY, Marshall SW, Harding HP, Jr, Guskiewicz KM. Nine-year risk of depression diagnosis increases with increasing self-reported concussions in retired professional football players. *Am J Sports Med*. 2012;40(10):2206–2212.

13. Guskiewicz KM, McCrea M, Marshall SW, et al. Cumulative effects associated with recurrent concussion in collegiate football players: The NCAA Concussion Study. *JAMA*. 2003;290(19):2549–2555.

14. Breedlove EL, Robinson M, Talavage TM, et al. Biomechanical correlates of symptomatic and asymptomatic neurophysiological impairment in high school football. *J Biomech*. 2012;45(7):1265–1272.

15. De Beaumont L, Tremblay S, Poirier J, Lassonde M, Theoret H. Altered bidirectional plasticity and reduced implicit motor learning in concussed athletes. *Cereb Cortex*. 2012;22(1):112–121.

16. Covassin T, Schatz P, Swanik CB. Sex differences in neuropsychological function and post-concussion symptoms of concussed collegiate athletes. *Neurosurgery*. 2007;61(2):345–350; discussion 350–341.

17. Wilk JE, Herrell RK, Wynn GH, Riviere LA, Hoge CW. Mild traumatic brain injury (concussion), post-traumatic stress disorder, and depression in US soldiers involved in combat deployments: Association with postdeployment symptoms. *Psychosom Med*. 2012;74(3):249–257.

18. Carlson KF, Kehle SM, Meis LA, et al. Prevalence, assessment, and treatment of mild traumatic brain injury and posttraumatic stress disorder: A systematic review of the evidence. *J Head Trauma Rehab*. 2011;26(2):103–115.

19. Ellemberg D, Henry LC, Macciocchi SN, Guskiewicz KM, Broglio SP. Advances in sport concussion assessment: From behavioral to brain imaging measures. *J Neurotrauma*. 2009;26(12):2365–2382.

20. Hicks RR, Fertig SJ, Desrocher RE, Koroshetz WJ, Pancrazio JJ. Neurological effects of blast injury. *J Trauma*. 2010;68(5):1257–1263.

21. Leung LY, Wei G, Shear DA, Tortella FC. The acute effects of hemorrhagic shock on cerebral blood flow, brain tissue oxygen tension, and spreading depolarization following penetrating ballistic-like brain injury. *J Neurotrauma*. 2013;30(14):1288–1298.

22. Liu L, Sun T, Liu Z, et al. Traumatic brain injury dysregulates microRNAs to modulate cell signaling in rat hippocampus. *PLoS One*. 2014;9(8):e103948.

23. Meissner L, Gallozzi M, Balbi M, et al. Temporal profile of microRNA expression in contused cortex after traumatic brain injury in mice. *J Neurotrauma*. 2016;33(8):713–720.

24. Sabirzhanov B, Stoica BA, Zhao Z, et al. miR-711 upregulation induces neuronal cell death after traumatic brain injury. *Cell Death Differ*. 2016;23(4):654–668.

25. Sabirzhanov B, Zhao Z, Stoica BA, et al. Downregulation of miR-23a and miR-27a following experimental traumatic brain injury induces neuronal cell death through activation of proapoptotic Bcl-2 proteins. *J Neurosci*. 2014;34(30):10055–10071.

26. Ge XT, Lei P, Wang HC, et al. miR-21 improves the neurological outcome after traumatic brain injury in rats. *Sci Rep*. 2014;4:6718.

27. Ge X, Han Z, Chen F, et al. MiR-21 alleviates secondary blood-brain barrier damage after traumatic brain injury in rats. *Brain Res*. 2015;1603:150–157.

28. Lv J, Zeng Y, Qian Y, Dong J, Zhang Z, Zhang J. MicroRNA let-7c-5p improves neurological outcomes in a murine model of traumatic brain injury by suppressing neuroinflammation and regulating microglial activation. *Brain Res*. 2018;1685:91–104.

29. Sun L, Liu A, Zhang J, et al. miR-23b improves cognitive impairments in traumatic brain injury by targeting ATG12-mediated neuronal autophagy. *Behav Brain Res*. 2018;340:126–136.

30. Sun L, Zhao M, Zhang J, et al. miR-144 promotes beta-amyloid accumulation-induced cognitive impairments by targeting ADAM10 following traumatic brain injury. *Oncotarget*. 2017;8(35):59181–59203.

31. Sun L, Zhao M, Wang Y, et al. Neuroprotective effects of miR-27a against traumatic brain injury via suppressing FoxO3a-mediated neuronal autophagy. *Biochem Biophys Res Commun*. 2017;482(4):1141–1147.

32. Harrison EB, Emanuel K, Lamberty BG, et al. Induction of miR-155 after brain injury promotes Type 1 interferon and has a neuroprotective effect. *Front Mol Neurosci.* 2017;10:228.

33. Martinez B, Peplow PV. MicroRNAs as diagnostic markers and therapeutic targets for traumatic brain injury. *Neural Regen Res.* 2017;12(11):1749–1761.

34. Yang T, Song J, Bu X, et al. Elevated serum miR-93, miR-191, and miR-499 are noninvasive biomarkers for the presence and progression of traumatic brain injury. *J Neurochem.* 2016;137(1):122–129.

35. Redell JB, Moore AN, Ward 3rd NH, Hergenroeder GW, Dash PK. Human traumatic brain injury alters plasma microRNA levels. *J Neurotrauma.* 2010;27(12):2147–2156.

36. Di Pietro V, Ragusa M, Davies D, et al. MicroRNAs as novel biomarkers for the diagnosis and prognosis of mild and severe traumatic brain injury. *J Neurotrauma.* 2017;34(11):1948–1956.

37. Aiguo W, Zhe Y, Gomez-Pinilla F. Vitamin E protects against oxidative damage and learning disability after mild traumatic brain injury in rats. *Neurorehabil Neural Repair.* 2010;24(3):290–298.

38. Conte V, Uryu K, Fujimoto S, et al. Vitamin E reduces amyloidosis and improves cognitive function in Tg2576 mice following repetitive concussive brain injury. *J Neurochem.* 2004;90(3):758–764.

39. Wu A, Molteni R, Ying Z, Gomez-Pinilla F. A saturated-fat diet aggravates the outcome of traumatic brain injury on hippocampal plasticity and cognitive function by reducing brain-derived neurotrophic factor. *Neuroscience.* 2003;119(2):365–375.

40. Wu A, Ying Z, Gomez-Pinilla F. Dietary curcumin counteracts the outcome of traumatic brain injury on oxidative stress, synaptic plasticity, and cognition. *Exp Neurol.* 2006;197(2):309–317.

41. Wu A, Ying Z, Gomez-Pinilla F. The salutary effects of DHA dietary supplementation on cognition, neuroplasticity, and membrane homeostasis after brain trauma. *J Neurotrauma.* 2011;28(10):2113–2122.

42. Tavazzi B, Vagnozzi R, Signoretti S, et al. Temporal window of metabolic brain vulnerability to concussions: Oxidative and nitrosative stresses—Part II. *Neurosurgery.* 2007;61(2):390–395; discussion 395–396.

43. Shultz SR, Bao F, Omana V, Chiu C, Brown A, Cain DP. Repeated mild lateral fluid percussion brain injury in the rat causes cumulative long-term behavioral impairments, neuroinflammation, and cortical loss in an animal model of repeated concussion. *J Neurotrauma.* 2012;29(2):281–294.

44. Hausmann R, Kaiser A, Lang C, Bohnert M, Betz P. A quantitative immunohistochemical study on the time-dependent course of acute inflammatory cellular response to human brain injury. *Int J Legal Med.* 1999;112(4):227–232.

45. Holmin S, Soderlund J, Biberfeld P, Mathiesen T. Intracerebral inflammation after human brain contusion. *Neurosurgery.* 1998;42(2):291–298; discussion 298–299.

46. Holmin S, Hojeberg B. In situ detection of intracerebral cytokine expression after human brain contusion. *Neurosci Lett.* 2004;369(2):108–114.

47. Beschorner R, Nguyen TD, Gozalan F, et al. CD14 expression by activated parenchymal microglia/macrophages and infiltrating monocytes following human traumatic brain injury. *Acta Neuropathol.* 2002;103(6):541–549.

48. Reger ML, Poulos AM, Buen F, Giza CC, Hovda DA, Fanselow MS. Concussive brain injury enhances fear learning and excitatory processes in the amygdala. *Biol Psychiatry.* 2012;71(4):335–343.

49. Fang WH, Wang DL, Wang F. Expression of c-myc protein on rats' brains after brain concussion. *Fa yi xue za zhi.* 2006;22(5):333–334.

50. Wang F, Li YH, Hu YL. A study on the expression of C-FOS protein after experimental rat brain concussion. *Fa yi xue za zhi.* 2003;19(1):8–9.

51. Hang CH, Chen G, Shi JX, Zhang X, Li JS. Cortical expression of nuclear factor kappaB after human brain contusion. *Brain Res.* 2006;1109(1):14–21.

52. Prasad KN, Cohrs RJ, Sharma OK. Decreased expressions of c-myc and H-ras oncogenes in vitamin E succinate induced morphologically differentiated murine B-16 melanoma cells in culture. *Biochem Cell Biol.* 1990;68(11):1250–1255.

53. Shen WH, Zhang CY, Zhang GY. Antioxidants attenuate reperfusion injury after global brain ischemia through inhibiting nuclear factor-kappa B activity in rats. *Acta Pharm Sinic.* 2003;24(11):1125–1130.

54. Gahm C, Holmin S, Mathiesen T. Nitric oxide synthase expression after human brain contusion. *Neurosurgery.* 2002;50(6):1319–1326.

55. Graham DI, McIntosh TK, Maxwell WL, Nicoll JA. Recent advances in neurotrauma. *J Neuropathol Exp Neurol.* 2000;59(8):641–651.

56. Rael LT, Bar-Or R, Mains CW, Slone DS, Levy AS, Bar-Or D. Plasma oxidation-reduction potential and protein oxidation in traumatic brain injury. *J Neurotrauma.* 2009;26(8):1203–1211.

57. Shao C, Roberts KN, Markesbery WR, Scheff SW, Lovell MA. Oxidative stress in head trauma in aging. *Free Radic Biol Med.* 2006;41(1):77–85.

58. Mikawa S, Kinouchi H, Kamii H, et al. Attenuation of acute and chronic damage following traumatic brain injury in copper, zinc-superoxide dismutase transgenic mice. *J Neurosurg.* 1996;85(5):885–891.
59. Petronilho F, Feier G, de Souza B, et al. Oxidative stress in brain according to traumatic brain injury intensity. *J Surg Res.* 2009;164(2):316–320.
60. Tavazzi B, Signoretti S, Lazzarino G, et al. Cerebral oxidative stress and depression of energy metabolism correlate with severity of diffuse brain injury in rats. *Neurosurgery.* 2005;56(3):582–589; discussion 582–589.
61. Singh IN, Sullivan PG, Hall ED. Peroxynitrite-mediated oxidative damage to brain mitochondria: Protective effects of peroxynitrite scavengers. *J Neurosci Res.* 2007;85(10):2216–2223.
62. Huttemann M, Lee I, Kreipke CW, Petrov T. Suppression of the inducible form of nitric oxide synthase prior to traumatic brain injury improves cytochrome c oxidase activity and normalizes cellular energy levels. *Neuroscience.* 2008;151(1):148–154.
63. Louin G, Marchand-Verrecchia C, Palmier B, Plotkine M, Jafarian-Tehrani M. Selective inhibition of inducible nitric oxide synthase reduces neurological deficit but not cerebral edema following traumatic brain injury. *Neuropharmacology.* 2006;50(2):182–190.
64. Ansari MA, Roberts KN, Scheff SW. Oxidative stress and modification of synaptic proteins in hippocampus after traumatic brain injury. *Free Radic Biol Med.* 2008;45(4):443–452.
65. Lima FD, Souza MA, Furian AF, et al. Na+,K+-ATPase activity impairment after experimental traumatic brain injury: Relationship to spatial learning deficits and oxidative stress. *Behav Brain Res.* 2008;193(2):306–310.
66. Bai XY, Ma Y, Ding R, Fu B, Shi S, Chen XM. miR-335 and miR-34a promote renal senescence by suppressing mitochondrial antioxidative enzymes. *J Am Soc Nephrol.* 2011;22(7):1252–1261.
67. Varma S, Janesko KL, Wisniewski SR, et al. F2-isoprostane and neuron-specific enolase in cerebrospinal fluid after severe traumatic brain injury in infants and children. *J Neurotrauma.* 2003;20(8):781–786.
68. Bayir H, Kagan VE, Tyurina YY, et al. Assessment of antioxidant reserves and oxidative stress in cerebrospinal fluid after severe traumatic brain injury in infants and children. *Pediatr Res.* 2002;51(5):571–578.
69. Ragan DK, McKinstry R, Benzinger T, Leonard JR, Pineda JA. Alterations in cerebral oxygen metabolism after traumatic brain injury in children. *J Cerebr Blood F Met.* 2013;33(1):48–52.
70. Darwish RS, Amiridze N, Aarabi B. Nitrotyrosine as an oxidative stress marker: Evidence for involvement in neurologic outcome in human traumatic brain injury. *J Traum.* 2007;63(2):439–442.
71. Darwish RS, Amiridze NS. Detectable levels of cytochrome C and activated caspase-9 in cerebrospinal fluid after human traumatic brain injury. *Neurocrit Care.* 2010;12(3):337–341.
72. Emmerling MR, Morganti-Kossmann MC, Kossmann T, et al. Traumatic brain injury elevates the Alzheimer's amyloid peptide A beta 42 in human CSF. A possible role for nerve cell injury. *Ann N Y Acad Sci.* 2000;903:118–122.
73. Pappolla MA, Chyan YJ, Omar RA, et al. Evidence of oxidative stress and in vivo neurotoxicity of beta-amyloid in a transgenic mouse model of Alzheimer's disease: A chronic oxidative paradigm for testing antioxidant therapies in vivo. *Am J Pathol.* 1998;152(4):871–877.
74. Butterfield DA. Amyloid beta-peptide (1-42)-induced oxidative stress and neurotoxicity: Implications for neurodegeneration in Alzheimer's disease brain. A review. *Free Radic Res.* 2002;36(12):1307–1313.
75. Butterfield DA, Castegna A, Lauderback CM, Drake J. Evidence that amyloid beta-peptide-induced lipid peroxidation and its sequelae in Alzheimer's disease brain contribute to neuronal death. *Neurobiol Aging.* 2002;23(5):655–664.
76. Qi XL, Xiu J, Shan KR, et al. Oxidative stress induced by beta-amyloid peptide(1–42) is involved in the altered composition of cellular membrane lipids and the decreased expression of nicotinic receptors in human SH-SY5Y neuroblastoma cells. *Neurochem Int.* 2005;46(8):613–621.
77. Yu GF, Jie YQ, Wu A, Huang Q, Dai WM, Fan XF. Increased plasma 8-iso-prostaglandin F2alpha concentration in severe human traumatic brain injury. *Clinica Chimica Acta.* 2013;421:7–11.
78. Clausen F, Marklund N, Lewen A, Enblad P, Basu S, Hillered L. Interstitial F(2)-isoprostane 8-iso-PGF(2alpha) as a biomarker of oxidative stress after severe human traumatic brain injury. *J Neurotrauma.* 20 2012;29(5):766–775.
79. Nayak CD, Nayak DM, Raja A, Rao A. Erythrocyte indicators of oxidative changes in patients with graded traumatic head injury. *Neurol India.* 2008;56(1):31–35.
80. Hohl A, Gullo Jda S, Silva CC, et al. Plasma levels of oxidative stress biomarkers and hospital mortality in severe head injury: A multivariate analysis. *J Critical Care.* 2012;27(5):523 e511–e529.
81. Lin C, Wang N, Shen ZP, Zhao ZY. Plasma copeptin concentration and outcome after pediatric traumatic brain injury. *Peptides.* 2013;42:43–47.

82. Manevich Y, Hutchens S, Halushka PV, et al. Peroxiredoxin VI oxidation in cerebrospinal fluid correlates with traumatic brain injury outcome. *Free Radic Biol Med.* 2014;72:210–221.

83. Yen HC, Chen TW, Yang TC, Wei HJ, Hsu JC, Lin CL. Levels of F2-isoprostanes, F4-neuroprostanes, and total nitrate/nitrite in plasma and cerebrospinal fluid of patients with traumatic brain injury. *Free Radic Res.* 2015;49(12):1419–1430.

84. Dong XQ, Yu WH, Zhang ZY, et al. Serum thioredoxin and in-hospital major adverse events after traumatic brain injury. *Clinica Chimica Acta.* 2017;469:75–80.

85. Robertson CL, Scafidi S, McKenna MC, Fiskum G. Mitochondrial mechanisms of cell death and neuroprotection in pediatric ischemic and traumatic brain injury. *Exp Neurol.* 2009;218(2):371–380.

86. Mazzeo AT, Beat A, Singh A, Bullock MR. The role of mitochondrial transition pore, and its modulation, in traumatic brain injury and delayed neurodegeneration after TBI. *Exp Neurol.* 2009;218(2):363–370.

87. Opii WO, Nukala VN, Sultana R, et al. Proteomic identification of oxidized mitochondrial proteins following experimental traumatic brain injury. *J Neurotrauma.* 2007;24(5):772–789.

88. Sharma P, Benford B, Li ZZ, Ling GS. Role of pyruvate dehydrogenase complex in traumatic brain injury and Measurement of pyruvate dehydrogenase enzyme by dipstick test. *J Emerg Trauma Shock.* 2009;2(2):67–72.

89. Dai W, Cheng HL, Huang RQ, Zhuang Z, Shi JX. Quantitative detection of the expression of mitochondrial cytochrome c oxidase subunits mRNA in the cerebral cortex after experimental traumatic brain injury. *Brain Res.* 2009;1251:287–295.

90. Gilmer LK, Roberts KN, Joy K, Sullivan PG, Scheff SW. Early mitochondrial dysfunction after cortical contusion injury. *J Neurotrauma.* 2009;26(8):1271–1280.

91. Singh IN, Sullivan PG, Deng Y, Mbye LH, Hall ED. Time course of posttraumatic mitochondrial oxidative damage and dysfunction in a mouse model of focal traumatic brain injury: Implications for neuroprotective therapy. *J Cereb Blood Flow Metab.* 2006;26(11):1407–1418.

92. Readnower RD, Pandya JD, McEwen ML, Pauly JR, Springer JE, Sullivan PG. Post-injury administration of the mitochondrial permeability transition pore inhibitor, NIM811, is neuroprotective and improves cognition after traumatic brain injury in rats. *J Neurotrauma.* 2011;28(9):1845–1853.

93. Mustafa AG, Singh IN, Wang J, Carrico KM, Hall ED. Mitochondrial protection after traumatic brain injury by scavenging lipid peroxyl radicals. *J Neurochem.* 2010;114(1):271–280.

94. Conley YP, Okonkwo DO, Deslouches S, et al. Mitochondrial polymorphisms impact outcomes after severe traumatic brain injury. *J Neurotrauma.* 2014;31(1):34–41.

95. Aygok GA, Marmarou A, Fatouros P, Kettenmann B, Bullock RM. Assessment of mitochondrial impairment and cerebral blood flow in severe brain injured patients. *Acta Neurochir Suppl.* 2008;102:57–61.

96. Belli A, Sen J, Petzold A, et al. Extracellular N-acetylaspartate depletion in traumatic brain injury. *J Neurochem.* 2006;96(3):861–869.

97. Pandya JD, Pauly JR, Nukala VN, et al. Post-injury administration of mitochondrial uncouplers increases tissue sparing and improves behavioral outcome following traumatic brain injury in rodents. *J Neurotrauma.* 2007;24(5):798–811.

98. Chen XR, Besson VC, Palmier B, Garcia Y, Plotkine M, Marchand-Leroux C. Neurological recovery-promoting, antiinflammatory, and anti-oxidative effects afforded by fenofibrate, a PPAR alpha agonist, in traumatic brain injury. *J Neurotrauma.* 2007;24(7):1119–1131.

99. Maier B, Lehnert M, Laurer HL, Mautes AE, Steudel WI, Marzi I. Delayed elevation of soluble tumor necrosis factor receptors p75 and p55 in cerebrospinal fluid and plasma after traumatic brain injury. *Shock.* 2006;26(2):122–127.

100. Bermpohl D, You Z, Lo EH, Kim HH, Whalen MJ. TNF alpha and Fas mediate tissue damage and functional outcome after traumatic brain injury in mice. *J Cereb Blood Flow Metab.* 2007;27(11):1806–1818.

101. Tuzgen S, Tanriover N, Uzan M, et al. Nitric oxide levels in rat cortex, hippocampus, cerebellum, and brainstem after impact acceleration head injury. *Neurol Res.* 2003;25(1):31–34.

102. Clausen F, Hanell A, Bjork M, et al. Neutralization of interleukin-1beta modifies the inflammatory response and improves histological and cognitive outcome following traumatic brain injury in mice. *Eur J Neurosci.* 2009;30(3):385–396.

103. Shohami E, Gallily R, Mechoulam R, Bass R, Ben-Hur T. Cytokine production in the brain following closed head injury: Dexanabinol (HU-211) is a novel TNF-alpha inhibitor and an effective neuroprotectant. *J Neuroimmunol.* 1997;72(2):169–177.

104. Trembovler V, Beit-Yannai E, Younis F, Gallily R, Horowitz M, Shohami E. Antioxidants attenuate acute toxicity of tumor necrosis factor-alpha induced by brain injury in rat. *J Interferon Cytokine Res.* 1999;19(7):791–795.

105. Lloyd E, Somera-Molina K, Van Eldik LJ, Watterson DM, Wainwright MS. Suppression of acute proinflammatory cytokine and chemokine upregulation by postinjury administration of a novel small molecule improves long-term neurologic outcome in a mouse model of traumatic brain injury. *J Neuroinflammation.* 2008;5:28.
106. Wei HH, Lu XC, Shear DA, et al. NNZ-2566 treatment inhibits neuroinflammation and pro-inflammatory cytokine expression induced by experimental penetrating ballistic-like brain injury in rats. *J Neuroinflammation.* 2009;6:19.
107. Wu H, Mahmood A, Lu D, et al. Attenuation of astrogliosis and modulation of endothelial growth factor receptor in lipid rafts by simvastatin after traumatic brain injury. *J Neurosurg.* 2009;113(3):591–597.
108. Colin-Gonzalez AL, Orozco-Ibarra M, Chanez-Cardenas ME, et al. Heme oxygenase-1 (HO-1) upregulation delays morphological and oxidative damage induced in an excitotoxic/pro-oxidant model in the rat striatum. *Neuroscience.* 2013;231:91–101.
109. Donkin JJ, Nimmo AJ, Cernak I, Blumbergs PC, Vink R. Substance P is associated with the development of brain edema and functional deficits after traumatic brain injury. *J Cereb Blood Flow Metab.* 2009;29(8):1388–1398.
110. Woodcock T, Morganti-Kossmann MC. The role of markers of inflammation in traumatic brain injury. *Front Neurol.* 2013;4:18.
111. Frugier T, Morganti-Kossmann MC, O'Reilly D, McLean CA. In situ detection of inflammatory mediators in post mortem human brain tissue after traumatic injury. *J Neurotrauma.* 2010;27(3):497–507.
112. Ramlackhansingh AF, Brooks DJ, Greenwood RJ, et al. Inflammation after trauma: Microglial activation and traumatic brain injury. *Ann Neurol.* 2011;70(3):374–383.
113. Skandsen T, Kvistad KA, Solheim O, Strand IH, Folvik M, Vik A. Prevalence and impact of diffuse axonal injury in patients with moderate and severe head injury: A cohort study of early magnetic resonance imaging findings and 1-year outcome. *J Neurosurg.* 2010;113(3):556–563.
114. Lin Y, Wen L. Inflammatory response following diffuse axonal injury. *Int J Med Sci.* 2013;10(5):515–521.
115. Lucas SM, Rothwell NJ, Gibson RM. The role of inflammation in CNS injury and disease. *Br J Pharmacol.* 2006;147(Suppl 1):S232–S240.
116. Goodman JC, Van M, Gopinath SP, Robertson CS. Pro-inflammatory and pro-apoptotic elements of the neuroinflammatory response are activated in traumatic brain injury. *Acta Neurochir Suppl.* 2008;102:437–439.
117. Hutchinson PJ, O'Connell MT, Rothwell NJ, et al. Inflammation in human brain injury: Intracerebral concentrations of IL-1alpha, IL-1beta, and their endogenous inhibitor IL-1ra. *J Neurotrauma.* 2007;24(10):1545–1557.
118. You Z, Yang J, Takahashi K, et al. Reduced tissue damage and improved recovery of motor function after traumatic brain injury in mice deficient in complement component C4. *J Cereb Blood Flow Metab.* 2007;27(12):1954–1964.
119. Hein AM, O'Banion MK. Neuroinflammation and memory: The role of prostaglandins. *Mol Neurobiol.* 2009;40(1):15–32.
120. Dietrich WD, Chatzipanteli K, Vitarbo E, Wada K, Kinoshita K. The role of inflammatory processes in the pathophysiology and treatment of brain and spinal cord trauma. *Acta Neurochir Suppl.* 2004;89:69–74.
121. Potts MB, Koh SE, Whetstone WD, et al. Traumatic injury to the immature brain: Inflammation, oxidative injury, and iron-mediated damage as potential therapeutic targets. *NeuroRx.* 2006;3(2):143–153.
122. Hall ED, Detloff MR, Johnson K, Kupina NC. Peroxynitrite-mediated protein nitration and lipid peroxidation in a mouse model of traumatic brain injury. *J Neurotrauma.* 2004;21(1):9–20.
123. Gahm C, Holmin S, Wiklund PN, Brundin L, Mathiesen T. Neuroprotection by selective inhibition of inducible nitric oxide synthase after experimental brain contusion. *J Neurotrauma.* 2006;23(9):1343–1354.
124. Minambres EC, Cemborain A, Sanchez-Velasco P, et al. Correlation between transcranial interleukin-6 gradient and outcome in patients with acute brain injury. *Crit Care Med.* 2003;31:33–38.
125. Xiao GM, Wei J. Effects of beta-Aescin on the expression of nuclear factor-kappaB and tumor necrosis factor-alpha after traumatic brain injury in rats. *J Zhejiang Univ Sci B.* 2005;6(1):28–32.
126. Venetsanou K, Vlachos K, Moles A, Fragakis G, Fildissis G, Baltopoulos G. Hypolipoproteinemia and hyperinflammatory cytokines in serum of severe and moderate traumatic brain injury (TBI) patients. *Eur Cytokine Netw.* 2007;18(4):206–209.
127. Buttram SD, Wisniewski SR, Jackson EK, et al. Multiplex assessment of cytokine and chemokine levels in cerebrospinal fluid following severe pediatric traumatic brain injury: Effects of moderate hypothermia. *J Neurotrauma.* 2007;24(11):1707–1717.

128. Gopinath SP, Valadka AB, Goodman JC, Robertson CS. Extracellular glutamate and aspartate in head injured patients. *Acta Neurochir Suppl.* 2000;76:437–438.

129. Rao VL, Baskaya MK, Dogan A, Rothstein JD, Dempsey RJ. Traumatic brain injury downregulates glial glutamate transporter (GLT-1 and GLAST) proteins in rat brain. *J Neurochem.* 1998;70(5):2020–2027.

130. Yi JH, Hazell AS. Excitotoxic mechanisms and the role of astrocytic glutamate transporters in traumatic brain injury. *Neurochem Int.* 2006;48(5):394–403.

131. Goodrich GS, Kabakov AY, Hameed MQ, Dhamne SC, Rosenberg PA, Rotenberg A. Ceftriaxone treatment after traumatic brain injury restores expression of the glutamate transporter, GLT-1, reduces regional gliosis, and reduces posttraumatic seizures in the rat. *J Neurotrauma.* 2013;30(16):1434–1441.

132. Hinzman JM, Thomas TC, Quintero JE, Gerhardt GA, Lifshitz J. Disruptions in the regulation of extracellular glutamate by neurons and glia in the rat striatum two days after diffuse brain injury. *J Neurotrauma.* 2012;29(6):1197–1208.

133. Hascup ER, Hascup KN, Stephens M, et al. Rapid microelectrode measurements and the origin and regulation of extracellular glutamate in rat prefrontal cortex. *J Neurochem.* 2010;115(6):1608–1620.

134. Globus MY, Alonso O, Dietrich WD, Busto R, Ginsberg MD. Glutamate release and free radical production following brain injury: Effects of posttraumatic hypothermia. *J Neurochem.* 1995;65(4):1704–1711.

135. Panter SS, Faden AI. Pretreatment with NMDA antagonists limits release of excitatory amino acids following traumatic brain injury. *Neurosci Lett.* 1992;136(2):165–168.

136. Obrenovitch TP, Urenjak J. Is high extracellular glutamate the key to excitotoxicity in traumatic brain injury? *J Neurotrauma.* 1997;14(10):677–698.

137. Zlotnik A, Leibowitz A, Gurevich B, et al. Effect of estrogens on blood glutamate levels in relation to neurological outcome after TBI in male rats. *Intensive Care Med.* 2012;38(1):137–144.

138. Movsesyan VA, Faden AI. Neuroprotective effects of selective group II mGluR activation in brain trauma and traumatic neuronal injury. *J Neurotrauma.* 2006;23(2):117–127.

139. Allen JW, Ivanova SA, Fan L, Espey MG, Basile AS, Faden AI. Group II metabotropic glutamate receptor activation attenuates traumatic neuronal injury and improves neurological recovery after traumatic brain injury. *J Pharmacol Exp Ther.* 1999;290(1):112–120.

140. Balk SJ. Ultraviolet radiation: A hazard to children and adolescents. *Pediatrics.* 2011;127(3):e791–e817.

141. Yi JH, Hoover R, McIntosh TK, Hazell AS. Early, transient increase in complexin I and complexin II in the cerebral cortex following traumatic brain injury is attenuated by N-acetylcysteine. *J Neurotrauma.* 2006;23(1):86–96.

142. Bullock R, Zauner A, Woodward JJ, et al. Factors affecting excitatory amino acid release following severe human head injury. *J Neurosurg.* 1998;89(4):507–518.

143. Yamamoto T, Rossi S, Stiefel M, et al. CSF and ECF glutamate concentrations in head injured patients. *Acta Neurochir Suppl.* 1999;75:17–19.

144. Koura SS, Doppenberg EM, Marmarou A, Choi S, Young HF, Bullock R. Relationship between excitatory amino acid release and outcome after severe human head injury. *Acta Neurochir Suppl.* 1998;71:244–246.

145. Stover JF, Morganti-Kosmann MC, Lenzlinger PM, Stocker R, Kempski OS, Kossmann T. Glutamate and taurine are increased in ventricular cerebrospinal fluid of severely brain-injured patients. *J Neurotrauma.* 1999;16(2):135–142.

146. Stover JF, Unterberg AW. Increased cerebrospinal fluid glutamate and taurine concentrations are associated with traumatic brain edema formation in rats. *Brain Res.* 2000;875(1–2):51–55.

147. Chamoun R, Suki D, Gopinath SP, Goodman JC, Robertson C. Role of extracellular glutamate measured by cerebral microdialysis in severe traumatic brain injury. *J Neurosurg.* 2010;113(3):564–570.

148. Mellergard P, Sjogren F, Hillman J. The cerebral extracellular release of glycerol, glutamate, and FGF2 is increased in older patients following severe traumatic brain injury. *J Neurotrauma.* 2012;29(1):112–118.

149. Timofeev I, Carpenter KL, Nortje J, et al. Cerebral extracellular chemistry and outcome following traumatic brain injury: A microdialysis study of 223 patients. *Brain.* 2011;134(Pt 2):484–494.

150. Robertson CL, Bell MJ, Kochanek PM, et al. Increased adenosine in cerebrospinal fluid after severe traumatic brain injury in infants and children: Association with severity of injury and excitotoxicity. *Crit Care Med.* 2001;29(12):2287–2293.

151. Grossetete M, Phelps J, Arko L, Yonas H, Rosenberg GA. Elevation of matrix metalloproteinases 3 and 9 in cerebrospinal fluid and blood in patients with severe traumatic brain injury. *Neurosurgery.* 2009;65(4):702–708.

152. Roberts DJ, Jenne CN, Leger C, et al. Association between the cerebral inflammatory and matrix metalloproteinase responses after severe traumatic brain injury in humans. *J Neurotrauma.* 2013;30(20):1727–1736.

153. Ates O, Cayli S, Altinoz E, et al. Neuroprotection by resveratrol against traumatic brain injury in rats. *Mol Cell Biochem.* 2007;294(1–2):137–144.

154. Sonmez U, Sonmez A, Erbil G, Tekmen I, Baykara B. Neuroprotective effects of resveratrol against traumatic brain injury in immature rats. *Neurosci Lett.* 2007;420(2):133–137.

155. Toklu HZ, Hakan T, Biber N, Solakoglu S, Ogunc AV, Sener G. The protective effect of alpha lipoic acid against traumatic brain injury in rats. *Free Radic Res.* 2009;43(7):658–667.

156. Chen G, Shi J, Hu Z, Hang C. Inhibitory effect on cerebral inflammatory response following traumatic brain injury in rats: A potential neuroprotective mechanism of N-acetylcysteine. *Mediators Inflamm.* 2008;2008:716458.

157. Yi JH, Hazell AS. N-acetylcysteine attenuates early induction of heme oxygenase-1 following traumatic brain injury. *Brain Res.* 2005;1033(1):13–19.

158. Beni SM, Kohen R, Reiter RJ, Tan DX, Shohami E. Melatonin-induced neuroprotection after closed head injury is associated with increased brain antioxidants and attenuated late-phase activation of NF-kappaB and AP-1. *FASEB J.* 2004;18(1):149–151.

159. Afaq F, Zaid MA, Khan N, Dreher M, Mukhtar H. Protective effect of pomegranate-derived products on UVB-mediated damage in human reconstituted skin. *Exp Dermatol.* 2009;18(6):553–561.

160. Xia J, Duan Q, Ahmad A, et al. Genistein inhibits cell growth and induces apoptosis through upregulation of miR-34a in pancreatic cancer cells. *Curr Drug Targets.* 2012;13(14):1750–1756.

161. Wu A, Ying Z, Gomez-Pinilla F. Vitamin E protects against oxidative damage and learning disability after mild traumatic brain injury in rats. *Neurorehabil Neural Repair.* 2009;24(3):290–298.

162. Xiong Y, Shie FS, Zhang J, Lee CP, Ho YS. Prevention of mitochondrial dysfunction in posttraumatic mouse brain by superoxide dismutase. *J Neurochem.* 2005;95(3):732–744.

163. Tsuru-Aoyagi K, Potts MB, Trivedi A, et al. Glutathione peroxidase activity modulates recovery in the injured immature brain. *Ann Neurol.* 2009;65(5):540–549.

164. Wu A, Ying Z, Gomez-Pinilla F. Dietary omega-3 fatty acids normalize BDNF levels, reduce oxidative damage, and counteract learning disability after traumatic brain injury in rats. *J Neurotrauma.* 2004;21(10):1457–1467.

165. Al Moutaery K, Al Deeb S, Ahmad Khan H, Tariq M. Caffeine impairs short-term neurological outcome after concussive head injury in rats. *Neurosurgery.* 2003;53(3):704–711; discussion 711–702.

166. Dong W, Yang B, Wang L, et al. Curcumin plays neuroprotective roles against traumatic brain injury partly via Nrf2 signaling. *Toxicol Appl Pharmacol.* 018;346:28–36.

167. Dai W, Wang H, Fang J, et al. Curcumin provides neuroprotection in model of traumatic brain injury via the Nrf2-ARE signaling pathway. *Brain Res Bull.* 2018;140:65–71.

168. Dohi K, Satoh K, Mihara Y, et al. Alkoxyl radical-scavenging activity of edaravone in patients with traumatic brain injury. *J Neurotrauma.* 2006;23(11):1591–1599.

169. Gottshall K, Hoffer, ME, Balough, BJ. Use of antioxidants micronutrient compounds in vestibular rehabilitation after operational head trauma or blast injury. Paper presented at: Barany International Balance MeetingJune, 2006; Stockholm, Sweden.

170. Prasad KN. Simultaneous activation of Nrf2 and elevation of dietary and endogenous antioxidants for prevention and improved managment of Parkinson's disease. In: Bondy SCC, ed. *Inflammation, Aging and Oxidative Stress.* New York: Springer; 2016:277–301.

171. Prasad KN. Oxidative stress and pro-inflammatory cytokines may act as one of signals for regulating microRNAs expression in Alzheimer's disease. *Mech Ageing Dev.* 2017;162:63–71.

172. Vile GF, Winterbourn CC. Inhibition of adriamycin-promoted microsomal lipid peroxidation by beta-carotene, alpha-tocopherol, and retinol at high and low oxygen partial pressures. *FEBS Lett.* 1988;238(2):353–356.

173. Niki E. Interaction of ascorbate and alpha-tocopherol. *Ann N Y Acad Sci.* 1987;498:186–199.

174. Wu H, Kong L, Tan Y, et al. C66 ameliorates diabetic nephropathy in mice by both upregulating NRF2 function via increase in miR-200a and inhibiting miR-21. *Diabetologia.* 2016;59:1558–1568.

175. Jaramillo MC, Zhang DD. The emerging role of the Nrf2-Keap1 signaling pathway in cancer. *Genes Dev.* 2013;27(20):2179–2191.

176. Williamson TP, Johnson DA, Johnson JA. Activation of the Nrf2-ARE pathway by siRNA knockdown of Keap1 reduces oxidative stress and provides partial protection from MPTP-mediated neurotoxicity. *Neurotoxicology.* 2012;33(3):272–279.

177. Itoh K, Chiba T, Takahashi S, et al. An Nrf2/small Maf heterodimer mediates the induction of phase II detoxifying enzyme genes through antioxidant response elements. *Biochem Biophys Res Commun.* 1997;236(2):313–322.

178. Hayes JD, Chanas SA, Henderson CJ, et al. The Nrf2 transcription factor contributes both to the basal expression of glutathione S-transferases in mouse liver and to their induction by the chemopreventive synthetic antioxidants, butylated hydroxyanisole, and ethoxyquin. *Biochem Soc Trans*. 2000;28(2):33–41.

179. Chan K, Han XD, Kan YW. An important function of Nrf2 in combating oxidative stress: Detoxification of acetaminophen. *Proc Natl Acad Sci USA*. 2001;98(8):4611–4616.

180. Ramsey CP, Glass CA, Montgomery MB, et al. Expression of Nrf2 in neurodegenerative diseases. *J Neuropathol Exp Neurol*. 2007;66(1):75–85.

181. Chen PC, Vargas MR, Pani AK, et al. Nrf2-mediated neuroprotection in the MPTP mouse model of Parkinson's disease: Critical role for the astrocyte. *Proc Natl Acad Sci USA*. 2009;106(8):2933–2938.

182. Lastres-Becker I, Ulusoy A, Innamorato NG, et al. Alpha-synuclein expression and Nrf2 deficiency cooperate to aggravate protein aggregation, neuronal death and inflammation in early-stage Parkinson's disease. *Hum Mol Genet*. 2012;21(14):3173–3192.

183. Xi YD, Yu HL, Ding J, et al. Flavonoids protect cerebrovascular endothelial cells through Nrf2 and PI3K from beta-amyloid peptide-induced oxidative damage. *Curr Neurovasc Res*. 2012;9(1):32–41.

184. Suh JH, Shenvi SV, Dixon BM, et al. Decline in transcriptional activity of Nrf2 causes age-related loss of glutathione synthesis, which is reversible with lipoic acid. *Proc Natl Acad Sci USA*. 2004;101(10):3381–3386.

185. Trujillo J, Chirino YI, Molina-Jijon E, Anderica-Romero AC, Tapia E, Pedraza-Chaverri J. Renoprotective effect of the antioxidant curcumin: Recent findings. *Redox Biol*. 2013;1(1):448–456.

186. Steele ML, Fuller S, Patel M, Kersaitis C, Ooi L, Munch G. Effect of Nrf2 activators on release of glutathione, cysteinylglycine, and homocysteine by human U373 astroglial cells. *Redox Biol*. 2013;1(1):441–445.

187. Kode A, Rajendrasozhan S, Caito S, Yang SR, Megson IL, Rahman I. Resveratrol induces glutathione synthesis by activation of Nrf2 and protects against cigarette smoke-mediated oxidative stress in human lung epithelial cells. *Am J Physiol Lung Cell Mol Physiol*. 2008;294(3):L478–L488.

188. Gao L, Wang J, Sekhar KR, et al. Novel n-3 fatty acid oxidation products activate Nrf2 by destabilizing the association between Keap1 and Cullin3. *J Biol Chem*. 2007;282(4):2529–2537.

189. Saw CL, Yang AY, Guo Y, Kong AN. Astaxanthin and omega-3 fatty acids individually and in combination protect against oxidative stress via the Nrf2-ARE pathway. *Food Chem Toxicol*. 2013;62:869–875.

190. Song J, Kang SM, Lee WT, Park KA, Lee KM, Lee JE. Glutathione protects brain endothelial cells from hydrogen peroxide-induced oxidative stress by increasing nrf2 expression. *Exp Neurobiol*. 2014;23(1):93–103.

191. Ji L, Liu R, Zhang XD, et al. N-acetylcysteine attenuates phosgene-induced acute lung injury via upregulation of Nrf2 expression. *Inhal Toxicol*. 2010;22(7):535–542.

192. Choi HK, Pokharel YR, Lim SC, et al. Inhibition of liver fibrosis by solubilized coenzyme Q10: Role of Nrf2 activation in inhibiting transforming growth factor-beta1 expression. *Toxicol Appl Pharmacol*. 2009;240(3):377–384.

193. Bai H, Liu R, Chen HL, et al. Enhanced antioxidant effect of caffeic acid phenethyl ester and Trolox in combination against radiation induced-oxidative stress. *Chem Biol Interact*. 25 2014;207:7–15.

194. Cui L, Jeong H, Borovecki F, Parkhurst CN, Tanese N, Krainc D. Transcriptional repression of PGC-1alpha by mutant huntingtin leads to mitochondrial dysfunction and neurodegeneration. *Cell*. 2006;127(1):59–69.

195. Li XH, Li CY, Lu JM, Tian RB, Wei J. Allicin ameliorates cognitive deficits ageing-induced learning and memory deficits through enhancing of Nrf2 antioxidant signaling pathways. *Neurosci Lett*. 2012;514(1):46–50.

196. Bergstrom P, Andersson HC, Gao Y, et al. Repeated transient sulforaphane stimulation in astrocytes leads to prolonged Nrf2-mediated gene expression and protection from superoxide-induced damage. *Neuropharmacology*. 2011;60(2–3):343–353.

197. Wruck CJ, Gotz ME, Herdegen T, Varoga D, Brandenburg LO, Pufe T. Kavalactones protect neural cells against amyloid beta peptide-induced neurotoxicity via extracellular signal-regulated kinase 1/2-dependent nuclear factor erythroid 2-related factor 2 activation. *Mol Pharmacol*. 2008;73(6):1785–1795.

198. Jin W, Wang H, Yan W, et al. Disruption of Nrf2 enhances upregulation of nuclear factor-kappaB activity, proinflammatory cytokines, and intercellular adhesion molecule-1 in the brain after traumatic brain injury. *Mediators Inflamm*. 2008;2008:725174.

199. Jin W, Wang H, Yan W, et al. Role of Nrf2 in protection against traumatic brain injury in mice. *J Neurotrauma*. 2009;26(1):131–139.

200. Lu XY, Wang HD, Xu JG, Ding K, Li T. Deletion of Nrf2 exacerbates oxidative stress after traumatic brain injury in mice. *Cell Mol Neurobiol.* 2015;35(5):713–721.

201. Song SM, Park YS, Lee A, et al. Concentrations of blood vitamin A, C, E, coenzyme Q10 and urine cotinine related to cigarette smoking exposure. *Korean J Lab Med.* 2009;29(1):10–16.

202. Galan P, Viteri FE, Bertrais S, et al. Serum concentrations of beta-carotene, vitamins C and E, zinc and selenium are influenced by sex, age, diet, smoking status, alcohol consumption, and corpulence in a general French adult population. *Eur J Clin Nutr.*2005;59(10):1181–1190.

203. Adhikari D, Baxi J, Risal S, Singh PP. Oxidative stress and antioxidant status in cancer patients and healthy subjects, a case-control study. *Nepal Med Coll J.*2005;7(2):112–115.

204. Li W, Khor TO, Xu C, et al. Activation of Nrf2-antioxidant signaling attenuates NFkappaB-inflammatory response and elicits apoptosis. *Biochem Pharmacol.* 2008;76(11):1485–1489.

205. Kim J, Cha YN, Surh YJ. A protective role of nuclear factor-erythroid 2-related factor-2 (Nrf2) in inflammatory disorders. *Mutat Res.* 2010;690(1–2):12–23.

206. Abate A, Yang G, Dennery PA, Oberle S, Schroder H. Synergistic inhibition of cyclooxygenase-2 expression by vitamin E and aspirin. *Free Radic Biol Med.* 2000;29(11):1135–1142.

207. Devaraj S, Tang R, Adams-Huet B, et al. Effect of high-dose alpha-tocopherol supplementation on biomarkers of oxidative stress and inflammation and carotid atherosclerosis in patients with coronary artery disease. *Am J Clin Nutr.* 2007;86(5):1392–1398.

208. Fu Y, Zheng S, Lin J, Ryerse J, Chen A. Curcumin protects the rat liver from CCl4-caused injury and fibrogenesis by attenuating oxidative stress and suppressing inflammation. *Mol Pharmacol.* 2008;73(2):399–409.

209. Lee HS, Jung KK, Cho JY, et al. Neuroprotective effect of curcumin is mainly mediated by blockade of microglial cell activation. *Pharmazie.* 2007;62(12):937–942.

210. Rahman S, Bhatia K, Khan AQ, et al. Topically applied vitamin E prevents massive cutaneous inflammatory and oxidative stress responses induced by double application of 12-O-tetradecanoylphorbol-13-acetate (TPA) in mice. *Chem Biol Interact.* 2008;172(3):195–205.

211. Suzuki YJ, Aggarwal BB, Packer L. Alpha-lipoic acid is a potent inhibitor of NF-kappa B activation in human T cells. *Biochem Biophys Res Commun.* 1992;189(3):1709–1715.

212. Zhu J, Yong W, Wu X, et al. Anti-inflammatory effect of resveratrol on TNF-alpha-induced MCP-1 expression in adipocytes. *Biochem Biophys Res Commun.* 2008;369(2):471–477.

213. Chang Y, Huang SK, Wang SJ. Coenzyme Q10 inhibits the release of glutamate in rat cerebrocortical nerve terminals by suppression of voltage-dependent calcium influx and mitogen-activated protein kinase signaling pathway. *J Agric Food Chem.* 2012;60(48):11909–11918.

214. Schubert D, Kimura H, Maher P. Growth factors and vitamin E modify neuronal glutamate toxicity. *Proc Natl Acad Sci USA.* 1992;89(17):8264–8267.

215. Sandhu JK, Pandey S, Ribecco-Lutkiewicz M, et al. Molecular mechanisms of glutamate neurotoxicity in mixed cultures of NT2-derived neurons and astrocytes: Protective effects of coenzyme Q10. *J Neurosci Res.* 2003;72(6):691–703.

216. Yang TT, Wang SJ. Pyridoxine inhibits depolarization-evoked glutamate release in nerve terminals from rat cerebral cortex: A possible neuroprotective mechanism? *J Pharmacol Exp Ther.* 2009;331(1):244–254.

217. Hung KL, Wang CC, Huang CY, Wang SJ. Cyanocobalamin, vitamin B12, depresses glutamate release through inhibition of voltage-dependent Ca^{2+} influx in rat cerebrocortical nerve terminals (synaptosomes). *Eur J Pharmacol.* 2009;602(2–3):230–237.

218. Olanow CW, Arendash GW. Metals and free radicals in neurodegeneration. *Curr Opin Neurol.* 1994;7(6):548–558.

219. Prasad KN, Kumar B, Yan XD, Hanson AJ, Cole WC. Alpha-tocopheryl succinate, the most effective form of vitamin E for adjuvant cancer treatment: A review. *J Am Coll Nutr.* 2003;22(2):108–117.

220. Bayir H, Adelson PD, Wisniewski SR, et al. Therapeutic hypothermia preserves antioxidant defenses after severe traumatic brain injury in infants and children. *Crit Care Med.* 2009;37(2):689–695.

221. Butte NF, Fox MK, Briefel RR, et al. Nutrient intakes of US infants, toddlers, and preschoolers meet or exceed dietary reference intakes. *J Am Diet Assoc.* 2010;110 (12 suppl):S27–S37.

222. Acharya MM, Lan ML, Kan VH, et al. Consequences of ionizing radiation-induced damage in human neural stem cells. *Free Radic Biol Med.* 2010;49(12):1846–1855.

223. Grasso G, Sfacteria A, Meli F, Fodale V, Buemi M, Iacopino DG. Neuroprotection by erythropoietin administration after experimental traumatic brain injury. *Brain Res.* 2007;1182:99–105.

224. Xiong Y, Chopp M, Lee CP. Erythropoietin improves brain mitochondrial function in rats after traumatic brain injury. *Neurol Res.* 2009;31(5):496–502.

225. Sharma HS, Patnaik R, Patnaik S, Mohanty S, Sharma A, Vannemreddy P. Antibodies to serotonin attenuate closed head injury induced blood brain barrier disruption and brain pathology. *Ann N Y Acad Sci.* 2007;1122:295–312.
226. Zhang B, West EJ, Van KC, et al. HDAC inhibitor increases histone H3 acetylation and reduces microglia inflammatory response following traumatic brain injury in rats. *Brain Res.* 2008;1226:181–191.
227. Foley K, Kast RE, Altschuler EL. Ritonavir and disulfiram have potential to inhibit caspase-1 mediated inflammation and reduce neurological sequelae after minor blast exposure. *Med Hypotheses.* 2009;72(2):150–152.
228. Hakan T, Toklu HZ, Biber N, et al. Effect of COX-2 inhibitor meloxicam against traumatic brain injury-induced biochemical, histopathological changes, and blood-brain-barrier permeability. *Neurol Res.* 2009;32(6):629–635.
229. Chen X, Choi IY, Chang TS, et al. Pretreatment with interferon-gamma protects microglia from oxidative stress via upregulation of Mn-SOD. *Free Radic Biol Med.* 2009;46(8):1204–1210.

14 Micronutrients in Prevention and Improvement of the Standard Therapy in HIV/AIDS

INTRODUCTION

The emergence of pathogenic human immunodeficiency virus (HIV) has markedly alarmed public and health professionals alike throughout the world. Similar viruses have been found in monkeys. These viruses may have coexisted with their respective hosts throughout the entire evolutionary processes and maintained their species specificity. The presence of genetic variants of viruses within the host suggests that these viruses can be mutated. Mutations may occur spontaneously or may be induced by increased oxidative stress in the host due to adverse environmental and dietary conditions that generate excessive amounts of free radicals. Some mutated forms of virus may acquire aggressive traits and kill the host; whereas, other mutated forms may infect different species and may become pathogenic in the new host.

Although most HIV-infected persons progress to acquired immunodeficiency syndrome (AIDS), some do not. This implies that the immune system of some individuals is competent enough to mount a defensive response against HIV infection. The role of the immune system in HIV infection is further supported by the fact that micronutrient deficiency and illicit drugs that are known to impair immune function increase the risk of HIV infection. This may be due to the fact that micronutrient deficiency increased the levels of oxidative stress that can induce inflammation in the individuals. Increased oxidative stress and inflammation are also associated with the progression of HIV infection. The current prevention strategy has emphasized on safe sex by using condom, and use of clean needled for intravenous (IV) drug users. Micronutrients such as dietary and endogenous antioxidants that reduce oxidative stress and inflammation, and play prominent role in stimulating host's immune function have not drawn adequate attention for reducing the risk of HIV infection or slowing down the rate of progression of HIV to AIDS.

The introduction of highly active anti-retroviral therapy (HAART) has improved the survival time of patients with AIDS, but it has failed to affect the risk of developing dementia, and it is very toxic. Low-dose HAART is also used in reducing the risk of transmission of virus from the infected to uninfected persons with limited success. Antiviral therapy also increases oxidative stress; therefore, the use of antioxidants in combination with HAART appears to be one of the rational choices for improving the efficacy of HAART in patients with AIDS. Unfortunately, most previous studies utilized a single antioxidant in combination with HAART, and they produced inconsistent results with respect to producing clinical outcomes better than HAART alone. In rare cases, where more than one antioxidant was used in combination with HAART, only dietary antioxidants were used. For optimal effects, it would be essential to utilize multiple micronutrients including both dietary and endogenous antioxidants.

This chapter describes the history, prevalence, incidence, and cost of HIV infection and presents evidence for the role of increased oxidative stress and inflammation in HIV infection and progression to AIDS. In order to optimally reduce oxidative stress and inflammation, it is essential to increase the levels of antioxidant enzymes and dietary and endogenous antioxidants. The levels of antioxidants can be increased by supplementation, but increasing the levels of antioxidant enzymes requires an activation of Nrf2, a nuclear transcription factor. This chapter discusses agents that activate Nrf2, and proposes a mixture of micronutrients that would enhance the levels of antioxidant enzymes by activating Nrf2 as well enhance the levels of dietary and endogenous antioxidants. Clinical studies with the proposed micronutrient mixture alone, or in combination of antiviral therapy (ART), are proposed in order to evaluate its effectiveness in reducing the progression of HIV infection and improving the outcomes of ART.

HISTORY, PREVALENCE, INCIDENCE, AND COST OF HIV/AIDS

HISTORY OF HIV/AIDS

The first case of unusual defect in the immune system was detected among gay men in the USA in 1981. In 1982, Acquired Immunodeficiency Syndrome (AIDS) was defined, and HIV was isolated in 1983. The main types of HIV are HIV-1 and HIV-2, HIV-2 being less transmissible and less pathogenic. There are several subtypes of HIV-1, and genetic recombination of subtypes results in the generation of mosaic and recombinant viruses. Certain recombinant strains of HIV are present in the circulating blood. The prevalence of specific subtype of HIV or their recombinants varies depending upon the region of the world. It has been shown that HIV primarily kills cells of immune system (CD4 lymphocytes and macrophages that play a key defensive role in viral infection). HIV infection thus results in the progressive decline in the function of immune system. This then makes the host more susceptible to additional infections such as esophageal candidiasis; HIV infection eventually progresses to AIDS.

PREVALENCE OF HIV INFECTION

Prevalence of HIV infection among US population aged 13 years and older appear to increase from 1 million in 2004 to 1.2 million in 2016, an increase of about 20%; however, it dropped from 39.6 to 36.7 million during the same period in the world (CDC, 2005 and 2018).

INCIDENCE OF HIV INFECTION

Except in 2006, the incidence of HIV infection remains stable around 40,000 new cases per year in the USA as described below.

Incidence of HIV infection among US population aged 13 and over

Year	Number of new cases
2004	44,000
2006	56,300
2010	41,800
2015	38,500
2016	39,782

Data were summarized from CDC report, 2005 and CDC. Estimated HIV Incidence and Prevalence in the United States 2010–2015. HIV Surveillance Supplemental Report, 2018.

In 2016, approximately 18,160 cases of HIV infection stage 3 (AIDS) were diagnosed in the USA. Globally, 1.8 million new cases of HIV infection were diagnosed. About 35 million people died of AIDS-related diseases since the start of the epidemic. Sub-Saharan Africa has about 10% of world's population, but about 65% of them are infected with HIV (CDC, 2005). The exact reasons for the difference in HIV infection rate between the USA and the Sub-Saharan populations are unknown; however, the higher prevalence of micronutrient deficiency that can adversely affect the immune function may in part account for the increased rates of HIV infection in Sub-Saharan populations.

Based on the study published in 2008,[1] the Centers for Disease Control and Prevention (CDC) estimated that in 2006, 56,300 new cases of HIV infection occurred in the USA, and about 50% of them were found in gay and bisexual men. The incidence of this infection among blacks/African Americans was 7 times higher than that found among whites. This increase in incidence of HIV infection was primarily due to improved detection technique rather than new infection. The annual incidence of about 40,000 remained stable since 1992. In 2007, new cases of HIV estimated to 35,934 (26,355 male and 9,579 female). The difference in incidence between male and female appears to be about 3-fold. Estimated number of deaths due to HIV/AIDS was 14,105 in adults and 5 in children under the age of 13 years. These studies suggest that the incidence rate of HIV infection did not increase in the USA as predicted earlier by some experts in the field.

COST OF TREATING HIV INFECTION

Annual cost of treating HIV/AIDS patients in 2010 dollars is $23,000 per person, and lifetime treatment cost is about $379,668 per person (CDC, 2017). In 2001, the annual estimated economic loss (including productive losses) among the USA population was about $18.2 billion, out of which direct medical cost alone was estimated to be about $9.2 billion.

ROLE OF IMMUNE FUNCTION IN HIV INFECTION

The immune status of the host is one of the most important determining factors in HIV infection. This is evidenced by the fact HIV infection does not progress to AIDS in some infected individuals. The primary cellular target of HIV is the immune cell. In addition, micronutrient deficiency and illicit drugs that are known to impair immune function also increase the risk of HIV infection, and the rate of progression of HIV infection to AIDS.

MICRONUTRIENT DEFICIENCY IMPAIRS IMMUNE FUNCTION

Micronutrient deficiency can increase oxidative stress and inflammation that could damage the immune system, and thereby, makes the individuals more susceptible to HIV infection. It can also increase the toxicity of antiviral drugs, mortality, disease progression, and the risk of maternal-fetal transmission of HIV. Indeed, the deficiency of antioxidants and other micronutrients is a common feature of adults and children with HIV/AIDS. The deficiency of micronutrients includes selenium, vitamin E, vitamin A, beta-carotene, lycopene, glutathione, coenzyme Q10, vitamin C, vitamin B-6, vitamin B-12, and Zn.[2–7] Micronutrient deficiency, which includes selenium, lycopene, beta-carotene, retinol, vitamin A, and vitamin E, has also been reported in children with HIV infection.[8,9] Low plasma levels of antioxidants in pregnant women were associated with increased risks of fetal death and HIV transmission through the intrapartum route.[10]

Other than the poor diet, the mechanisms of nutritional deficiency associated with HIV infection and/or AIDS are not fully understood. One study showed that individuals infected with HIV or patients with AIDS exhibit increased excretion of vitamin A and vitamin E.[11] The malabsorption may account for deficiency of some nutrients such as selenium and beta-carotene.[12] Furthermore, HIV-1 encodes for one of the human glutathione peroxidase; and therefore, its replication may cause deficiency of glutathione, selenium, cysteine, glutamine, and tryptophan.[13] Increased oxidative stress in HIV-infected individuals can also deplete antioxidant levels in the body. Therefore, a preventive strategy to protect immune function by correcting micronutrient deficiency may be one of the rational choices for reducing the rate of HIV infection.

The consequences of these nutritional deficiencies have been also investigated. For example, low serum levels of selenium in HIV-infected population is associated with loss of CD4+ cells, increased levels of markers of cytokines (interleukin-8), and soluble tumor necrosis factor receptors (sTNFR).[14] Selenium deficiency causes adverse effect on immune function, and thereby making the individuals more susceptible to HIV infection.[15] Malnutrition and selenium deficiency increase the risk of mycobacterial infection in illicit drug abusers as well as in HIV-infected individuals.[16] Low serum levels of vitamin B-12 are associated with increased neurological abnormalities and more rapid progression of HIV infection to AIDS and an increase in AZT-induced bone marrow toxicity.[17] Vitamin A deficiency is associated with increased mortality and more rapid disease progression and increased maternal-fetal transmission.[17] Thus, micronutrient deficiency plays a central role in enhancing the rate of progression of HIV infection to AIDS, the risk of AIDS-related neurological deficits, mortality, maternal-fetal transmission, as well as AZT-induced toxicity to bone marrow.

ILLICIT DRUGS IMPAIR IMMUNE FUNCTION

According to CDC about 70% of HIV infection occurs among drug users suggesting that these illicit drugs may play an important role in increasing the risk of HIV infection. Illicit drugs such as Ecstasy are one of the agents that suppress immune function.[18–22] They also enhance the progression of HIV infection to AIDS.[21] The illicit drugs may also increase the activation of microglia in the brain that may contribute to dementia in some HIV-infected individuals.[23] The use of intravenous drug may impair short- and long-term CD4 cell recovery in HIV-positive patients during active antiviral therapy.[24] Several clinical observations, neuroimaging, and neuropathological studies suggested that the use of illicit drugs enhanced the adverse effects of HIV infection on the central nervous system. The investigations on cell culture models support this conclusion. Furthermore, the intravenous injection of illicit drugs is also a risk factor for acquiring HIV infection, the incidence of which continues to rise among IV drug users even in countries with access to antiviral therapy.[25] Thus, a preventive strategy that is based on protecting the immune system and brain against the adverse effects of illicit drugs may be one of the rational choices for reducing the rate of HIV infection and dementia.

EVIDENCE FOR INCREASED OXIDATIVE STRESS ENHANCING THE PROGRESSION OF HIV INFECTION

Many conditions can induce increased oxidative stress in the body. They include micronutrient deficiency[2–9] and illicit drugs.[18–23] HIV infection also increased oxidative stress in humans and animal models. This is supported by the observation that high oxidative stress was found in patients with AIDS[3,26]. Additionally, increased oxidative stress in human erythrocytes was observed in asymptomatic patient infected with HIV and patients with AIDS.[27] Oxidative stress activates HIV replication in vitro by enhancing the levels of NF-kB. Another cytokine TNF-alpha also increases the replication of HIV by generating hydroxyl free radicals and causes apoptosis.[28]

Damage to the blood-brain-barrier (BBB) contributes to the development of HIV-associated dementia. Treatment of brain microvascular endothelial cells (BMECs) with a HIV protein Tat1-72 increased the levels of oxidative stress and decreased the levels of glutathione, NF-kB, and activator protein-1 (AP-1). Injection of Tat1-72 into mouse hippocampus induced elevated levels of monocyte chemoattractant protein1 (MCP-1) mRNA.[29] Studies on the autopsied samples of the frontal cortex showed that increased nuclear and mitochondrial DNA damage (8-hydroxydeoxyguanosine, a marker of oxidative of DNA) were associated with HIV-related cognitive dysfunction.[30] Increased levels of ceramide, sphingomyelin, and 4-hydroxynonenal (4-HNNE) were found in patients with HIV encephalitis. It was further demonstrated that enhanced levels of 4-HNE and ceramide were associated with progressing HIV dementia, while increased level of sphingomyelin was associated with inactive HIV dementia.[31] The plasma and lymphocytes from HIV-infected patients had reduced levels of thiols and increased levels of oxidized products showing the involvement of oxidative stress in the progression of HIV infection.[32] High levels of mtDNA damage (8-hydroxydeoxyguanosine) were associated with the lateral ventricular enlargement and reduced volume of hippocampus, palladium, and total subcortical gray matter. These changes in the brain volume and mtDNA damage contribute to cognitive dysfunction.[33] Supernatant obtained from human primary macrophages (M/M) infected by HIV induced oxidative stress and apoptosis in human astroglia cells in culture.[34] Pretreatment of astrocytes with a SOD mimetic M40401 prevented HIV-induced oxidative stress and apoptosis. These results suggest that apoptosis in astocytes was related to over-production of superoxide anions and not by HIV infection.

HIV-viral protein gp120 induced apoptosis by increasing oxidative stress that contributes to the HIV associated cognitive dysfunction.[35] The levels of heme oxygenase-1 (HO-1), an antioxidant enzyme, were lower in HIV infected individuals with cognitive dysfunction than in control subjects. This implies that Nrf2 activation becomes resistant to increased oxidative stress. Reduced level of HO-1 was associated with the release of glutamate from both HIV-infected and immune-activated macrophages.[36] The amounts of vitamin C, alpha-tocopherol, beta-carotene, and selenium were lower, while the levels of lipid peroxides, breath pentane, and ethane output were higher in HIV-infected patients than in control subjects.[37] The levels of oxidative stress in the plasma were higher in HIV patients who consumed alcohol than in those who did not consume alcohol.[38] Mild to moderate tobacco smoking enhanced progression of HIV infection by increasing oxidative stress in the plasma and monocytes.[39] HIV infection enhanced hepatitis C virus (HCV)-associated liver damage by increasing oxidative stress.[40] Increased oxidative stress acts as a predictor for mortality in HIV-infected patients.[41]

HIV viral protein reverse transcriptase (RT) also increased oxidative stress in human embryonic kidney cells (HEK293).[42] Red blood cell counts significantly decreased in HIV patients on HAART, compared to HIV patients without HAART, and HIV patients coinfected with tuberculosis. In addition, the levels of MDA were higher in HIV patients who were not on HAART compared to those patients on HAART. All patients with HIV infection had decreased level of glutathione compared to uninfected control subjects.[43]

These studies suggest that increased oxidative stress is one of the major initiators of HIV infection, probably by impairing the immune function. In the autopsied brain samples from AIDS patients with dementia, the levels of 3-nitrotyrosine, a marker of oxidative damage, was elevated in comparison to those observed in the autopsied brain samples from the uninfected, nondemented persons.[44] This result suggests that simultaneous production of nitric oxide and superoxide anion increases the levels of peroxynitrite that may contribute to the neuropathology of HIV-1 infection. In cats, feline immunodeficiency virus increased the levels of oxidative stress during acute phase of viral infection.[45] These studies suggest that increased oxidative stress occurs during HIV infection and its progression.

EVIDENCE FOR INCREASED INFLAMMATION ENHANCING THE PROGRESSION OF HIV INFECTION

The main features of HIV infection include chronic immune activation and products of inflammation including cytokines.[46] Pro-inflammatory cytokines released during inflammatory reactions are also associated with the HIV infection.[14] Increased oxidative stress and pro-inflammatory cytokines can further impair immune function and thereby increasing the susceptibility of the individuals to HIV infection. Both free radicals and TNF-alpha activate NF-kappa-B that is required for HIV proliferation.[47,48]

HIV infection caused depletion of CD4-T cells, chronic inflammation, and changes in cellular metabolism. Antiviral therapy did not attenuate inflammation fully leading to increased risk of non-AIDS events.[49] Combination ART has allowed HIV-infected people to live longer and healthier lives. HIV-infected individuals are often coinfected with cytomegalovirus (CMV). Both viruses can cause inflammation-related morbidities.[50] Cytokine driven chronic immune activation precedes the development of non-Hodgkin lymphoma.[51] ART-induced serious non-AIDS events that are major causes of morbidity and mortality in HIV-infected individuals are considered due to persistent immune activation.[52] It is very interesting to note that despite suppression of HIV replication, immune activation and inflammation continue to persist.[53] Among HIV infected individuals, increased levels of inflammation biomarkers IL-6 and hsCRP persisted, despite suppression of HIV replication. Plasma markers of inflammation that predict morbidity and mortality were strongly associated with monocyte activation and migration, modestly associated with T-cell maturation. These markers were not associated with CD+ T-cell activation.[54] Antiviral therapy did not significantly reduce inflammation that contributes to the renal disease,[55] cardiovascular disease,[56] and bone loss[57] in HIV-infected individuals. Residual inflammation that persists after HAART contributes to HIV reservoir.[58] The existence viral reservoir makes difficult to cure HIV infection. Increased levels of inflammation markers IL-6 and TNF-alpha receptor-1 were associated with enhanced risk of frailty and mortality among aging HIV-infected and uninfected IV drug users.[59]

The studied discussed above suggest that increased oxidative stress and inflammatory reactions play an important role in determining the rate of the progression of the HIV infection. They also play an important role in the development of complications associated with AIDS including cognitive dysfunction and increased rate of myocardial infarction.[2,16,60,61] Therefore, attenuation of oxidative stress and inflammation should be considered as one of the crucial strategies for reducing the risk and progression of HIV/AIDS.

EVIDENCE FOR MICRONUTRIENTS REDUCING PROGRESSION OF HIV INFECTION

Some studies have reported that supplementation with one or two antioxidants improved health outcomes, such as enhanced immune function, reduced the rate of progression of the disease, oxidative damage, and inflammation in the HIV/AIDS patients.[48,62,63] For example, vitamin E and selenium also produce some beneficial effects in a mouse model of AIDS.[64] Selenium supplementation decreased progression of HIV infection by reducing viral load and improving CD4 counts.[65] Selenium supplementation also inhibited abnormally high levels of pro-inflammatory cytokines (TNF-alpha and IL-8) in HIV/AIDS disease, which is often associated with neurological abnormalities, Kaposi sarcoma, wasting syndrome, and increased viral replication.[2] In addition, alpha-lipoic acid, N-acetylcysteine, selenium, and alpha-tocopheryl succinate inhibited HIV replication by reducing activation of NF-kappa B that is required for HIV replication.[48,62,63,66] In Botswana, supplementation with glutathione and amino acids (cysteine, tryptophan, and glutamine) reversed AIDS in 99% of patient. Vitamin E supplementation protected T-lymphocytes of HIV-infected patients from apoptosis by suppressing the expression of CD95L (a physiological ligand that stimulates CD95, a death receptor) that is involved in this mechanism of cell death.[67] Low concentration of beta-carotene is a common observation in patients with HIV/AIDS, and it can predict mortality rate. Supplementation with micronutrients and natural mixed carotenoids may improve the survival rates by correcting the deficiency.[68] A short-term supplementation with beta-carotene may increase CD4+ cell count in patient with AIDS.[69] In addition, beta-carotene (60 mg/day) supplementation showed an objective and subjective improvement in patients with AIDS, but it did not affect lymphadenopathy.[70] Higher doses of beta-carotene in combination with hyperthermia were effective even in patients with advanced AIDS. Alpha-tocopheryl succinate inhibited HIV replication and reduced the toxicity of AZT in lymphocytes in vitro.[66] Supplementation with vitamin A, vitamin C, vitamin E, beta-carotene, vitamin B6, and vitamin B12 retarded the development of immune dysfunction.[4] Supplementation with beta-carotene and selenium improved immunological function and decreased lipid peroxidation.[12] Supplementation with beta-carotene (5,450 IU of vitamin A), vitamin C (250 mg), vitamin E (100 IU), selenium (100 µg), coenzyme Q10 (50 mg) improved some parameters of oxidative stress, but did not decrease the viral load.[71] On the other hand, supplementation with high doses of NAC and vitamin C for 60 days in HIV patients with advanced immunodeficiency can reduce viral load and improve immunological function.[72] Supplementation with curcumin and its analogs prevent HIV infection and replication.[73]

Supplementation with multiple vitamins to HIV-infected women during pregnancy and lactation resulted in better health of their children than those not taking vitamins.[74] Anemia is a frequent complication among HIV-infected individuals and is associated with faster disease progression and mortality. Supplementation with multiple vitamins in women during pregnancy and in the postpartum period provided a significant improvement in hematological status among HIV-infected women and their children.[75] This is interesting to note that certain antioxidants inhibit viral replication the mechanism of which is different from that of antiviral drugs. Antioxidants inhibit viral replication by reducing activation of NF-kappa B, whereas antiviral drugs decreased it by inhibiting reverse transcriptase activity. Therefore, the combination of two should reduce viral load more than that produced by the individual agents.

Supplementation with high-dose or low-dose multivitamin (vitamin B complex, vitamin C, and vitamin E) in combination with HAART had no effect on disease progression or death, but it increased the levels of alanine transaminase.[76] Analysis of 33 trials with 10,325 participants suggested that supplementation with micronutrients had no significant benefits in patients with HIV. The author suggested micronutrient supplementation in case of deficiency.[77]

POTENTIAL REASONS FOR INCONSISTENT RESULTS WITH MICRONUTRIENTS IN PATIENTS WITH HIV/AIDS

The failure to yield consistent beneficial effects in patients with HIV infection may be due to the fact that most studies have utilized single micronutrients, some utilized multivitamins without comprehensive dietary and endogenous antioxidants. Some potentials causes are described here: (a) antioxidants show differential subcellular distribution and different mechanisms of action; therefore, a single antioxidant cannot protect all parts of the cell; (b) a single antioxidant in a high internal oxidative environment in high-risk patients is oxidized and can then itself act as a prooxidant rather than as an antioxidant; (c) the body protects against oxidative damage by elevating antioxidant enzymes, and dietary and endogenous antioxidants; (d) antioxidants neutralize free radicals by donating electrons to those molecules with unpaired electron, whereas antioxidant enzymes destroy free radicals by catalysis, converting them to harmless molecules such as water and oxygen. Therefore, both of these agents should be enhanced to achieve substantial protection against oxidative damage; (e) the affinity of different antioxidants for free radicals differs, depending upon their solubility; (f) both the aqueous and lipid compartments of the cell need to be protected together. Water-soluble antioxidants such as vitamin C and glutathione protect molecules in the aqueous environment of the cells, whereas lipid soluble antioxidants such as vitamin A and vitamin E protect molecules in the lipid compartment; (g) vitamin E is more effective in quenching free radicals in a reduced oxygenated cellular environment, whereas vitamin C and alpha-tocopherol are more effective in a higher oxygenated environment of the cells[78]; (h) vitamin C is important for recycling the oxidized form of alpha-tocopherol to the antioxidant form[79]; (i) antioxidants produce cell protective proteins by altering the expression of different microRNAs.[80] For example, some antioxidants can activate Nrf2 by upregulating miR-200a that inhibits its target protein Keap1, whereas others activate Nrf2 by downregulating miR-21 that binds with 3'-UTR Nrf2 mRNA.[81]

The use of a single micronutrient or randomly selected multiple micronutrients without scientific rationales is not expected to produce optimal protection against oxidative stress and inflammation, which contribute to the progression of HIV infection. For this reason, it is proposed that an elevation of the levels of antioxidant enzymes and dietary and endogenous antioxidants may be essential for simultaneously reducing oxidative stress and inflammation. Oral supplementation can increase the levels of dietary and endogenous antioxidants; however, elevation of the levels of antioxidant enzymes requires an activation of Nrf2. Therefore, it is essential to understand the regulation of activation of Nrf2.

ACTIVATION OF Nrf2 (NUCLEAR FACTOR-ERYTHROID-2-RELATED FACTOR 2)

Nrf2

The nuclear transcriptional factor, Nrf2 (nuclear factor-erythroid-2-related factor 2) belongs to the Cap 'n' Collar (CNC) family that contains a conserved basic leucine zipper (bZIP) transcriptional factor.[82] Under physiological condition, Nrf2 is associated with Kelch-like ECH associated protein 1 (Keap1), which acts as an inhibitor of Nrf2.[83] Keap1 protein serves as an adaptor to link Nrf2 to the ubiquitin ligase CuI-Rbx1 complex for degradation by proteasomes and maintains the steady levels of Nrf2 in the cytoplasm. Nrf2-keap1 complex is primarily located in the cytoplasm; Keap1 acts as a sensor for ROS/electrophilic stress.

ACTIVATION OF Nrf2 DURING ACUTE OXIDATIVE STRESS

During acute oxidative stress, ROS is required to activate Nrf2, which then dissociates itself from Keap1-CuI-Rbx1 complex and translocates in the nucleus where it heterodimerizes with a small Maf protein, binds with ARE leading to increased expression of target genes coding for several cytoprotective enzymes including antioxidant enzymes.[84–86]

FAILURE OF ROS TO ACTIVATE Nrf2 DURING CHRONIC OXIDATIVE STRESS

During chronic oxidative stress, Nrf2 becomes resistant to ROS,[87–89] suggesting that activation of Nrf2 by a ROS-independent mechanism exists. This is evidenced by the fact that increased chronic oxidative stress occurs despite the presence of Nrf2 in patients with HIV infection. The question arises as to how to activate ROS-resistant Nrf2 in these patients.

ANTIOXIDANTS ACTIVATE ROS-RESISTANT Nrf2

Some examples are vitamin E and genistein,[90] alpha-lipoic acid,[91] curcumin,[92] resveratrol,[93,94] omega-3-fatty acids,[95,96] glutathione,[97] NAC,[98] and coenzyme Q10.[99] Several plant-derived phytochemicals, such as epigallocatechin-3-gallate, carestol, kahweol, cinnamonyl-based compounds, zerumbone, lycopene and carnosol,[82,100,101] genistein,[90] allicin, a major organosulfur compound found in garlic,[102] sulforaphane, a organosulfur compound, found in cruciferous vegetables,[103] and kavalactones (methysticin, kavain, and yangonin).[104] The reasons for the activation of ROS-resistant Nrf2 by antioxidants are not known.

BINDING OF Nrf2 WITH ARE IN THE NUCLEUS

An activation of Nrf2 alone is not sufficient to increase the levels of antioxidant enzymes. Activated Nrf2 must bind with the ARE in the nucleus for increasing the expression of target genes coding for antioxidant enzymes. This binding ability of Nrf2 with the ARE was impaired in old rats and this defect was restored by supplementation with alpha-lipoic acid.[91] It is unknown whether the binding ability of Nrf2 with ARE is impaired in patients with HIV infection.

Nrf2 IN PATIENTS WITH HIV INFECTION

No studies have been performed on the expression of Nrf2 in the autopsied brain tissues of HIV/AIDS patients. Oxidative stress plays an important role in HIV associated neurocognitive disorders. HIV envelope protein gp120 induces apoptosis in human astrocytes in culture by increasing the levels of markers of oxidative stress and inflammation. This acute oxidative stress activates Nrf2 that is a transient adaptive protective response to ROS. Oxidative damage is more severe in the absence of Nrf2 than in the presence of Nrf2.[35,105] The fact that increased levels of oxidative stress and inflammation markers are found in patients with HIV infection/AIDS suggests that Nrf2 has become resistant to ROS. Studies should be performed on the levels of Nrf2 in the autopsied brain tissues as well as peripheral tissues.

REDUCING OXIDATIVE STRESS LEVEL IN HIV-INFECTED PEOPLE

Activation of Nrf2 may not be sufficient to optimally reduce oxidative stress, because antioxidants compounds are also decreased during chronic oxidative stress[106–108]; therefore, their levels must also be simultaneously elevated.

REDUCING INFLAMMATION LEVEL IN HIV-INFECTED PEOPLE

Activation of Nrf2[109,110] and some individual antioxidant compounds reduced chronic inflammation.[111–117]

PROPOSED MICRONUTRIENT MIXTURE FOR REDUCING OXIDATIVE STRESS AND INFLAMMATION LEVELS IN PATIENTS WITH HIV INFECTION

A comprehensive micronutrient mixture containing multiple dietary antioxidants (vitamin A, natural mixed carotenoids, vitamin C, vitamin E succinate, vitamin E acetate, selenomethionine, curcumin, resveratrol), endogenous antioxidants (alpha-lipoic acid, L-carnitine, and coenzyme Q10), a synthetic antioxidant N-acetylcysteine (NAC), vitamin D3, omega-3-fatty acids, all B-vitamins, and mineral zinc, is proposed. This mixture of micronutrients may optimally reduce oxidative stress and chronic inflammation by simultaneously enhancing the levels of antioxidant enzymes through activation of the Nrf2/ARE pathway, and elevation of the levels of antioxidants.

No iron, copper, or manganese would be included in this micronutrient mixture, because these trace minerals are known to interact with vitamin C to produce free radicals. These trace minerals are absorbed from the intestinal tract more in the presence of antioxidants than in their absence that could results in increased body stores of free forms of these minerals after a long-term consumption. Increased iron stores have been linked to increased risk of some neurodegenerative diseases.[118] In case of iron deficiency anemia, iron supplement can be administered until the anemia is corrected, but it may be given a few hours after micronutrient consumption. No heavy metals such as zirconium and molybdenum would be added because of their potential neurotoxicity after long-term consumption.

The recommended micronutrient supplements should be taken daily orally divided into two doses, one-half in the morning and the other-half in the evening with meal. This is because the biological half-lives of micronutrients are highly variable, which can create high levels of fluctuations in the tissue levels of micronutrients. A 2-fold difference in the levels of certain micronutrients such as alpha-tocopheryl succinate can cause a marked difference in the expression of gene profiles.[119] In order to maintain relatively steady levels of micronutrients in the body, the proposed micronutrients should be taken twice a day.

TOXICITY OF INGREDIENTS IN PROPOSED MICRONUTRIENT MIXTURE

Only a few antioxidants at very high doses are considered toxic. Vitamin A at doses of 10,000 IU or more per day can cause birth defects in pregnant women, and beta-carotene at doses 50 mg or more can produce bronzing of the skin that is reversible on discontinuation. Vitamin C as ascorbic acid at high doses (10 grams or more per day) can cause diarrhea in some individuals. Vitamin E at high doses (2,000 IU or more per day) can induce clotting defects after long-term consumption. Vitamin B6 at high doses (50 mg or more per day) may produce peripheral neuropathy, and selenium at doses 400 µg or more per day can cause skin and liver toxicity after long-term consumption.

All ingredients present in the proposed micronutrient mixture are safe and come under category of "food supplement" and therefore do not require FDA approval for their use.

PRIMARY PREVENTION AGAINST HIV INFECTION

Primary prevention refers to a strategy that would reduce the risk of HIV infection in normal uninfected populations. Although the primary prevention strategy appears to be the most rational for reducing the risk of HIV infection, an adequate attention has not been paid to this approach. At present, there are no specific recommendations for the primary prevention. Since the immune system is considered one of the primary targets for HIV infection, the use of proposed micronutrient mixture that would improve immune function appears to be one of the rational choices for primary prevention. In addition, avoiding the consumption of illicit drugs that impairs immune function, using clean needles for illicit drugs that would reduce the risk of transmission from HIV infected individuals to uninfected individuals, and safe sex for adults, may also help in reducing the risk of HIV infection throughout the world. The proposed strategy for primary prevention is cheap and nontoxic and easy to implement and could markedly reduce the risk of HIV infection in individuals especially those who are malnourished and those who regularly consume illicit drugs. Vaccines against HIV infection that are currently in the development phase could be of great help in the primary prevention strategy. Until then, the proposed strategy could be useful in prevention HIV infection. This strategy should be tested by well-designed clinical studies in subjects who have a high risk of developing HIV infection, such as malnourished individuals and individuals taking illicit drugs.

SECONDARY PREVENTION FOR REDUCING THE PROGRESSION OF HIV INFECTION

Secondary prevention refers to a strategy that would reduce the rate of progression of HIV infection in adults who were diagnosed with HIV infection but had not received antiviral therapy. Daily supplementation with the proposed micronutrient mixture may also be useful in reducing the progression of HIV infection in these individuals.

TREATMENTS OF HIV/AIDS

The evolution of antiviral therapy for the treatments of HIV/AIDS has led to the development of HAART that includes combination of three or more classes of antiviral drugs. They represent nucleoside and nucleotide reverse transcriptase inhibitors (nNRTI), non-nucleoside nucleotide reverse transcriptase inhibitors (NNRTI), protease inhibitors, integrase inhibitors, and entry inhibitors. NNRTI inhibits reverse transcriptase by incorporating themselves into the newly synthesized viral DNA preventing its function; nNRTI inhibits reverse transcriptase directly by binding to the enzyme and prevents further transcription of viruses; protease inhibitor stops the viral replication by inhibiting activity of protease, which is needed to complete the final assembly of HIV; integrase inhibitor inhibits enzyme integrase, which is responsible for integration of viral DNA into the DNA of infected cells, and thus stops virus production, and entry inhibitors help to prevent the virus from entering and infecting cells.

HAART has been useful in increasing the survival time of HIV/AIDS patients and slowing the rate of disease progression; but it has largely failed to produce any beneficial effect on HIV-related dementia.[120] At present, there is no effective treatment for HIV dementia. It has been reported that patients with apolipoprotein E (ApoE) 4 allele are more susceptible to oxidative damage-induced dementia.[120] The introduction of HAART has decreased HIV-associated oral lesions, but the incidence of oral warts and HIV-associated salivary gland disease increased in Brazil.[121] In addition, HAART increased oxidative stress that caused toxicities including metabolic bone diseases such as osteopenia and osteoporosis,[122] distal sensory polyneuropathy, cataracts, retinitis, cystoids macular edema,[123] and hyperlipidemia.[124] Some patients are forced to discontinue antiviral drugs because of toxicity. In addition, some HIV-infected individuals cannot tolerate antiviral drugs; some of them cannot afford these drugs financially. The introduction of HAART into HIV-infected people of Nicaragua has increased the death rate.[125] This could have been, in part, due to a nutritional deficiency that is common in developing countries. Therefore, additional approaches to improve the efficacy and reduce the toxicity of HAART are needed.

ANTIVIRAL THERAPY IN REDUCING THE RISK OF TRANSMISSION FROM MOTHER TO INFANTS

HIV transmission from mother to child during pregnancy, delivery, or breastfeeding, is referred to as prenatal transmission. This mode of transmission is the most common route of HIV infection in children in the USA. Most of the children with AIDS are from the minority ethnic groups.[126] Antiviral therapy administered to HIV-positive mother during pregnancy, labor and delivery, as well as during an elective cesarean and then to the newborn, can reduce the rate of prenatal HIV transmission to 2% or less.[127] If antiviral therapy to the HIV-positive mother is started during labor and delivery, the rate of HIV transmission to the newborn can be decreased to less than 10%.[128] Although the rate of HIV infection was markedly decreased in newborns by antiviral therapy to their mothers during pregnancy, labor, and delivery, the subsequent health status of these children has not been evaluated. In view of the fact that antiviral therapy even at low doses have potential to produce some late adverse health effect in children because this therapy is known to increase oxidative stress. Antioxidants that are known to reduce oxidative stress in combination with antiviral therapy could be useful in reducing the potential harmful effects of this therapy in children. The multiple micronutrients such as proposed in the section of Primary Prevention at lower doses may be useful in reducing the risk of prenatal transmission. Indeed, certain micronutrients may also reduce the rate of pre-natal transmission of HIV. A well-designed clinical study in which only one micronutrient (vitamin A containing 30 mg beta-carotene and 5000 IU preformed vitamin A) or multiple micronutrients containing two dietary antioxidants (500 mg vitamins C and 30 mg E), B-vitamins (20 mg B1, 20 mg B2, 25 mg B6, 100 mg niacin, 50 µg B12), and 0.8 mg folic acid were administered orally to immunologically and nutritionally compromised Tanzanian breastfeeding mothers. Some beneficial effects included reduced vertical transmission of HIV through breastfeeding to children and child mortality was observed.[129,130] Micronutrient treatment of during pregnancy improved body weight of fetuses and immune function, and lowered viral load and hypertension was observed.[131]

PROPOSED MICRONUTRIENT MIXTURE IN COMBINATION WITH ANTIVIRAL DRUGS

Since most antiviral drugs can increase oxidative stress and are very toxic, supplementation with the proposed micronutrient mixture multiple micronutrients may improve the efficacy of the antiviral therapy in patients with HIV/AIDS. Indeed, alpha-tocopheryl succinate reduced the toxicity of AZT in lymphocyte culture.[66] Vitamin C and vitamin E supplementation reduced AZT-induced cardiac damage in mice.[132] The coadministration of antioxidants and AZT increases the therapeutic potential of AZT.[133]

In contrast to laboratory studies, clinical trials with one or two antioxidants in combination with antiviral therapy have produced inconsistent results varying from no effects to beneficial effects. In a randomized-placebo-controlled trial in which 49 HIV-positive patients participated, supplementation with dl-alpha-tocopheryl acetate (800 IU/day and vitamin C (1000 mg/day) was administered orally for a period of 3 months. The results showed that supplementation reduced oxidative stress compared to placebo control. In addition, a trend towards a reduction in viral load was observed in supplemented group.[134] A review on the efficacy of micronutrients supplementation in HIV-positive patients taking HAART has concluded that supplementation did not improve the efficacy of HAART.[135] In a randomized, double-blind, placebo-controlled trial with HIV-positive patients receiving antiviral therapy, supplementation with NAC alone for 180 days did not improve the efficacy of antiviral therapy.[136] In a prospective, double-blind, placebo-controlled trial, 40 HIV-positive patients taking HAART were randomized to receive micronutrients or placebo twice daily for 12 weeks. The results showed that micronutrients supplementation significantly improved CD4+ lymphocyte counts in patients taking HAART.[137]

CONCLUSIONS

Emergence of pathogenic HIV has greatly alarmed health professionals throughout the world. Although most HIV-infected persons progress to AIDS, some do not. This implies that the immune system of some individuals is competent enough to mount a defensive response against HIV. The role of immune system in HIV infection is further supported by the fact that micronutrient deficiency and illicit drugs that are known to impair immune function increase the risk of HIV infection. However, the current primary prevention strategy has not emphasized the importance of stimulating immune system for reducing the risk of HIV infection. The increased oxidative stress and chronic inflammation appear to increase the risk of HIV infection as well as enhance the progression of the disease by impairing immune function and allowing replication of HIV virus. Therefore, attenuation of oxidative damage and inflammatory events may prevent the HIV Infection and its progression. Previous studies using single micronutrients or randomly selected a few micronutrients have produced inconsistent results. I have proposed that elevation of the levels of antioxidant enzymes and dietary and endogenous antioxidants is essential for optimally and simultaneously reducing oxidative stress, inflammation, and improving immune function. The levels of dietary and endogenous antioxidants can be increased by supplementation, but increasing the levels of antioxidant enzymes requires an activation of Nrf2. During chronic oxidative stress found in HIV-infected individuals, Nrf2 becomes resistant to ROS; however, certain antioxidants activate ROS-resistant Nrf2. A mixture of micronutrients that would activate the Nrf2/ARE pathway and elevate the levels of dietary and endogenous antioxidants is proposed for primary and secondary prevention of HIV infection. The introduction of highly active anti-retroviral therapy (HAART) has improved the survival time of patients with AIDS, but it has failed to affect the risk of developing dementia, and it is very toxic. Low-dose HAART is also used in preventing the transmission of virus from the infected- to uninfected persons with limited success. The proposed micronutrient mixture in combination antiviral therapy may improve the effectiveness of antiviral therapy by decreasing the viral load and reducing side effects. Clinical studies with the proposed micronutrient mixture should be initiated to test its efficacy in prevention, and in combination with antiviral therapy in improved management of HIV-infected patients. In the meanwhile, those individuals who are at high risk for HIV infection, and those patients with HIV infection with or without antiviral drugs may like to adopt the proposed micronutrient preparations in consultations with their doctors.

REFERENCES

1. 1994–2004 TDoDs. *Lessoned Learned and New Challenges: Worshop.* Washington DC: National Academic Press; 2008.
2. Baum MK, Miguez-Burbano MJ, Campa A, Shor-Posner G. Selenium and interleukins in persons infected with human immunodeficiency virus type 1. *J Infect Dis.* 2000;182 Suppl 1:S69–73.
3. Favier A, Sappey C, Leclerc P, Faure P, Micoud M. Antioxidant status and lipid peroxidation in patients infected with HIV. *Chem Biol Interact.* 1994;91(2–3):165–180.

4. Liang B, Chung S, Araghiniknam M, Lane LC, Watson RR. Vitamins and immunomodulation in AIDS. *Nutrition.* 1996;12(1):1–7.

5. Patrick L. Nutrients and HIV: Part 2: vitamins A and E, zinc, B-vitamins, and magnesium. *Altern Med Rev.* 2000;5(1):39–51.

6. Ullrich R, Schneider T, Heise W, et al. Serum carotene deficiency in HIV-infected patients. Berlin Diarrhoea/Wasting Syndrome Study Group. *AIDS.* 1994;8(5):661–665.

7. Dworkin BM. Selenium deficiency in HIV infection and the acquired immunodeficiency syndrome (AIDS). *Chem Biol Interact.* 1994;91(2–3):181–186.

8. Omene JA, Easington CR, Glew RH, Prosper M, Ledlie S. Serum beta-carotene deficiency in HIV-infected children. *J Natl Med Assoc.* 1996;88(12):789–793.

9. Periquet BA, Jammes NM, Lambert WE, et al. Micronutrient levels in HIV-1-infected children. *AIDS.* 1995;9(8):887–893.

10. Kupka R, Garland M, Msamanga G, Spiegelman D, Hunter D, Fawzi W. Selenium status, pregnancy outcomes, and mother-to-child transmission of HIV-1. *J Acquir Immune Defic Syndr.* 2005;39(2):203–210.

11. Jordao Junior AA, Silveira S, Figueiredo JF, Vannucchi H. Urinary excretion and plasma vitamin E levels in patients with AIDS. *Nutrition.* 1998;14(5):423–426.

12. Patrick L. Nutrients and HIV: Part 1—Beta carotene and selenium. *Altern Med Rev.* 1999;4(6):403–413.

13. Foster HD. How HIV-1 causes AIDS: Implications for prevention and treatment. *Med Hypotheses.* 2004;62(4):549–553.

14. Look MP, Rockstroh JK, Rao GS, Kreuzer KA, Spengler U, Sauerbruch T. Serum selenium versus lymphocyte subsets and markers of disease progression and inflammatory response in human immunodeficiency virus-1 infection. *Biol Trace Elem Res.* 1997;56(1):31–41.

15. Rayman MP, Rayman MP. The argument for increasing selenium intake. *Proc Nutr Soc.* 2002;61(2):203–215.

16. Shor-Posner G, Miguez MJ, Pineda LM, et al. Impact of selenium status on the pathogenesis of mycobacterial disease in HIV-1-infected drug users during the era of highly active antiretroviral therapy. *J Acquir Immune Defic Syndr.* 2002;29(2):169–173.

17. Tang AM, Smit E. Selected vitamins in HIV infection: A review. *AIDS Patient Care STDS.* 1998;12(4):263–273.

18. Friedman H, Newton C, Klein TW. Microbial infections, immunomodulation, and drugs of abuse. *Clin Microbiol Rev.* 2003;16(2):209–219.

19. Lugoboni F, Quaglio G, Pajusco B, et al. Immunogenicity, reactogenicity, and adherence to a combined hepatitis A and B vaccine in illicit drug users. *Addiction.* 2004;99(12):1560–1564.

20. Conner TJ. Methyllenedioxymethamphetamine (MDMA, Ectasy): A stressor on the immune system. *Immnunology.* 2004;111:357–367.

21. Nair MP, Schwartz SA, Mahajan SD, et al. Drug abuse and neuropathogenesis of HIV infection: Role of DC-SIGN and IDO. *J Neuroimmunol.* 2004;157(1–2):56–60.

22. Nair MP, Mahajan S, Hewitt R, Whitney ZR, Schwartz SA. Association of drug abuse with inhibition of HIV-1 immune responses: Studies with long-term of HIV-1 non-progressors. *J Neuroimmunol.* 2004;147(1–2):21–25.

23. Arango JC, Simmonds P, Brettle RP, Bell JE. Does drug abuse influence the microglial response in AIDS and HIV encephalitis? *AIDS.* 2004;18 Suppl 1:S69–S74.

24. Dronda F, Zamora J, Moreno S, et al. CD4 cell recovery during successful antiretroviral therapy in naive HIV-infected patients: The role of intravenous drug use. *AIDS.* 2004;18(16):2210–2212.

25. Anthony IC, Arango JC, Stephens B, Simmonds P, Bell JE. The effects of illicit drugs on the HIV infected brain. *Front Biosci.* 2008;13:1294–1307.

26. Greenspan HC. The role of reactive oxygen species, antioxidants, and phytopharmaceuticals in human immunodeficiency virus activity. *Med Hypotheses.* 1993;40(2):85–92.

27. Repetto M, Reides C, Gomez Carretero ML, Costa M, Griemberg G, Llesuy S. Oxidative stress in blood of HIV infected patients. *Clin Chim Acta.* 1996;255(2):107–117.

28. Baruchel S, Wainberg MA. The role of oxidative stress in disease progression in individuals infected by the human immunodeficiency virus. *J Leukoc Biol.* 1992;52(1):111–114.

29. Toborek M, Lee YW, Pu H, et al. HIV-Tat protein induces oxidative and inflammatory pathways in brain endothelium. *J Neurochem.* 2003;84(1):169–179.

30. Zhang Y, Wang M, Li H, et al. Accumulation of nuclear and mitochondrial DNA damage in the frontal cortex cells of patients with HIV-associated neurocognitive disorders. *Brain Res.* 2012;1458:1–11.

31. Sacktor N, Haughey N, Cutler R, et al. Novel markers of oxidative stress in actively progressive HIV dementia. *J Neuroimmunol.* 2004;157(1–2):176–184.

32. Walmsley SL, Winn LM, Harrison ML, Uetrecht JP, Wells PG. Oxidative stress and thiol depletion in plasma and peripheral blood lymphocytes from HIV-infected patients: Toxicological and pathological implications. *AIDS.* 1997;11(14):1689–1697.

33. Kallianpur KJ, Gerschenson M, Mitchell BI, et al. Oxidative mitochondrial DNA damage in peripheral blood mononuclear cells is associated with reduced volumes of hippocampus and subcortical gray matter in chronically HIV-infected patients. *Mitochondrion.* 2016;28:8–15.

34. Mollace V, Salvemini D, Riley DP, et al. The contribution of oxidative stress in apoptosis of human-cultured astroglial cells induced by supernatants of HIV-1-infected macrophages. *J Leukoc Biol.* 2002;71(1):65–72.

35. Reddy PV, Gandhi N, Samikkannu T, et al. HIV-1 gp120 induces antioxidant response element-mediated expression in primary astrocytes: Role in HIV associated neurocognitive disorder. *Neurochem Int.* 2012;61(5):807–814.

36. Ambegaokar SS, Kolson DL. Heme oxygenase-1 dysregulation in the brain: Implications for HIV-associated neurocognitive disorders. *Curr HIV Res.* 2014;12(3):174–188.

37. Allard JP, Aghdassi E, Chau J, Salit I, Walmsley S. Oxidative stress and plasma antioxidant micronutrients in humans with HIV infection. *Am J Clin Nutr.* 1998;67(1):143–147.

38. Ande A, Sinha N, Rao PS, et al. Enhanced oxidative stress by alcohol use in HIV+ patients: Possible involvement of cytochrome P450 2E1 and antioxidant enzymes. *AIDS Res Ther.* 2015;12:29.

39. Ande A, McArthur C, Ayuk L, et al. Effect of mild-to-moderate smoking on viral load, cytokines, oxidative stress, and cytochrome P450 enzymes in HIV-infected individuals. *PLoS One.* 2015;10(4):e0122402.

40. Huang X, Liang H, Fan X, Zhu L, Shen T. Liver damage in patients with HCV/HIV coinfection is linked to HIV-related oxidative stress. *Oxid Med Cell Longev.* 2016;2016:8142431.

41. Masia M, Padilla S, Fernandez M, et al. Oxidative stress predicts all-cause mortality in HIV-infected patients. *PLoS One.* 2016;11(4):e0153456.

42. Isaguliants M, Smirnova O, Ivanov AV, et al. Oxidative stress induced by HIV-1 reverse transcriptase modulates the enzyme's performance in gene immunization. *Hum Vaccin Immunother.* 2013;9(10):2111–2119.

43. Awodele O, Olayemi SO, Nwite JA, Adeyemo TA. Investigation of the levels of oxidative stress parameters in HIV and HIV-TB coinfected patients. *J Infect Dev Ctries.* 2012;6(1):79–85.

44. Boven LA, Gomes L, Hery C, et al. Increased peroxynitrite activity in AIDS dementia complex: Implications for the neuropathogenesis of HIV-1 infection. *J Immunol.* 1999;162(7):4319–4327.

45. Aldrich TK, Gustave J, Hall CB, et al. Lung function in rescue workers at the World Trade Center after 7 years. *N Engl J Med.* 2010;362(14):1263–1272.

46. Nixon DE, Landay AL. Biomarkers of immune dysfunction in HIV. *Curr Opin HIV AIDS.* 2010;5(6):498–503.

47. Reznick AZ, Cross CE, Hu ML, et al. Modification of plasma proteins by cigarette smoke as measured by protein carbonyl formation. *Biochem J.* 1992;286 (Pt 2):607–611.

48. Suzuki YJ, Packer L. Inhibition of NF-kappa B activation by vitamin E derivatives. *Biochem Biophys Res Commun.* 1993;193(1):277–283.

49. Aounallah M, Dagenais-Lussier X, El-Far M, et al. Current topics in HIV pathogenesis, part 2: Inflammation drives a Warburg-like effect on the metabolism of HIV-infected subjects. *Cytokine Growth Factor Rev.* 2016;28:1–10.

50. Freeman ML, Lederman MM, Gianella S. Partners in crime: The role of CMV in immune dysregulation and clinical outcome during HIV infections. *Curr HIV/AIDS Rep.* 2016;13(1):10–19.

51. Vendrame E, Hussain SK, Breen EC, et al. Serum levels of cytokines and biomarkers for inflammation and immune activation, and HIV-associated non-Hodgkin B-cell lymphoma risk. *Cancer Epidemiol Biomarkers Prev.* 2014;23(2):343–349.

52. Hsu DC, Sereti I. Serious Non-AIDS events: Therapeutic targets of immune activation and chronic inflammation in HIV infection. *Drugs.* 2016;76(5):533–549.

53. Bricaire F, Valantin MA. Inflammation and HIV. *Bull Acad Natl Med.* 2011;195(3):531–542; discussion 543–534.

54. Wilson EM, Singh A, Hullsiek KH, et al. Monocyte-activation phenotypes are associated with biomarkers of inflammation and coagulation in chronic HIV infection. *J Infect Dis.* 2014;210(9):1396–1406.

55. Gupta SK, Kitch D, Tierney C, et al. Markers of renal disease and function are associated with systemic inflammation in HIV infection. *HIV Med.* 2015;16(10):591–598.

56. Beltran LM, Rubio-Navarro A, Amaro-Villalobos JM, Egido J, Garcia-Puig J, Moreno JA. Influence of immune activation and inflammatory response on cardiovascular risk associated with the human immunodeficiency virus. *Vasc Health Risk Manag.* 2015;11:35–48.

57. Ofotokun I, McIntosh E, Weitzmann MN. HIV: Inflammation and bone. *Curr HIV/AIDS Rep.* 2012;9(1):16–25.

58. Massanella M, Fromentin R, Chomont N. Residual inflammation and viral reservoirs: Alliance against an HIV cure. *Curr Opin HIV AIDS.* 2016;11(2):234–241.

59. Piggott DA, Varadhan R, Mehta SH, et al. Frailty, inflammation, and mortality among persons aging with HIV infection and injection drug use. *J Gerontol A Biol Sci Med Sci.* 2015;70(12):1542–1547.

60. Mollace V, Nottet HS, Clayette P, et al. Oxidative stress and neuroAIDS: Triggers, modulators, and novel antioxidants. *Trends Neurosci.* 2001;24(7):411–416.

61. Turchan J, Pocernich CB, Gairola C, et al. Oxidative stress in HIV demented patients and protection ex vivo with novel antioxidants. *Neurology.* 2003;60(2):307–314.

62. Harakeh S, Jariwalla RJ, Pauling L. Suppression of human immunodeficiency virus replication by ascorbate in chronically and acutely infected cells. *Proc Natl Acad Sci USA.* 1990;87(18):7245–7249.

63. Hori K, Hatfield D, Maldarelli F, Lee BJ, Clouse KA. Selenium supplementation suppresses tumor necrosis factor alpha-induced human immunodeficiency virus type 1 replication *in vitro. AIDS Res Hum Retroviruses.* 1997;13(15):1325–1332.

64. Tan JS, Wang JJ, Flood V, Rochtchina E, Smith W, Mitchell P. Dietary antioxidants and the long-term incidence of age-related macular degeneration: The Blue Mountains eye study. *Ophthalmology.* 2008;115(2):334–341.

65. Hurwitz BE, Klaus JR, Llabre MM, et al. Suppression of human immunodeficiency virus type 1 viral load with selenium supplementation: A randomized controlled trial. *Arch Intern Med.* 2007;167(2):148–154.

66. Gogu SR, Lertora JJ, George WJ, Hyslop NE, Agrawal KC. Protection of zidovudine-induced toxicity against murine erythroid progenitor cells by vitamin E. *Exp Hematol.* 1991;19(7):649–652.

67. Li-Weber M, Weigand MA, Giaisi M, et al. Vitamin E inhibits CD95 ligand expression and protects T cells from activation-induced cell death. *J Clin Invest.* 2002;110(5):681–690.

68. Ly JV, Zavala JA, Donnan GA. Neuroprotection and thrombolysis: Combination therapy in acute ischaemic stroke. *Expert Opin Pharmacother.* 2006;7(12):1571–1581.

69. Fryburg DA, Mark RJ, Griffith BP, Askenase PW, Patterson TF. The effect of supplemental beta-carotene on immunologic indices in patients with AIDS: A pilot study. *Yale J Biol Med.* 1995;68(1–2):19–23.

70. Santamaria L, Bianchi-Santamaria A, dell'Orti M. Carotenoids in cancer, mastalgia, and AIDS: Prevention and treatment: An overview. *J Environ Pathol Toxicol Oncol.* 1996;15(2–4):89–95.

71. Batterham M, Gold J, Naidoo D, et al. A preliminary open label dose comparison using an antioxidant regimen to determine the effect on viral load and oxidative stress in men with HIV/AIDS. *Eur J Clin Nutr.* 2001;55(2):107–114.

72. Muller F, Svardal AM, Nordoy I, Berge RK, Aukrust P, Froland SS. Virological and immunological effects of antioxidant treatment in patients with HIV infection. *Eur J Clin Invest.* 2000;30(10):905–914.

73. Prasad S, Tyagi AK. Curcumin and its analogues: A potential natural compound against HIV infection and AIDS. *Food Funct.* 2015;6(11):3412–3419.

74. Fawzi WW, Msamanga GI, Wei R, et al. Effect of providing vitamin supplements to human immunodeficiency virus-infected, lactating mothers on the child's morbidity and CD4+ cell counts. *Clin Infect Dis.* 2003;36(8):1053–1062.

75. Fawzi WW, Msamanga GI, Kupka R, et al. Multivitamin supplementation improves hematologic status in HIV-infected women and their children in Tanzania. *Am J Clin Nutr.* 2007;85(5):1335–1343.

76. Isanaka S, Mugusi F, Hawkins C, et al. Effect of high-dose vs standard-dose multivitamin supplementation at the initiation of HAART on HIV disease progression and mortality in Tanzania: A randomized controlled trial. *JAMA.* 2012;308(15):1535–1544.

77. Visser ME, Durao S, Sinclair D, Irlam JH, Siegfried N. Micronutrient supplementation in adults with HIV infection. *Cochrane Database Syst Rev.* 2017;5:CD003650.

78. Vile GF, Winterbourn CC. Inhibition of adriamycin-promoted microsomal lipid peroxidation by beta-carotene, alpha-tocopherol, and retinol at high and low oxygen partial pressures. *FEBS Lett.* 1988;238(2):353–356.

79. Niki E. Interaction of ascorbate and alpha-tocopherol. *Ann N Y Acad Sci.* 1987;498:186–199.

80. Prasad KN. Oxidative stress and pro-inflammatory cytokines may act as one of signals for regulating microRNAs expression in Alzheimer'sdisease. *Mech Ageing Dev.* 2017;162:63–71.

81. Wu H, Kong L, Tan Y, et al. C66 ameliorates diabetic nephropathy in mice by both upregulating NRF2 function via increase in miR-200a and inhibiting miR-21. *Diabetologia.* 2016;59:1558–1568.

82. Jaramillo MC, Zhang DD. The emerging role of the Nrf2-Keap1 signaling pathway in cancer. *Genes Dev.* 2013;27(20):2179–2191.

83. Williamson TP, Johnson DA, Johnson JA. Activation of the Nrf2-ARE pathway by siRNA knockdown of Keap1 reduces oxidative stress and provides partial protection from MPTP-mediated neurotoxicity. *Neurotoxicology.* 2012;33(3):272–279.

84. Itoh K, Chiba T, Takahashi S, et al. An Nrf2/small Maf heterodimer mediates the induction of phase II detoxifying enzyme genes through antioxidant response elements. *Biochem Biophys Res Commun.* 1997;236(2):313–322.

85. Hayes JD, Chanas SA, Henderson CJ, et al. The Nrf2 transcription factor contributes both to the basal expression of glutathione S-transferases in mouse liver and to their induction by the chemopreventive synthetic antioxidants, butylated hydroxyanisole, and ethoxyquin. *Biochem Soc Trans.* 2000;28(2):33–41.

86. Chan K, Han XD, Kan YW. An important function of Nrf2 in combating oxidative stress: Detoxification of acetaminophen. *Proc Natl Acad Sci USA.* 2001;98(8):4611–4616.

87. Ramsey CP, Glass CA, Montgomery MB, et al. Expression of Nrf2 in neurodegenerative diseases. *J Neuropathol Exp Neurol.* 2007;66(1):75–85.

88. Chen PC, Vargas MR, Pani AK, et al. Nrf2-mediated neuroprotection in the MPTP mouse model of Parkinson's disease: Critical role for the astrocyte. *Proc Natl Acad Sci USA.* 2009;106(8):2933–2938.

89. Lastres-Becker I, Ulusoy A, Innamorato NG, et al. Alpha-synuclein expression and Nrf2 deficiency cooperate to aggravate protein aggregation, neuronal death, and inflammation in early-stage Parkinson's disease. *Hum Mol Genet.* 2012;21(14):3173–3192.

90. Xi YD, Yu HL, Ding J, et al. Flavonoids protect cerebrovascular endothelial cells through Nrf2 and PI3K from beta-amyloid peptide-induced oxidative damage. *Curr Neurovasc Res.* 2012;9(1):32–41.

91. Suh JH, Shenvi SV, Dixon BM, et al. Decline in transcriptional activity of Nrf2 causes age-related loss of glutathione synthesis, which is reversible with lipoic acid. *Proc Natl Acad Sci USA.* 2004;101(10):3381–3386.

92. Trujillo J, Chirino YI, Molina-Jijon E, Anderica-Romero AC, Tapia E, Pedraza-Chaverri J. Renoprotective effect of the antioxidant curcumin: Recent findings. *Redox Biol.* 2013;1(1):448–456.

93. Steele ML, Fuller S, Patel M, Kersaitis C, Ooi L, Munch G. Effect of Nrf2 activators on release of glutathione, cysteinylglycine and homocysteine by human U373 astroglial cells. *Redox Biol.* 2013;1(1):441–445.

94. Kode A, Rajendrasozhan S, Caito S, Yang SR, Megson IL, Rahman I. Resveratrol induces glutathione synthesis by activation of Nrf2 and protects against cigarette smoke-mediated oxidative stress in human lung epithelial cells. *Am j Physiol Lung Cell Mol Physiol.* 2008;294(3):L478–L488.

95. Gao L, Wang J, Sekhar KR, et al. Novel n-3 fatty acid oxidation products activate Nrf2 by destabilizing the association between Keap1 and Cullin3. *J Biol Chem.* 2007;282(4):2529–2537.

96. Saw CL, Yang AY, Guo Y, Kong AN. Astaxanthin and omega-3 fatty acids individually and in combination protect against oxidative stress via the Nrf2-ARE pathway. *Food Chem Toxicol.* 2013;62:869–875.

97. Song J, Kang SM, Lee WT, Park KA, Lee KM, Lee JE. Glutathione protects brain endothelial cells from hydrogen peroxide-induced oxidative stress by increasing nrf2 expression. *Exp Neurobiol.* 2014;23(1):93–103.

98. Ji L, Liu R, Zhang XD, et al. N-acetylcysteine attenuates phosgene-induced acute lung injury via upregulation of Nrf2 expression. *Inhal Toxicol.* 2010;22(7):535–542.

99. Choi HK, Pokharel YR, Lim SC, et al. Inhibition of liver fibrosis by solubilized coenzyme Q10: Role of Nrf2 activation in inhibiting transforming growth factor-beta1 expression. *Toxicol Appl Pharmacol.* 2009;240(3):377–384.

100. Bai H, Liu R, Chen HL, et al. Enhanced antioxidant effect of caffeic acid phenethyl ester and Trolox in combination against radiation induced-oxidative stress. *Chem Biol Interact.* 2014;207:7–15.

101. Cui L, Jeong H, Borovecki F, Parkhurst CN, Tanese N, Krainc D. Transcriptional repression of PGC-1alpha by mutant huntingtin leads to mitochondrial dysfunction and neurodegeneration. *Cell.* 2006;127(1):59–69.

102. Li XH, Li CY, Lu JM, Tian RB, Wei J. Allicin ameliorates cognitive deficits ageing-induced learning and memory deficits through enhancing of Nrf2 antioxidant signaling pathways. *Neurosci Lett.* 2012;514(1):46–50.

103. Bergstrom P, Andersson HC, Gao Y, et al. Repeated transient sulforaphane stimulation in astrocytes leads to prolonged Nrf2-mediated gene expression and protection from superoxide-induced damage. *Neuropharmacology.* 2011;60(2–3):343–353.

104. Wruck CJ, Gotz ME, Herdegen T, Varoga D, Brandenburg LO, Pufe T. Kavalactones protect neural cells against amyloid beta peptide-induced neurotoxicity via extracellular signal-regulated kinase 1/2-dependent nuclear factor erythroid 2-related factor 2 activation. *Mol Pharmacol.* 2008;73(6):1785–1795.

105. Reddy PV, Agudelo M, Atluri VS, Nair MP. Inhibition of nuclear factor erythroid 2-related factor 2 exacerbates HIV-1 gp120-induced oxidative and inflammatory response: Role in HIV associated neuro-cognitive disorder. *Neurochem Res.* 2012;37(8):1697–1706.

106. Song SM, Park YS, Lee A, et al. Concentrations of blood vitamin A, C, E, coenzyme Q10, and urine cotinine related to cigarette smoking exposure. *Korean J Lab Med.* 2009;29(1):10–16.

107. Galan P, Viteri FE, Bertrais S, et al. Serum concentrations of beta-carotene, vitamins C and E, zinc and selenium are influenced by sex, age, diet, smoking status, alcohol consumption, and corpulence in a general French adult population. *Eur J Clin Nutr.* 2005;59(10):1181–1190.

108. Adhikari D, Baxi J, Risal S, Singh PP. Oxidative stress and antioxidant status in cancer patients and healthy subjects, a case-control study. *Nepal Med Coll J.* 2005;7(2):112–115.

109. Li W, Khor TO, Xu C, et al. Activation of Nrf2-antioxidant signaling attenuates NFkappaB-inflammatory response and elicits apoptosis. *Biochem Pharmacol.* 2008;76(11):1485–1489.

110. Kim J, Cha YN, Surh YJ. A protective role of nuclear factor-erythroid 2-related factor-2 (Nrf2) in inflammatory disorders. *Mutat Res.* 2010;690(1–2):12–23.

111. Abate A, Yang G, Dennery PA, Oberle S, Schroder H. Synergistic inhibition of cyclooxygenase-2 expression by vitamin E and aspirin. *Free Radic Biol Med.* 2000;29(11):1135–1142.

112. Devaraj S, Tang R, Adams-Huet B, et al. Effect of high-dose alpha-tocopherol supplementation on biomarkers of oxidative stress and inflammation and carotid atherosclerosis in patients with coronary artery disease. *Am J Clin Nutr.* 2007;86(5):1392–1398.

113. Fu Y, Zheng S, Lin J, Ryerse J, Chen A. Curcumin protects the rat liver from CCl$_4$-caused injury and fibrogenesis by attenuating oxidative stress and suppressing inflammation. *Mol Pharmacol.* 2008;73(2):399–409.

114. Lee HS, Jung KK, Cho JY, et al. Neuroprotective effect of curcumin is mainly mediated by blockade of microglial cell activation. *Pharmazie.* 2007;62(12):937–942.

115. Rahman S, Bhatia K, Khan AQ, et al. Topically applied vitamin E prevents massive cutaneous inflammatory and oxidative stress responses induced by double application of 12-O-tetradecanoylphorbol-13-acetate (TPA) in mice. *Chem Biol Interact.* 2008;172(3):195–205.

116. Suzuki YJ, Aggarwal BB, Packer L. Alpha-lipoic acid is a potent inhibitor of NF-kappa B activation in human T cells. *Biochem Biophys Res Commun.* 1992;189(3):1709–1715.

117. Zhu J, Yong W, Wu X, et al. Anti-inflammatory effect of resveratrol on TNF-alpha-induced MCP-1 expression in adipocytes. *Biochem Biophys Res Commun.* 2008;369(2):471–477.

118. Olanow CW, Arendash GW. Metals and free radicals in neurodegeneration. *Curr Opin Neurol.* 1994;7(6):548–558.

119. Prasad KN, Kumar B, Yan XD, Hanson AJ, Cole WC. Alpha-tocopheryl succinate, the most effective form of vitamin E for adjuvant cancer treatment: A review. *J Am Coll Nutr.* 2003;22(2):108–117.

120. Steiner J, Haughey N, Li W, et al. Oxidative stress and therapeutic approaches in HIV dementia. *Antioxid Redox Signal.* 2006;8(11–12):2089–2100.

121. Ferreira S, Noce C, Junior AS, et al. Prevalence of oral manifestations of HIV infection in Rio De Janeiro, Brazil from 1988 to 2004. *AIDS Patient Care STDS.* 2007;21(10):724–731.

122. Pan G, Yang Z, Ballinger SW, McDonald JM. Pathogenesis of osteopenia/osteoporosis induced by highly active anti-retroviral therapy for AIDS. *Ann N Y Acad Sci.* 2006;1068:297–308.

123. Thorne JE, Jabs DA, Kempen JH, et al. Causes of visual acuity loss among patients with AIDS and cytomegalovirus retinitis in the era of highly active antiretroviral therapy. *Ophthalmology.* 2006;113(8):1441–1445.

124. Benesic A, Zilly M, Kluge F, et al. Lipid lowering therapy with fluvastatin and pravastatin in patients with HIV infection and antiretroviral therapy: Comparison of efficacy and interaction with indinavir. *Infection.* 2004;32(4):229–233.

125. Matute AJ, Delgado E, Amador JJ, Hoepelman AI. The epidemiology of clinically apparent HIV infection in Nicaragua. *Eur J Clin Microbiol Infect Dis.* 2008;27(2):105–108.

126. Davis RR, Kuo MW, Stanton SG, Canlon B, Krieg E, Alagramam KN. N-Acetyl L-cysteine does not protect against premature age-related hearing loss in C57BL/6J mice: A pilot study. *Hear Res.* 2007;226(1–2):203–208.

127. Weber T, Dalen H, Andera L, et al. Mitochondria play a central role in apoptosis induced by alpha-tocopheryl succinate, an agent with antineoplastic activity: Comparison with receptor-mediated pro-apoptotic signaling. *Biochemistry.* 2003;42(14):4277–4291.

128. Wade NA, Birkhead GS, Warren BL, et al. Abbreviated regimens of zidovudine prophylaxis and perinatal transmission of the human immunodeficiency virus. *N Engl J Med.* 1998;339(20):1409–1414.

129. Fawzi WW, Msamanga GI, Hunter D, et al. Randomized trial of vitamin supplements in relation to transmission of HIV-1 through breastfeeding and early child mortality. *AIDS*. 2002;16(14):1935–1944.
130. Fawzi WW, Msamanga GI, Spiegelman D, et al. A randomized trial of multivitamin supplements and HIV disease progression and mortality. *N Engl J Med*. 2004;351(1):23–32.
131. Merchant AT, Msamanga G, Villamor E, et al. Multivitamin supplementation of HIV-positive women during pregnancy reduces hypertension. *J Nutr*. 2005;135(7):1776–1781.
132. de la Asuncion JG, Del Olmo ML, Gomez-Cambronero LG, Sastre J, Pallardo FV, Vina J. AZT induces oxidative damage to cardiac mitochondria: Protective effect of vitamins C and E. *Life Sci*. 2004;76(1):47–56.
133. Romero-Alvira D, Roche E. The keys of oxidative stress in acquired immune deficiency syndrome apoptosis. *Med Hypotheses*. 1998;51(2):169–173.
134. Allard JP, Aghdassi E, Chau J, et al. Effects of vitamins E and C supplementation on oxidative stress and viral load in HIV-infected subjects. *AIDS*. 1998;12(13):1653–1659.
135. Drain PK, Kupka R, Mugusi F, Fawzi WW. Micronutrients in HIV-positive persons receiving highly active antiretroviral therapy. *Am J Clin Nutr*. 2007;85(2):333–345.
136. Treitinger A, Spada C, Masokawa IY, et al. Effect of N-acetyl-L-cysteine on lymphocyte apoptosis, lymphocyte viability, TNF-alpha, and IL-8 in HIV-infected patients undergoing anti-retroviral treatment. *Braz J Infect Dis*. 2004;8(5):363–371.
137. Kaiser JD, Campa AM, Ondercin JP, Leoung GS, Pless RF, Baum MK. Micronutrient supplementation increases CD4 count in HIV-infected individuals on highly active antiretroviral therapy: A prospective, double-blinded, placebo-controlled trial. *J Acquir Immune Defic Syndr*. 2006;42(5):523–528.

15 Improved Management of Autism Spectrum Disorder (ASD) by Micronutrients

INTRODUCTION

Autism spectrum disorder (ASD) refers to a group of complex brain development disorders. This includes autistic disorders and Asperger's syndrome (AS). The symptoms of AS are generally milder than classical autism. The symptoms of ASD and attention deficit hyperactivity (ADHD) syndrome overlap. The exact causes of ASD are poorly understood; however, environmental and genetic factors are considered contributing agents. Among biochemical abnormalities, increased oxidative stress, inflammation, and glutamate initiate and promote the progression of ASD. Therefore, simultaneous attenuation of these biochemical defects may reduce the risk of developing ASD, and in combination with standard care, improve the management of this disease.

This chapter describes prevalence, cost, environmental and genetic factors, major symptoms, and brain pathology and presents evidence to show that increased oxidative stress, inflammation, and glutamate are involved in development and progression of ASD. It proposes a hypothesis that in order to simultaneously reduce the above biochemical defects, it is essential to increase the levels of antioxidant enzymes, dietary and endogenous antioxidants, and prevent the release and toxicity of glutamate. This chapter also suggests a mixture of micronutrients that may simultaneously attenuate these biochemical abnormalities involved in ASD, and thereby prevent and, in combination with standard therapy, improve the management of this disorder.

PREVALENCE AND COST OF ASD

PREVALENCE

The prevalence of ASD in the USA is increasing. In 2000, the prevalence per 1000 children was 6.7% (age 4.5 to 9.9 years); in 2008 it was 11.3% (age 4.8 to 21.2 years); and in 2012 it was 14.6% (age 8.2 to 24.6 years).[1] ASD occurs in all racial, ethnic, and socioeconomic groups. Prevalence of ASD is about 4.5 times more among boys (1 in 42 children) than among girls (1 in 189 children).

COST

In the USA, the total annual direct and indirect cost of management of children with ASD is about $11.5–$60.9 billion (in 2011 US dollars). In 2013, the cost of supporting individuals with ASD with intellectual disability during his or her lifespan was $2.4 million; whereas it was $1.4 million for those with ASD without intellectual disabilities.[2]

ENVIRONMENTAL AND GENETIC FACTORS

ENVIRONMENTAL FACTORS

Environmental and genetic factors contribute to the etiology of ASD. Environmental factors include exposure to organic pollutants, such as dichlorodiphenyltrichloroethane (DDT), polychlorinated biphenyls (PCBs), and polybrominated diphenyl ethers (PBDEs), and emerging chemicals of concern such as phthalates and bisphenol A (BPA), toxic waste sites, air pollutants, pesticides, herbicides, glyphosate, heavy metals (mercury and lead), and aluminum used in vaccines as an adjuvant.[3,4] Analysis of previous studies suggests that exposure to environmental toxins during preconception, gestation, and early childhood was associated with the development of ASD in 92% of cases.[3,5] However, environmental sources such as consumption of fish and thimerosal, a mercury-containing preservative used in the vaccines, have drawn significant attention. It was suggested that exposure to mercury from thimerosal increased the risk of developing ASD.[6–8] Other studies suggested that there was no relationship between exposure to thimerosal-containing ethylmercury in the vaccine and appearance of ASD.[9–11] Thus, the safety of ethylmercury in the vaccine remains controversial; therefore, prudent strategy would be to remove organic mercury from the vaccine until further clinical studies are performed. A recent review has addressed this controversies and explained potential mechanisms of actions of organic mercury involving increased oxidative stress.[12]

The results of a Danish National Birth Cohort Study revealed that the use of acetaminophen during pregnancy was associated with increased risk of ASD with hyperkinetic symptoms by 2-fold.[13] Consumption of acetaminophen enhanced the toxicity of oxidative stress and inflammation in babies and small children and thereby enhances the risk of developing autism.[14]

HEALTH CONDITIONS

Health risk factors during prenatal and perinatal include 35 years or older mother, low birth weight, multiple gestations, prematurity, vaginal bleeding, prolonged labor, and hypoxia are associated with a higher risk of ASD in offspring.[15] Prenatal and perinatal exposure to respiratory distress and other markers of hypoxia were associated with increased risk of ASD in males, whereas appearance of jaundice was associated with increased risk of ASD in females.[16]

Another new concept is emerging suggesting that compositional alterations in the gut microbiota induced by bacterial infection or chronic antibiotic treatment may contribute to autistic behavior.[17] The gut microbiota regulate gastrointestinal physiology, immune function, and certain brain functions through butyric acid, a 4-carbon fatty acid (an inhibitor of histone decetylase), generated during fermentation of primarily soluble fibers by the microbiota (Prasad and Bondy, unpublished). Therefore, changes in the composition or amounts of microbiota may increase the risk of developing ASD. It was further suggested that the gut microbiota acts as an interface between environmental and genetic risk factors associated with ASD.[18]

GENETIC FACTORS

Many gene defects have been associated with ASD. They include common polygenic risk, de novo single nucleotide variants, and rare inherited variants, which confer heterogeneity and complexity of ASD.[19] Copy variants in genes regulating synapse formation and intrasynaptic connections, and polymorphisms in genes encoding prosocial peptide system-oxytocin and vasopressin are associated with ASD.[20] Polymorphisms in genes PON1, glutathione S-transferase (GSTM1 and GSTP1), delta aminolevulinic acid dehydratase, and the metal regulatory transcriptional factor 1 may increase the susceptibility to environmental toxins.[5] Sleep disruption is commonly observed in children with ASD was associated with two melatonin pathway genes that showed decreased expression of acetylserotonin O-methyltransferase (ASMT) and cytochrome P450 1A2 (CYP1A2).[21] Several clinical studies have revealed that supplementation with melatonin improved sleeping pattern, including longer sleep duration, less nighttime awakening, and quicker sleep onset in patients with ASD.[22] In addition, improvements in sleeping pattern were noted when other sleep medication failed.

TABLE 15.1

Major Symptoms of Autism Spectrum Disorder

Difficulty in Speech/Communication	Difficulty in Social Skills
1. Talking in sentences	Ignore others
2. Explaining needs	Uncooperative attitude
3. Carrying on conversation	Avoid eye-to-eye contact
4. Asking meaningful questions	Avoid friendship with others
5. Repeating sentences	Poor interactions with parents
6. Communicating to others	No meaningful smile
Difficulty in Sensory/Mental Awareness	**Difficulty in Behavior/Health**
7. Responding to questions	Aggressive behavior
8. No awareness of danger	Anxious and fearful
9. Unusual facial expression	Injury to self or others
10. Not following Instructions	Poor sleep quality
11. Does not initiate activities	Rigid routines
12. Does not asks questions	Low energy levels
13. Not interested in activities	Obsessive speech
14. Poor class performance	Sitting quietly

MAJOR SYMPTOMS OF ASD

The major symptoms of ASD include abnormalities in speech/communication, social skill, sensory/mental awareness, and behavior/health. They are described in detail in Table 15.1.

In order to develop strategies for prevention and improved management of ASD, it is essential to identify critical cellular defects that contribute to the development and progression of ASD. Analysis of published studies to be discussed later in this chapter suggests that increased oxidative stress, inflammation, and glutamate may play an important role in the initiation and progression of ASD. The question arises how to reduce these cellular defects at the same time.

BRAIN CHANGES IN ASD

Evidence for neurodegeneration in the brain of patients with ASD includes loss of neurons, activated microglia and astrocytes, pro-inflammatory cytokines, and oxidative stress.[23] Damage in the amygdala, temporal and frontal cortexes, hippocampus, and cerebellum was associated with the behavior impairments in ASD.[24] In the autopsied samples of Broadman area 21 (BA21) of temporal cortex of patients with ASD, the activities of mitochondrial respiratory chain protein complexes, complex 1 and complex IV, and mitochondrial Mn-dependent antioxidant enzyme superoxide dismutase 2 (SOD2) decreased. In addition, enhanced oxidative damage was also observed.[25]

The symptoms of ASD appear to remain the same or worsened from childhood into adulthood, Using neuroimaging technique, it was demonstrated that mean value of cortical white matter decreased, whereas mean ventricular volume increased in ASD. Reduction in regional mean volumes occurs in ASD during adolescence and adulthood. The mean volume of many brain structures continued to decline as patients with ASD grow older.[26] Quantitative analysis of in vivo MRI brain scans showed that and periventricular and deep subcortical white matter hypointensity (WMH) volume were increased in ASD, and that increase in periventricular WMH was associated with a higher degree of repetitive behaviors and restricted interest, but it was not associated with age.[27] It was further shown that age-related reduction in gray matter and white matter in parietal and inferior temporal regions of the brain and age-related enhancement in gray matter in frontal and anterior-temporal regions of the brain occur in ASD.[28] Analysis of autopsied brain samples of adult patients with ASD showed that amygdala had reduced number of neurons. The average non-neuronal cell numbers and volume did not differ between ASD and control cases. A few patients with ASD exhibited increased activation of microglia. In adult patients with ASD, there were fewer oligodendrocytes in the amygdala compared to control cases. These changes in the brain structures may be linked to altered connectivity or impaired communication associated with ASD.[29] Bilateral decreased in gray matter volume extending from the thalamus to the cerebellum, anterior medial temporal lobes, and orbitofrontal regions was observed in patients with ASD. Furthermore, the severity of ASD was associated with decreased gray matter volume in prefrontal cortex, inferior parietal, and temporal regions. Similar relationships between gray matter volume and age were observed suggesting that changes in gray matter occur throughout the lifespan of ASD patients.[30] Self-injurious behaviors, one of the symptoms of ASD, appears to be related to changes in the somatosensory cortical and subcortical regions and their supporting white matter.[31]

MicroRNAs IN ASD

MicroRNAs

MicroRNAs (miRs) are evolutionarily conserved small noncoding single-stranded RNAs of approximately 22 nucleotides in length, and are present in all living organisms including humans.[32–35] The biogenesis of miRs is very complex and involves multiple biochemical steps. The majority of miRs are transcribed by RNA polymerase II (Pol II), while some are transcribed by RNA polymerase III (Pol III) from the noncoding region of the DNA to produce primary miRs (pri-miRs). Pri-miRs undergo a nuclear cleavage by ribonuclease III Drosa to generate precursor-miRs (pre-miRs) that migrate to the cytoplasm where they are further cleaved by ribonuclease III Dicer to ultimately form mature single-stranded miRs with the help of another protein argonaute (Ago)[34,36–38] Each microRNA binds to its complimentary sequences in the 3′-untranslated region (3′-UTR) of the mRNA, promotes degradation of the mRNA transcript, and prevents translation of the message of protein. In this manner, miRs regulate the translation of proapoptotic or antiapoptotic proteins from their respective mRNAs, depending upon whether they receive damaging or protective signal. The expression of some miroRNAs may also be altered in response to the disease state.

MicroRNAs IN SERUM

In the serum of ASD patients, the expression of miR-151a-3p, miR-181b-5p, miR-320a, miR-328, miR-433, miR-489, miR-572, and miR-663a was downregulated, whereas the expression of miR-101-3p, miR-106b-5p, miR-130a-3p, miR-195-5p, and miR-19b-3p was upregulated.[39] Another study reported that 11 miRs were overexpressed and 29 miRs were downregulated in the serum of ASD patients. The target genes for these microRNAs were alpha 1C subunit of voltage-dependent calcium channel, L type (CACNA1C), beta 1C subunit of voltage-dependent calcium channel, L type (CACNAB1), and other genes like cytoplasmic ribonuclease type III (Dicer).[40] It was suggested that serum levels of miR-424-5p, miR-197-5p, miR-328-3p, miR-500a-5p, miR-619-5p, miR-3135a, miR-664a-3p, and miR-365a-3p might be useful as potential biomarkers for ASD in children.

MicroRNAs IN SALIVA

In the saliva of adults with ASD, 14 microRNAs were differentially expressed compared with control subjects.[41] These microRNAs are expressed in developing brain, and therefore, any alterations in the expression of one or more miRs may interfere with the development of brain. Sexual dimorphism in expression of noncoding RNAs that include p1w1interacting RNAs (piRNAs), small nucleolar RNAs (snoRNAs), transcribed ultraconserved regions (T-UCRs), and large intergenic non-coding RNAs), and miRNAs occurred in the temporal cortex and in the different regions of ASD patients.[42] There are two microRNAs, miR-219 and miR-338, which promote differentiation of oligodendrocytes, and miR-125, which promotes differentiation of neurons, and miR-488, which increases anxiety. Putative targets of these miRs are immune-related mRNAs and mRNAs that control brain cell differentiation in both sexes.

MicroRNAs in Autopsied Brain Samples

In autopsied cerebellar cortex samples of ASD patients, the expression of 9 miRs were altered.[43] These miRs target mRNA of neurexin and SHANK3. Abnormalities in these proteins are linked with ASD. In the autopsied brain samples of ASD patients, the expression of miR-142-5p, miR-142-3p, miR-451a, miR-144-3p, and miR-21-5p were upregulated. In addition, the promoter region of the miR-142 was hypomethylated, suggesting that epigenetics is an important factor in dysregulation of microRNA. These miRs target mRNAs destined to be translated into proteins involved in synaptic function. Further analysis revealed that miR-451a and miR-21-5p target mRNA for oxytocin receptor (OXTR). Overexpression of miR-21-5p reduces the levels of OXTR by binding with 3'-UTR OXTR mRNA.[44] In autopsied brain samples of ASD patients, the expression of miR-4753-5p and miR-1 in the superior temporal sulcus (STS), and miR-664-3p, miR-4709-3p, miR-4742-3p, and miR-297 in the primary auditory cortex (PAC) was differently expressed compared with controls.[45] MicroRNAs in each brain region targeted mRNAs that are involved in making cell cycle protein and canonical signaling pathways, including P13-Akt that are implicated in ASD. MicroRNAs impaired immune pathways only in the STS. Small non-coding RNAs (snoRNAs) and pre-miR were also differentially expressed in ASD patients compare with control subjects.

MicroRNAs in Cell Culture

In the lymphoblast cell lines from monozygotic twins with ASD, the expression of two microRNAs has-miR-29b and has-miR-219-5p that target inhibitor of DNA binding protein 3 (ID3) and polio-like kinase2 (PLK2), respectively, were altered.[46]

MicroRNAs in Animals

Animal study revealed that overexpression of miR-124a was associated with decreased levels of its target BDNF mRNA. Overexpression of this microRNA in denate gyrus enhanced repetitive behaviors, social impairment, and anxiety without any effect on locomotor activity in rats.[47] In valproic acid-induced rat model of ASD, increased expression of miR-181c and miR-30d was associated with reduced levels of proteins that are involved in the development of brain.[48] Selective inhibition of miR-181c decreased neurite outgrowth and branching leading to reduction in synaptic density in the primary amigdala neurons in culture.

The studies discussed above suggest that dysregulation of microRNAs may be involved in the etiology of ASD. These microRNAs target mRNAs that are responsible for producing proteins involved in brain development including synaptic functions.

EVIDENCE FOR INCREASED OXIDATIVE STRESS IN ASD

Human Studies

Analysis of published studies suggests that increased oxidative stress play an important role in the initiation and progression of ASD. The urinary levels of total antioxidant capacity were lower and the levels of hexanoyl-lysine (HEL), a marker of oxidative damage, were higher in patients with

ASD than in control healthy subjects suggesting the presence of increased oxidative stress in these patients.[49] In the Chinese children with ASD, the serum levels of superoxide dismutase (SOD) were lower than in healthy control children.[50] Plasma levels of two carbonylated proteins, complement component C8 alpha chain and Ig kappa chain C were elevated in children with ASD in comparison to those found in normal children.[51] The levels of plasma protein dityrosine, a marker of oxidative damage of protein, were increased in patients with ASD, whereas the levels of thiamine pyrophosphate that is needed for generating energy by mitochondria are reduced in patients with ASD.[52] Urine levels of markers of oxidative damage (lipid peroxidation and 4-hydroxynonenal, oxidative stress index, and protein carbonyls) were elevated, whereas the levels of antioxidant excreted in the urine were decreased.[53] Increased nitration of sulfur proteins, and decreased levels of enzymatic and non-enzymatic antioxidants in hairs and nail samples were found in children with ASD compared with normal children.[54] Plasma levels of 8-isoprostane, a marker of oxidative damage, and cysteinyl-leukotrienes, a marker of inflammation were elevated in children with ASD.[55] Increased oxidative stress, mitochondrial dysfunction, inflammation, and impaired immune function were found in patients with ASD.[56] Serum levels of thioredoxin, a marker of oxidative stress, were elevated in children with ASD compared with control children.[57] Reduction in the levels of glutathione was associated with ASD. This was further confirmed by experiment in which the activities of glutathione peroxidase, glutathione-S-transferase were decreased in the autopsied cerebellum tissues of patients with ASD compare to those found in control cases.[58] Buccal swab analysis showed that extensive impairment of mitochondrial respiratory complexes activities occurred in children with ASD.[59] In the autopsied samples of temporal lobe of patients with ASD, mitochondrial dysfunction and oxidative DNA damage levels were increased.[25] Increased mitochondrial DNA deletion and enhanced oxidative stress, and reduced complexes activities were found in autopsied brain tissues of patients with ASD.[60] In the tissue homogenates of autopsied brain samples of children with ASD, the rate of transport of mitochondrial AGC (aspartate/glutamate carrier) was higher than control subjects.[61] Rise in the AGC transport was blocked by a calcium chelator. The levels of calcium in the neocortical were higher than in control cases. In addition, the expression of AGC1, the predominant AGC isoform in the brain, and cytochrome c were elevated in children with ASD.

The levels of 3-nitrosine (3-NT) and neurotrophin-3 (NT-3) increased in the cerebella of ASD patients. Distribution of these markers of oxidative damage varies from one region of the brain to the other. For example, in one of the two case of ASD involving an older patient, the brain regions with highest levels of 3-NT included the orbitofrontal cortex, Wernicke's area, cerebellar vermis, cerebellar hemisphere, and pons. These areas of the brain control speech processing, sensory and motor coordination, emotional and social behavior, and memory. On the other hand, the levels of 3-NT enhanced in the cerebellar hemispheres and putamen in both ASD patients. Furthermore, increased levels of NT-3 were found in the cerebellar hemisphere in both patients with ASD. Higher levels of NT-3 were also present in the dorsolateral prefrontal cortex in the older patient, and in the Wernicke's area and cingulated gyrus in the younger patients.[24] Increased oxidative stress contributes to the shortening of telomere length.[62] Therefore, it is not surprising that analysis of saliva samples from children with ASD show shortening of telomere length; however, it is surprising that older siblings and parents of children with ASD also exhibit shortening of the length of telomere compared to families with history of ASD.[63]

Cell Culture Models

Mitochondrial dysfunction is associated with ASD; and oxidative stress induced this abnormality in the lymphoblastoid cell lines (LCLs) derived from children with ASD.[64] ASD LCLs showed higher ATP-dependent respiration, higher respiratory capacity, and greater glycolysis and glycolytic reserve than sibling LCLs. Exposure to acute oxidative stress induced greater changes in these parameters in ASD LCLs compared to in sibling or control LCLs.[65] These data show that ASD patients and their unaffected sibling share some mitochondrial dysfunction and redox abnormalities.

Expression of genes for SIRT1 (Silent mating type information regulation 2 homolog 1, a NAD-dependent deacetylase) and PGC-1 alpha (perixome proliferator-activated receptor gamma coactivator 1-alpha that regulates mitochondrial biogenesis and respiration rate for energy production) were downregulated at RNA and protein levels in ASD patients and immortalized ASD lymphoblastoid cell lines (LCLs), and the intracellular levels of ROS, mitochondrial ROS, and apoptosis were enhanced in ASD LCLs. Furthermore, translocation of cytochrome c and DIABLO (a protein promoting apoptosis) from the mitochondria to the cytosol occurred in ASD LCLs. Over expression of PGC-1 alpha upregulated expression of the SIRT1/PGC-1 alpha axis genes and reduced translocation of cytochrome c and DIABLO to the cytosol, and inhibited the production of ROS and apoptosis in these ASD cells.[66]

EVIDENCE FOR INCREASED INFLAMMATION IN ASD

The levels of pro-inflammatory cytokine IL-8 were elevated in the plasma of ASD children in comparison to control healthy children.[67] Plasma levels of pro-inflammatory cytokines, such as IL-1ß, IL-6, IL-8, IL-12p40, IL-5, IL-1RA, IL-12(p70), IL-13, IL-17, and GRO-alpha (growth regulated oncogene-alpha), a cytokine, were higher in ASD children than in normal healthy control.[68–70] Granulocytes of children with ASD exhibited impaired oxidative phosphorylation, immune response and antioxidant defense in comparison to those found in normal children.[71] The levels of several markers of inflammation together with increased lipid peroxidation were found in the plasma of patients with ASD.[72] Plasma levels of 8-isoprostane, a marker of oxidative damage, and cysteinyl leukotrienes that stimulates pro-inflammatory cytokines, were elevated in children with ASD.[55]

IMBALANCES BETWEEN NEURONAL EXCITATION AND INHIBITION

Studies on animal research, genetics, and autopsied brain tissues suggest that imbalances between neuronal excitation and inhibition may be involved in ASD symptoms. Analysis of previous studies revealed higher blood levels of glutamate in ASD patients.[73]

HUMAN STUDIES

Using a magnetic resonance spectroscopy (MRS) technique, it was found that the levels of n-acetyl-aspartate, glutamate, and glutamine decreased in the cingulated cortex of adult patients with ASD.[74] Using a proton magnetic resonance spectroscopy (pMRS), it was demonstrated that the levels of glutamate and glutamine were elevated in the midline pregenual anterior cingulate of children with ASD compared to controls.[75] This study shows that increased neuronal excitation over neuronal inhibition occurred in children with ASD that is opposite to that observed in adults with ASD who exhibit reduced levels of glutamate and glutamine. Using a pMRS technique, it was found that children with ASD had higher levels of glutamate, glutamine, n-acetyl-aspartate, and creatine than the control subjects. The levels of these parameters did not differ in parents of children with ASD compared to those in controls.[76] The increased levels of glutamate and glutamine in the auditory cortex is consistent with previous imaging data in the hippocampus and frontal lobe, and suggest that increased cortical excitability may be associated with some of the symptoms of ASD in children, whereas increased levels of n-acetyl-aspartate and creatine may reflect defects in brain metabolism in ASD patients. Using the same technique, higher glutamine levels and lower gamma-aminobutyric acid/creatine levels were found in the anterior cingulate cortex of children with ASD, and they were associated with lower IQ and higher impairments in social cognition.[77] Increased levels of glutamate were found in the midline anterior cingulated cortex of children with ASD or obsessive compulsive disorder (OCD) compared with controls by a pMRS technique. The concentration of glutamate in the anterior cingulate cortex appears to be associated with the severity of OCD.[78] Using MRS technique, it was demonstrated that the levels of glutamate/creatine increased in the putamen.[79]

Using a pMRS technique, it was demonstrated that ASD children of 3–4 years showed lower concentrations of n-acetyl-aspartate, choline and creatine in the gray matter and white matter; however, no such changes were observed in children of 9–10 years. In children of age 3–4 years with idiopathic developmental delay (DD), the levels of n-acetyl-aspartate decreased in both gray matter and white matter, the levels of n-acetyl-aspartate remained low in the DD group of 9–10 years compared with control subjects.[80]

Using a pMRS technique, it was observed that the levels of GABA were lower in the auditory cortex of children with ASD than in control subjects, suggesting an impaired inhibitory transmission in ASD.[81] The levels of GABA were lower in the anterior cingulated cortex and striatum in ASD children with primary complex stereotypies compared with controls by using pMRS technique.[82]

In the autopsied mainly cerebellum samples from patients with ASD, the mRNA levels of several genes, including excitatory amino acid transporter 1 and glutamate receptor AMPA 1 were increased.[83] In the autopsied brain samples, the levels of Fragile X mental retardation protein (FMRP) and GABA (A) receptor beta 3 (GABARbeta3) decreased in the vermis of adult patients with ASD, whereas the levels of metabotropic glutamate receptor 5 (mGluR5) increased in the vermis of children with ASD.[84]

USE OF SINGLE ANTIOXIDANTS IN THE MANAGEMENT OF ASD

HUMAN STUDIES

Oral supplementation with high doses of N-acetylcysteine (NAC) reduced irritability in children with ASD.[85] In another study, NAC treatment enhanced glutathione levels, but no significant improvement in social interaction.[86] After 10 days of treatment, NAC in combination with risperidone (a drug used in ASD treatment) reduced irritability and hyperactivity more than that observed in risperidone treatment alone.[87] Oral supplementation with NAC failed to produce any benefit in children ASD.[88] Thus, treatment with NAC alone produced inconsistent beneficial effect in children with ASD.

Treatment with coenzyme Q10 improved symptoms of ASD Children, such as communication with parents, verbal communication with others, and playing games of children. Mitochondrial dysfunction is associated with ASD; and oxidative stress induced this abnormality in the lymphoblastoid cell lines derived from children with ASD.[64] Supplement with coenzyme Q10 also improved seeping pattern, verbal communication, and reduced food rejection behaviors.[89]

Treatment with sulforaphane, a phytochemical derived from broccoli sprout extract, caused substantial reduction in Aberrant Behavior Checklist (ABC) and Social Responsiveness Scale (SRS) compared with placebo control. In addition, ASD patients receiving sulforaphane showed improvement in social interaction, abnormal behavior, and verbal communication.[90]

Supplementation with methyl B12 improved symptoms of ASD in children with ASD compared with controls.[85]

There appears to be an association between reduction in melatonin levels and the severity of autistic behavior. Supplementation with melatonin improved sleep patterns, including longer sleep duration, less nighttime awakenings, and quicker onset of sleep.[22]

ANIMAL STUDIES

In the propanoic acid-induced rat model of ASD, supplementation with curcumin and resveratrol improved symptoms of ASD by reducing oxidative and nitrosylative stress.[91,92] Using the same rat model of ASD, it was demonstrated that resveratrol treatment restored symptoms to normal levels by reducing oxidative stress, mitochondrial dysfunction, TNF-α, and MMP-9.[92] In a valproic acid-induced mice model of ASD, treatment with astaxanthin improved behavioral disorder and reduced oxidative damage in the brain and liver.[93] In valproic acid-induced rat model of autism, supplementation with NAC prevented repetitive and stereotypic behavior and reduced oxidative stress,[94] and administration of docosahexaenoic acid (DHA) protected hippocampal neurons and improved learning ability and memory.[95] Chronic NAC treatment restored valproic acid-induced dysfunction in social interaction, and reduced anxiety symptom in rats.[96]

Maternal administration of Polyriboinosinix-polyribocytidilic acid (poly(I:C)) produces some symptoms that are related to ASD and other neurodevelopment disorders in mice.[97] Prenatal administration of VitaminD3 prevented behavioral abnormalities induced by Poly(I:C) but has no effect on the levels of pro-inflammatory cytokines in juvenile mice. This study suggests the mechanisms of protection by vitamin D3 may not involve reduction in inflammation. Deficiency in Vitamin D was found in patients with ASD, but deficiency in folic acid and omega-3-fatty acids was inclusive.[98]

The above animal studies suggest potential value of antioxidants in improving the symptoms of ASD. Human studies with most individual antioxidants improved some, but not most symptoms of ASD. Since patients with ASD exhibit multiple abnormal behaviors, it is not possible to expect to improve the most or all symptoms associated with ASD with one micronutrient (antioxidant or B-vitamin). Since increased oxidative stress and inflammation are involved in the development and progression of ASD, simultaneous reduction of these two events may help in reducing the rate of progression of this mental disorder.

STUDIES WITH INDIVIDUAL ANTIOXIDANTS IN HUMAN NEURODEGENERATIVE DISEASES

Treatment with individual antioxidants such as vitamin E[99,100] and curcumin[101] do not improve cognitive function, whereas alpha-lipoic acid,[102] vitamin E,[103] and omega-3-fatty acids[104,105] produce transient and limited improvement in cognitive function only in early phases of Alzheimer's disease (AD). In the case of Parkinson's disease, high doses of coenzyme Q10 produce some transient improvements in some symptoms.[106] The reasons for individual antioxidants producing no effect or transient beneficial effects may have been for several reasons: (a) antioxidants show differential subcellular distribution and different mechanisms of action; therefore, a single antioxidant cannot protect all parts of the cell; (b) a single antioxidant in a high internal oxidative environment of patients with neurodegenerative diseases is oxidized and can then itself act as a prooxidant rather than as an antioxidant; (c) the body protects against oxidative damage by elevating antioxidant enzymes, and dietary and endogenous antioxidants; (d) antioxidants neutralize free radicals by donating electrons to those molecules with unpaired electron, whereas antioxidant enzymes destroy free radicals by catalysis, converting them to harmless molecules such as water and oxygen. Therefore, both of these events need to be enhanced in concert to achieve substantial therapeutic gain; (e) the affinity of different antioxidants for free radicals differs, depending upon their lipophilicity; (f) both the aqueous and lipid components of the cell need to be protected together. Water-soluble antioxidants such as vitamin C and glutathione protect molecules in the aqueous environment of the cells, whereas lipid soluble antioxidants such as vitamin A and vitamin E protect molecules in the lipid compartment; (g) vitamin E is more effective in quenching free radicals in a reduced oxygenated cellular environment, whereas vitamin C and alpha-tocopherol are more effective in a higher oxygenated environment of the cells[107]; (h) vitamin C is important for recycling the oxidized form of alpha-tocopherol to the antioxidant form at the lipid/aqueous interface[108]; (i) antioxidants produce cell protective proteins by altering the expression of different microRNAs.[109] For example, some antioxidants can activate Nrf2 by upregulating miR-200a that inhibits its target protein Keap1, whereas others activate Nrf2 by downregulating miR-21 that binds with 3′-UTR Nrf2 mRNA.[110]

These studies suggest that use of a single micronutrient in prevention or improved management of human neurodegenerative diseases is not expected to yield any beneficial effects. For this reason, a mixture of micronutrients that can simultaneously reduce oxidative stress and inflammation by enhancing the levels of antioxidant enzymes through the activation of Nrf2 pathway together with dietary and endogenous antioxidants for AD and PD has been suggested.[109,111] The same suggestion is proposed for the improved management of ASD. Oral supplementation can increase the levels of dietary and endogenous antioxidants; however, elevation of the levels of antioxidant enzymes requires an activation of Nrf2. Therefore, it is essential to understand the regulation of activation of Nrf2.

REGULATION OF ACTIVATION OF Nrf2

REACTIVE OXYGEN SPECIES (ROS) ACTIVATES Nrf2

Normally, during acute oxidative stress, ROS is needed to activate Nrf2 which then dissociates itself from Keap1-Cul-Rbx1 complex and translocates in the nucleus where it heterodimerizes with a small Maf protein, and binds with the ARE (antioxidant response element), leading to increased expression of target genes coding for several cytoprotective enzymes including antioxidant enzymes.[112–114] In this manner, activation of Nrf2 increases the levels of cytoprotective enzymes including antioxidant enzymes and phase-2-detoxifying enzymes.[115,116]

BINDING OF Nrf2 WITH ARE IN THE NUCLEUS

Activation of Nrf2 alone may not be sufficient to increase the levels of antioxidant enzymes. Activated Nrf2 must bind with antioxidant response element (ARE) in the nucleus for increasing the expression of its target genes. This binding ability of Nrf2 with ARE was impaired in aged rats and this defect was restored by supplementation with alpha-lipoic acid.[117] It is unknown whether the binding ability of Nrf2 with ARE is impaired in ASD.

EXISTENCE OF ROS-RESISTANT Nrf2

Activation of Nrf2 by ROS becomes impaired in ASD. This is evidenced by the fact that increased oxidative stress occurs in ASD despite the presence of Nrf2. Only one animal study showed that administration of valproic acid into Nrf2 knockout mice during an early development caused more severe damage to neurons, and greater learning ability, memory deficits, and behavior impairments compared to the valproic acid-treated wild-type mice.[118] This study demonstrate importance of Nrf2 in neuroprotection in ASD.

ANTIOXIDANTS ACTIVATE ROS-RESISTANT Nrf2

Activation of Nrf2 becomes unresponsive to ROS in ASD. Some dietary antioxidants and phytochemicals can activate Nrf2 without requiring ROS. These include vitamin C[119,120] vitamin E,[121] endogenous antioxidants such as alpha-lipoic acid,[117] and coenzyme Q10,[122] synthetic antioxidant N-acetylcysteine (NAC),[123] omega-3-fatty acids,[124,125] and phytochemicals such as curcumin[126] and resveratrol.[127,128]

L-CARNITINE ACTIVATES Nrf2 BY A ROS-DEPENDENT MECHANISM

Treatment with L-carnitine activates Nrf2 by a ROS-dependent mechanism,[129] probably by generating transient ROS.

ACTIVATION OF Nrf2 BY MicroRNAs

The complex of Keap1-Nrf2 in the cytoplasm prevents activation of Nrf2. Over-expression of miR-200a reduced Keap-1 levels allowing Nrf2 to migrate to the nucleus where it binds to the ARE that enhanced the transcription of target cytoprotective genes including antioxidant enzymes.[130] Increased oxidative stress enhanced the expression of miR-153 that reduced the expression of Nrf2 by binding to its 3'-UTR region of Nrf2 mRNA.[131] Mutation in miR-153 restored the oxidative stress-induced reduction in Nrf2 activity.

SUPPRESSION OF CHRONIC INFLAMMATION

The activation of Nrf2 also suppresses chronic inflammation.[115,116] Some antioxidant compounds also reduce markers of chronic inflammation.[132–137]

INHIBITION OF RELEASE AND TOXICITY OF GLUTAMATE

In ASD patients, increased excitatory neurotransmission is observed because of increased release of glutamate. Release of glutamate was blocked by antioxidants, such as vitamin E,[138] tempol, a superoxide dismutase mimetic, and edaravone, a synthetic antioxidant,[139] quercetin,[140] glutathione and vitamin E,[141] alpha-lipoic acid,[142] and coenzyme Q10.[143] In addition to antioxidants, vitamin B6,[144] vitamin B12,[145] and vitamin B2 (riboflavin)[146] also reduce release of glutamate. Antioxidants such as alpha-tocopherol[147] and coenzyme Q10[148] also protected neurons against glutamate-induced degeneration and death.

DRUG TREATMENT IN HUMAN ASD

The ASD is very complex brain development disorder involving different areas of the brain exhibiting multiple symptoms varying from behavior impairment to cognitive dysfunction. Therefore, it is not possible to develop a single drug that attenuates all or most symptoms of the disease. This could be only possible if increased oxidative stress and chronic inflammation that initiate and promote the ASD are reduced. For acute cases, it would be rationale to use a particular drug that can improve one or more specific symptoms together with the agents that can simultaneously reduce oxidative stress and chronic inflammation. Commonly used FDA-approved drugs include[149]:

Antipsychotic drugs: Risperidone, fluphenazine, and clozapine for improving behavior problems, such as irritability and aggression

Antidepression drugs: Sertraline, Citalopram, and Fluoxetine (also called Prozac), (a serotonin reuptake inhibitor), Venlafaxine (a serotonin and norepinephrine inhibitor) for improving depressive disorder, anxiety disorder, panic disorder, and obsessive compulsive disorder

Psychotropic drugs: Aripiprazole (also called Abilify) for treatment of irritability

Mild CNS stimulant: Methylphenidate (also called Ritalin, and concerta) for treating attention deficits and hyperactivity

Cognitive disorder: Memantine (also called Nameda), an antigonist of glutamate receptor NMDA, Rivastigmine, an inhibitor of acetylcholinesterase, for treating cognitive dysfunction

Insomnia: Mirtazapine (also called Remeron), antidepression, and melatonin secreted by the pineal gland, for treating insomnia

Aggression: Haloperidol(also called Haldol), a selective dopamine D2 receptor antigonist, for treating aggression

Social functioning: Oxytocin (also called Pitocin), a hormone to regulate lactation and parturition, for improving social functioning

Antiepileptic drugs: for treatment of seizures (10%–30% of children develop seizures)

Lithium: for the treatment of mood disorders

Guanfacine for the treatment of hyperactivity and impulsiveness

Lurasidone: An antipsychotic drug for the treatment of irritability and anger

Other treatment approaches include behavior and communication treatments, speech therapy, dietary modifications, and complementary and alternative medicines. None of these therapies have shown any significant benefits (mayoclinic.org/disease/autism-spectrum-disorder/diagnosis-treatment/drc-20352934).

DRUG TREATMENT IN ANIMAL ASD MODELS

Using the valproic acid-induced rat model of ASD, it was demonstrated that administration of Fingolimod, a immunomodulating FDA approved drug primarily for the treatment multiple sclerosis (MS), improved social behavior, spatial learning, and memory. These improvements were associated with a reduction in neuronal loss, and apoptosis of pyramidal cells in hippocampal CA1 regions, inhibition of microglia activation, lowering the levels of pro-inflammatory cytokines, such as IL-1b, and IL-6 in the hippocampus and markers of oxidative stress, reduction in the levels of Bax and caspase-3 proteins and enhancement of the expression of Bcl2 in the hippocampus.[150]

PROPOSED MIXTURE OF MICRONUTRIENTS FOR IMPROVED MANAGEMENT OF ASD

Based on the studies discussed above, a mixture of micronutrients containing vitamin A, mixed carotenoids, vitamin C, α-tocopheryl acetate, α-tocopheryl succinate, vitamin D3, alpha-lipoic acid, N-acetylcysteine, coenzyme Q10, L-carnitine, omega-3-fatty acids, curcumin, resveratrol, all B-vitamins, selenomethionine, and zinc, but without iron, copper, manganese, or heavy metals such as molybdenum and zirconium for the prevention or delaying the onset of symptoms is proposed. The inclusion of iron, copper, and manganese is not suggested, because these trace minerals, although essential for many biological reactions, can combine with vitamin C and generate excessive amounts of free radicals. Furthermore, these minerals are absorbed from the intestine better in the presence of antioxidants than in their absence that could increase body store of free iron, copper, and manganese after long-term consumption. The body has no significant mechanisms of excretion of these trace minerals. Slight increase in the body store of free forms of these minerals can increase the risk of most chronic diseases. Heavy metals were not included because the body has no mechanisms of excretion of these heavy metals. Consequently, their levels in the body would increase after long-term consumption. High levels of heavy metals could interfere with the function of organs including the brain.

It is expected that the proposed micronutrient mixture would increase the levels of antioxidant enzymes by activating the Nrf2 pathway. This together with enhancement of dietary and endogenous antioxidants, and B-vitamins could lead to simultaneously reduction in oxidative stress, chronic inflammation, and glutamate levels in ASD.

This mixture of micronutrients, in combination with standard treatment, may be useful for enhancing the management of ASD. Preclinical and clinical studies are needed to substantiate the potential role of proposed mixture of micronutrients for the improved management of ASD.

CONCLUSIONS

Autism spectrum disorder (ASD) refers to a group of complex brain development disorders that include autistic disorders and Asperger's syndrome (AS). This disorder is characterized by abnormalities in multiple areas of the brain and exhibit multiple defects in speech/communication, social skill, sensory/mental awareness, and behavior/health. Environmental and genetic factors contribute to the development of ASD. The current standard treatment is considered unsatisfactory because one or two drugs may not affect multiple abnormal symptoms that are associated with ASD. Among initial and early biochemical abnormalities, increased oxidative stress, inflammation, and glutamate initiate and promote the progression of ASD. Therefore, simultaneous attenuation these biochemical defects may reduce the risk of developing ASD, and in combination with standard care, improve the management of this disease. In order to reduce these biochemical abnormalities, it is essential to increase the levels of antioxidant enzymes and dietary and endogenous antioxidants, and reduce the release and toxicity of glutamate. The levels of antioxidants can be increased and glutamate by supplementation, but enhancing the levels of antioxidant enzymes requires an activation of Nrf2.

A mixture of micronutrients that would achieve the above goal is proposed. This mixture of micronutrients in combination with standard therapy may improve the management of ASD.

REFERENCES

1. CDC Data and Statistics on Autism Spectrum Disorder, 2017.
2. Buescher AV, Cidav Z, Knapp M, Mandell DS. Costs of autism spectrum disorders in the United Kingdom and the United States. *JAMA Pediatr.* 2014;168(8):721–728.
3. Ye BS, Leung AOW, Wong MH. The association of environmental toxicants and autism spectrum disorders in children. *Environ Pollut.* 2017;227:234–242.
4. Sealey LA, Hughes BW, Sriskanda AN, et al. Environmental factors in the development of autism spectrum disorders. *Environ Int.* 2016;88:288–298.
5. Rossignol DA, Genuis SJ, Frye RE. Environmental toxicants and autism spectrum disorders: A systematic review. *Transl Psychiatry.* 2014;4:e360.
6. Geier DA, Geier MR. A comparative evaluation of the effects of MMR immunization and mercury doses from thimerosal-containing childhood vaccines on the population prevalence of autism. *Med Sci Monit.* 2004;10(3):PI33–PI39.
7. Geier DA, Hooker BS, Kern JK, King PG, Sykes LK, Geier MR. A two-phase study evaluating the relationship between thimerosal-containing vaccine administration and the risk for an autism spectrum disorder diagnosis in the United States. *Transl Neurodegener.* 2013;2(1):25.
8. Geier DA, Kern JK, Geier MR. Increased risk for an atypical autism diagnosis following Thimerosal-containing vaccine exposure in the United States: A prospective longitudinal case-control study in the vaccine safety datalink. *J Trace Elem Med Biol.* 2017;42:18–24.
9. Gadad BS, Li W, Yazdani U, et al. Administration of thimerosal-containing vaccines to infant rhesus macaques does not result in autism-like behavior or neuropathology. *Proc Natl Acad Sci USA.* 2015;112(40):12498–12503.
10. Curtis B, Liberato N, Rulien M, et al. Examination of the safety of pediatric vaccine schedules in a non-human primate model: Assessments of neurodevelopment, learning, and social behavior. *Environ Health Perspect.* 2015;123(6):579–589.
11. Price CS, Thompson WW, Goodson B, et al. Prenatal and infant exposure to thimerosal from vaccines and immunoglobulins and risk of autism. *Pediatrics.* 2010;126(4):656–664.
12. Morris G, Puri BK, Frye RE, Maes M. The putative role of environmental mercury in the pathogenesis and pathophysiology of autism spectrum disorders and subtypes. *Mol Neurobiol.* 2017;55:1–23.
13. Liew Z, Ritz B, Virk J, Olsen J. Maternal use of acetaminophen during pregnancy and risk of autism spectrum disorders in childhood: A Danish national birth cohort study. *Autism Res.* 2016;9(9):951–958.
14. Parker W, Hornik CD, Bilbo S, et al. The role of oxidative stress, inflammation, and acetaminophen exposure from birth to early childhood in the induction of autism. *J Int Med Res.* 2017;45(2):407–438.
15. Maramara LA, He W, Ming X. Pre- and perinatal risk factors for autism spectrum disorder in a New Jersey cohort. *J Child Neurol.* 2014;29(12):1645–1651.
16. Froehlich-Santino W, Londono Tobon A, Cleveland S, et al. Prenatal and perinatal risk factors in a twin study of autism spectrum disorders. *J Psychiatr Res.* 2014;54:100–108.
17. Li Q, Zhou JM. The microbiota-gut-brain axis and its potential therapeutic role in autism spectrum disorder. *Neuroscience.* 2016;324:131–139.
18. Vuong HE, Hsiao EY. Emerging roles for the gut microbiome in autism spectrum disorder. *Biol Psychiatry.* 2017;81(5):411–423.
19. Robinson EB, Neale BM, Hyman SE. Genetic research in autism spectrum disorders. *Curr Opin Pediatr.* 2015;27(6):685–691.
20. Rybakowski F, Chojnicka I, Dziechciarz P, et al. The role of genetic factors and pre- and perinatal influences in the etiology of autism spectrum disorders—Indications for genetic referral. *Psychiatr Pol.* 2016;50(3):543–554.
21. Veatch OJ, Pendergast JS, Allen MJ, et al. Genetic variation in melatonin pathway enzymes in children with autism spectrum disorder and comorbid sleep onset delay. *J Autism Dev Disord.* 2015;45(1):100–110.
22. Rossignol DA, Frye RE. Melatonin in autism spectrum disorders. *Curr Clin Pharmacol.* 2014;9(4):326–334.

23. Kern JK, Geier DA, Sykes LK, Geier MR. Evidence of neurodegeneration in autism spectrum disorder. *Transl Neurodegener.* 2013;2(1):17.

24. Sajdel-Sulkowska EM, Xu M, McGinnis W, Koibuchi N. Brain region-specific changes in oxidative stress and neurotrophin levels in autism spectrum disorders (ASD). *Cerebellum.* 2011;10(1):43–48.

25. Tang G, Gutierrez Rios P, Kuo SH, et al. Mitochondrial abnormalities in temporal lobe of autistic brain. *Neurobiol Dis.* 2013;54:349–361.

26. Lange N, Travers BG, Bigler ED, et al. Longitudinal volumetric brain changes in autism spectrum disorder ages 6–35 years. *Autism Res.* 2015;8(1):82–93.

27. Blackmon K, Ben-Avi E, Wang X, et al. Periventricular white matter abnormalities and restricted repetitive behavior in autism spectrum disorder. *Neuroimage Clin.* 2016;10:36–45.

28. DeRamus TP, Kana RK. Anatomical likelihood estimation meta-analysis of grey and white matter anomalies in autism spectrum disorders. *Neuroimage Clin.* 2015;7:525–536.

29. Morgan JT, Barger N, Amaral DG, Schumann CM. Stereological study of amygdala glial populations in adolescents and adults with autism spectrum disorder. *PLoS One.* 2014;9(10):e110356.

30. Osipowicz K, Bosenbark DD, Patrick KE. Cortical changes across the autism lifespan. *Autism Res.* 2015;8(4):379–385.

31. Duerden EG, Card D, Roberts SW, et al. Self-injurious behaviours are associated with alterations in the somatosensory system in children with autism spectrum disorder. *Brain Struct Funct.* 2014;219(4):1251–1261.

32. Lee RC, Feinbaum RL, Ambros V. The C. elegans heterochronic gene lin-4 encodes small RNAs with antisense complementarity to lin-14. *Cell.* 1993;75(5):843–854.

33. Wightman B, Ha I, Ruvkun G. Posttranscriptional regulation of the heterochronic gene lin-14 by lin-4 mediates temporal pattern formation in C. elegans. *Cell.* 1993;75(5):855–862.

34. Macfarlane LA, Murphy PR. MicroRNA: Biogenesis, function and role in cancer. *Curr Genomics.* 2010;11(7):537–561.

35. Londin E, Loher P, Telonis AG, et al. Analysis of 13 cell types reveals evidence for the expression of numerous novel primate- and tissue-specific microRNAs. *Proc Natl Acad Sci USA.* 2015;112(10):E1106–E1115.

36. Denli AM, Tops BB, Plasterk RH, Ketting RF, Hannon GJ. Processing of primary microRNAs by the Microprocessor complex. *Nature.* 2004;432(7014):231–235.

37. Lee Y, Ahn C, Han J, et al. The nuclear RNase III Drosha initiates microRNA processing. *Nature.* 2003;425(6956):415–419.

38. Hutvagner G, McLachlan J, Pasquinelli AE, Balint E, Tuschl T, Zamore PD. A cellular function for the RNA-interference enzyme Dicer in the maturation of the let-7 small temporal RNA. *Science.* 2001;293(5531):834–838.

39. Mundalil Vasu M, Anitha A, Thanseem I, et al. Serum microRNA profiles in children with autism. *Mol Autism.* 2014;5:40.

40. kichukova TM, Popov, N.T., Ivanov, I.S., Vachev, T.I. Profile of circulating serum microRNAs in children with autism spectrum disorder using stem-loop qRT-PCR assay. *Folia Med (Plovdiv).* 2017;59:43–52.

41. Hicks SD, Ignacio C, Gentile K, Middleton FA. Salivary miRNA profiles identify children with autism spectrum disorder, correlate with adaptive behavior, and implicate ASD candidate genes involved in neurodevelopment. *BMC Pediatr.* 2016;16:52.

42. Schumann CM, Sharp FR, Ander BP, Stamova B. Possible sexually dimorphic role of miRNA and other sncRNA in ASD brain. *Mol Autism.* 2017;8:4.

43. Abu-Elneel K, Liu T, Gazzaniga FS, et al. Heterogeneous dysregulation of microRNAs across the autism spectrum. *Neurogenetics.* 2008;9(3):153–161.

44. Mor M, Nardone S, Sams DS, Elliott E. Hypomethylation of miR-142 promoter and upregulation of microRNAs that target the oxytocin receptor gene in the autism prefrontal cortex. *Mol Autism.* 2015;6:46.

45. Ander BP, Barger N, Stamova B, Sharp FR, Schumann CM. Atypical miRNA expression in temporal cortex associated with dysregulation of immune, cell cycle, and other pathways in autism spectrum disorders. *Mol Autism.* 2015;6:37.

46. Sarachana T, Zhou R, Chen G, Manji HK, Hu VW. Investigation of post-transcriptional gene regulatory networks associated with autism spectrum disorders by microRNA expression profiling of lymphoblastoid cell lines. *Genome Med.* 2010;2(4):23.

47. Bahi A. Sustained lentiviral-mediated overexpression of microRNA124a in the dentate gyrus exacerbates anxiety- and autism-like behaviors associated with neonatal isolation in rats. *Behav Brain Res.* 2016;311:298–308.

48. Olde Loohuis NF, Kole K, Glennon JC, et al. Elevated microRNA-181c and microRNA-30d levels in the enlarged amygdala of the valproic acid rat model of autism. *Neurobiol Dis.* 2015;80:42–53.

49. Yui K, Tanuma N, Yamada H, Kawasaki Y. Decreased total antioxidant capacity has a larger effect size than increased oxidant levels in urine in individuals with autism spectrum disorder. *Environ Sci Pollut Res Int.* 2017;24(10):9635–9644.

50. Wang L, Jia J, Zhang J, Li K. Serum levels of SOD and risk of autism spectrum disorder: A case-control study. *Int J Dev Neurosci.* 2016;51:12–16.

51. Feng C, Chen Y, Pan J, et al. Redox proteomic identification of carbonylated proteins in autism plasma: Insight into oxidative stress and its related biomarkers in autism. *Clin Proteomics.* 2017;14:2.

52. Anwar A, Marini M, Abruzzo PM, et al. Quantitation of plasma thiamine, related metabolites and plasma protein oxidative damage markers in children with autism spectrum disorder and healthy controls. *Free Radic Res.* 2016;50(supp 1):S85–S90.

53. Damodaran LP, Arumugam G. Urinary oxidative stress markers in children with autism. *Redox Rep.* 2011;16(5):216–222.

54. Lakshmi Priya MD, Geetha A. A biochemical study on the level of proteins and their percentage of nitration in the hair and nail of autistic children. *Clinica Chimica Acta.* 2011;412(11–12):1036–1042.

55. Qasem H, Al-Ayadhi L, El-Ansary A. Cysteinyl leukotriene correlated with 8-isoprostane levels as predictive biomarkers for sensory dysfunction in autism. *Lipids Health Dis.* 2016;15:130.

56. Rossignol DA, Frye RE. Evidence linking oxidative stress, mitochondrial dysfunction, and inflammation in the brain of individuals with autism. *Front Physiol.* 2014;5:150.

57. Zhang QB, Gao SJ, Zhao HX. Thioredoxin: A novel, independent diagnosis marker in children with autism. *Int J Dev Neurosci.* 2015;40:92–96.

58. Gu F, Chauhan V, Chauhan A. Impaired synthesis and antioxidant defense of glutathione in the cerebellum of autistic subjects: Alterations in the activities and protein expression of glutathione-related enzymes. *Free Radic Biol Med.* 2013;65:488–496.

59. Goldenthal MJ, Damle S, Sheth S, et al. Mitochondrial enzyme dysfunction in autism spectrum disorders; A novel biomarker revealed from buccal swab analysis. *Biomark Med.* 2015;9(10):957–965.

60. Hollis F, Kanellopoulos AK, Bagni C. Mitochondrial dysfunction in Autism Spectrum Disorder: Clinical features and perspectives. *Curr Opin Neurobiol.* 2017;45:178–187.

61. Palmieri L, Papaleo V, Porcelli V, et al. Altered calcium homeostasis in autism-spectrum disorders: Evidence from biochemical and genetic studies of the mitochondrial aspartate/glutamate carrier AGC1. *Mol Psychiatry.* 2010;15(1):38–52.

62. Prasad KN, Wu M, Bondy SC. Telomere shortening during aging: Attenuation by antioxidants and antiinflammatory agents. *Mech Ageing Dev.* 2017;164:61–66.

63. Nelson CA, Varcin KJ, Coman NK, De Vivo I, Tager-Flusberg H. Shortened telomeres in families with a propensity to autism. *J Am Acad Child Adolesc Psychiatry.* 2015;54(7):588–594.

64. Rose S, Frye RE, Slattery J, et al. Oxidative stress induces mitochondrial dysfunction in a subset of autism lymphoblastoid cell lines in a well-matched case control cohort. *PLoS One.* 2014;9(1):e85436.

65. Rose S, Bennuri SC, Wynne R, Melnyk S, James SJ, Frye RE. Mitochondrial and redox abnormalities in autism lymphoblastoid cells: A sibling control study. *FASEB J.* 2017;31(3):904–909.

66. Bu X, Wu, Lu X, et al. Role of SIRT1/PGC-1alpha in mitochondrial oxidative stress in autistic spectrum disorder. *Neuropsychiatr Dis Treat.* 2017;13:1633–1645.

67. Tonhajzerova I, Ondrejka I, Mestanik M, et al. Inflammatory activity in autism spectrum disorder. *Adv Exp Med Biol.* 2015;861:93–98.

68. Ashwood P, Krakowiak P, Hertz-Picciotto I, Hansen R, Pessah I, Van de Water J. Elevated plasma cytokines in autism spectrum disorders provide evidence of immune dysfunction and are associated with impaired behavioral outcome. *Brain Behav Immun.* 2011;25(1):40–45.

69. Jyonouchi H, Geng L, Davidow AL. Cytokine profiles by peripheral blood monocytes are associated with changes in behavioral symptoms following immune insults in a subset of ASD subjects: An inflammatory subtype? *J Neuroinflammation.* 2014;11:187.

70. Suzuki K, Matsuzaki H, Iwata K, et al. Plasma cytokine profiles in subjects with high-functioning autism spectrum disorders. *PLoS One.* 2011;6(5):e20470.

71. Napoli E, Wong S, Hertz-Picciotto I, Giulivi C. Deficits in bioenergetics and impaired immune response in granulocytes from children with autism. *Pediatrics.* 2014;133(5):e1405–e1410.

72. Cortelazzo A, De Felice C, Guerranti R, et al. Expression and oxidative modifications of plasma proteins in autism spectrum disorders: Interplay between inflammatory response and lipid peroxidation. *Proteomics Clin Appl.* 2016;10(11):1103–1112.

73. Zheng Z, Zhu T, Qu Y, Mu D. Blood glutamate levels in autism spectrum disorder: A systematic review and metaanalysis. *PLoS One.* 2016;11(7):e0158688.

74. Tebartz van Elst L, Maier S, Fangmeier T, et al. Disturbed cingulate glutamate metabolism in adults with high-functioning autism spectrum disorder: Evidence in support of the excitatory/inhibitory imbalance hypothesis. *Mol Psychiatry.* 2014;19(12):1314–1325.

75. Bejjani A, O'Neill J, Kim JA, et al. Elevated glutamatergic compounds in pregenual anterior cingulate in pediatric autism spectrum disorder demonstrated by 1H MRS and 1H MRSI. *PLoS One.* 2012;7(7):e38786.

76. Brown MS, Singel D, Hepburn S, Rojas DC. Increased glutamate concentration in the auditory cortex of persons with autism and first-degree relatives: A (1)H-MRS study. *Autism Res.* 2013;6(1):1–10.

77. Cochran DM, Sikoglu EM, Hodge SM, et al. Relationship among glutamine, gamma-aminobutyric acid, and social cognition in autism spectrum disorders. *J Child Adolesc Psychopharmacol.* 2015;25(4):314–322.

78. Naaijen J, Zwiers MP, Amiri H, et al. Fronto-striatal glutamate in autism spectrum disorder and obsessive compulsive disorder. *Neuropsychopharmacology.* 2017;42(12):2456–2465.

79. Doyle-Thomas KA, Card D, Soorya LV, Wang AT, Fan J, Anagnostou E. Metabolic mapping of deep brain structures and associations with symptomatology in autism spectrum disorders. *Res Autism Spectr Disord.* 2014;8(1):44–51.

80. Corrigan NM, Shaw DW, Estes AM, et al. Atypical developmental patterns of brain chemistry in children with autism spectrum disorder. *JAMA Psychiatry.* 2013;70(9):964–974.

81. Rojas DC, Singel D, Steinmetz S, Hepburn S, Brown MS. Decreased left perisylvian GABA concentration in children with autism and unaffected siblings. *Neuroimage.* 2014;86:28–34.

82. Harris AD, Singer HS, Horska A, et al. GABA and glutamate in children with primary complex motor stereotypies: An 1H-MRS study at 7T. *AJNR Am J Neuroradiol.* 2016;37(3):552–557.

83. Purcell AE, Jeon OH, Zimmerman AW, Blue ME, Pevsner J. Postmortem brain abnormalities of the glutamate neurotransmitter system in autism. *Neurology.* 2001;57(9):1618–1628.

84. Fatemi SH, Folsom, T.D., Kneeland, R.E., Liesch, S.B. Metabotropic glutamate receptor 5 upregulation in children with autism is associated with underexpression of both fragile X mental retardation protein and GABA receptor beta3 in adults with autism. *Anat Rec (Hoboken).* 2011;294:1635–1645.

85. Hardan AY, Fung LK, Libove RA, et al. A randomized controlled pilot trial of oral N-acetylcysteine in children with autism. *Biol Psychiatry.* 2012;71(11):956–961.

86. Wink LK, Adams R, Wang Z, et al. A randomized placebo-controlled pilot study of N-acetylcysteine in youth with autism spectrum disorder. *Mol Autism.* 2016;7:26.

87. Nikoo M, Radnia H, Farokhnia M, Mohammadi MR, Akhondzadeh S. N-acetylcysteine as an adjunctive therapy to risperidone for treatment of irritability in autism: A randomized, double-blind, placebo-controlled clinical trial of efficacy and safety. *Clin Neuropharmacol.* 2015;38(1):11–17.

88. Dean OM, Gray KM, Villagonzalo KA, et al. A randomised, double blind, placebo-controlled trial of a fixed dose of N-acetyl cysteine in children with autistic disorder. *Aust N Z J Psychiatry.* 2017;51(3):241–249.

89. Gvozdjakova A, Kucharska J, Ostatnikova D., Babinska K., Nakladal D, Creane FL. Ubiquinol improves symptoms in children with autism. *Oxid Med Cell Longev.* 2014;2014.

90. Singh K, Connors SL, Macklin EA, et al. Sulforaphane treatment of autism spectrum disorder (ASD). *P Natl Acad Sci USA.* 2014;111(43):15550–15555.

91. Bhandari R, Kuhad A. Neuropsychopharmacotherapeutic efficacy of curcumin in experimental paradigm of autism spectrum disorders. *Life Sci.* 2015;141:156–169.

92. Bhandari R, Kuhad A. Resveratrol suppresses neuroinflammation in the experimental paradigm of autism spectrum disorders. *Neurochem Int.* 2017;103:8–23.

93. Al-Amin MM, Rahman MM, Khan FR, Zaman F, Mahmud Reza H. Astaxanthin improves behavioral disorder and oxidative stress in prenatal valproic acid-induced mice model of autism. *Behav Brain Res.* 2015;286:112–121.

94. Zhang Y, Cui W, Zhai Q, Zhang T, Wen X. N-acetylcysteine ameliorates repetitive/stereotypic behavior due to its antioxidant properties without activation of the canonical Wnt pathway in a valproic acid-induced rat model of autism. *Mol Med Rep.* 2017;16(2):2233–2240.

95. Gao J, Wang X, Sun H, et al. Neuroprotective effects of docosahexaenoic acid on hippocampal cell death and learning and memory impairments in a valproic acid-induced rat autism model. *Int J Dev Neurosci.* 2016;49:67–78.

96. Chen YW, Lin HC, Ng MC, et al. Activation of mGluR2/3 underlies the effects of N-acetylcystein on amygdala-associated autism-like phenotypes in a valproate-induced rat model of autism. *Front Behav Neurosci.* 2014;8:219.

97. Vuillermot S, Luan W, Meyer U, Eyles D. Vitamin D treatment during pregnancy prevents autism-related phenotypes in a mouse model of maternal immune activation. *Mol Autism.* 2017;8:9.

98. Modabbernia A, Velthorst E, Reichenberg A. Environmental risk factors for autism: An evidence-based review of systematic reviews and meta-analyses. *Mol Autism.* 2017;8:13.

99. Isaac MG, Quinn R, Tabet N. Vitamin E for Alzheimer's disease and mild cognitive impairment. *Cochrane Database Syst Rev.* 2008;2008(3):CD002854.

100. Farina N, Isaac MG, Clark AR, Rusted J, Tabet N. Vitamin E for Alzheimer's dementia and mild cognitive impairment. *Cochrane Database Syst Rev.* 2012;11:CD002854.

101. Hamaguchi T, Ono K, Yamada M. Review: Curcumin and Alzheimer's disease. *CNS Neurosci Ther.* 2010;16(5):285–297.

102. Hager K, Kenklies M, McAfoose J, Engel J, Munch G. Alpha-lipoic acid as a new treatment option for Alzheimer's disease—A 48 month follow-up analysis. *J Neural Transm Suppl.* 2007(72):189–193.

103. Dysken MW, Sano M, Asthana S, et al. Effect of vitamin E and memantine on functional decline in Alzheimer disease: The TEAM-AD VA cooperative randomized trial. *JAMA.* 2014;311(1):33–44.

104. Fiala M, Terrando N, Dalli J. Specialized pro-resolving mediators from omega-3 fatty acids improve amyloid-beta phagocytosis and regulate inflammation in patients with minor cognitive impairment. *J Alzheimers Dis.* 2015;48(2):293–301.

105. Chiu CC, Su KP, Cheng TC, et al. The effects of omega-3 fatty acids monotherapy in Alzheimer's disease and mild cognitive impairment: A preliminary randomized double-blind placebo-controlled study. *Prog Neuropsychopharmacol Biol Psychiatry.* 2008;32(6):1538–1544.

106. Shults CW, Oakes D, Kieburtz K, et al. Effects of coenzyme Q10 in early Parkinson disease: Evidence of slowing of the functional decline. *Arch Neurol.* 2002;59(10):1541–1550.

107. Vile GF, Winterbourn CC. Inhibition of adriamycin-promoted microsomal lipid peroxidation by beta-carotene, alpha-tocopherol, and retinol at high and low oxygen partial pressures. *FEBS Lett.* 1988;238(2):353–356.

108. Niki E. Interaction of ascorbate and alpha-tocopherol. *Ann N Y Acad Sci.* 1987;498:186–199.

109. Prasad KN. Oxidative stress and pro-inflammatory cytokines may act as one of signals for regulating MicroRNAs expression in Alzheimer's disease. *Mech Ageing Dev.* 2017;162:63–71.

110. Wu H, Kong L, Tan Y, et al. C66 ameliorates diabetic nephropathy in mice by both upregulating Nrf2 function via increase in miR-200a and inhibiting miR-21. *Diabetologia.* 2016;59:1558–1568.

111. Prasad KN. Simultaneous activation of Nrf2 and elevation of antioxidant compounds for reducing oxidative stress and chronic inflammation in human Alzheimer's disease. *Mech Ageing Dev.* 2016;153:41–47.

112. Itoh K, Chiba T, Takahashi S, et al. An Nrf2/small Maf heterodimer mediates the induction of phase II detoxifying enzyme genes through antioxidant response elements. *Biochem Biophys Res Commun.* 1997;236(2):313–322.

113. Williamson TP, Johnson DA, Johnson JA. Activation of the Nrf2-ARE pathway by siRNA knockdown of Keap1 reduces oxidative stress and provides partial protection from MPTP-mediated neurotoxicity. *Neurotoxicology.* 2012;33(3):272–279.

114. Jaramillo MC, Zhang DD. The emerging role of the Nrf2-Keap1 signaling pathway in cancer. *Genes Dev.* 2013;27(20):2179–2191.

115. Li W, Khor TO, Xu C, et al. Activation of Nrf2-antioxidant signaling attenuates NFkappaB-inflammatory response and elicits apoptosis. *Biochem Pharmacol.* 2008;76(11):1485–1489.

116. Kim J, Cha YN, Surh YJ. A protective role of nuclear factor-erythroid 2-related factor-2 (Nrf2) in inflammatory disorders. *Mutat Res.* 2010;690(1–2):12–23.

117. Suh JH, Shenvi SV, Dixon BM, et al. Decline in transcriptional activity of Nrf2 causes age-related loss of glutathione synthesis, which is reversible with lipoic acid. *Proc Natl Acad Sci USA.* 2004;101(10):3381–3386.

118. Furnari MA, Saw CL, Kong AN, Wagner GC. Altered behavioral development in Nrf2 knockout mice following early postnatal exposure to valproic acid. *Brain Res Bull.* 2014;109:132–142.

119. Mostafavi-Pour Z, Ramezani F, Keshavarzi F, Samadi N. The role of quercetin and vitamin C in Nrf2-dependent oxidative stress production in breast cancer cells. *Oncol Lett.* 2017;13(3):1965–1973.

120. Katsuyama Y, Tsuboi T, Taira N, Yoshioka M, Masaki H. 3-O-Laurylglyceryl ascorbate activates the intracellular antioxidant system through the contribution of PPAR-gamma and Nrf2. *J Dermatol Sci.* 2016;82(3):189–196.

121. Xi YD, Yu HL, Ding J, et al. Flavonoids protect cerebrovascular endothelial cells through Nrf2 and PI3K from beta-amyloid peptide-induced oxidative damage. *Curr Neurovasc Res.* 2012;9(1):32–41.

122. Choi HK, Pokharel YR, Lim SC, et al. Inhibition of liver fibrosis by solubilized coenzyme Q10: Role of Nrf2 activation in inhibiting transforming growth factor-beta1 expression. *Toxicol Appl Pharmacol.* 2009;240(3):377–384.

123. Ji L, Liu R, Zhang XD, et al. N-acetylcysteine attenuates phosgene-induced acute lung injury via upregulation of Nrf2 expression. *Inhal Toxicol.* 2010;22(7):535–542.

124. Gao L, Wang J, Sekhar KR, et al. Novel n-3 fatty acid oxidation products activate Nrf2 by destabilizing the association between Keap1 and Cullin3. *J Biol Chem.* 2007;282(4):2529–2537.

125. Saw CL, Yang AY, Guo Y, Kong AN. Astaxanthin and omega-3 fatty acids individually and in combination protect against oxidative stress via the Nrf2-ARE pathway. *Food Chem Toxicol.* 2013;62:869–875.

126. Trujillo J, Chirino YI, Molina-Jijon E, Anderica-Romero AC, Tapia E, Pedraza-Chaverri J. Renoprotective effect of the antioxidant curcumin: Recent findings. *Redox Biol.* 2013;1(1):448–456.

127. Steele ML, Fuller S, Patel M, Kersaitis C, Ooi L, Munch G. Effect of Nrf2 activators on release of glutathione, cysteinylglycine, and homocysteine by human U373 astroglial cells. *Redox Biol.* 2013;1(1):441–445.

128. Kode A, Rajendrasozhan S, Caito S, Yang SR, Megson IL, Rahman I. Resveratrol induces glutathione synthesis by activation of Nrf2 and protects against cigarette smoke-mediated oxidative stress in human lung epithelial cells. *Am J Physiol. Lung Cell Mol Physiol.* 2008;294(3):L478–L488.

129. Zambrano S, Blanca AJ, Ruiz-Armenta MV, et al. The renoprotective effect of L-carnitine in hypertensive rats is mediated by modulation of oxidative stress-related gene expression. *Eur J Nutr.* 2013;52(6):1649–1659.

130. Eades G, Yang M, Yao Y, Zhang Y, Zhou Q. miR-200a regulates Nrf2 activation by targeting Keap1 mRNA in breast cancer cells. *J Biol Chem.* 2011;286(47):40725–40733.

131. Narasimhan M, Riar AK, Rathinam ML, Vedpathak D, Henderson G, Mahimainathan L. Hydrogen peroxide responsive miR153 targets Nrf2/ARE cytoprotection in paraquat induced dopaminergic neurotoxicity. *Toxicol Lett.* 2014;228(3):179–191.

132. Abate A, Yang G, Dennery PA, Oberle S, Schroder H. Synergistic inhibition of cyclooxygenase-2 expression by vitamin E and aspirin. *Free Radic Biol Med.* 2000;29(11):1135–1142.

133. Fu Y, Zheng S, Lin J, Ryerse J, Chen A. Curcumin protects the rat liver from CCl4-caused injury and fibrogenesis by attenuating oxidative stress and suppressing inflammation. *Mol Pharmacol.* 2008;73(2):399–409.

134. Lee HS, Jung KK, Cho JY, et al. Neuroprotective effect of curcumin is mainly mediated by blockade of microglial cell activation. *Pharmazie.* 2007;62(12):937–942.

135. Rahman S, Bhatia K, Khan AQ, et al. Topically applied vitamin E prevents massive cutaneous inflammatory and oxidative stress responses induced by double application of 12-O-tetradecanoylphorbol-13-acetate (TPA) in mice. *Chem Biol Interact.* 2008;172(3):195–205.

136. Suzuki YJ, Aggarwal BB, Packer L. Alpha-lipoic acid is a potent inhibitor of NF-kappa B activation in human T cells. *Biochem Biophys Res Commun.* 1992;189(3):1709–1715.

137. Zhu J, Yong W, Wu X, et al. Anti-inflammatory effect of resveratrol on TNF-alpha-induced MCP-1 expression in adipocytes. *Biochem Biophys Res Commun.* 2008;369(2):471–477.

138. Barger SW, Goodwin ME, Porter MM, Beggs ML. Glutamate release from activated microglia requires the oxidative burst and lipid peroxidation. *J Neurochem.* 2007;101(5):1205–1213.

139. Dohare P, Hyzinski-Garcia MC, Vipani A, et al. The neuroprotective properties of the superoxide dismutase mimetic tempol correlate with its ability to reduce pathological glutamate release in a rodent model of stroke. *Free Radic Biol Med.* 2014;77:168–182.

140. Lu CW, Lin TY, Wang SJ. Quercetin inhibits depolarization-evoked glutamate release in nerve terminals from rat cerebral cortex. *Neurotoxicology.* 2013;39:1–9.

141. Hurtado O, De Cristobal J, Sanchez V, et al. Inhibition of glutamate release by delaying ATP fall accounts for neuroprotective effects of antioxidants in experimental stroke. *FASEB J.* 2003;17(14):2082–2084.

142. Santos PS, Campelo LM, Freitas RL, Feitosa CM, Saldanha GB, Freitas RM. Lipoic acid effects on glutamate and taurine concentrations in rat hippocampus after pilocarpine-induced seizures. *Arquivos de neuro-psiquiatria.* 2011;69(2B):360–364.

143. Chang Y, Huang SK, Wang SJ. Coenzyme Q10 inhibits the release of glutamate in rat cerebrocortical nerve terminals by suppression of voltage-dependent calcium influx and mitogen-activated protein kinase signaling pathway. *J Agric Food Chem.* 2012;60(48):11909–11918.

144. Yang TT, Wang SJ. Pyridoxine inhibits depolarization-evoked glutamate release in nerve terminals from rat cerebral cortex: A possible neuroprotective mechanism? *J Pharmacol Exp Ther.* 2009;331(1):244–254.

145. Hung KL, Wang CC, Huang CY, Wang SJ. Cyanocobalamin, vitamin B12, depresses glutamate release through inhibition of voltage-dependent Ca^{2+} influx in rat cerebrocortical nerve terminals (synaptosomes). *Eur J Pharmacol.* 2009;602(2–3):230–237.

146. Wang SJ, Wu WM, Yang FL, Hsu GS, Huang CY. Vitamin B2 inhibits glutamate release from rat cerebrocortical nerve terminals. *Neuroreport.* 2008;19(13):1335–1338.

147. Behl C, Davis J, Cole GM, Schubert D. Vitamin E protects nerve cells from amyloid beta protein toxicity. *Biochem Biophys Res Commun.* 1992;186(2):944–950.

148. Sandhu JK, Pandey S, Ribecco-Lutkiewicz M, et al. Molecular mechanisms of glutamate neurotoxicity in mixed cultures of NT2-derived neurons and astrocytes: Protective effects of coenzyme Q10. *J Neurosci Res.* 2003;72(6):691–703.

149. LeClerc S, Easley D. Pharmacological therapies for autism spectrum disorder: A review. *Pharm Ther.* 2015;40(6):389–397.

150. Wu H, Wang X, Gao J, et al. Fingolimod (FTY720) attenuates social deficits, learning and memory impairments, neuronal loss, and neuroinflammation in the rat model of autism. *Life Sci.* 2017;173:43–54.

16 Micronutrients in the Management of Prion Disease

INTRODUCTION

Prion diseases are a group of rare, progressive, transmissible, incurable, and fatal neurodegenerative diseases. They are characterized by transmissible spongiform encephalopathy (TSE) and are found in mammals, including humans. In 1730's, the symptoms of prion disease were known as scrapie in sheep and goat. In 1957, a transmissible neurological disease called Kuru, similar to Creutzfeldt-Jakob disease (CJD), was identified in the Fore tribe of Papua, New Guinea.[1] Extracts from the autopsied brain samples of individuals with Kuru when administered into chimpanzees led to similar brain pathology.[2] A similar cross-species infectivity was found in the United Kingdom following an outbreak of "mad cow disease." In 1982, Dr. Stanley Prusiner of the University of California School of Medicine, San Francisco, proposed the term "prion" because pathogenic misfolded normal prion proteins caused this disease. He isolated an infective agent from the brain of sheep with scrapie and bovine spongiform encephalopathy (BSE) in cattle that causes neurodegeneration in sheep and goats.[3] A similar infectious agent was isolated from brains of victims of the genetic diseases Creutzfeldt-Jakob disease (CJD) and Gerstmann-Sträussler-Scheinker syndrome (GSS). In 2012, a novel idea suggested that neurodegenerative diseases such as Alzheimer's disease (AD) and Parkinson's disease could be considered a prion disease.[4] This view was questioned because the similarity between beta-sheet of Aβ peptides of AD and their aggregation characteristics and the characteristics of PrPsc in producing neurodegeneration is not sufficient to support this suggestion.[5] Beta-sheet Aβ peptide of AD does not replicate, but PrPsc of prion disease does.

This chapter briefly describes the incidence, types of prion disease, modes of transmission, and pathological changes in the brain and discusses factors facilitating the transition of normal prion protein (PrPc) to infectious prion protein (PrPsc). It presents evidence to show that increased oxidation of PrPc is one of the factors that initiate the transition of PrPc to PrPsc and describes PrPsc-induced inflammation that contributes to the progression of prion disease. This chapter proposes a novel idea that in order to reduce oxidative stress and inflammation at the same time, it is essential to increase the levels of antioxidant enzyme by activating the Nrf2 pathway as well as dietary and endogenous antioxidants. It also proposes a mixture of micronutrients that would activate Nrf2 and enhance the levels of antioxidants and improve the management of human prion disease.

INCIDENCE OF PRION DISEASE

The annual incidence of prion disease Creutzfeldt-Jakob disease (CJD) in the USA is about 1 case/million persons[6] or about 300 cases per year (National Institute of neurological Disorders and Stroke, 2017). Generally, the symptoms appear at age of about 60 years, and about 90% of patients die within a year.

TYPES OF PRION DISEASE

This disease is grouped into 4 categories, sporadic CJD (sCJD), variant CJD (vCJD), familial (fCJD), and iatrogenic CJD. Sporadic CJD, the most common form (about 85%), results from spontaneous conversion of PrPc to PrPsc, rather than from PrPsc infection from external sources.[7,8] One of the largest clusters of familial CJD (fCJD) is found in Libyan Jews. The clinical and pathological features of CJD in this community are similar to those observed in sCJD, but the incidence of this disease is 100 times higher than in the general population.[9] The fCJD in this community is linked to the E200K mutation (substitution of glutamate for lysine at codon 200) in PRNP gene. Another fCJD linked to the mutation in which a substitution of valine (V) for glycine (G) at codon 114 (G114V) is found in Chinese patients.[10] In the USA, fCJD represents about 5%–10% of prion disease. Sporadic CJD occurs mostly in older individuals with rapid progression of dementia leading to death within a year, whereas variant CJD (vCJD) is found in younger individuals with slower progression of the disease.[11,12] Mode of transmission of sCJD is uncertain. Variant CJD can be transmitted from person to person by consumption of infected meat, medical procedures such as blood transfusion, and contaminated dental tools.[13,14] Transmission of vCJD through medical/surgical treatment produces iatrogenic CJD. The skin of patients with sCJD contained about 10^3–10^5-fold lower PrPsc than the brain. When skin homogenates from sCJD patients were inoculated into transgenic mice, all developed prion disease, suggesting the iatrogenic sCJD transmission may occur via skin.[15]

One of the early clinical features of sCJD is progressive dementia, whereas in vCJD, it is progressive psychiatry disorders. Human prion diseases include sCJD, vCJD, fCJD, GSS, Kuru, and fatal Familial Insomnia (FFI), whereas animal prion diseases include bovine spongiform encephalitis (BSE), chronic wasting disease (CWD), scrapie, transmissible mink encephalitis, and feline spongiform encephalitis.

MODES OF TRANSMISSION OF PRION DISEASE TO THE BRAIN

Normal prion protein (PrPc) is expressed on the surface membranes of all cells including neurons and is coded by the gene PRNP located on the chromosome 20 at position 13.[16,17] The infectious PrPsc is misfolded and its beta-sheet conformation can act as a template for the conversion of normal PrPc to PrPsc leading to the formation of insoluble aggregates causing transmissible spongiform encephalopathy (TSE) in mammals.

The migration of PrPsc from the periphery to the brain is very complex. Following oral ingestion of infective agents or blood transfusion from infected individuals, the replication and accumulation of PrPsc occur within the secondary lymphoid organs from where PrPsc enters the brain via peripheral nerves. PrPsc continue to replicate and form aggregates that cause neurodegeneration and ultimately death of the host. Mononuclear phagocytes play an important role in the pathogenesis of prion disease. Some phagocytes may help PrPsc to enter lymphoid tissues where they propagate, whereas others may remove them by phagocytosis. It was observed that an intact splenic marginal zone allows the rapid delivery of PrPsc into B-lymphocyte follicles where they replicate upon the follicular dendritic cells before entering the brain. PrPsc continue to replicate into the brain leading to inflammatory events that contribute to the progression of disease.[18]

PATHOLOGICAL CHANGES IN THE BRAIN

The pathological changes in the brain of CJD patients are also complex, depending upon the type of mutation in PRPN gene and regions of the brain. The extent of vacuolation (spongiform change) and deposition of PrPsc differ in various regions of the brain. The density of vacuolation was highest in the occipital cortex and cerebellum and lowest in the dentate gyrus, whereas the amounts of deposition of PrPsc were similar in the cortex and cerebellum, but they were absent in the dentate gyrus.[19] The clinical changes in CJD patients consist of rapid progressive cognitive dysfunction, diffusion-weighted magnetic resonance imaging (DWI) hyperintensity, myoclonus, periodic sharp-wave complexes on electroencephalogram, and akinetic mutism state. Pathological alterations in the brain included spongiform changes in the gray matter, gliosis, and neuropil rarefaction, followed by neuronal loss.[20] This study further reveals that changes in the levels of spongiform occurred several months before gliosis and the emergence of symptoms.

SYMPTOMS OF PRION DISEASE

The symptoms of sCJD are characterized by rapid progressive dementia. Earlier symptoms include muscular incoordination, impaired memory, judgment, thinking, and vision. Individuals with CJD may suffer from insomnia, depression, or unusual sensation. These symptoms are progressive. Individuals may develop myoclonus, a disease of involuntary jerky movement, and may become blind. They eventually are unable to move or speak and then enter a coma. Pneumonia and other infections often precipitate death. The symptoms of vCJD is characterized by the early onset of progressive psychiatric disorders, and longer period incubation period (CDC, 2017).

FACTORS FACILITATING CONVERSION OF PrPc TO PrPsc AND MECHANISMS OF PROLIFERATION OF PrPsc

EFFECT OF MUTATIONS IN PRNP GENE

Mutations in prion gene PRNP coding for PrPc can produce infective PrPsc. More than 30 mutations in PRNP gene coding for normal prion protein are associated with familial prion disease[21] of which E200K-associated familial CJD is the most common.[22] These can trigger conformational change in normal α-helix structure of PrPc converting it to the abnormal β-sheet structure of PrPsc leading to the formation of intracellular aggregates that are not susceptible to proteolytic degradation and are toxic. Such aggregates can grow and extend between cells. They thus become infectious resembling bacteria and viruses.[23] However, unlike bacteria and viruses, they have no nucleic acids.[24,25] The mechanisms of transition from PrPc to PrPsc structure and replication of PrPsc are not well understood. They are likely to involve interaction between PrPc and PrPsc at the cell surface. The newly formed PrPsc structure can accumulate as intracellular aggregates or at the cell surface.[23] This procedure of transition from PrPc to PrPsc repeated many times leads to a chain reaction and an exponential increase in the number of PrPsc.[26] In the familial variant of prion disease, spontaneous generation of PrPsc may be due to selective migration of mutant PrPc to the acidic environment of the lysosome that facilitate the conversion of PrPc to PrPsc.[27] A substantial degree of conversion of PrPc to PrPsc is likely to occur in the endosomal/lysosomal system in all prionoses.

ROLE OF EXOSOMES

Exosomes, membranous vesicles secreted into the extracellular spaces, may serve as shuttles for the transport of PrPsc into uninfected tissue. Ceramide and endosomal sorting complex required for transport (ESCRT-0) play an important role in the biogenesis of exosomes; therefore, they may play a role in the formation, release, and spread of PrPsc. Silencing HRS-ESCRT-0, a subunit hepatocyte growth factor-regulated tyrosine kinase substrate (HRS) of (ESCRT-0), markedly reduces the adoption of a PrPsc configuration. Depletion of ESCRT-1 complex subunit tsg101 (tumor susceptibility gene101) or reduction in the production of ceramide significantly decreases the release of PrPsc.[28,29] These results suggest that ESCRT-dependent pathways play an important role in the formation and release of PrPsc. Increased levels of PrPsc induce endoplasmic reticulum (ER) stress and lead to an activated unfolded protein response (UPR). A major chaperone protein of the ER, GRP78/Bip decreases ER stress levels and reduces apoptosis. Reduction in levels of GRP78 accelerates the progression of prion disease.[30] In the acquired prion disease, infection is initially propagated in the lymphoid tissue before invading and spreading in the brain. Cultured medium of infected neuronal cells contains PrPsc within the exosomes and this can initiate propagation of PrPsc configuration in uninfected cells.[31] After infection with sheep PrPsc, both PrPc and PrPsc are released into the extracellular environment where they are associated with exosomes.[32] Plasminogen markedly stimulates propagation of the PrPsc format in a dose-dependent manner by increasing the rate of generation of this transmissible agent.[33]

Effects on Polymorphisms of PNRP Gene

Polymorphisms in the PrPc gene (PNRP) strongly influence susceptibility to prion disease.[34] The PrPc allele PrP^{VRQ} is present in significant number in scrapie-infected cells, whereas the other allele PrP^{ARR} is found only in healthy sheep. Two other alleles PrP^{ARQ} and PrP^{ARH} are present in both infected and uninfected sheep cells in similar number. Rov cells (derived from RK13 cell line of normal rabbit kidney epithelial cells) expressing an ovine PrPc allele PRP^{VRQ} are very sensitive to sheep prion transmission and replication, whereas Rov cells expressing Prpc allele PrP^{ARR} are resistant to prion infection.[35]

Polymorphism of the human PRNP gene, methionine (M)/valine (V) at codon129 and glutamic acid (E)/lysine (K) at codon219 affect the sensitivity of host to prison disease. In patients with scud and cud, 129M/M homozygote is overexpressed. Although 219E/K heterozygosity provides protection against the development of sCJD, this genotype does not confer the same protection in acquired forms (iatrogenic and vCJD) or genetic forms (genetic CJD and Gerstmann-Sträussler-Scheinker syndrome).[36] A mutation at codon 178 (Asp178/Aspn) is associated with fatal familial insomnia and familial CJD disease, depending upon the presence of Met or val at codon129. Polymorphic variants D178N/M129 and D178N/V129 have a high rate of conversion of PrPc to PrPsc (at acidic pH) and to thioflavin T-positive amyloid fibrils (at neutral pH). This rate of this conversion by D178N variant is markedly dependent upon the M/V polymorphism at codon129. No such observation was made for the wild-type protein.[37]

The sequence of steps whereby the normal structure and function of prion protein (PrPc) can be subverted to infectious prion protein (PrPsc) that eventually leads to spongiform encephalopathy is summarized in Figure 16.1.

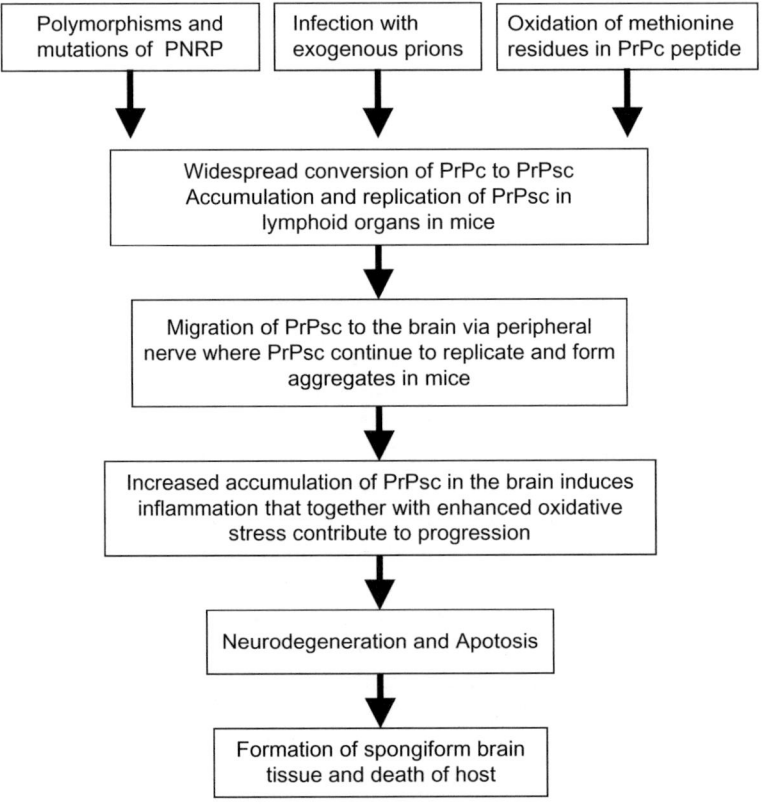

FIGURE 16.1　Onset and progression of prion toxicity.

EFFECTS OF INCREASED OXIDATIVE STRESS

Increased oxidative stress is likely to play a central role in the initiation and progression of neuro-degenerative diseases including familial, sporadic and infectious forms of prion disease. Several studies suggest that oxidative events may be one of the important factors in conversion of normal prion protein (PrPc) to misfolded infective protein PrPsc. Increased lipid peroxidation is one of the earliest signs of oxidative damage in regions of the brain infected with the PrPsc.[38] In patients with CJD, the levels of lipid peroxidation are increased in the cerebral spinal fluid (CSF) and plasma, while the levels of polyunsaturated fatty acids are decreased in the plasma alone. In addition, the levels of ascorbate are reduced in both plasma and CSF, and alpha-tocopherol levels decreased in the CSF. Thus, increased oxidative stress may play an important role in the pathogenesis of CJD.[39] In sporadic CJD, serum levels of the antioxidant uric acid are decreased.[40]

OXIDATION OF METHIONINE RESIDUES IN PrPc

Oxidation of methionine residues in PrPc may be responsible for conformational change from the α-helical form of PrPc to beta sheets of PrPsc and this may be a factor determining the rate and progression of familial CJD.[21] Oxidation of methionine 213 (Met213) and Met 205/206 converted PrPc to a PrPsc.[21] Oxidation of PrPc destabilizes the helical core of PrPc (Met205, Met212, Val209, Val160, and Tyr156), and this can facilitate the structural transition from PrPc to a PrPsc.[41] Loss of antioxidant defense systems may then contribute to the development and progression of prion disease.[42] In fatal familial insomnia (FFI), associated with mutation in the D178N/129M gene, methionine oxidation also converts PrPc to a PrPsc.[43] Oxidation of methionine residues (Met 206 and Met 213) in Helix-3 appears to be an early biochemical defect that allows the conversion of PrPc to protease resistant PrPsc in familial CJD.[44,45] Mutations in the G114v and A116V genes lie in the hydrophobic domain of PrPc. Cells expressing these mutations when exposed to PrPsc result in formation of relatively a protease digestible PrPsc structure that is still highly neurotoxic. Thus, infective PrPsc does not have to be always protease-resistant.[46] These studies suggest that increased oxidative stress may be one of the early events in conversion of PrPc to PrPsc.

EFFECTS OF PrPsc-INDUCED INFLAMMATION IN THE BRAIN

Activation of immune cells in the brain appears to be one of earliest events in the development of prion disease. Increased accumulation of PrPsc causes inflammatory events leading to dysfunctional neurons and eventually neuronal death.[47] In the PrPsc infected brain, activated microglia accumulate in the vicinity of abnormal prion aggregates. They release inflammatory cytokines such as IL-1β that are likely to play an important role in the pathogenesis of prion disease.[48] The role of microglia in inducing inflammatory events within the brain has been recently reviewed.[49] The distribution of PrPsc in the neurons, astroglia, and microglia in the brain is related to the type of the originating PrPsc strain. Strain 22L of PrPsc primarily accumulates in the astroglia, whereas strain ME7 is mainly localized in the neurons and neuropil.[50] In the preceding report, expressions of all 90 genes that regulate neuroinflammation were found to be similarly upregulated in all three strains of PrPsc tested. This correlated with the activation of both astroglia and microglia that occurs in the early phase of the disease prior to the development of vascular pathology or clinical symptoms. Aggregated misfolded prion proteins induce inflammation, and this is likely to contribute to spongiform degeneration of the brain.[51] Infection of a mouse brain with PrPsc upregulates several genes associated with inflammation.[52] Infection with PrPsc releases a pro-inflammatory cytokine IL-1β by activating the inflammasomes that participate in the progression of the prion disease.[53] In CJD, such increased levels of IL-1β contribute to the death of neurons.[54] In human prion disease, inflammation-regulated expression of miR-146 was enhanced. This may form the basis of irreversible progressive neurodegeneration in the brain.[55,56] In a puzzling contrast to the increased induction of inflammatory genes by PrPsc in the brain, lymphoid tissues of sheep infected with PrPsc exhibit reduced expression of inflammatory genes. This is, however, not a progressive phenomenon.[57] Increased intracellular accumulation of Ca^{2+} is present in the brain of CJD and activation of the calpain-cathepsin axis occurs at the preclinical stage of the disease.[58] It may then be that excessive levels of free ionic calcium might also have a role in the pathogenesis of this disease.

A synthetic peptide homologous to the region 106–126 of PrPc exhibits many features of PrPsc including the ability to produce apoptosis of neurons.[59] This peptide is toxic to the cells expressing PrPc but not to the cells with PrPc knocked out. Thus normal PrPc mediates the toxicity of PrP106–126.[60] PrP106–126 also enhances the expression of inducible nitric oxide (iNOS), pro-inflammatory cytokines IL-1β and TNF-alpha, and activated NF-kB in mouse macrophages. Inhibition of NF-kB blocked these effects of PrP106–126 on markers of inflammation.[61]

A PrPc fragment containing amino acids 90–231 also causes neuropathological changes similar to that produced by pathogenic prion protein PrPsc in microglia culture. Microglia activation led to that release of prostaglandin E2 (PGE2) and nitric oxide (NO), in amounts toxic to neurons. Conditioned medium from PrP90–231 treated microglia when added to the mesencephalic neurons also induced degeneration. Celecoxib, an inhibitor of COX 2, prevented PrP90–231-induced activation of microglia cells, and release of PGE2 and NO. However, Ketoprofen, a specific inhibitor of COX1 was ineffective.[62] These results suggest that PrPsc-induced inflammatory events play an important role in the progression of prion disease in the brain.

The findings discussed above suggest that Increased oxidative stress and chronic inflammation can be involved in the initiation and progression of prion disease. These two biochemical defects are likely to play a central role at different stages of the disease. While increased oxidative stress converts PrPc to PrPsc and promote conversion of PrP to PrPsc in peripheral tissue, progressive accumulation of PrPsc may induce inflammatory events in the brain. These events then may accelerate the progression of the disease.

MECHANISMS OF NEUROTOXICITY

The mechanisms of neurotoxicity are highly complex; therefore, in vitro models using toxic prion peptides have been used to study this. Prion peptide PrP106-126 peptide that induces neuropathology similar to that of PrPsc appears to produce neurotoxicity by multiple pathways. It activates microglia that release reactive oxygen species (ROS) and pro-inflammatory cytokines.[63] It also increases Ca^{2+} uptake through voltage-sensitive Ca^{2+} channels, and thus activates NMDA receptors leading to cell death.[64] Other mechanisms of toxicity were investigated by generating the β-sheet state of oligomeric PrPsc through protein misfolding cyclic amplification from recombinant full-length in hamster, human, rabbit, and mutated rabbit PrPc. These β-sheet oligomers are toxic to primary mouse cortical neurons independent of the presence of PrPc in the neurons. The mechanisms of toxicity produced by these beta-oligomers involve elevation of levels of proapoptotic proteins such as Bcl2, Bax, and caspase-3.[65] Another mechanism was suggested by the beta-amyloid of Alzheimer's disease that has beta-sheet configuration similar to that of PrPsc. This is suspected to cause neuronal death by generation of prooxidant free radicals.[66–68] It is likely that PrPsc-induced prion aggregates also induce neuronal death by this mechanism. This is further substantiated by reports, to be discussed in the subsequent section, in which antioxidants prevent the progression of prion diseases in both cell culture and intact animals.

MicroRNAs IN PRION DISEASE

MicroRNAs (miRs) are evolutionarily conserved small noncoding single-stranded RNAs of approximately 22 nucleotides in length, and are present in all living organisms including humans.[69–72] The biogenesis of miRs is very complex and involves multiple biochemical steps. The majority of miRs are transcribed by RNA polymerase II (Pol II), while some are transcribed by RNA polymerase

III (Pol III) from the noncoding region of the DNA to produce primary miRs (pri-miRs). Pri-miRs undergo a nuclear cleavage by ribonuclease III Drosa to generate precursor-miRs (pre-miRs) that migrate to the cytoplasm where they are further cleaved by ribonuclease III Dicer to ultimately form mature single-stranded miRs with the help of another protein argonaute (Ago)[71,73–75] Each microRNA binds to its complimentary sequences in the 3′-untranslated region (3′-UTR) of the mRNA, promotes degradation of the mRNA transcript, and prevents translation of the message of protein. In this manner, miRs regulate the translation of proapoptotic or antiapoptotic proteins from their respective mRNAs, depending upon whether they receive damaging or protective signal.

MicroRNAs are involved in the pathogenesis of other neurodegenerative diseases such as Alzheimer's disease (AD)[76] and Parkinson's disease (PD).[77] Reactive oxygen species (ROS) and pro-inflammatory cytokines that play a major role in the initiation and progression of these disease alter the expression of miRs in neuronal and neuron-glial culture were investigated.

Since increased oxidative stress and chronic inflammation are also found in prion disease, alterations in the expression of miRs leading to degenerative changes may occur in the brain; however, only limited studies have been performed. Using mice infected with pathogenic scrapie, it was demonstrated that miRs, which were upregulated in the asymptomatic phase were different from those that were upregulated in the symptomatic phase. In addition, certain miRs that were downregulated in the symptomatic phase were not expressed in the asymptomatic phase[78] (Table 16.1). The expression of miR-146 was upregulated by pro-inflammatory cytokines, Aβ peptides and oxidative stress. The upregulation of *has*-miR-342-3p and has-miR-494 was also observed in the brain of bovine spongiform encephalopathy (BSE)–infected macaques. The expression of *has*-342-3p was increased the autopsied brain samples of human sCJD as well as from scrapie-infected mice.[79] Synthetic dual microRNAs (DmiR) suppressed the expression of PrPc in PrPsc-infected differentiated C2C12 cell culture (immortal cell line from mouse skeletal myoblast) and primary mixed neuronal and glial cell culture and slowed the replication of PrPsc.[80] Upregulated miR-342-3p and miR-21-5p were found in scrapie-infected animals.[81] None of these studies identified the potential protein targets; therefore, it is difficult to explain the significance of alterations in the expression of miRs in prion disease. It is unknown whether changes in the expression of microRNAs are due to alterations in their transcription, processing by Drosa in the nucleus and Dicer in the cytoplasm or stability. Because of the involvement of increased oxidative stress and inflammation in prion disease, it is possible that changes in the expression of miRs may increase apoptotic and inflammatory pathways to cause degeneration in the brain.

TABLE 16.1
Alterations in Expression of MicroRNAs in Synaptoneurosomas of Mice Infected with Pathogenic Scrapie (PrPsc)

Asymptomatic Stage	Symptomatic Stage
Upregulated	**Upregulated**
miR-124a-3p, miR-136-5p	miR-146a-5p, miR-142-3p, miR-143-3p
miR-376a-3p	miR-145a-5p, miR-150-5p, miR-451a, miR-let-7b, miR-320
	Downregulated
	miR-200a-3p, miR-200b-3p, miR-200c-3p
	miR-141-3p, miR-429-3p, miR-182-5p
	miR-183-5p

Note: Alterations in the expression of microRNAs in prion disease could be due to alterations in their transcription, processing by Drosa in the nucleus and Dicer in the cytoplasm or stability.

STUDIES WITH INDIVIDUAL ANTIOXIDANTS AND PHYTOCHEMICALS IN MODELS OF PRION DISEASES

Since increased oxidative stress is one of the factors in conversion of PrPc to PrPsc and since antioxidant reduce oxidative stress, loss of antioxidant defense system may be considered as one of the primary events for allowing conversion of PrPc to PrPsc. Several antioxidants and phytochemicals have shown promise for the delay and mitigation of the devastating consequences of prion disease in cell culture and animal models. Some of these are enumerated.

Members of the peroxiredoxin class of enzymes are all antioxidants and peroxiredoxin 6 (Prdx6) protects human neuroblastoma cells (SK-N-SH) against oxidative stress caused by H_2O_2, hydroperoxides, or peroxynitrite.[82] In mice infected with prion disease, the overexpression of Prdx6 protects against oxidative damage, reduces severity of behavioral deficits, and diminishes progression of neuropathology. This increases the survival time in comparison to parallel treatment of mice with knockout of Prdx6.[82]

Phytochemicals such as baicalein, the dried root of *Scutellaria baicalensis* (known as Huang-quin in traditional Chinese medicine) protects human neuroblastoma cells in culture against development of prion disease induced by the human PrPc fragment containing amino acids 106–126 (PrP106–126) that induces neuropathological changes similar to those produced by PrPsc. This protective effect of baicalein that was correlated with inhibition of ROS and restoration of mitochondrial functions may have been affected by way of modulation of phosphorylation of JNK (c-Jun N-terminal kinase).[83]

Treatment with melatonin prevented PrP106–126-induced damage to human neuroblastoma cells (SH-SY5Y). Melatonin activates beta-catenin and this may account for some of its antioxidant activity. An inhibitor of beta-catenin blocked the protective effect of melatonin.[84]

Resveratrol has both antioxidant and anti-inflammatory activity. Treatment of neuronal cells with resveratrol attenuates PrP106–126 induced cell death by activating autophagy that prevented mitochondrial dysfunction and translocation of pro-apoptotic protein Bax to the mitochondria and cytochrome C release.[85] Resveratrol treatment also prevents PrP106–126-induced neuronal death by activating SIRT1.[86]

Rutin is a bioflavonoid known to possess antioxidant and anti-inflammatory properties. Treatment of dopaminergic neurons with rutin prevents PrP106–126-induced neuronal death by increasing the production of neurotropic factors and reducing activation of apoptotic pathways.[87]

An extract of pomegranate seed oil in nanodroplet form that exhibits antioxidant activity, delayed the manifestation of prion disease when administered to an asymptomatic genetic mouse model of prion disease.[88]

Treatment of neuronal PC12 cells in culture with PrP106–126 peptide decreases intracellular levels of glutathione, superoxide dismutase activity, depolarizes the mitochondrial membrane, and increases the activity of caspase-3. These effects of the toxic peptide are all reduced in the presence of a synthetic antioxidant edaravone.[89]

Epigallocatechin gallate (EGCG) and gallocatechin gallate are the primary polyphenols in green tea and are antioxidants. They induce conformational changes in PrP to produce a detergent insoluble form that is distinct from the PrPsc sheet structure. This form of insoluble PrP is rapidly internalized from the plasma membrane and degraded by lysosomes. In scrapie-infected cells, treatment with EGCG prevents proliferation of abnormal prion configurations.[90] EGCG thus appears to have the potential to block the progression of prion disease.

Treatment of a mouse model of prion disease with a potent Mn-SOD/catalase mimetic, EUK-189, improves survival time, and this is correlated with reduced oxidative and nitrosylative events and lessened spongiform changes.[91]

Administration of dimethylsulfoxide (DMSO) a solvent that exhibits antioxidant activity, to scrapie-infected hamsters significantly prolongs the period of disease latency, and delays the accumulation of PrPsc-induced aggregates in the brain.[92]

These studies provide indirect support for both the role of increased oxidative stress in the development and progression of prion disease, and for the possibility of therapeutic antioxidant and anti-inflammatory measures, as suggested for other neurodegenerative disease.[93,94]

The effects of antioxidants on non-neuronal cells are mediated via alterations in the expression of miRs that inhibit proapoptotic and inflammatory pathways.[76] Since antioxidants and phytochemicals protect against the prion disease in cell culture and animal models, it is likely that they may also influence the expression of miRs in neuronal cells. No such data are available on prion model.

STUDIES WITH INDIVIDUAL ANTIOXIDANTS IN OTHER NEURODEGENERATIVE DISEASES

Since increased oxidative stress and inflammation are involved in the development and progression of prion disease, simultaneous reduction of these two events may help in lessening the rate of progression of this disease. In order to address this issue, there are a few reports discussed earlier on the treatment of prion disease with antioxidants and phytochemicals in experimental models but not in humans. However, Alzheimer's disease (AD) has been more studied in this context. This may be relevant as AD also involves some similar pathological changes such as formation of indigestible β-sheet aggregates and dementia. Reports on AD treatment using a single antioxidant as a test compound have not been promising. Vitamin E[95,96] and curcumin[97] do not improve cognitive function, whereas alpha-lipoic acid,[98] vitamin E,[99] and omega-3-fatty acids[100,101] produce transient and limited improvement in cognitive function, benefits confined to early phases of the disease (AD). In the case of Parkinson's disease, high doses of coenzyme Q10[102] produce some transient improvement. The reasons for individual antioxidants producing no effect or transient beneficial effects may have been for several reasons: (a) antioxidants show differential subcellular distribution and different mechanisms of action; therefore, a single antioxidant cannot protect all parts of the cell; (b) a single antioxidant in a high internal oxidative environment of patients with neurodegenerative diseases is oxidized and can then itself act as a prooxidant rather than as an antioxidant; (c) the body protects against oxidative damage by elevating antioxidant enzymes, and dietary and endogenous antioxidants. Antioxidants neutralize free radicals by donating electrons to those with unpaired electron, whereas antioxidant enzymes destroy free radicals by catalysis, converting them to harmless molecules such as water and oxygen. Perhaps both of these events need to be enhanced in concert to achieve substantial gain; (d) the affinity of different antioxidants for free radicals differs, depending upon their lipophilicity; (e) both the aqueous and lipid components of the cell need to be protected together. Water-soluble antioxidants such as vitamin C and glutathione protect molecules in the aqueous environment of the cells, whereas lipid soluble antioxidants such as vitamin A and vitamin E protect molecules in the lipid compartment; (f) Vitamin E is more effective in quenching free radicals in a reduced oxygenated cellular environment, whereas vitamin C and alpha-tocopherol are more effective in a higher oxygenated environment of the cells[103]; (g) vitamin C is important for recycling the oxidized form of alpha-tocopherol to the antioxidant form at the lipid/aqueous interface[104]; (h) antioxidants produce cell protective proteins by altering the expression of different microRNAs.[76] For example, some antioxidants can activate Nrf2 by upregulating miR-200a that inhibits its target protein Keap1, whereas others activate Nrf2 by downregulating miR-21 that binds with 3'-UTR Nrf2 mRNA.[105]

These studies suggest that use of a single micronutrient in prevention or improved management of human neurodegenerative diseases is not expected to yield any beneficial effects. For this reason, a mixture of micronutrients that can simultaneously reduce oxidative stress and inflammation by enhancing the levels of antioxidant enzymes through the activation of Nrf2 pathway together with dietary and endogenous antioxidants for other neurodegenerative diseases has been suggested.[76,94] The same suggestion is proposed for the management of prion disease. Oral supplementation can increase the levels of dietary and endogenous antioxidants; however, elevation of the levels of anti-oxidant enzymes requires an activation of Nrf2. Therefore, it is essential to understand the regulation of activation of Nrf2.

REGULATION OF ACTIVATION OF Nrf2

REACTIVE OXYGEN SPECIES (ROS) ACTIVATES Nrf2

Normally, during acute oxidative stress, ROS is needed to activate Nrf2 which then dissociates itself from Keap1-Cul-Rbx1 complex and translocates in the nucleus where it heterodimerizes with a small Maf protein, and binds with the ARE (antioxidant response element) leading to increased expression of target genes coding for several cytoprotective enzymes including antioxidant enzymes.[106–108] In this manner, activation of Nrf2 increases the levels of cytoprotective enzymes including antioxidant enzymes and phase-2-detoxifying enzymes.[109,110]

BINDING OF Nrf2 WITH ARE IN THE NUCLEUS

Activation of Nrf2 alone may not be sufficient to increase the levels of antioxidant enzymes. Activated Nrf2 must bind with antioxidant response element (ARE) in the nucleus for increasing the expression of its target genes. This binding ability of Nrf2 with ARE was impaired in aged rats and this defect was restored by supplementation with alpha-lipoic acid.[111] It is unknown whether the binding ability of Nrf2 with ARE is impaired in prion disease.

EXISTENCE OF ROS-RESISTANT Nrf2 IN PRION DISEASE

Activation of Nrf2 by ROS becomes impaired in prion disease. This is evidenced by the fact that increased oxidative stress occurs in prion disease despite the presence of Nrf2.[112]

ANTIOXIDANTS ACTIVATE OF ROS-RESISTANT Nrf2

Activation of Nrf2 becomes unresponsive to ROS in prion disease.[112] Antioxidants activate Nrf2 without the need for ROS. Some examples are listed here.

The occurrence of persistent heightened levels of oxidative stress in PrPsc-infected cells or animals, suggests that ROS-dependent mechanisms of activation have been overwhelmed. Some dietary antioxidants can activate Nrf2 without requiring elevation of ROS. These include vitamin C,[113,114] vitamin E,[115] endogenous antioxidants such as alpha-lipoic acid[111] and coenzyme Q10,[116] synthetic antioxidant N-acetylcysteine (NAC),[117] omega-3-fatty acids,[118,119] and phytochemicals such as curcumin[120] and resveratrol.[121,122]

L-CARNITINE ACTIVATES Nrf2 BY A ROS-DEPENDENT MECHANISM

Treatment with L-carnitine activates Nrf2 by a ROS-dependent mechanism,[123] probably by generating transient ROS.

ACTIVATION OF Nrf2 BY MicroRNAs

The complex of Keap1-Nrf2 in the cytoplasm prevents activation of Nrf2. Overexpression of miR-200a reduced Keap-1 levels allowing Nrf2 to migrate to the nucleus where it binds to the ARE that enhanced the transcription of target cytoprotective genes including antioxidant enzymes.[124] Increased oxidative stress enhanced the expression of miR-153 and reduced the expression of Nrf2 by binding to its 3'-UTR region of Nrf2 mRNA.[125] Mutation in miR-153 restored the oxidative stress-induced reduction in Nrf2 activity.

SUPPRESSION OF CHRONIC INFLAMMATION

The activation of Nrf2 also suppresses chronic inflammation.[109,110] Some antioxidant compounds also reduce inflammation.[126–131]

PROPOSED MIXTURE OF MICRONUTRIENTS IN PREVENTION AND IMPROVED MANAGEMENT OF PRION DISEASE

Based on the studies discussed above, a mixture of micronutrients containing vitamin A, mixed carotenoids, vitamin C, α-tocopheryl acetate, α-tocopheryl succinate, vitamin D3, alpha-lipoic acid, N-acetylcysteine, coenzyme Q10, L-carnitine, omega-3-fatty acids, curcumin, resveratrol, all B-vitamins, selenomethionine, and zinc, but without iron, copper, manganese, or heavy metals such as molybdenum and zirconium for the prevention or delaying the onset of symptoms is proposed. The inclusion of iron, copper, and manganese is not suggested, because these trace mineral, although essential for many biological reactions, can combine with vitamin C and generate excessive amounts of free radicals. Furthermore these minerals are absorbed from the intestine better in the presence of antioxidants than in their absence that could increase body store of free iron, copper and manganese after a long-term consumption. The body has no significant mechanisms of excretion of these trace minerals. Slight increase in the body store of free forms of these minerals can increase the risk of most chronic diseases. Heavy metals were not included because the body has no mechanisms of excretion of these heavy metals. Consequently, their levels in the body would increase after long-term consumption. High levels of heavy metals could interfere with the function of organs, including the brain.

It is expected that the proposed micronutrient mixture would increase the levels of antioxidant enzymes by activating the Nrf2 pathway. This together with enhancement of dietary and endogenous antioxidants could lead to simultaneously reduction in oxidative stress, chronic inflammation in prion disease. This micronutrient mixture in combination with standard therapy, may improve the management of this disease.

PREVENTION OF PRION DISEASE

The suggested micronutrients mixture may reduce the risk of developing prion disease in individuals who have been infected with PrPsc but has not developed the symptoms of the disease.

IMPROVED MANAGEMENT OF PRION DISEASE

This mixture of micronutrients, in combination with standard care, may also be useful in decreasing the rate of progression of the disease. At present there is no effective drug treatment for the prion disease.

Preclinical and clinical studies are needed to substantiate the potential role of proposed mixture of micronutrients in prevention and improved management of prion disease.

CONCLUSIONS

Prion diseases are a group of transmissible, incurable, fatal, progressive neurodegenerative diseases. Studies suggest that increased oxidative stress is one of the factors that initiate conversion PrPc to PrPsc in the lymphoid organs where the accumulation and replication of PrPsc takes place, leading to abnormal protein accessing first the peripheral nerves and then the central nervous system. This then effects neurodegenerative changes leading to dementia, and ultimately death. Enhanced accumulation of PrPsc induces inflammation that contributes to the progression of prion disease. Since some antioxidants and phytochemicals prevent or slow the development and progression of the disease in cell culture and in animal models, a mixture of micronutrients that can simultaneously reduce oxidative stress and inflammation is proposed.

REFERENCES

1. Gajdusek DC, Zigas V. Degenerative disease of the central nervous system in New Guinea. The endemic occurrence of "KURU" in the native population. *New Eng J Med.* 1957;257:974–978.
2. Gibbs CJ, Gajdusek DC, Asher DM, Alpers MP, Beck E, Daniel PM, et al. Creutzfeldt-Jakob disease (spongioform encephalopathy): Transmission to chimpanzee. *Science.* 1968;161:388–389.
3. Prusiner SB. Novel proteinaceous infectious particles cause scrapie. *Science.* 1982;216(4542):136–144.
4. Prusiner SB. Cell biology. A unifying role for prions in neurodegenerative diseases. *Science.* 2012;336(6088):1511–1513.
5. Lahiri DK. Prions: A piece of the puzzle? *Science.* 2012;337(6099):1172.
6. Holman RC, Belay ED, Christensen KY, et al. Human prion diseases in the United States. *PLoS One.* 2010;5(1):e8521.
7. Parchi P, Giese A, Capellari S, et al. Classification of sporadic Creutzfeldt-Jakob disease based on molecular and phenotypic analysis of 300 subjects. *Ann Neurol.* 1999;46(2):224–233.
8. Hsiao K, Meiner Z, Kahana E, et al. Mutation of the prion protein in Libyan Jews with Creutzfeldt-Jakob disease. *N Engl J Med.* 1991;324(16):1091–1097.
9. Meiner Z, Gabizon R, Prusiner SB. Familial Creutzfeldt-Jakob disease. Codon 200 prion disease in Libyan Jews. *Medicine (Baltimore).* 1997;76(4):227–237.
10. Shi Q, Zhang BY, Gao C, et al. The diversities of PrP(Sc) distributions and pathologic changes in various brain regions from a Chinese patient with G114V genetic CJD. *Neuropathology.* 2012;32(1):51–59.
11. Belay ED. Transmissible spongiform encephalopathies in humans. *Annu Rev Microbiol.* 1999;53:283–314.
12. Valleron AJ, Boelle PY, Will R, Cesbron JY. Estimation of epidemic size and incubation time based on age characteristics of vCJD in the United Kingdom. *Science.* 2001;294(5547):1726–1728.
13. Belay ED, Sejvar JJ, Shieh WJ, et al. Variant Creutzfeldt-Jakob disease death, United States. *Emerg Infect Dis.* 2005;11(9):1351–1354.
14. Ghosh S. Mechanism of intestinal entry of infectious prion protein in the pathogenesis of variant Creutzfeldt-Jakob disease. *Adv Drug Deliv Rev.* 2004;56(6):915–920.
15. Orru CD, Yuan J, Appleby BS, et al. Prion seeding activity and infectivity in skin samples from patients with sporadic Creutzfeldt-Jakob disease. *Sci Transl Med.* 2017;9(417).
16. Robakis NK, Sawh PR, Wolfe GC, Rubenstein R, Carp RI, Innis MA. Isolation of a cDNA clone encoding the leader peptide of prion protein and expression of the homologous gene in various tissues. *Proc Natl Acad Sci USA.* 1986;83(17):6377–6381.
17. Sparkes RS, Simon M, Cohn VH, et al. Assignment of the human and mouse prion protein genes to homologous chromosomes. *Proc Natl Acad Sci USA.* 1986;83(19):7358–7362.
18. Bradford BM, Crocker PR, Mabbott NA. Peripheral prion disease pathogenesis is unaltered in the absence of sialoadhesin (Siglec-1/CD169). *Immunology.* 2014;143(1):120–129.
19. Armstrong RA, Cairns NJ, Lantos PL. Quantification of the vacuolation (spongiform change) and prion protein deposition in 11 patients with sporadic Creutzfeldt-Jakob disease. *Acta Neuropathol.* 2001;102(6):591–596.
20. Iwasaki Y. Creutzfeldt-Jakob disease. *Neuropathology.* 2017;37(2):174–188.
21. Wang Z, Feng B, Xiao G, Zhou Z. Roles of methionine oxidation in E200K prion protein misfolding: Implications for the mechanism of pathogenesis in E200K linked familial Creutzfeldt-Jakob disease. *Biochim Biophys Acta.* 2016;1864(4):346–358.
22. Kovacs GG, Seguin J, Quadrio I, et al. Genetic Creutzfeldt-Jakob disease associated with the E200K mutation: Characterization of a complex proteinopathy. *Acta Neuropathol.* 2011;121(1):39–57.
23. Grassmann A, Wolf H, Hofmann J, Graham J, Vorberg I. Cellular aspects of prion replication in vitro. *Viruses.* 2013;5(1):374–405.
24. Basler K, Oesch B, Scott M, et al. Scrapie and cellular PrP isoforms are encoded by the same chromosomal gene. *Cell.* 1986;46(3):417–428.
25. Chesebro B, Race R, Wehrly K, et al. Identification of scrapie prion protein-specific mRNA in scrapie-infected and uninfected brain. *Nature.* 1985;315(6017):331–333.
26. Rigter A, Priem J, Timmers-Parohi D, Langeveld JP, van Zijderveld FG, Bossers A. Prion protein self-peptides modulate prion interactions and conversion. *BMC Biochem.* 2009;10:29.
27. Ashok A, Hegde RS. Selective processing and metabolism of disease-causing mutant prion proteins. *PLoS Pathog.* 2009;5(6):e1000479.
28. Vilette D, Laulagnier K, Huor A, et al. Efficient inhibition of infectious prions multiplication and release by targeting the exosomal pathway. *Cell Mol Life Sci.* 2015;72(22):4409–4427.

29. Guo BB, Bellingham SA, Hill AF. Stimulating the release of exosomes increases the intercellular transfer of prions. *J Biol Chem.* 2016;291(10):5128–5137.

30. Park KW, Eun Kim G, Morales R, et al. The endoplasmic reticulum chaperone GRP78/BiP modulates prion propagation in vitro and in vivo. *Sci Rep.* 2017;7:44723.

31. Vella LJ, Sharples RA, Lawson VA, Masters CL, Cappai R, Hill AF. Packaging of prions into exosomes is associated with a novel pathway of PrP processing. *J Pathol.* 2007;211(5):582–590.

32. Fevrier B, Vilette D, Archer F, et al. Cells release prions in association with exosomes. *Proc Natl Acad Sci USA.* 2004;101(26):9683–9688.

33. Mays CE, Ryou C. Plasminogen: A cellular protein cofactor for PrPSc propagation. *Prion.* 2011;5(1):22–27.

34. Bossers A, Belt P, Raymond GJ, Caughey B, de Vries R, Smits MA. Scrapie susceptibility-linked polymorphisms modulate the in vitro conversion of sheep prion protein to protease-resistant forms. *Proc Natl Acad Sci USA.* 1997;94(10):4931–4936.

35. Sabuncu E, Petit S, Le Dur A, et al. PrP polymorphisms tightly control sheep prion replication in cultured cells. *J Virol.* 2003;77(4):2696–2700.

36. Kobayashi A, Teruya K, Matsuura Y, et al. The influence of PRNP polymorphisms on human prion disease susceptibility: An update. *Acta Neuropathol.* 2015;130(2):159–170.

37. Apetri AC, Vanik DL, Surewicz WK. Polymorphism at residue 129 modulates the conformational conversion of the D178N variant of human prion protein 90–231. *Biochemistry.* 2005;44(48):15880–15888.

38. Brazier MW, Lewis V, Ciccotosto GD, et al. Correlative studies support lipid peroxidation is linked to PrP(res) propagation as an early primary pathogenic event in prion disease. *Brain Res Bull.* 2006;68(5):346–354.

39. Arlt S, Kontush A, Zerr I, et al. Increased lipid peroxidation in cerebrospinal fluid and plasma from patients with Creutzfeldt-Jakob disease. *Neurobiol Dis.* 2002;10(2):150–156.

40. Chen S, He S, Shang JK, et al. Serum uric acid and lipid profiles in sporadic Creutzfeldt-Jakob disease. *Clin Biochem.* 2016;49(3):292–294.

41. Younan ND, Nadal RC, Davies P, Brown DR, Viles JH. Methionine oxidation perturbs the structural core of the prion protein and suggests a generic misfolding pathway. *J Biol Chem.* 2012;287(34):28263–28275.

42. Brown DR. Neurodegeneration and oxidative stress: Prion disease results from loss of antioxidant defence. *Folia Neuropathol.* 2005;43(4):229–243.

43. Feng B, Wang Z, Liu T, et al. Methionine oxidation accelerates the aggregation and enhances the neurotoxicity of the D178N variant of the human prion protein. *Biochim Biophys Acta.* 2014;1842(12 Pt A):2345–2356.

44. Canello T, Frid K, Gabizon R, et al. Oxidation of helix-3 methionines precedes the formation of PK-resistant PrP. *PLoS Pathog.* 2010;6(7):e1000977.

45. Colombo G, Meli M, Morra G, Gabizon R, Gasset M. Methionine sulfoxides on prion protein helix-3 switch on the alpha-fold destabilization required for conversion. *PLoS One.* 2009;4(1):e4296.

46. Coleman BM, Harrison CF, Guo B, et al. Pathogenic mutations within the hydrophobic domain of the prion protein lead to the formation of protease-sensitive prion species with increased lethality. *J Virol.* 2014;88(5):2690–2703.

47. Crespo I, Roomp K, Jurkowski W, Kitano H, del Sol A. Gene regulatory network analysis supports inflammation as a key neurodegeneration process in prion disease. *BMC Syst Biol.* 2012;6:132.

48. Shi F, Yang L, Kouadir M, et al. The NALP3 inflammasome is involved in neurotoxic prion peptide-induced microglial activation. *J Neuroinflammation.* 2012;9:73.

49. Obst J, Simon E, Mancuso R, Gomez-Nicola D. The role of microglia in prion diseases: A paradigm of functional diversity. *Front Aging Neurosci.* 2017;9:207.

50. Carroll JA, Striebel JF, Rangel A, et al. Prion strain differences in accumulation of PrPSc on neurons and glia are associated with similar expression profiles of neuroinflammatory genes: Comparison of three prion strains. *PLoS Pathog.* 2016;12(4):e1005551.

51. Hu PP, Huang CZ. Prion protein: Structural features and related toxicity. *Acta Biochim Biophys Sin (Shanghai).* 2013;45(6):435–441.

52. Carroll JA, Striebel JF, Race B, Phillips K, Chesebro B. Prion infection of mouse brain reveals multiple new upregulated genes involved in neuroinflammation or signal transduction. *J Virol.* 2015;89(4):2388–2404.

53. Shi F, Kouadir M, Yang Y. NALP3 inflammasome activation in protein misfolding diseases. *Life Sci.* 2015;135:9–14.

54. Van Everbroeck B, Dewulf E, Pals P, Lubke U, Martin JJ, Cras P. The role of cytokines, astrocytes, microglia, and apoptosis in Creutzfeldt-Jakob disease. *Neurobiol Aging.* 2002;23(1):59–64.

55. Saba R, Gushue S, Huzarewich RL, et al. MicroRNA 146a (miR-146a) is over-expressed during prion disease and modulates the innate immune response and the microglial activation state. *PLoS One.* 2012;7(2):e30832.

56. Lukiw WJ, Dua P, Pogue AI, Eicken C, Hill JM. Upregulation of micro RNA-146a (miRNA-146a), a marker for inflammatory neurodegeneration, in sporadic Creutzfeldt-Jakob disease (sCJD) and Gerstmann-Sträussler-Scheinker (GSS) syndrome. *J Toxicol Environ Health A.* 2011;74(22–24):1460–1468.

57. Gossner AG, Hopkins J. The effect of PrP(Sc) accumulation on inflammatory gene expression within sheep peripheral lymphoid tissue. *Vet Microbiol.* 2015;181(3–4):204–211.

58. Llorens F, Thune K, Sikorska B, et al. Altered Ca2+ homeostasis induces Calpain-Cathepsin axis activation in sporadic Creutzfeldt-Jakob disease. *Acta Neuropathol Commun.* 2017;5(1):35.

59. Forloni G, Angeretti N, Chiesa R, et al. Neurotoxicity of a prion protein fragment. *Nature.* 1993;362(6420):543–546.

60. Fioriti L, Quaglio E, Massignan T, et al. The neurotoxicity of prion protein (PrP) peptide 106–126 is independent of the expression level of PrP and is not mediated by abnormal PrP species. *Mol Cell Neurosci.* 2005;28(1):165–176.

61. Lu Y, Liu A, Zhou X, et al. Prion peptide PrP106-126 induces inducible nitric oxide synthase and proinflammatory cytokine gene expression through the activation of NF-kappaB in macrophage cells. *DNA Cell Biol.* 2012;31(5):833–838.

62. Villa V, Thellung S, Corsaro A, et al. Celecoxib inhibits prion protein 90-231-mediated proinflammatory responses in microglial cells. *Mol Neurobiol.* 2016;53(1):57–72.

63. Brown DR, Schmidt B, Kretzschmar HA. Role of microglia and host prion protein in neurotoxicity of a prion protein fragment. *Nature.* 1996;380(6572):345–347.

64. Brown DR, Herms JW, Schmidt B, Kretzschmar HA. PrP and beta-amyloid fragments activate different neurotoxic mechanisms in cultured mouse cells. *Eur J Neurosci.* 1997;9(6):1162–1169.

65. Yuan Z, Yang L, Chen B, et al. Protein misfolding cyclic amplification induces the conversion of recombinant prion protein to PrP oligomers causing neuronal apoptosis. *J Neurochem.* 2015;133(5):722–729.

66. Butterfield DA, Hensley K, Harris M, Mattson M, Carney J. Beta-amyloid peptide free radical fragments initiate synaptosomal lipoperoxidation in a sequence-specific fashion: Implications to Alzheimer's disease. *Biochem Biophys Res Commun.* 1994;200(2):710–715.

67. Butterfield DA, Bush AI. Alzheimer's amyloid beta-peptide (1-42): Involvement of methionine residue 35 in the oxidative stress and neurotoxicity properties of this peptide. *Neurobiol Aging.* 2004;25(5):563–568.

68. Varadarajan S, Yatin S, Kanski J, Jahanshahi F, Butterfield DA. Methionine residue 35 is important in amyloid beta-peptide-associated free radical oxidative stress. *Brain Res Bull.* 1999;50(2):133–141.

69. Lee RC, Feinbaum RL, Ambros V. The C. elegans heterochronic gene lin-4 encodes small RNAs with antisense complementarity to lin-14. *Cell.* 1993;75(5):843–854.

70. Wightman B, Ha I, Ruvkun G. Posttranscriptional regulation of the heterochronic gene lin-14 by lin-4 mediates temporal pattern formation in C. elegans. *Cell.* 1993;75(5):855–862.

71. Macfarlane LA, Murphy PR. MicroRNA: Biogenesis, function and role in cancer. *Curr Genomics.* 2010;11(7):537–561.

72. Londin E, Loher P, Telonis AG, et al. Analysis of 13 cell types reveals evidence for the expression of numerous novel primate- and tissue-specific microRNAs. *Proc Natl Acad Sci USA.* 2015;112(10):E1106–E1115.

73. Denli AM, Tops BB, Plasterk RH, Ketting RF, Hannon GJ. Processing of primary microRNAs by the microprocessor complex. *Nature.* 2004;432(7014):231–235.

74. Lee Y, Ahn C, Han J, et al. The nuclear RNase III Drosha initiates microRNA processing. *Nature.* 2003;425(6956):415–419.

75. Hutvagner G, McLachlan J, Pasquinelli AE, Balint E, Tuschl T, Zamore PD. A cellular function for the RNA-interference enzyme Dicer in the maturation of the let-7 small temporal RNA. *Science.* 2001;293(5531):834–838.

76. Prasad KN. Oxidative stress and proinflammatory cytokines may act as one of signals for regulating microRNAs expression in Alzheimer's disease. *Mech Ageing Dev.* 2017;162:63–71.

77. Prasad KN. Oxidative stress, proinflammatory cytokines, and antioxidants regulate expression levels of microRNAs in Parkinson's disease. *Curr Aging Sci.* 2017;10(3):177–184.

78. Boese AS, Saba R, Campbell K, et al. MicroRNA abundance is altered in synaptoneurosomes during prion disease. *Mol Cell Neurosci.* 2016;71:13–24.

79. Montag J, Hitt R, Opitz L, Schulz-Schaeffer WJ, Hunsmann G, Motzkus D. Upregulation of miRNA hsa-miR-342-3p in experimental and idiopathic prion disease. *Mol Neurodegener.* 2009;4:36.

80. Kang SG, Kim C, Aiken J, Yoo HS, McKenzie D. Dual microRNA to cellular prion protein inhibits propagation of pathogenic prion protein in cultured cells. *Mol Neurobiol.* 2018;55(3):2384–2396.

81. Sanz Rubio D, Lopez-Perez O, de Andres Pablo A, et al. Increased circulating microRNAs miR-342-3p and miR-21-5p in natural sheep prion disease. *J Gen Virol.* 2017;98(2):305–310.

82. Asuni AA, Guridi M, Sanchez S, Sadowski MJ. Antioxidant peroxiredoxin 6 protein rescues toxicity due to oxidative stress and cellular hypoxia in vitro, and attenuates prion-related pathology in vivo. *Neurochem Int.* 2015;90:152–165.

83. Moon JH, Park SY. Baicalein prevents human prion protein-induced neuronal cell death by regulating JNK activation. *Int J Mol Med.* 2015;35(2):439–445.

84. Jeong JK, Lee JH, Moon JH, Lee YJ, Park SY. Melatonin-mediated beta-catenin activation protects neuron cells against prion protein-induced neurotoxicity. *J Pineal Res.* 2014;57(4):427–434.

85. Jeong JK, Moon MH, Bae BC, et al. Autophagy induced by resveratrol prevents human prion protein-mediated neurotoxicity. *Neurosci Res.* 2012;73(2):99–105.

86. Seo JS, Moon MH, Jeong JK, et al. SIRT1, a histone deacetylase, regulates prion protein-induced neuronal cell death. *Neurobiol Aging.* 2012;33(6):1110–1120.

87. Na JY, Kim S, Song K, Kwon J. Rutin alleviates prion peptide-induced cell death through inhibiting apoptotic pathway activation in dopaminergic neuronal cells. *Cell Mol Neurobiol.* 2014;34(7):1071–1079.

88. Mizrahi M, Friedman-Levi Y, Larush L, et al. Pomegranate seed oil nanoemulsions for the prevention and treatment of neurodegenerative diseases: The case of genetic CJD. *Nanomedicine.* 2014;10(6):1353–1363.

89. Pan YH, Wang YC, Zhang LM, Duan SR. Protective effect of edaravone against PrP106-126-induced PC12 cell death. *J Biochem Mol Toxicol.* 2010;24(4):235–241.

90. Rambold AS, Miesbauer M, Olschewski D, et al. Green tea extracts interfere with the stress-protective activity of PrP and the formation of PrP. *J Neurochem.* 2008;107(1):218–229.

91. Brazier MW, Doctrow SR, Masters CL, Collins SJ. A manganese-superoxide dismutase/catalase mimetic extends survival in a mouse model of human prion disease. *Free Radic Biol Med.* 2008;45(2):184–192.

92. Shaked GM, Engelstein R, Avraham I, Kahana E, Gabizon R. Dimethyl sulfoxide delays PrP sc accumulation and disease symptoms in prion-infected hamsters. *Brain Res.* 2003;983(1–2):137–143.

93. Prasad KN, Bondy SC. Inhibition of early upstream events in prodromal Alzheimer's disease by use of targeted antioxidants. *Curr Aging Sci.* 2014;7(2):77–90.

94. Prasad KN. Simultaneous activation of Nrf2 and elevation of antioxidant compounds for reducing oxidative stress and chronic inflammation in human Alzheimer's disease. *Mech Ageing Dev.* 2016;153:41–47.

95. Isaac MG, Quinn R, Tabet N. Vitamin E for Alzheimer's disease and mild cognitive impairment. *Cochrane Database Syst Rev.* 2008(3):CD002854.

96. Farina N, Isaac MG, Clark AR, Rusted J, Tabet N. Vitamin E for Alzheimer's dementia and mild cognitive impairment. *Cochrane Database Syst Rev.* 2012;11:CD002854.

97. Hamaguchi T, Ono K, Yamada M. Review: Curcumin and Alzheimer's disease. *CNS Neurosci Ther.* 2010;16(5):285–297.

98. Hager K, Kenklies M, McAfoose J, Engel J, Munch G. Alpha-lipoic acid as a new treatment option for Alzheimer's disease: A 48 month follow-up analysis. *J Neural Transm Suppl.* 2007(72):189–193.

99. Dysken MW, Sano M, Asthana S, et al. Effect of vitamin E and memantine on functional decline in Alzheimer disease: The TEAM-AD VA cooperative randomized trial. *JAMA.* 2014;311(1):33–44.

100. Fiala M, Terrando N, Dalli J. Specialized pro-resolving mediators from omega-3 fatty acids improve amyloid-beta phagocytosis and regulate inflammation in patients with minor cognitive impairment. *J Alzheimers Dis.* 2015;48(2):293–301.

101. Chiu CC, Su KP, Cheng TC, et al. The effects of omega-3 fatty acids monotherapy in Alzheimer's disease and mild cognitive impairment: A preliminary randomized, double-blind, placebo-controlled study. *Prog Neuropsychopharmacol Biol Psychiatry.* 2008;32(6):1538–1544.

102. Shults CW, Oakes D, Kieburtz K, et al. Effects of coenzyme Q10 in early Parkinson disease: Evidence of slowing of the functional decline. *Arch Neurol.* 2002;59(10):1541–1550.

103. Vile GF, Winterbourn CC. Inhibition of adriamycin-promoted microsomal lipid peroxidation by beta-carotene, alpha-tocopherol and retinol at high and low oxygen partial pressures. *FEBS Lett.* 1988;238(2):353–356.

104. Niki E. Interaction of ascorbate and alpha-tocopherol. *Ann N Y Acad Sci.* 1987;498:186–199.

105. Wu H, Kong L, Tan Y, et al. C66 ameliorates diabetic nephropathy in mice by both upregulating Nrf2 function via increase in miR-200a and inhibiting miR-21. *Diabetologia.* 2016;59:1558–1568.

106. Itoh K, Chiba T, Takahashi S, et al. An Nrf2/small Maf heterodimer mediates the induction of phase II detoxifying enzyme genes through antioxidant response elements. *Biochem Biophys Res Commun.* 1997;236(2):313–322.

107. Williamson TP, Johnson DA, Johnson JA. Activation of the Nrf2-ARE pathway by siRNA knockdown of Keap1 reduces oxidative stress and provides partial protection from MPTP-mediated neurotoxicity. *Neurotoxicology.* 2012;33(3):272–279.

108. Jaramillo MC, Zhang DD. The emerging role of the Nrf2-Keap1 signaling pathway in cancer. *Genes Dev*. 2013;27(20):2179–2191.

109. Li W, Khor TO, Xu C, et al. Activation of Nrf2-antioxidant signaling attenuates NFkappaB-inflammatory response and elicits apoptosis. *Biochem Pharmacol*. 2008;76(11):1485–1489.

110. Kim J, Cha YN, Surh YJ. A protective role of nuclear factor-erythroid 2-related factor-2 (Nrf2) in inflammatory disorders. *Mutat Res*. 2010;690(1–2):12–23.

111. Suh JH, Shenvi SV, Dixon BM, et al. Decline in transcriptional activity of Nrf2 causes age-related loss of glutathione synthesis, which is reversible with lipoic acid. *Proc Natl Acad Sci USA*. 2004;101(10):3381–3386.

112. Cichon AC, Brown DR. Nrf-2 regulation of prion protein expression is independent of oxidative stress. *Mol Cell Neurosci*. 2014;63:31–37.

113. Mostafavi-Pour Z, Ramezani F, Keshavarzi F, Samadi N. The role of quercetin and vitamin C in Nrf2-dependent oxidative stress production in breast cancer cells. *Oncol Lett*. 2017;13(3):1965–1973.

114. Katsuyama Y, Tsuboi T, Taira N, Yoshioka M, Masaki H. 3-O-Laurylglyceryl ascorbate activates the intracellular antioxidant system through the contribution of PPAR-gamma and Nrf2. *J Dermatol Sci*. 2016;82(3):189–196.

115. Xi YD, Yu HL, Ding J, et al. Flavonoids protect cerebrovascular endothelial cells through Nrf2 and PI3K from beta-amyloid peptide-induced oxidative damage. *Curr Neurovasc Res*. 2012;9(1):32–41.

116. Choi HK, Pokharel YR, Lim SC, et al. Inhibition of liver fibrosis by solubilized coenzyme Q10: Role of Nrf2 activation in inhibiting transforming growth factor-beta1 expression. *Toxicol Appl Pharmacol*. 2009;240(3):377–384.

117. Ji L, Liu R, Zhang XD, et al. N-acetylcysteine attenuates phosgene-induced acute lung injury via up-regulation of Nrf2 expression. *Inhal Toxicol*. 2010;22(7):535–542.

118. Gao L, Wang J, Sekhar KR, et al. Novel n-3 fatty acid oxidation products activate Nrf2 by destabilizing the association between Keap1 and Cullin3. *J Biol Chem*. 2007;282(4):2529–2537.

119. Saw CL, Yang AY, Guo Y, Kong AN. Astaxanthin and omega-3 fatty acids individually and in combination protect against oxidative stress via the Nrf2-ARE pathway. *Food Chem Toxicol*. 2013;62:869–875.

120. Trujillo J, Chirino YI, Molina-Jijon E, Anderica-Romero AC, Tapia E, Pedraza-Chaverri J. Renoprotective effect of the antioxidant curcumin: Recent findings. *Redox Biol*. 2013;1(1):448–456.

121. Steele ML, Fuller S, Patel M, Kersaitis C, Ooi L, Munch G. Effect of Nrf2 activators on release of glutathione, cysteinylglycine, and homocysteine by human U373 astroglial cells. *Redox Biol*. 2013;1(1):441–445.

122. Kode A, Rajendrasozhan S, Caito S, Yang SR, Megson IL, Rahman I. Resveratrol induces glutathione synthesis by activation of Nrf2 and protects against cigarette smoke-mediated oxidative stress in human lung epithelial cells. *Am J Physiol Lung Cell Mol Physiol*. 2008;294(3):L478–L488.

123. Zambrano S, Blanca AJ, Ruiz-Armenta MV, et al. The renoprotective effect of L-carnitine in hypertensive rats is mediated by modulation of oxidative stress-related gene expression. *Eur J Nutr*. 2013;52(6):1649–1659.

124. Eades G, Yang M, Yao Y, Zhang Y, Zhou Q. miR-200a regulates Nrf2 activation by targeting Keap1 mRNA in breast cancer cells. *J Biol Chem*. 2011;286(47):40725–40733.

125. Narasimhan M, Riar AK, Rathinam ML, Vedpathak D, Henderson G, Mahimainathan L. Hydrogen peroxide responsive miR153 targets Nrf2/ARE cytoprotection in paraquat induced dopaminergic neurotoxicity. *Toxicol Lett*. 2014;228(3):179–191.

126. Abate A, Yang G, Dennery PA, Oberle S, Schroder H. Synergistic inhibition of cyclooxygenase-2 expression by vitamin E and aspirin. *Free Radic Biol Med*. 2000;29(11):1135–1142.

127. Fu Y, Zheng S, Lin J, Ryerse J, Chen A. Curcumin protects the rat liver from CCl4-caused injury and fibrogenesis by attenuating oxidative stress and suppressing inflammation. *Mol Pharmacol*. 2008;73(2):399–409.

128. Lee HS, Jung KK, Cho JY, et al. Neuroprotective effect of curcumin is mainly mediated by blockade of microglial cell activation. *Pharmazie*. 2007;62(12):937–942.

129. Rahman S, Bhatia K, Khan AQ, et al. Topically applied vitamin E prevents massive cutaneous inflammatory and oxidative stress responses induced by double application of 12-O-tetradecanoylphorbol-13-acetate (TPA) in mice. *Chem Biol Interact*. 2008;172(3):195–205.

130. Suzuki YJ, Aggarwal BB, Packer L. Alpha-lipoic acid is a potent inhibitor of NF-kappa B activation in human T cells. *Biochem Biophys Res Commun*. 1992;189(3):1709–1715.

131. Zhu J, Yong W, Wu X, et al. Anti-inflammatory effect of resveratrol on TNF-alpha-induced MCP-1 expression in adipocytes. *Biochem Biophys Res Commun*. 2008;369(2):471–477.

17 Micronutrients for Improved Management of Huntington's Disease

INTRODUCTION

Huntington's disease (HD) is a progressive, fatal, dominant, hereditary, incurable neurodegenerative disease of the brain in which primarily the striatum and cortex that are involved in regulating movement, intellect, and emotions are gradually destroyed. This disease is characterized by jerking, uncontrollable movements of the limbs, trunk, and face (chorea), progressive loss of cognitive functions, and the development of psychiatric problems. Muscle rigidity progresses at a rapid rate, leading to akinesia (loss of control of voluntary muscle movements).

The wild-type huntingtin protein plays an important role in neurogenesis, development, and survival of neurons in the brain, especially in those areas of brain most affected in HD, such as the cortex and striatum. In the wild-type huntingtin gene, the number of trinucleotide CAG (cytosine, adenine, and guanosine), coding for glutamine varies from 1 to 34 repeats. The huntingtin gene is located on the chromosome 4p 16.3.

In 1993, it was discovered that an autosomal dominant mutation in the wild-type huntingtin gene contains expansion of repeats of the trinucleotide CAG coding region. The number of triplet CAG repeats in the pathological HD gene varies from 35 to over 140. Translation of this mutated huntingtin gene leads to the enlargement of the polyglutamine tract in the N-terminus of the huntingtin protein.[1] Individuals carrying 39–60 CAG repeats exhibit late-onset HD; whereas individuals carrying more than 60 CAG repeats exhibit earlier onset of HD.[2–4] The larger the number of triplet CAG repeats, the earlier the onset of the symptoms of disease. Dominant heritable mutations are generally lethal during embryogenesis or at birth because of normal natural selection pressure; however, in case of HD, this dominant mutation escapes the normal selection pressure, because the deleterious effects of this genetic mutation do not appear until adulthood.

Each child of an HD parent has a 50% chance of inheriting the mutated HD gene. The child carrying an HD gene develops the symptoms of disease at an age that can vary, generally between 30 and 50 years. The disease progresses over 10–25 years, and patients ultimately become unable to take care of themselves. Juvenile HD generally appears before the age of 20 and progresses rapidly.

Despite research of several decades, there are no effective means of delaying the onset or progression of symptoms of HD. Current therapies involving drugs, physical therapy, speech therapy and psychotherapy offer minimal beneficial effects, and there is no cure for this disease. Using animal models and human HD, some biochemical defects have been identified. They include increased oxidative stress, mitochondrial dysfunction, chronic inflammation, elevated glutamate and glutamate receptors activation, enhanced levels of gamma-aminobutyric acid (GABA) receptors, reduced levels of receptors for dopamine and cannabinoids, transcriptional dysregulation, and posttranslational modification of the abnormal HD protein. Among these defects, increased oxidative stress occurs before the onset of other cellular defects. These issues are discussed in detail later in this chapter.

In an attempt to reduce oxidative stress, several antioxidants have been used individually in animal models of HD (to be discussed in detail later in this chapter). They include vitamin C, N-acetylcysteine (NAC), alpha-lipoic acid, coenzyme Q10, L-carnitine, lycopene and epigallocatechin, melatonin, curcumin, resveratrol, *Ginkgo biloba* extract, and nicotinamide (vitamin B3).

Each of these studies measured different biochemical parameters and HD symptoms. These neurological symptoms, motor function, cognitive function, energy metabolism, and survival improved somewhat, depending upon the type of vitamin. Vitamin treatment also reduced oxidative stress, brain atrophy, gliosis, and formation of HD protein aggregates.

In contrast to animal studies, the use of a single antioxidant produced very little or no beneficial effects in humans. A human study on 73 patients with HD showed that treatment with d-alpha-tocopherol (vitamin E) had no effect on neurological or neuropsychiatric symptoms; however, some temporary improvements of neurological symptoms were observed during the early phase of the disease.[5] Administration of coenzyme Q10 was also ineffective in improving any neurological symptoms or slowing down the progression of the disease in humans.[6] The reasons of this discrepancy between the effects of micronutrients in animal HD models and Human HD are discussed later in this chapter.

This chapter briefly presents incidence and cost, signs and symptoms, brain pathology, and receptor abnormalities in HD and presents evidence in support of a hypothesis that increased oxidative stress, chronic inflammation, and glutamate levels are one of the early events that initiate and promote neurodegeneration and neuronal death in HD. It proposes that in order to simultaneously decrease the above biochemical defects, a concurrent elevation of the levels of antioxidant enzymes together with dietary and endogenous antioxidants may be necessary. This chapter also suggests a mixture of micronutrients that may simultaneously attenuate these biochemical abnormalities involved in HD, and thereby, prevent or delay, and in combination with standard therapy, improve the management of this disease.

INCIDENCE, PREVALENCE, AND COST OF HD

INCIDENCE AND PREVALENCE

It is estimated that the incidence of HD in the USA is about 1,550 cases per year. The prevalence of this disease in the USA, Europe, and Australia is 5–7 cases/100,000 individuals, whereas in the Asia, it is only 0.4/100,000.[7] The reasons for this difference in prevalence of HD are unknown. From the studies in the USA, Australia, and Western Europe, it is estimated that the prevalence of HD increases 15%–20% every decade.[8]

COST

Average annual cost of treating patients (evenly distributed by stage early/middle/late) was $4,947–$22,582, whereas it was $3,257–$37,495 for Medicaid patients (late stage).[9]

SIGNS AND SYMPTOMS

In most cases of HD, symptoms appear in young adult life and become progressively worse. Signs and symptoms include movement disorders, cognitive dysfunction, and psychiatric problems. The sequence of their appearance varies from one individual to another (http://www.healthcommunities.com/huntington-disease/symptoms.shtml). Uncontrolled movement or tics in the fingers, feet, face, or trunk, which become more intense when the individuals are anxious or disturbed, characterize the movement disorders. As the disease progresses, other symptoms, such as clumsiness, jaw clenching (bruxism), loss of coordination and balance, slurred speech, difficulty in swallowing, uncontrolled continual muscular contractions (dystonia), and walking difficulties leading to stumbling and falling appear. Weight loss is commonly associated with HD.

The cognitive dysfunctions are characterized by the progressive loss of memory and ability to concentrate, answer questions, and recognize familiar objects. These cognitive dysfunctions generally appear later in the course of the disease.

The major psychiatric problems include depression, which appears early during progression of HD. The symptoms of depression include hostility, irritability, lack of energy, and inability to enjoy pleasures of life. Some individuals may develop manic-depression or bipolar disorder during the course of the disease. Others may exhibit psychotic behaviors, such as delusions, hallucinations, unprovoked aggression, and paranoia.

PATHOLOGY OF THE BRAIN IN HD

HUMAN STUDIES

Damage to the striatum appears early and becomes severe at a later stage of the disease. Other regions of the brain, such as the cortex, thalamus, and subthalamus also show degenerative changes at a later stage. Within the striatum, the median spiny projection neurons selectively degenerate in HD while interneurons are relatively spared.[10] The cerebellum of all HD patients showed significant atrophy and loss of Purkinje cells and neurons.[11] It has been suggested that degeneration of the cerebellum may contribute to some of the symptoms of HD, such as impaired rapid alternating movements, fine motor skills, dysarthria, ataxia, and postural stability. Analysis of autopsied brain samples of HD patients showed that loss of neurons occurred from the substantia nigra, pontine nuclei, reticulotegmental nucleus of the pons, superior and inferior olives, and from the area of the excitatory burst neurons for horizontal saccades, raphe interpositus nucleus, and vestibular nuclei.[12] During preclinical stage, individuals carrying mutated Huntington's disease gene are symptom-free despite the presence of neurodegeneration in the brain. Studies by functional imaging of the brain showed an evidence for neuronal compensation in preclinical stage of HD in which functional reorganization in the brain occurred in order to preserve motor and cognitive functions.[13] The number of nerve cells decreased in the Brodmann's primary visual area 17 (BA17) of HD patients. Neuronal loss was most pronounced in the outer pyramidal layer III, the inner granular layers IVa and IVc, and in the multiform layer of VI of BA17 of HD patients.[14] Neuronal loss in the anterior cingulated cortex was associated with mood symptoms profiles of HD patients, whereas neuronal loss in the primary motor cortex was associated with motor symptoms.[15] Another study demonstrated that loss of neurons and pyramidal cells occurred in the entire cortical regions. The number of neuronal loss varied markedly within the same brain and between patients with HD. In addition, neuronal loss in the primary sensory and secondary visual cortices was associated with impaired motor symptoms, whereas neuronal loss in the frontal, parietal, and temporal lobes was associated with motor and mood symptoms of HD.[16,17]

ANIMAL STUDIES

Both chemical- and genetic-induced animal models of HD are used to investigate the mechanisms of HD and to identify potential targets for the development of novel agents for the treatment of HD. Quinolinic acid, an NMDA (N-methyl-D-aspartate) receptor agonist, and 3-nitropropionic acid (3-NP), an inhibitor of mitochondrial dehydrogenase, induced changes in the striatum similar to those observed in human HD. Administration of quinolinic acid directly into the striatum region of the rat brain produced some biochemical, morphological, and behavioral characteristics of HD. The biochemical changes after quinolinate treatment included elevated activity of NADPH oxidase that catalyzes superoxide anion production in the striatal neurons. Treatment with Apocynin, a specific inhibitor of NADPH oxidase, decreased lipid peroxidation, circling behavior, and histological changes in the brain after quinolinate administration (60). Quinolinic acid and 3-NP also increased oxidative and nitrosylative stress that may contribute to the neurodegeneration (61, 62).

Several genetic mouse models of HD have been developed in recent years. These HD mice mimic the neuropathology and symptoms similar to those observed in human HD. Transgenic HD mouse models expressing short N-terminals fragments (R6/1 and R6/2) or full length HD gene (YAC128) exhibited rapid effects on gene expression in the striatal neurons similar to those observed in human HD.[18]

RECEPTOR ABNORMALITIES IN HD

DOPAMINE RECEPTORS

It appears that striatal neurons expressing dopamine receptors degenerate in patients with HD. This is due to the activation of dopamine receptors D1 and D2 that causes aggregation of HD proteins. Using neuroblastoma cells with a dopamine D1 receptor expressing huntingtin genes with a 25 and a 103 triplet repeat of CAG, it was demonstrated that nuclear and cytoplasmic HD protein aggregated.[19] Low doses of selective dopamine D1 receptor agonists increased the aggregation of HD protein in the nucleus but decreased the number of aggregates in the cytoplasm.[19] The presence of these aggregates in the nucleus may induce transcriptional deregulation by binding to the histone.

Dopamine D2 receptor agonists also increased HD protein aggregation and this was blocked by a dopamine D2 receptors antagonist. The combination of ascorbate and dopamine D2 antagonist was more effective in reducing the formation of HD protein aggregates and neuronal death in the striatum than the individual agents (Charvin, 2005 #2577). In transgenic rats expressing HD gene, chronic treatment with haloperidol, an antagonist of dopamine D2 receptor, protected striatal neurons, suggesting that activation of dopamine D2 receptors contributes to HD protein aggregation and neurodegeneration in the brain.[20]

Cortical dopamine dysfunction has been found in both symptomatic and asymptomatic patients with HD. Using a radioactive dopamine D2 receptor agonist ^{11}C-raclopride in PET (positron emission tomography) on 16 symptomatic and 11 asymptomatic patients with HD, 62.5% of symptomatic and 64.5% of asymptomatic patients showed reduced binding of dopamine D2 receptors, suggesting the loss of dopamine neurons.[21] This study was confirmed by another study in which a reduction in binding of dopamine D2 receptors in the striatum of patients with HD was observed. The severity of clinical symptoms of the disease, such as chorea and cognitive dysfunction, were correlated with degree of reduction in the binding of dopamine D2 receptors.[22] Another study utilizing PET technology and using a radioactive ^{11}C-raclopride and [11]C(R)-PK11195, markers of microglia activation in asymptomatic and symptomatic HD patients revealed that significant loss of dopamine D2 receptors occurred in the hypothalamus of patients with HD.[23] Dopamine release was also reduced in transgenic HD model rats, and this contributed to the motor deficiency as evidenced by gait disturbances in these animals.[24]

CANNABINOID RECEPTORS

Cannabinoid receptors CB1 and CB2 are reduced in the key areas of the HD brain, such as the striatum and cortex. Loss of CB1 receptors was observed at the early stage of HD in the autopsied brain samples of patients with HD.[25] This was confirmed by the PET, using a novel CB1 ligand N-[2-(3-cyano-phenyl)-3-(4-(2-^{18}F-fluorethoxy)phenyl)-1-methylpropyl-2-(5-methyl-2-pyridyloxyl)-2-methylproponamide in 20 symptomatic HD patients and 14 healthy subjects. Levels of CB1 receptors decreased throughout the gray matter of the cerebellum, cerebellum, and brainstem.[26] Thus, upregulation of CB1 receptors may be of protective value. Indeed, upregulation of CB1 receptors slowed progression of the disease in transgenic R6/1 HD mice.[27] Deletion of CB1 receptors aggravated the symptoms and caused neurodegeneration in transgenic HD mice.[28] Furthermore, administration of an endogenous cannabinoid receptor agonist delta-9-tetrahydrocannabinol prevented the effect of deletion of CB1 receptors in these mice. Therefore agonists of CB1 receptors may be useful in improving the symptoms of HD. Indeed, administration of CB1 agonist WIN 55,212-2 prevented the development of HD phenotype in quinolinate rat model of HD. This effect of a CB1 receptor agonist was blocked by the corresponding antagonist AM251.[29]

In a rat model of HD, an agonist of CB2 receptor prevented the death of striatal neurons.[30] CB2 receptors are present in small amounts in the stratum, but they are abundantly located in microglia and astrocytes, suggesting that glial cells mediate protective effects of agonists of CB2 receptors. Activation of CB2 receptors also reduced the levels of tumor necrosis factor–alpha (TNF-alpha). Activated peripheral immune cells and brain microglia are present in asymptomatic HD patients, and they increase with the progression of disease. Activation of cannabin receptor CB2 reduced immune activation. This is shown by the fact that deletion of CB2 receptor in HD mouse model accelerates the onset of motor deficits and increased their severity. Treatment of mice with a CB2 receptor agonist extended lifespan, and suppressed motor deficits, synapse loss, and brain inflammation, while a peripherally restricted CB2 receptor antagonist blocks these effects.[31] Furthermore, treatment with a CB2 receptor agonist reduced blood levels of IL-6 that was elevated in HD mice. Treatment with an antibody against IL-6 also improved motor function in these mice. However, in contrast to the beneficial effects of activation of cannabinoid receptors on improving some symptoms in rat HD models, treatment with a CB1 receptor agonist delta-9-tetrahydrocannabinol (THC) or CB2 receptor agonist HU210 did not alter the progression of motor deficits in a mouse model of HD (R6/1). HU210 treated HD animals actually had increased seizure events and an increased level of ubiquitinated aggregates in the striatum. In such mice, treatment with THC or HU210 had no significant effect on the ligand binding of CB1, dopamine D1 and D2 receptors, and serotonin 5HT2A or GABA (A) receptors.[32]

ADENOSINE RECEPTORS

Treatment with an adenosine A (2A) receptor agonist improved some of symptoms in the mouse HD model (R6/2).[33] Activation of A2ARs may be protective value at least in this model. If this were the case, then deletion of A2ARs should enhance the symptoms of HD. Indeed, genetic deletion of A2ARs in a transgenic HD mouse model (N171-82Q) aggravated motor performance and reduced survival.[34]

TRANSCRIPTIONAL DEREGULATION IN HD

HISTONE DEACETYLATION

Histone acetylation and deacetylation regulate gene transcription. Acetylation of histone at specific residues increases transcription of genes, whereas deacetylation of histones suppresses transcriptional activity that has been implicated in the pathogenesis of HD. In animal models of HD, expression of HD gene decreases the activity of histone acetyl transferase. This enzyme is responsible for deacetylation of histone leading to inhibition of the transcriptional activity that causes neurodegeneration in the brain. Inhibitors of histone deacetylase (HDAC) produce some beneficial effects in several animal models of HD[35]; however, their therapeutic value is limited by their toxicity. Chronic oral administration of a novel pimelic diphenylamide HDAC inhibitor, HDACi 4b, at the beginning and after the onset of motor deficits, significantly improved motor performance, overall appearance, and body weight in a transgenic HD mice model. These changes were associated with reduction in striatal atrophy and brain shrinkage. Alterations in gene expression caused by HD protein were prevented by the treatment with HDACi 4b.[36]

Mitogen- and stress-activated kinase (MSK-1), a nuclear protein kinase, involved in chromatin remodeling through histone H3 phosphorylation, was reduced in the striatum of patients with HD and animal models of HD.[37] Restoring MSK-1 expression in the striatal neurons in culture prevented HD protein-induced neuronal degeneration and death. Furthermore, deletion of MSK-1 gene in wild-type mice led to spontaneous striatal degeneration and increased sensitivity of striatal neurons to the mitochondrial neurotoxin 3-NP. Overexpression of MSK-1 upregulated PGC-1 alpha, suggesting the neuroprotective effect of MSK-1 is mediated through increased expression of this gene.

Wild-type huntingtin protein is present primarily in the cytoplasm, whereas N-terminal fragments produced by the cleavage of HD protein are present in both the cytoplasm and the nucleus. These HD protein fragments form insoluble aggregates. The nuclear deposits of insoluble HD protein fragments may cause transcriptional deregulation that may contribute to the degeneration and death of neurons.[38] Repressor element-1-silencing transcription factor (REST) is considered an inhibitory regulator of genes through the transcriptional regulation of miRNAs in the nerve cells. In HD, REST was translocated from the cytoplasm to the nucleus causing repression of genes, such as BDNF.[39] Reduced transcription of BDNF may contribute to the progression of HD.

PRE-TRANSLATIONAL MODIFICATION OF PROTEINS IN HD

MicroRNAs

MicroRNAs (miRs) regulate the translation of mRNAs transcripts into proteins. MicroRNAs are evolutionarily conserved small noncoding single-stranded RNAs of approximately 22 nucleotides in length, and are present in all living organisms, including humans.[40–43] The biogenesis of miRs is very complex and involves multiple biochemical steps. The majority of miRs are transcribed by RNA polymerase II (Pol II), while some are transcribed by RNA polymerase III (Pol III) from the noncoding region of the DNA to produce primary miRs (pri-miRs). Pri-miRs undergo a nuclear cleavage by ribonuclease III Drosa to generate precursor-miRs (pre-miRs) that migrate to the cytoplasm where they are further cleaved by ribonuclease III Dicer to ultimately form mature single-stranded miRs with the help of another protein argonaute (Ago)[42,44–46] Each microRNA binds to its complimentary sequences in the 3′-untranslated region (3′-UTR) of the mRNA, promotes degradation of the mRNA transcript, and prevents translation of the message of protein. In this manner, miRs regulate the translation of pro-apoptotic or anti-apoptotic proteins from their respective mRNAs, depending upon whether they receive damaging (from increased ROS and pro-inflammatory cytokines) or protective signal (from antioxidants). The expression of some microRNAs may also be altered in response to the disease state.

MicroRNAs in Brain Cell Pathology and Protection

MicroRNAs play an important role in the pathogenesis of HD. Seventy five miRs were identified in the autopsied samples of the pre-frontal cortex (Brodmann area 9). Among them, five miRs (miR-10b-3p, miR-10b-5p, miR-196a-5p, miR-196b-5p, and miR-106a-5p) that were associated with CAG-length-adjusted age of onset of the symptoms, the expression of miR-10b-5p was most prominent.[47] Furthermore, the association between miR-10b-5p and striatal involvement was independent of cortical involvement.

Cell cycle progression is delayed in S-phase and G2/M phase, and enhanced apoptosis in a cell culture model of HD (STsdh (Q111)/Hdh (Q111) striatal cells compared with control cells (STsdh (Q7)/Hdh (Q7).[48] Furthermore, decreased expression of miR-432, miR-146a, and miR-19a increased the levels of PCNA (proliferating nuclear antigen), CHEK1 (check point1), and CCNA2 (cyclin A2) in the primary cortical neurons expressing mutant N-terminal huntingtin protein (HTT), R6/2 mice, an animal model of HD, and HD cell model of striatum (STsdh (Q111)/Hdh (Q111). Increased expression of the above microRNAs in these striatal cells may prevent cell-cycle arrest and apoptosis.

MicroRNAs located in the HOX gene clusters play an important role in the pathogenesis of HD. Some of them are discussed here.[49] Ectopic overexpression of miR-10b-5p in neuronal cell line expressing a full length human huntingtin protein containing 73 CAG repeats (PC12 HTT-Q73) increased the survival of the cells, suggesting that increased expression of this microRNA may be a protective response. Furthermore, the association between huntingtin CAG repeats size, onset age, and age at death with the expression of specific miR was established as follow:

1. Huntingtin CAG repeat size, onset age, and age at death were independently and inversely related to miR-10b-5p expression.
2. Huntingtin CAG repeats size and onset age were independently and inversely related to miR-196a-5p expression.
3. Onset age was inversely related to miR-196b-5p expression.
4. Age at death was inversely related to miR-615-3p expression.

Expression of miR-24 decreased in the mouse model of HD and in patients with HD.[50] Furthermore, overexpression of miR-124 decreased the rate of progression of HD, increased striatal neurogenesis, and improved motor performance in the mouse model of HD. Expression of miR-196a attenuated striatum pathological changes in the mouse model of HD.[51] In addition, miR-196a enhanced neurite outgrowth in neuroblastoma cells in culture, suggesting that this microRNA improved the cytoskeleton structures of the cells. Overexpression of this microRNA also reduced the levels and aggregation of mutant Huntington protein in vitro and slowed down progression of pathological changes in the brain of transgenic HD model mice.[52] Overexpression of miR-22 reduced degeneration of primary striatal and cortical neurons in culture exposed to mutated human huntingtin protein fragments (Htt171-82Q) and in primary culture of striatal cells treated with 3-NP.[53] This microRNA reduced caspase activation and the levels of proapoptotic protein mitogen-activated protein kinase 14/p38 (MAPK114/p38).

Transgenic HD mouse models (YAC128 and R6/2) and 3-nitropropionic acid (3-NP)-induced rat HD model revealed abnormal biogenesis of microRNAs that was age-dependent. For example, at 5 months, increased expression of nuclear Drosha that cleaves primary miR to form pre-miR was associated with enhanced expression of dominant miRs; whereas, at 12 months, decreased expression of Dicer that cleaves pre-miR to form mature miR was associated with reduced expression of miRs in YAC128 mice.[54] In 10 week-old R6/2 mice, decreased expression of Drosha was associated with reduced expression of dominant miRs. Expressions of 9 miRs (miR-22, miR-29c, miR-128, miR-132, miR-138, miR-218, miR-222, miR-344, and miR-674) were downregulated in 12-month-old YAC128 and 10-week-old R6/2 mice. Similar dynamic changes in the profiles of miRs were observed in 3NP-treated rats.

The expression of miR-128 was downregulated in the brain of an HD monkey model at the time of birth as well as in asymptomatic and symptomatic animals with HD. This microRNA also regulated the expression of huntingtin protein and huntingtin interaction protein 1 (HIP1).[55] Overexpression of miR-214 caused downregulation of beta catenin protein levels in HD cell model (STHdhQ111/Q111). The reduction in the levels of beta-catenin was independent of proteasome.[56] The levels of miR-27a and multidrug resistant protein-1 (MDR-1) decreased in the brain of mouse HD model (R6/2). Overexpression of miR-27a decreased aggregation of mutated huntingtin protein and increased the levels of MDR-1 protein. Knocking down of MDR-1 by siRNA increased the aggregation of mutated huntingtin protein.[57]

Four miRs (miR-214, miR-150, miR-146a, and miR-125b) targeted human and mouse huntingtin protein. Overexpression of these microRNAs reduced the aggregation of mutated huntingtin protein in mouse cells.[58]

MicroRNAs in Plasma

The plasma levels of has-miR-34b were elevated in asymptomatic individuals carrying HD gene.[59] The plasma levels of 13 miRs (miR-877-5p, miR-223-3p, miR-233-5p, miR-30d-5p, miR-128, miR-22-5p, miR-222-3p, miR-338-3p, miR-130b-3p, miR-425-5p, miR-628-3p, miR-361-5p, and miR-942) were significantly elevated in patients with HD compared with control subjects.[60] Furthermore, the expression of miR-100-5p was elevated, and the expression of miR-641 and miR-330-3p were decreased when HD patients were rearranged by Total Functional Capacity, suggesting that stage of the disease can modify the expression of certain miRs.

POST-TRANSLATIONAL MODIFICATION OF PROTEINS IN HD

Post-translational modification of proteins by the lipid palmitate is needed for the correct targeting and functioning of certain proteins, including huntingin protein. Palmitoylation of proteins is regulated by two functionally opposing enzymes palmitoyl acyltransferases, which add palmitate to proteins, and acyl protein thioesterases, which remove palmitate from proteins. This process of palmitate is important for the development of synapses and synaptic activity in the brain. Wild-type huntingin protein is palmitoylated by huntingtin-interacting protein-14 (HIP-14), which exhibits palmitate acyltransferase activity.[61] If the interaction between HD protein and HIP-14 is reduced, the palmitoylation of HD protein is decreased leading to increased protein aggregations and neuronal toxicity. Conversely, overexpression of HIP-14 can increase palmitoylation and this markedly reduced HD protein aggregation. This study suggests that palmitoylation by HIP-14 plays a role in the pathogenesis of HD. This was further supported by the study in which deletion of HIP-14 caused development of HD pathology and behavioral features in mice.[62] Huntingtin-interacting protein-14 like (HIP-14L) is a paralog (as a result of gene duplication that may acquire different function) of HIP-14. Both HIP-14 and HIP-14L are essential for palmitoylation of huntingin protein. HIP-14L-deficient mice have reduced palmitoylation of the HIP-14L substrate SNAP25 (synaptosomal-associated protein-25), early onset of motor deficits, and widespread and progressive neurodegeneration in the brain.[63]

EVIDENCE FOR INCREASED OXIDATIVE STRESS AS AN EARLY EVENT IN THE ONSET OF HD SYMPTOMS

Increased markers of oxidative stress, mitochondrial dysfunction and chronic inflammation have been repeatedly observed in the autopsied brain samples of HD patients[64]; however, it is difficult to conclude whether these biochemical defects are the cause or the consequence of the disease. Strongest support for the proposed hypotheses comes from the asymptomatic individuals carrying the mutated HD gene and animal models of HD.

Studies on Asymptomatic and Symptomatic Individuals

Analysis of markers of oxidative stress in 19 HD patients, 47 age- and sex-matched control subjects, 11 asymptomatic individuals carrying HD genes revealed that increased plasma levels of lipid peroxidation and reduced levels of glutathione were present in both asymptomatic and symptomatic patients with HD compared with control subjects.[65] Similar changes in the levels of markers of oxidative stress were observed in 11 asymptomatic individuals carrying HD gene compared to those of 22 age- and sex-matched healthy subjects who were not HD gene carriers. These results suggest that increased oxidative stress occurs prior to the onset of HD symptoms in asymptomatic individuals carrying HD gene.[66] The activities of proteolytic aminopeptidases decreased in the plasma of asymptomatic individual carrying HD gene and patients with HD[67] Peptidases cause release of glutamate and aspartate from the proteins, thus increasing their concentrations. Elevated levels of these excitatory neurotransmitters can increase oxidative stress in the brain and cause neuronal degeneration and death. Appearance of increased markers of oxidative stress and glutamate levels in asymptomatic individuals carrying HD gene provides an opportunity to intervene with micronutrients that can simultaneously reduce these cellular defects.

In a study involving 16 HD patients, markers of oxidative stress, such as leukocyte 8-hydroxy-deoxyguanosine (8-OHdG) and plasma malondialdehyde (MDA), were increased relative to 36 age- and gender-matched controls, while the activities of erythrocyte Cu/Zn superoxide dismutase (Cu/Zn-SOD) and glutathione peroxidase were reduced in HD patients compared to those in healthy controls.[68] Plasma MDA levels were significantly correlated with the severity of the disease. An increased extent of mitochondrial DNA defects was also observed in the autopsied brain samples of HD patients, possibly induced by HD protein.

Postmortem analysis of brain tissues from HD patients showed that activities of oxidative phosphorylation enzymes were impaired and that this was confined to the basal ganglia.[69] In addition, the levels of markers of oxidative stress increased in the caudate of HD brain. These results suggest that increased oxidative stress contribute to the progression of HD. Therefore, intervention of antioxidants may decrease the rate of progression of HD.

AGGREGATION OF HD PROTEIN

Protein aggregation is one of the early events in the initiation of neurodegeneration in HD. HD protein is present in the form of N-terminal fragments, oligomers, and polymers primarily in the striatum and cortex. Oligomers are mostly soluble; however, N-terminal fragments, polymers, and other proteins attach with each other and form the insoluble aggregates that are toxic to neurons.[70] The aggregated form of HD protein components produces reactive oxygen species (ROS) and treatment with MW7 antibody to HD protein inhibited HD protein aggregation and also reduced ROS production.[71] The treatment of antioxidants could also reduce aggregation of HD proteins.

STUDIES ON ANIMAL MODELS OF HD

Using a transgenic HD mouse model, caspase-1 and caspase-3 were found to be transcriptionally upregulated and activated. The degree of activation of caspases correlated with the progression of this disease in HD mice.[72] Similar observations were made in autopsied brain samples of HD patients. Activation of caspase-2 cleaves HD protein selectively at amino acid 552, and fragmented HD proteins become aggregated. The aggregated form of HD protein causes selective neuronal cell death in the striatum and cortex of autopsied brain samples of human HD as well as in HD mouse model expressing full length HD gene (YAC72 mice).[73] Inhibitors of caspase delayed the onset of symptoms in the transgenic HD mouse model. Treatment of animals with quinolinic acid- and 3-NP increased oxidative stress and induced HD-like changes in the brain.[74,75] HD protein also activates microglia causing the release of pro-inflammatory cytokines and reactive oxygen species (ROS).

STUDIES ON CELL CULTURE MODELS OF HD

Increased oxidative stress is one of the factors causing aggregation of HD protein that contributes to neuronal cell death.[76] Oxidative events also inhibited proteasome function in neurons expressing HD gene. Furthermore, overexpression of Cu/Zn-superoxide dismutase (SOD1) reversed the oxidative stress-induced proteasome inhibition, HD protein aggregation, and death of neuronal cells in culture.[76]

MITOCHONDRIAL DYSFUNCTION IN ASYMPTOMATIC AND SYMPTOMATIC INDIVIDUALS CARRYING HD GENE

A study on 16 HD patients, 4 asymptomatic individuals carrying the HD gene and 20 healthy controls revealed that 2 genes involved in regulating mitochondrial functions, aconitase-2 (ACO-2) and 3-oxoacid CoA transferase-1 (OXCT-1), were downregulated in peripheral leukocytes of asymptomatic and symptomatic patients with HD.[77] These changes can reduce mitochondrial efficiency and would enhance the formation of free radicals during oxidative phosphorylation of proteins. HD protein accumulates in the mitochondria and causes the mitochondrial dysfunction associated with the progression of HD.[78] HD protein may bind to the respiratory chains complexes and thus inhibits mitochondrial energy production, one of the characteristic features of HD. Mitochondrial dysfunction as evidenced by decreased activities of complexes II, III, and IV in the striatum of HD patients has been consistently observed.[79]

In patients with HD, the number of mitochondria in spiny striatal neurons decreased. In addition, mitochondrial transcriptional factor A and peroxisome proliferator-activated receptor-co-activator gamma-1alpha (PGC-1 alpha), a key transcriptional regulator of energy metabolism and mitochondrial biogenesis, were reduced with increasing in the severity of disease.[80] These results suggest that mitochondrial dysfunction plays an important role in the pathogenesis of HD.[81] Aspects of mitochondrial dysfunction include reduction of Ca2+ buffering capacity, loss of membrane potential, and decreased expression of oxidative phosphorylation enzymes,[82] as well as increased production of reactive oxygen species.

EVIDENCE FOR INCREASED CHRONIC INFLAMMATION IN HD

STUDIES ON ASYMPTOMATIC AND SYMPTOMATIC INDIVIDUALS

If oxidative damage fails to heal, chronic inflammation sets in motion. Therefore, chronic inflammation, together with increased oxidative stress participates in the pathogenesis of HD and is associated with subclinical progression of the disease. Microglia activation is associated with elevated levels of translocator protein (TSPO) which was measured by PET (positron emission tomography), using a tracer[11] C (R)-PK11195. The results showed that increased TSPO levels were associated with increased plasma levels of IL-1β in the cortical, basal ganglia, and thalamus regions of asymptomatic individuals carrying mutated huntingtin gene.[83] Another study also showed an increase in microglia activation in asymptomatic HD carriers.[84] Atrophy in the sensorimotor striatum, substantia nigra, orbitofrontal, and anterior prefrontal cortex was also found in asymptomatic HD patients. Plasma levels of IL-6 were already elevated in asymptomatic individuals carrying HD gene 16 years before the onset of symptoms of the disease and monocytes from the subjects expressing HD gene were hyperactive in response to stimulation.[85] Furthermore, cerebrospinal fluid from HD patients exhibited increased immune activation. These results suggest that immune activation mediated by microglia plays a role in the pathogenesis of HD.

Pro-inflammatory cytokines accumulate in the serum of asymptomatic individuals carrying HD gene, and their levels correlate with disease progression. The IkB kinase ß (IKKß) is a regulator of inflammation in the brain. Oxidative stress-induced damage to DNA activates IKKß that triggers caspase-dependent cleavage of wild-type and HD protein causing increased accumulation of oligomeric fragments.[86] The N-terminal fragments of HD protein directly bind to and activate IKKß, which cleaves HD protein to form insoluble oligomeric fragments that are toxic to neurons. Thus, DNA damage as well as N-terminal fragments of HD protein activates IKKß, which cleaves full-length HD proteins to increase the levels of N-terminal fragments that are neurotoxic. Elevated IKKß activity is present in the brain of mouse model of HD, but is confined to the striatum in the asymptomatic mice carrying HD protein. Inhibitors of IKKB prevented the toxicity of HD protein fragments in the striatum.[75,86] Thus, increased presence pro-inflammatory cytokines is one of the early events that contribute to the progression of HD.

Activated microglia is present in the area of neuronal loss in the autopsied brain samples. They produce excessive amounts of neurotoxic factors, such as free radicals, pro-inflammatory cytokines, and prostaglandins. Reduction in binding of dopamine D2 receptors and performance on the Unified Huntington Disease Scale Score were correlated.[87] Using the same PET technique as described previously in asymptomatic HD patients, microglial activation was an early event in pathogenesis of HD and was associated with subclinical progression of disease.[84] In addition, atrophy in the sensorimotor striatum, substantia nigra, orbitofrontal, and anterior prefrontal cortex were found in asymptomatic HD patients. In addition, binding of dopamine D2/D3 receptors was reduced and activation of microglia increased in these patients. These abnormalities progressively increased in symptomatic HD patients. It was concluded that activation of microglia occurs in the areas of brain responsible for cognitive function.[88] The number of activated microglia increased in the vicinity of neurons expressing HD protein in corticostriatal slices and primary neuronal cultures. Increased levels of interleukin-6 (IL-6) and complement protein 1q occurred as neurodegeneration progressed.[89]

Treatment with verapamil or diltiazem, drugs approved by the FDA for other conditions, improved motor functions in humans and also reduced oxidative damage and markers of pro-inflammatory cytokines (TNF-alpha, IL-6 and caspase-3) in the HD rat model.[90]

Blood levels of pro-inflammatory cytokines IL-23 and the soluble human leukocyte antigen-G (sHLA-G) were increased in the most advanced cases of HD and there was a significant correlation between IL-23 and the severity of the disease.[91]

STUDIES ON ANIMAL MODELS OF HD

Treatment of a rat model of HD (quinolinic acid-induced HD) with a selective inhibitor of cyclooxygenase-2 (COX-2) celecoxib markedly improved behavior and biochemical changes in the brain of HD rats, suggesting that activation of immune active cells like microglia may contribute to the pathogenesis of HD.[92]

INCREASED GLUTAMATE LEVELS AND GLUTAMATE RECEPTOR ACTIVATION IN HD

Glutamate release contributes to the pathogenesis of HD. Activation of mGluR2/3 autoreceptors present in the corticostrital terminals reduces the release of glutamate. In HD mouse model (R6/2), daily subcutaneous injection of LY379268, a mGluR2/3 receptor agonist, produced no adverse effects in wild-type mice; however, in HD mice, it increased the survival by 11%, improved motor functions (activity, speed, endurance, and gait), and enhanced the survival of cortical and striatal neurons by 15%–20%. Furthermore, deficits of motor neuron function were greater in male HD mice than in female, and beneficial effect of LY379268 was greater in male than in female.[93] The protective effect of LY379268 is mediated via upregulating the expression of brain-derived neurotrophic factor (BDNF) in the cerebral cortex and hippocampus of mice.

Glutamate-mediated excitotoxicity is one of the mechanisms involved in the loss of striatal neurons in patients with HD. Treatment of striatal precursor cell line expressing full-length wild-type huntingtin gene (STHdh (Q7/Q7) or HD gene (STHdh (Q111/Q111) with N-methyl-D-aspartate (NMDA) agonist caused early death in cells expressing HD gene compared to that in cells expressing wild-type huntingtin gene.[94] Using a HD mouse model (YAC128), it was demonstrated that the striatal neurons exhibited enhanced sensitivity to excitotoxicity before the onset of HD phenotypes in the brain.[95]

Stimulation of N-methyl-D-aspartate (NMDA) receptor by glutamate has been implicated in neuronal damaged observed in HD. Neurons expressing high levels of NMDA receptors are lost from the striatum of individuals at their early stage of the disease because of the toxicity of glutamate. This is substantiated by the observations, which showed that administration of NMDA receptor agonist into the striatum of rodents or nonhuman primates induced HD phenotypes in the brain.[96]

As the diseases progressed, reduced dopamine and glutamate transmission were observed.[97] Loss of dopaminergic and glutamatergic neurons may account for the loss of their transmission in HD. Impairment of dopamine and glutamate transmission in HD suggests that restoring the balance between dopamine and glutamate transmission to a normal level may be useful in improving some of the symptoms of HD.[97]

The levels of glutamate in the extracellular fluid are increased in HD brain. This could be due to a decrease in the glutamate transporter protein-1-dependednt uptake of glutamate. The two major glutamate transporter proteins, glutamate transporter-1 (GLT-1) and glutamate-aspartate transporter

(GLAST) are primarily located in the astrocytes of adult brain and play an important role in maintaining physiological extracellular levels of glutamate. Release of ascorbate from the striatum into the extracellular fluid is reduced together with the reduction in GLT-1 dependent uptake of glutamate in mouse HD model (R6/2).[98] Levels of ascorbate decrease and the levels of glutamate increase in the extracellular fluid of striatal neurons. The reduction in ascorbate levels and enhancement of glutamate would contribute to degeneration and death of the striatal neurons. Thus, reduction in the function of glutamate transporter proteins may contribute to degeneration of striatal neurons by decreasing the levels of vitamin C and increasing the levels of glutamate. Injection of vitamin C restored extracellular levels of vitamin C in R6/2 mice to the levels in wild-type mice and normalized neuronal function in the striatum of HD mice.[98]

GABA RECEPTORS IN ASYMPTOMATIC AND SYMPTOMATIC INDIVIDUALS

Gamma-aminobutyric acid (GABA) receptors were elevated in symptomatic and asymptomatic HD patients.[99] In a chemical (quinolinic acid)-induced rat model of HD, elevated levels of GABA (B1) and GABA(B2) receptors were present in the striatal neurons as well as in the astrocytes.[100] Using transgenic HD model mice (R6/1 and R6/2), increases in spontaneous GABAergic synaptic currents and postsynaptic receptor function occurred in parallel to progressive decreases in glutamatergic inputs to GABAergic medium-sized spiny projection neurons.[101] Such changes may lead to impaired control of movement. It was also was found that GABA (A) receptor regulated trafficking function is impaired probably due to loss of GABA receptors.[102] Reduced inhibitory synaptic transmission may contribute to the loss of normal excitatory/inhibitory equilibrium, causing increased excitotoxicity in neurons in the HD brain.

USE OF SINGLE ANTIOXIDANTS, PHYTOCHEMICALS, AND B-VITAMINS IN THE MANAGEMENT OF HD

ALPHA-TOCOPHEROL (VITAMIN E)

In a clinical study involving 73 patients with HD, it was found that treatment with *d*-alpha-tocopherol had no effect on neurological or neuropsychiatric symptoms; however, some beneficial effects on neurological symptoms were observed during the early course of the disease.[5]

VITAMIN C

Using transgenic mouse HD model R6/2, it was shown that injection of vitamin C (ascorbate) at the beginning of the onset of symptoms restored striatal release of ascorbate improved neurological motor signs without altering overall motor activity.[103]

N-ACETYLCYSTEINE (NAC)

Since mitochondrial dysfunction is present in HD, the efficacy of NAC in improving mitochondrial function in rat HD model (induced by the treatment with 3-nitropropionic acid) was tested.[104] Rats treated with 3-nitropropionic acid (3-NP) exhibited inhibition of brain mitochondrial complexes II, IV, and V, but not of complex I in the striatum. As expected, increased production of ROS and lipid peroxidation were observed in brain mitochondria of 3-NP treated rats. In addition, increased cytosolic cytochrome c levels, mitochondrial swelling, and increased expression of caspase-3 and p53 were observed in the brain of NP-3 treated animals. Neuropathological changes included neurodegneration and gliosis and were associated with motor and cognitive deficits. Treatment with NAC reversed 3-NP-induced mitochondrial dysfunctions and deficits in motor and cognitive functions.

ALPHA-LIPOIC ACID

Treatment with alpha-lipoic acid increased the survival of transgenic mouse HD models (R6/2 and N-171-82Q).[105]

COENZYME Q10

Using transgenic mice HD model (expression of HD protein with approximately 120 trinucleotide repeats), it was demonstrated that mice fed with 0.2% and 0.6% of coenzyme Q10 in chow improved early behavior deficits and normalized some transcriptional deficits without altering the levels of HD protein aggregates in the striatum.[106] It was noted that coenzyme Q10 at a low dose was more effective than that observed at a high dose. Treatment of wild-type mice with a low-dose coenzyme Q10 (0.2%) induced motor deficits. This deleterious effect of coenzyme Q10 may be unique to mice since no harmful effects of even high doses of coenzyme Q10 have been observed in humans.

In another study using transgenic mouse model of HD (R6/2), it was demonstrated that brain levels of coenzyme Q9 and coenzyme Q10 were lower in R6/2 mice than in wild-type mice. Oral administration of coenzyme Q10 increased the levels of coenzyme Q10 in plasma and of coenzyme Q9 and coenzyme Q10 and adenosine triphosphate (ATP) in the brain of R6/2 mice. Treatment with high doses of coenzyme Q10 significantly extended survival of R6/2 mice in a dose-dependent manner, and improved motor deficits, reduced weight loss, brain atrophy, and HD protein aggregates.[107]

A combination of coenzyme Q10 and creatine produced an additive protective effect in improving motor performance and extending survival of transgenic R6/2 HD mice.[108]

L-CARNITINE

Using chemical-induced HD animal models (rats treated with quinolinic acid or 3-NP), it was demonstrated that treatment with L-carnitine prevented quinolinic acid-induced motor deficits and 3-NP-induced hypokinetic pattern (impaired movements).[109] L-carnitine treatment also reduced quinolinic acid-induced gliosis and 3-NP-induced brain damage. Using transgenic mouse HD model (N171-82Q), it was shown that administration of L-carnitine increased survival of HD mice, and improved motor function as well as reduced neuronal loss and the number of HD protein aggregates. It was suggested that the protective effect of L-carnitine was due to reduction in oxidative damage.[110]

LYCOPENE AND EPIGALLOCATECHIN

Using 3-NP-induced rat HD model, it was demonstrated that treatment with lycopene and epigallocatechin improved memory deficits and restored glutathione levels and glutathione-S-transferase activity in the striatum, hippocampus, and cortex areas of the brain. Furthermore, pretreatment with arginine (produced nitric oxide) increased the effectiveness of lycopene and epigallocatechin in protecting neuronal damage.[111]

MELATONIN

This hormone is secreted by the pineal gland and is necessary for sleep. Melatonin also exhibits antioxidant activity. A study has reported that supplementation with melatonin delayed the onset and mortality in a transgenic mouse model of HD.[112] Loss of type 1-melatonin receptors (MT1) has been found in human HD as well as in transgenic mouse HD model. It has been reported that high levels of MT1 receptors are present in the mitochondria from the brain of wild-type mice; however, in the transgenic mouse HD model, reduced levels of MT1 receptors were present.[112]

Treatment with melatonin inhibited mutated huntingtin protein-induced caspase activation and protected MT1 receptors expression, suggesting that protective effect of melatonin may be mediated through activation of MT1 receptors.

CURCUMIN

Curcumin is a naturally occurring phytochemicals with the ability to enter the blood-brain-barrier. The efficacy of curcumin in improving the symptoms of HD was tested in transgenic mouse HD model (expressing 140 repeats of trinucleotide). The results showed that HD mice fed with curcumin-containing diet since conception showed decreased aggregates of mutated huntingtin protein and increased striatal dopamine- and cAMP-regulated neuronal phosphoprotein (DARPP-32) and dopamine D1 receptor mRNAs, and prevented rearing deficits.[113] Although curcumin treatment impaired motor function in transgenic HD mice and wild-type mice in early study; however, in this study, curcumin treatment did not affect motor function, behavioral deficits, and muscle strength or food utilization in transgenic mice.

RESVERATROL

Using rat HD model (3-NP-induced HD phenotype), it was demonstrated that treatement with resveratrol before and after 3-NP treatment reduced motor and cognitive deficits by reducing oxidatitve stres.[114] Reduction in mitogen-activated protein kinase signaling pathway, particularly the Ras-extracellular signal-regulated kinase (ERK) cascade has been implicated in the pathogenesis of HD. Therefore, activation of ERK may be of therapeutic value in the management of HD. This hypothesis was tested in three HD models (PC-12, a neuronal cell line expressing HD gene, Drosophila expressing HD gene and R6/2 mouse HD model), using phytochemicals, such as resveratrol, which activate ERK. The results showed that activator of ERK reduced the harmful effects of HD protein in all three models.[115]

GINKGO BILOBA EXTRACT AND OLIVE OIL

Pre-treatment with *Ginkgo biloba* extract (EGb761) prevented 3-NP-induced motor deficits and elevated strital malondialdehyde (MDA) levels in rats.[116] Treatment with 3-NP upregulated the expression of striatal Bax gene and downregulated the expression of striatal Bcl-xl gene, upregulated the expression of striatal glyceraldehyde-3-pohosphate dehydrogenase (GAPDH), and inhibited succinate dehydrogenase enzyme activity. Pretreatment with (EGb-761) reversed the above changes in gene expression and enzyme activity involved in energy metabolism.

Treatment with extra-virgin olive oil prevented 3-NP-induced elevated levels of lipid peroxides and depletion of glutathione in the striatum of rats.[117] In addition, olive oil treatment also reversed 3-NP-induced inhibition of succinate dehydrogenase activity.

PROBUCOL

Probucol is known to exhibit antioxidant activity. Treatment with probucol prevented ROS formation and lipid peroxidation in all chemical-induced HD models (quinolinic acid; as an excitotoxic model, 3-NP; as an inhibitor of mitochondrial succinate dehydrogenase model, and combined model of quinolinic acid and 3-NP treatment), but it did not protect against 3-NP-induced mitochondrial dysfunctions.[118] Treatment with sodium succinate protected striatal slices only against 3-NP-induced mitochondrial dysfunctions. Treatment with a NMDA receptor antagonist MK-801 (also called Dizocilpine) protected mitochondrial dysfunctions in all HD models used in this study. These data suggest that a combination of NMDA receptor antigonist and an antioxidants may be more useful in reducing oxidatve stress and mitochondrial dysfunction than the individual agents.

B-Vitamins

Nicotinamide, a water soluble B3-vitamins, is an inhibitor of sirtuin1/class III NAD+-dependent histone deacetylase activity. Using the B6.HDR6/1 transgenic mouse model, it was demonstrated that treatment with nicotinamide increased mRNA levels of BDNF and Peroxisome proliferator-activated receptor gamma coactivator 1-alpha (PGC-1alpha). In addition, nicotinamide treatment enhanced protein levels of BDNF and activation of PGC-1alpha in HD mice. Furthermore, the above treatment improved motor function in HD mice even though there was no reduction in the levels of HD protein aggregates in the striatum or in the weight loss.[119]

Examination of autopsied samples human HD striatum showed increased levels carbonylation of proteins (a marker of protein oxidation). Oxidation of mitochondrial enzymes decreased catalytic activities, which reduced energy levels in HD, whereas oxidation of pyridoxal kinase and antiquitin-1 decreased the levels of pyridoxal 5-phosphate (vitamin B6). Using the Tet/HD94 conditional mouse HD model, it was shown that carbonylation (oxidation) of proteins in the striatum was dependent upon the expression of HD protein.[120] Vitamin B6 acts as a cofactor for several biological processes including transaminases, and synthesis of glutathione, GABA, and dopamine; therefore, the reduction in the levels of vitamin B6 in HD may be responsible for reduction in the levels of dopamine and GABA in this disease.

The above studies on animal and cell culture models of HD suggest potential value of antioxidants, phytochemicals and B-vitamins in reducing some symptoms of HD. Use of a single antioxidant, such as vitamin E and coenzyme Q10 produced no effect or caused transient benefit on some symptoms in an early phase of the disease.

The above studies on animal and cell culture models of HD suggest potential value of micronutrients in improving some symptoms of HD. Human studies with most individual antioxidants were not effective. Since increased oxidative stress, chronic inflammation, and glutamate are involved in the development and progression of HD, simultaneous reduction of these cellular events may help in delaying the onset of symptoms and reducing the rate of progression of this neurodegenerative disease.

STUDIES WITH INDIVIDUAL ANTIOXIDANTS IN OTHER HUMAN NEURODEGENERATIVE DISEASES

Treatment with individual antioxidants such as vitamin E[121,122] and curcumin[123] do not improve cognitive function, whereas alpha-lipoic acid,[124] vitamin E,[125] and omega-3-fatty acids[126,127] produce transient and limited improvement in cognitive function only in early phases of Alzheimer's disease (AD). In the case of Parkinson's disease, high doses of coenzyme Q10 produce transient improvements in some symptoms.[128] The reasons for individual antioxidants producing no effect or transient beneficial effects may have been for several reasons: (a) antioxidants show differential subcellular distribution and different mechanisms of action; therefore, a single antioxidant cannot protect all parts of the cell; (b) a single antioxidant in a high internal oxidative environment of patients with neurodegenerative diseases is oxidized and can then itself act as a prooxidant rather than as an antioxidant; (c) the body protects against oxidative damage by elevating antioxidant enzymes, and dietary and endogenous antioxidants levels. Antioxidants neutralize free radicals by donating electrons to those molecules with unpaired electron, whereas antioxidant enzymes destroy free radicals by catalysis, converting them to harmless molecules such as water and oxygen. Therefore, both of these events need to be enhanced to produce substantial therapeutic gain; (d) the affinity of different antioxidants for free radicals differs, depending upon their lipophilicity; (e) both the aqueous and lipid components of the cell need to be protected together. Water-soluble antioxidants such as vitamin C and glutathione protect molecules in the aqueous environment of the cells, whereas lipid soluble antioxidants such as vitamin A and vitamin E protect molecules in the lipid compartment; (f) vitamin E is more effective in quenching free radicals in a reduced oxygenated cellular environment, whereas vitamin C and α-tocopherol are more effective in a higher oxygenated environment of the cells[129]; (g) vitamin C is important for recycling the oxidized form of α-tocopherol to the antioxidant form at the lipid/aqueous interface[130]; and (h) antioxidants produce cell protective proteins by altering the expression of different microRNAs.[131] For example, some antioxidants can activate Nrf2 by upregulating miR-200a that inhibits its target protein Keap1, whereas others activate Nrf2 by downregulating miR-21 that binds with 3′-UTR Nrf2 mRNA.[132]

These studies suggest that use of a single micronutrient in prevention or improved management of human neurodegenerative diseases is not expected to yield any beneficial effects. For this reason, a mixture of micronutrients that can simultaneously reduce oxidative stress and inflammation by enhancing the levels of antioxidant enzymes through the activation of Nrf2 pathway together with dietary and endogenous antioxidants for Alzheimer's disease and Parkinson's disease has been suggested.[131,133] The same suggestion is proposed for the improved management of HD. Oral supplementation can increase the levels of dietary and endogenous antioxidants; however, elevation of the levels of antioxidant enzymes requires an activation of Nrf2. Therefore it is essential to understand the regulation of activation of Nrf2.

REGULATION OF ACTIVATION OF Nrf2

REACTIVE OXYGEN SPECIES (ROS) ACTIVATES Nrf2

Normally, during acute oxidative stress, ROS is needed to activate Nrf2, which then dissociates itself from the Keap1-CuI-Rbx1 complex and translocates in the nucleus, where it heterodimerizes with a small Maf protein and binds with the ARE (antioxidant response element) leading to increased expression of target genes coding for several cytoprotective enzymes including antioxidant enzymes.[134–136] In this manner, activation of Nrf2 increases the levels of cytoprotective enzymes including antioxidant enzymes and phase-2-detoxifying enzymes.[137,138]

BINDING OF Nrf2 WITH ARE IN THE NUCLEUS

Activation of Nrf2 alone may not be sufficient to increase the levels of antioxidant enzymes. Activated Nrf2 must bind with the ARE in the nucleus for increasing the expression of its target genes. This binding ability of Nrf2 with ARE was impaired in aged rats and this defect was restored by supplementation with alpha-lipoic acid.[139] It is unknown whether the binding ability of Nrf2 with ARE is impaired in HD.

EXISTENCE OF ROS-RESISTANT Nrf2

Activation of Nrf2 by ROS becomes impaired in HD. This is evidenced by the fact that increased oxidative stress occurs in HD despite the presence of Nrf2, and that Nrf2 deficient animals become more sensitive to chemical-induced HD phenotypes.

ANTIOXIDANTS ACTIVATE ROS-RESISTANT Nrf2

Activation of Nrf2 becomes unresponsive to ROS in HD. Some dietary antioxidants and phytochemicals can activate Nrf2 without requiring ROS. These include vitamin C[140,141] vitamin E,[142] endogenous antioxidants such as alpha-lipoic acid,[139] and coenzyme Q10,[143] synthetic antioxidant N-acetylcysteine (NAC),[144] omega-3-fatty acids,[145,146] and phytochemicals such as curcumin[147] and resveratrol.[148,149]

L-CARNITINE ACTIVATES Nrf2 BY A ROS-DEPENDENT MECHANISM

Treatment with L-carnitine activates Nrf2 by a ROS-dependent mechanism,[150] probably by generating transient ROS.

ACTIVATION OF Nrf2 BY MicroRNAs

The complex of Keap1-Nrf2 in the cytoplasm prevents activation of Nrf2. Overexpression of miR-200a reduced Keap-1 levels allowing Nrf2 to migrate to the nucleus where it binds to the ARE that enhanced the transcription of target cytoprotective genes including antioxidant enzymes.[151] Increased oxidative stress enhanced the expression of miR-153 that reduced the expression of Nrf2 by binding to its 3'-UTR region of Nrf2 mRNA.[152] Mutation in miR-153 restored the oxidative stress-induced reduction in Nrf2 activity.

Nrf2 IN HD

HD protein disrupted Nrf2 signaling pathway in the striatal neurons expressing the HD gene, and thus, contributed to mitochondrial dysfunction and enhanced sensitivity to oxidative stress.[153] Treatment of rats with 3-nitropropionic acid (3-NP) also caused a reduction in Nrf2 levels in the cytoplasm and the nucleus. Treatment of transgenic HD mouse models (R6/2 mice and YAC128 mice) with dimethylfumarate prevented weight loss, improved motor function, and protected neurons in the striatum and motor cortex. These effects appear to be mediated via Nrf2 signaling pathway.[154] Nrf2-deficient cells and Nrf2 knockout mice (Nrf2$^-$/Nrf2$^-$) are very sensitive to complex II mitochondrial inhibitors (3-NP and malonate) in causing degeneration of the striatal neurons. Intrastriatal transplantation of Nrf2 overexpressing astrocytes before treatments with 3-NP or malonate provided significant protection against damage produced by inhibitors of complex II.[155] Treatment of rat striatal slices with quinolinic acid induces oxidative damage. Nrf2 pathway is upregulated at an early stage presumably as an adaptive response to oxidative stress. Striatal slices from Nrf2$^-$/$^-$ mice were more sensitive to the deleterious effects of quinolinic acid than those obtained from Nrf2$^+$/$^+$ mice.[156] This implies that elevation of the Nrf2/ARE pathway could be of neuroprotective value in the treatment of HD.

SUPPRESSION OF OXIDATIVE STRESS BY Nrf2 AND ANTIOXIDANTS

Antioxidant-induced activation of Nrf2 would reduce oxidative stress by enhancing the levels of antioxidant enzymes, whereas antioxidants decrease oxidative stress by donation electrons to unpaired molecules.

SUPPRESSION OF CHRONIC INFLAMMATION BY Nrf2 AND ANTIOXIDANTS

The antioxidant-induced activation of Nrf2 also suppresses chronic inflammation.[137,138] Some antioxidants reduce markers of chronic inflammation.[157–162] They do so by decreasing the levels of pro-inflammatory cytokines and by reducing the activities of cyclooxygenase enzymes.

INHIBITION OF RELEASE AND TOXICITY OF GLUTAMATE BY ANTIOXIDANTS AND B-VITAMINS

In HD patients, imbalances between excitatory and inhibitory neurotransmission cause excitatory neurotransmission in HD patients. Release of glutamate was blocked by antioxidants, such as vitamin E,[163] tempol, a superoxide dismutase mimetic, and edaravone, a synthetic antioxidant,[164] quercetin,[165] glutathione and vitamin E,[166] alpha-lipoic acid,[167] and coenzyme Q10.[168] In addition to antioxidants, vitamin B6,[169] vitamin B12,[170] and vitamin B2 (riboflavin)[171] also reduce release of glutamate. Antioxidants such as α-tocopherol[172] and coenzyme Q10[173] also protected neurons against glutamate-induced degeneration and death.

PROPOSED MIXTURE OF MICRONUTRIENTS FOR IMPROVED MANAGEMENT OF HD

Based on the studies discussed above, a mixture of micronutrients containing vitamin A, mixed carotenoids, vitamin C, α-tocopheryl acetate, α-tocopheryl succinate, vitamin D3, alpha-lipoic acid, N-acetylcysteine, coenzyme Q10, L-carnitine, omega-3-fatty acids, curcumin, resveratrol, all B-vitamins, selenomethionine, and zinc, but without iron, copper, manganese, or heavy metals such as molybdenum and zirconium for the prevention or delaying the onset of symptoms is proposed. The inclusion of iron, copper, and manganese is not suggested, because these trace mineral, although essential for many biological reactions, can combine with vitamin C and generate excessive amounts of free radicals. Furthermore, these minerals are absorbed from the intestine better in the presence of antioxidants than in their absence that could increase body store of free iron, copper and manganese after a long-term consumption. The body has no significant mechanisms of excretion of these trace minerals. Slight increase in the body store of free forms of these minerals can increase the risk of most chronic diseases. Heavy metals were not included because the body has no mechanisms of excretion of these heavy metals. Consequently, their levels in the body would increase after long-term consumption. High levels of heavy metals could interfere with the function of organs including the brain.

It is expected that the proposed micronutrient mixture would increase the levels of antioxidant enzymes by activating the Nrf2 pathway. This together with enhancement of dietary and endogenous antioxidants, and B-vitamins could lead to simultaneously reduction in oxidative stress, chronic inflammation, and glutamate levels in HD. This micronutrient mixture then may prevent or delay the onset of HD symptoms, and in combination with standard therapy, may improve the management of this disease.

PREVENTION OR DELAYING THE ONSET OF SYMPTOMS BY PROPOSED MICRONUTRIENT MIXTURE?

It is often believed that the genetic basis of neurodegenerative diseases, such as HD cannot be prevented or delayed by any pharmacological and/or physiological means. Laboratory experiments on the genetic basis of another disease model (cancer) in *Drosophila melanogaster* (fruit fly) show that it may be possible to prevent or at least delay the onset of the genetic basis of human diseases.

The dominant HOP (TUM-1) mutation in the HOP Jak kinase causes leukemia-like cancer and other birth defects in female fruit flies. In collaboration with Dr. Bhattacharya et al. of NASA, Moffat Field, CA, it was found that whole-body irradiation of these flies with proton radiation dramatically increased the incidence of cancer compared to that of unirradiated flies. The question arose as to whether or not a preparation of multiple antioxidants can reduce the incidence of cancer, which is due to a specific gene defect. To test this possibility, a mixture of multiple dietary and endogenous antioxidants were fed to these flies through diet 7 days before proton irradiation and continued throughout the experimental period of 7 days after irradiation. The results showed that antioxidant treatment before and after irradiation blocked the proton radiation-induced cancer in fruit flies. This finding on fruit flies is of particular interest, because to my knowledge, this is a first demonstration in which genetic basis of a disease can be prevented by antioxidant treatment. This observation made on fruit flies cannot readily be extrapolated to humans. It is not known whether daily supplementation with antioxidants in asymptomatic individuals carrying HD gene can delay or prevent the appearance of disease symptoms. A clinical study is needed to test whether or not the proposed micronutrient mixture can prevent of or delay the onset of HD symptoms in humans.

PROPOSED MICRONUTRIENT MIXTURE IN COMBINATION WITH STANDARD TREATMENT

This proposed mixture of micronutrients, in combination with standard treatment, might be useful for enhancing the management of HD by reducing the progression of the disease. Preclinical and clinical studies are needed to substantiate the potential role of proposed mixture of micronutrients for the improved management of HD.

CURRENT TREATMENTS OF HD

The contents of this section are taken from the publication by Mayo Clinic Foundation for Medical Education and Research. At present, a combination of medications, psychotherapy, speech therapy, and physical therapy is used to manage the symptoms of HD. There are no drug treatments that can alter the course of HD in humans. The following groups of drugs are used in the treatment of HD in humans.

MOVEMENT DISORDER DRUGS

Tetrabenazine (Xenazine), an FDA-approved drug, suppresses chorea (jerking movements) associated with HD; however, serious side effects include the risk of worsening or triggering depression or other psychiatric problems, insomnia, drowsiness, nausea, and restlessness. These side effects limit the value of these drugs in the management of the symptoms of HD.

ANTIPSYCHOTIC DRUGS

Haloperidol (Haldol) and Clozapine can suppress chorea movements, but they can worsen involuntary contraction (dystonia) and muscle rigidity; therefore, they are not adequate for improving the symptoms of HD.

OTHER MEDICATIONS

Other drugs that can suppress chorea, dystonia, and muscle rigidity include antiseizure drugs, such as clonazepam (Klonopin) and antianxiety medications, such as diazepam (Valium). These drugs can alter consciousness and induce addiction and dependency.

MEDICATIONS FOR PSYCHIATRIC DISORDERS

Drugs to treat psychiatric disorders may vary depending upon the disorders and symptoms. Possible treatment drugs include the following.

ANTIDEPRESSANTS

Commonly used drugs include escitalopram (Lexapro), fluoxetine (Prozac, Sarafem), and sertraline (Zoloft). These drugs may also be useful in treating obsessive-compulsive disorder associated with HD. Some adverse side effects may include nausea, diarrhea, insomnia, and sexual problem.

MOOD-STABILIZING DRUGS

Drugs include lithium (Lithobid) and anticonvulsants, such as valporic acid (Depakene), divalproex (Depakote), and lamotrigine (Lamictal), which may be useful in the treatment of highs and lows associated with bipolar disorders. Common side effects include weight gain, tremor, and gastrointestinal problems. Periodic blood tests are needed because of toxicity of lithium on thyroid and kidney.

CLINICAL STUDIES WITH ADDITIONAL DRUGS IN HD

In a clinical study involving 6 patients with HD, the efficacy of Aripiprazole (AP), a dopamine D2 receptor partial agonist that is used to reduce schizophrenic symptoms, was compared with Tetrabenazine (TBZ), a dopamine depletor that is used to treat hyperkinesia, chorea, motor function, and functional disability in HD. The results showed that both drugs reduced chorea in a similar manner; however, AP caused less sedation and sleepiness than TBZ.[174] The sample size of this study was too small to make any conclusion. It is interesting to note that two drugs that have an opposite effect on the level of dopamine are used in this study.

In a randomized, double blind, placebo-controlled trial involving multicenter from 32 European countries, the efficacy of pridopidine, a dopaminergic stabilizer, was evaluated on motor function in patients with HD. The results showed that this drug did not affect non-motor endpoints, but some improvements in motor function were detected.[175] The drug at the dose of 90 mg/day was considered safe. A similar study with pridopidine was performed utilizing outpatient's neurological clinics at 27 sites in the USA and Canada on HD patients receiving 20 mg (N = 56), 45 mg (N = 55), 90 mg (N = 58), or placebo (N = 58) for a period of 12 weeks. The results showed that pridopidine treatment at a dose of 90 mg/day may improve some motor functions.[176]

PSYCHOTHERAPY

A psychiatrist, psychologist or social worker can provide psychotherapy. It is important to help a person with HD to manage behavioral problems, develop coping strategies, manage expectations during progress of the disease, and facilitate effective communication among family members.

SPEECH THERAPY

HD can markedly impair control of muscles of the mouth and throat that are essential for speech, eating, and swallowing. A speech therapist can help improve the ability of patients with HD to speak clearly and use communication devices correctly.

PHYSICAL THERAPY

A physical therapist can teach HD patients how to exercise safely and correctly in order to enhance muscle strength, flexibility, balance, and coordination. These exercises can help in maintaining mobility as long as possible and may reduce the risk of falls. The physical therapist can also provide instruction on appropriate posture and the use of supports to improve posture that may reduce the severity of some movement disorders. For those patients who may require a wheelchair or walker, a physical therapist can teach how to use these devices appropriately.

CONCLUSIONS

Huntington's disease (HD) is a progressive, fatal, dominant, hereditary, and incurable neurodegenerative disease of the brain. The striatum and cortex that are involved in movement, intellect, and emotions are gradually destroyed. This disease is characterized by an expansion of more than 35 repeats of the trinucleotide CAG (cytosine-adenine-guanosine) coding for glutamine in huntingtin gene. Evidence showed that among various cellular defects, increased oxidative stress, chronic inflammation, and glutamate levels play an important role in the pathogenesis of HD. The incidence and cost, signs and symptoms, brain pathology, receptor abnormalities, microRNAs role in pathogenesis, and regulation of activation of Nrf2 and Nrf2 in HD were discussed. The currently used standard therapy is briefly described. In order to simultaneously decrease the levels of oxidative stress, chronic inflammation, and glutamate levels, a concurrent elevation of the levels of antioxidant enzymes by activating the Nrf2 pathway together with dietary and endogenous antioxidants and B-vitamins may be necessary. A mixture of micronutrient that may simultaneously attenuate these biochemical abnormalities involved in HD, and thereby, prevent, and in combination with standard therapy, improve the management of this disease was proposed.

REFERENCES

1. MacDonald ME, Ambrose C.M, Duyao M.P, et al. A novel gene containing a trinucleotide repeat that is expanded and unstable on Huntington's disease chromosomes. *Cell.* 1993;72:971–983.
2. Snell RG, MacMillan JC, Cheadle JP, et al. Relationship between trinucleotide repeat expansion and phenotypic variation in Huntington's disease. *Nat Genet.* 1993;4(4):393–397.
3. Furtado S, Suchowersky O, Rewcastle B, Graham L, Klimek ML, Garber A. Relationship between trinucleotide repeats and neuropathological changes in Huntington's disease. *Ann Neurol.* 1996;39(1):132–136.
4. Ravina B, Romer M, Constantinescu R, et al. The relationship between CAG repeat length and clinical progression in Huntington's disease. *Mov Disord.* 2008;23(9):1223–1227.
5. Peyser CE, Folstein M, Chase GA, et al. Trial of d-alpha-tocopherol in Huntington's disease. *Am J Psychiat.* 1995;152(12):1771–1775.
6. Group HS. A random, placebo-controlled trial of coenzyme Q10 and remacemide in Huntington's disease. *Neurology.* 2001;14:397–404.
7. Pringsheim T, Wiltshire K, Day L, Dykeman J, Steeves T, Jette N. The incidence and prevalence of Huntington's disease: A systematic review and meta-analysis. *Mov Disord.* 2012;27(9):1083–1091.
8. Rawlins MD, Wexler NS, Wexler AR, et al. The prevalence of Huntington's disease. *Neuroepidemiology.* 2016;46(2):144–153.
9. Divino V, Dekoven M, Warner JH, et al. The direct medical costs of Huntington's disease by stage. A retrospective commercial and Medicaid claims data analysis. *J Med Econ.* 2013;16(8):1043–1050.
10. Sadri-Vakili G, Cha JH. Mechanisms of disease: Histone modifications in Huntington's disease. *Nat Clin Pract Neurol.* 2006;2(6):330–338.
11. Rub U, Hoche F, Brunt ER, et al. Degeneration of the cerebellum in Huntington's disease (HD): Possible relevance for the clinical picture and potential gateway to pathological mechanisms of the disease process. *Brain Pathol.* 2013;23(2):165–177.
12. Rub U, Hentschel M, Stratmann K, et al. Huntington's disease (HD): Degeneration of select nuclei, widespread occurrence of neuronal nuclear and axonal inclusions in the brainstem. *Brain Pathol.* 2014;24(3):247–260.
13. Papoutsi M, Labuschagne I, Tabrizi SJ, Stout JC. The cognitive burden in Huntington's disease: Pathology, phenotype, and mechanisms of compensation. *Mov Disord.* 2014;29(5):673–683.
14. Rub U, Seidel K, Vonsattel JP, et al. Huntington's Disease (HD): Neurodegeneration of Brodmann's Primary Visual Area 17 (BA17). *Brain Pathol.* 2015;25(6):701–711.
15. Thu DC, Oorschot DE, Tippett LJ, et al. Cell loss in the motor and cingulate cortex correlates with symptomatology in Huntington's disease. *Brain.* 2010;133(Pt 4):1094–1110.
16. Nana AL, Kim EH, Thu DC, et al. Widespread heterogeneous neuronal loss across the cerebral cortex in Huntington's disease. *J Huntingtons Dis.* 2014;3(1):45–64.
17. Mehrabi NF, Waldvogel HJ, Tippett LJ, Hogg VM, Synek BJ, Faull RL. Symptom heterogeneity in Huntington's disease correlates with neuronal degeneration in the cerebral cortex. *Neurobiol Dis.* 2016;96:67–74.
18. Kuhn A, Goldstein DR, Hodges A, et al. Mutant huntingtin's effects on striatal gene expression in mice recapitulate changes observed in human Huntington's disease brain and do not differ with mutant huntingtin length or wild-type huntingtin dosage. *Hum Mol Genet.* 2007;16(15):1845–1861.
19. Robinson P, Lebel M, Cyr M. Dopamine D1 receptor-mediated aggregation of N-terminal fragments of mutant huntingtin and cell death in a neuroblastoma cell line. *Neuroscience.* 2008;153(3):762–772.
20. Charvin D, Roze E, Perrin V, et al. Haloperidol protects striatal neurons from dysfunction induced by mutated huntingtin in vivo. *Neurobiol Dis.* 2008;29(1):22–29.
21. Pavese N, Politis M, Tai YF, et al. Cortical dopamine dysfunction in symptomatic and premanifest Huntington's disease gene carriers. *Neurobiol Dis.* 2010;37(2):356–361.

22. Esmaeilzadeh M, Farde L, Karlsson P, et al. Extrastriatal dopamine D(2) receptor binding in Huntington's disease. *Hum Brain Mapp.* 2011;32(10):1626–1636.

23. Politis M, Pavese N, Tai YF, Tabrizi SJ, Barker RA, Piccini P. Hypothalamic involvement in Huntington's disease: An in vivo PET study. *Brain.* 2008;131(Pt 11):2860–2869.

24. Ortiz AN, Osterhaus GL, Lauderdale K, et al. Motor function and dopamine release measurements in transgenic Huntington's disease model rats. *Brain Res.* 2012;1450:148–156.

25. Glass M, Dragunow M, Faull RL. The pattern of neurodegeneration in Huntington's disease: A comparative study of cannabinoid, dopamine, adenosine and GABA(A) receptor alterations in the human basal ganglia in Huntington's disease. *Neuroscience.* 2000;97(3):505–519.

26. Van Laere K, Casteels C, Dhollander I, et al. Widespread decrease of type 1 cannabinoid receptor availability in Huntington disease in vivo. *J Nucl Med.* 2010;51(9):1413–1417.

27. Glass M, van Dellen A, Blakemore C, Hannan AJ, Faull RL. Delayed onset of Huntington's disease in mice in an enriched environment correlates with delayed loss of cannabinoid CB1 receptors. *Neuroscience.* 2004;123(1):207–212.

28. Blazquez C, Chiarlone A, Sagredo O, et al. Loss of striatal type 1 cannabinoid receptors is a key pathogenic factor in Huntington's disease. *Brain.* 2011;134(Pt 1):119–136.

29. Pintor A, Tebano MT, Martire A, et al. The cannabinoid receptor agonist WIN 55,212-2 attenuates the effects induced by quinolinic acid in the rat striatum. *Neuropharmacology.* 2006;51(5):1004–1012.

30. Sagredo O, Gonzalez S, Aroyo I, et al. Cannabinoid CB2 receptor agonists protect the striatum against malonate toxicity: Relevance for Huntington's disease. *Glia.* 2009;57(11):1154–1167.

31. Bouchard J, Truong J, Bouchard K, et al. Cannabinoid receptor 2 signaling in peripheral immune cells modulates disease onset and severity in mouse models of Huntington's disease. *J Neurosci.* 2012;32(50):18259–18268.

32. Dowie MJ, Howard ML, Nicholson LF, Faull RL, Hannan AJ, Glass M. Behavioural and molecular consequences of chronic cannabinoid treatment in Huntington's disease transgenic mice. *Neuroscience.* 2010;170(1):324–336.

33. Martire A, Calamandrei G, Felici F, et al. Opposite effects of the A2A receptor agonist CGS21680 in the striatum of Huntington's disease versus wild-type mice. *Neurosci Lett.* 2007;417(1):78–83.

34. Mievis S, Blum D, Ledent C. A2A receptor knockout worsens survival and motor behaviour in a transgenic mouse model of Huntington's disease. *Neurobiol Dis.* 2011;41(2):570–576.

35. Sadri-Vakili G, Cha JH. Histone deacetylase inhibitors: A novel therapeutic approach to Huntington's disease (complex mechanism of neuronal death). *Curr Alzheimer Res.* 2006;3(4):403–408.

36. Thomas EA, Coppola G, Desplats PA, et al. The HDAC inhibitor 4b ameliorates the disease phenotype and transcriptional abnormalities in Huntington's disease transgenic mice. *Proc Natl Acad Sci USA.* 2008;105(40):15564–15569.

37. Martin E, Betuing S, Pages C, et al. Mitogen- and stress-activated protein kinase 1-induced neuroprotection in Huntington's disease: Role on chromatin remodeling at the PGC-1-alpha promoter. *Hum Mol Genet.* 2011;20(12):2422–2434.

38. Bithell A, Johnson R, Buckley NJ. Transcriptional dysregulation of coding and non-coding genes in cellular models of Huntington's disease. *Biochem Soc Trans.* 2009;37(Pt 6):1270–1275.

39. Buckley NJ, Johnson R, Zuccato C, Bithell A, Cattaneo E. The role of REST in transcriptional and epigenetic dysregulation in Huntington's disease. *Neurobiol Dis.* 2010;39(1):28–39.

40. Lee RC, Feinbaum RL, Ambros V. The C. elegans heterochronic gene lin-4 encodes small RNAs with antisense complementarity to lin-14. *Cell.* 1993;75(5):843–854.

41. Wightman B, Ha I, Ruvkun G. Posttranscriptional regulation of the heterochronic gene lin-14 by lin-4 mediates temporal pattern formation in C. elegans. *Cell.* 1993;75(5):855–862.

42. Macfarlane LA, Murphy PR. MicroRNA: Biogenesis, function and role in cancer. *Curr Genomics.* 2010;11(7):537–561.

43. Londin E, Loher P, Telonis AG, et al. Analysis of 13 cell types reveals evidence for the expression of numerous novel primate- and tissue-specific microRNAs. *Proc Natl Acad Sci USA.* 2015;112(10):E1106–E1115.

44. Denli AM, Tops BB, Plasterk RH, Ketting RF, Hannon GJ. Processing of primary microRNAs by the microprocessor complex. *Nature.* 2004;432(7014):231–235.

45. Lee Y, Ahn C, Han J, et al. The nuclear RNase III Drosha initiates microRNA processing. *Nature.* 2003;425(6956):415–419.

46. Hutvagner G, McLachlan J, Pasquinelli AE, Balint E, Tuschl T, Zamore PD. A cellular function for the RNA-interference enzyme Dicer in the maturation of the let-7 small temporal RNA. *Science.* 2001;293(5531):834–838.

47. Hoss AG, Labadorf A, Latourelle JC, et al. miR-10b-5p expression in Huntington's disease brain relates to age of onset and the extent of striatal involvement. *BMC Med Genomics.* 2015;8:10.

48. Das E, Jana NR, Bhattacharyya NP. Delayed cell cycle progression in STHdh(Q111)/Hdh(Q111) cells, a cell model for Huntington's disease mediated by microRNA-19a, microRNA-146a and microRNA-432. *Microrna.* 2015;4(2):86–100.

49. Hoss AG, Kartha VK, Dong X, et al. MicroRNAs located in the Hox gene clusters are implicated in Huntington's disease pathogenesis. *PLoS Genet.* 2014;10(2):e1004188.

50. Liu T, Im W, Mook-Jung I, Kim M. MicroRNA-124 slows down the progression of Huntington's disease by promoting neurogenesis in the striatum. *Neural Regen Res.* 2015;10(5):786–791.

51. Fu MH, Li CL, Lin HL, et al. The potential regulatory mechanisms of miR-196a in Huntington's disease through bioinformatic analyses. *PLoS One.* 2015;10(9):e0137637.

52. Cheng PH, Li CL, Chang YF, et al. miR-196a ameliorates phenotypes of Huntington disease in cell, transgenic mouse, and induced pluripotent stem cell models. *Am J Hum Genet.* 2013;93(2):306–312.

53. Jovicic A, Zaldivar Jolissaint JF, Moser R, Silva Santos Mde F, Luthi-Carter R. MicroRNA-22 (miR-22) overexpression is neuroprotective via general anti-apoptotic effects and may also target specific Huntington's disease-related mechanisms. *PLoS One.* 2013;8(1):e54222.

54. Lee ST, Chu K, Im WS, et al. Altered microRNA regulation in Huntington's disease models. *Exp Neurol.* 2011;227(1):172–179.

55. Kocerha J, Xu Y, Prucha MS, Zhao D, Chan AW. microRNA-128a dysregulation in transgenic Huntington's disease monkeys. *Mol Brain.* 2014;7:46.

56. Ghatak S, Raha S. Micro RNA-214 contributes to proteasome independent downregulation of beta catenin in Huntington's disease knock-in striatal cell model STHdhQ111/Q111. *Biochem Biophys Res Commun.* 2015;459(3):509–514.

57. Ban JJ, Chung JY, Lee M, Im W, Kim M. MicroRNA-27a reduces mutant hutingtin aggregation in an in vitro model of Huntington's disease. *Biochem Biophys Res Commun.* 2017;488(2):316–321.

58. Sinha M, Ghose J, Bhattarcharyya NP. Micro RNA -214,-150,-146a and-125b target Huntingtin gene. *RNA Biol.* 2011;8(6):1005–1021.

59. Gaughwin PM, Ciesla M, Lahiri N, Tabrizi SJ, Brundin P, Bjorkqvist M. Hsa-miR-34b is a plasma-stable microRNA that is elevated in pre-manifest Huntington's disease. *Hum Mol Genet.* 2011;20(11):2225–2237.

60. Diez-Planelles C, Sanchez-Lozano P, Crespo MC, et al. Circulating microRNAs in Huntington's disease: Emerging mediators in metabolic impairment. *Pharmacol Res.* 2016;108:102–110.

61. Yanai A, Huang K, Kang R, et al. Palmitoylation of huntingtin by HIP14 is essential for its trafficking and function. *Nat Neurosci.* 2006;9(6):824–831.

62. Young FB, Butland SL, Sanders SS, Sutton LM, Hayden MR. Putting proteins in their place: Palmitoylation in Huntington disease and other neuropsychiatric diseases. *Prog Neurobiol.* 2012;97(2):220–238.

63. Sutton LM, Sanders SS, Butland SL, et al. Hip14l-deficient mice develop neuropathological and behavioural features of Huntington disease. *Hum Mol Genet.* 2013;22(3):452–465.

64. Browne SE, Beal MF. Oxidative damage in Huntington's disease pathogenesis. *Antioxid Redox Signal.* 2006;8(11–12):2061–2073.

65. Klepac N, Relja M, Klepac R, Hecimovic S, Babic T, Trkulja V. Oxidative stress parameters in plasma of Huntington's disease patients, asymptomatic Huntington's disease gene carriers and healthy subjects: A cross-sectional study. *J Neurol.* 2007;254(12):1676–1683.

66. Hickey MA, Kosmalska A, Enayati J, et al. Extensive early motor and non-motor behavioral deficits are followed by striatal neuronal loss in knock-in Huntington's disease mice. *Neuroscience.* 2008;157(1):280–295.

67. Duran R, Barrero FJ, Morales B, Luna JD, Ramirez M, Vives F. Oxidative stress and plasma aminopeptidase activity in Huntington's disease. *J Neural Transm.* 2010;117(3):325–332.

68. Chen CM, Wu YR, Cheng ML, et al. Increased oxidative damage and mitochondrial abnormalities in the peripheral blood of Huntington's disease patients. *Biochem Biophys Res Commun.* 2007;359(2):335–340.

69. Browne SE, Bowling AC, MacGarvey U, et al. Oxidative damage and metabolic dysfunction in Huntington's disease: Selective vulnerability of the basal ganglia. *Ann Neurol.* 1997;41(5):646–653.

70. Hoffner G, Soues S, Djian P. Aggregation of expanded huntingtin in the brains of patients with Huntington disease. *Prion.* 2007;1(1):26–31.

71. Hands S, Sajjad MU, Newton MJ, Wyttenbach A. In vitro and in vivo aggregation of a fragment of huntingtin protein directly causes free radical production. *J Biol Chem.* 2011;286(52):44512–44520.

72. Sanchez Mejia RO, Friedlander RM. Caspases in Huntington's disease. *Neuroscientist.* 2001;7(6):480–489.

73. Hermel E, Gafni J, Propp SS, et al. Specific caspase interactions and amplification are involved in selective neuronal vulnerability in Huntington's disease. *Cell Death Differ.* 2004;11(4):424–438.

74. Borlongan CV, Koutouzis TK, Sanberg PR. 3-Nitropropionic acid animal model and Huntington's disease. *Neurosci Biobehav Rev.* 1997;21(3):289–293.

75. Moresco RM, Lavazza T, Belloli S, et al. Quinolinic acid induced neurodegeneration in the striatum: A combined in vivo and in vitro analysis of receptor changes and microglia activation. *Eur J Nucl Med Mol Imaging.* 2008;35(4):704–715.

76. Goswami A, Dikshit P, Mishra A, Mulherkar S, Nukina N, Jana NR. Oxidative stress promotes mutant huntingtin aggregation and mutant huntingtin-dependent cell death by mimicking proteasomal malfunction. *Biochem Biophys Res Co.* 2006;342(1):184–190.

77. Chang KH, Chen YC, Wu YR, Lee WF, Chen CM. Downregulation of genes involved in metabolism and oxidative stress in the peripheral leukocytes of Huntington's disease patients. *PLoS One.* 2012;7(9):e46492.

78. Browne SE. Mitochondria and Huntington's disease pathogenesis: Insight from genetic and chemical models. *Ann N Y Acad Sci.* 2008;1147:358–382.

79. del Hoyo P, Garcia-Redondo A, de Bustos F, et al. Oxidative stress in skin fibroblasts cultures of patients with Huntington's disease. *Neurochem Res.* 2006;31(9):1103–1109.

80. McGill JK, Beal MF. PGC-1alpha, a new therapeutic target in Huntington's disease? *Cell.* 2006;127(3):465–468.

81. Kim J, Moody JP, Edgerly CK, et al. Mitochondrial loss, dysfunction, and altered dynamics in Huntington's disease. *Hum Mol Genet.* 2010;19(20):3919–3935.

82. Damiano M, Galvan L, Deglon N, Brouillet E. Mitochondria in Huntington's disease. *Biochim Biophys Acta.* 2010;1802(1):52–61.

83. Politis M, Lahiri N, Niccolini F, et al. Increased central microglial activation associated with peripheral cytokine levels in premanifest Huntington's disease gene carriers. *Neurobiol Dis.* 2015;83:115–121.

84. Tai YF, Pavese N, Gerhard A, et al. Microglial activation in presymptomatic Huntington's disease gene carriers. *Brain.* 2007;130(Pt 7):1759–1766.

85. Bjorkqvist M, Wild EJ, Thiele J, et al. A novel pathogenic pathway of immune activation detectable before clinical onset in Huntington's disease. *J Exp Med.* 2008;205(8):1869–1877.

86. Khoshnan A, Patterson PH. The role of IkappaB kinase complex in the neurobiology of Huntington's disease. *Neurobiol Dis.* 2011;43(2):305–311.

87. Pavese N, Gerhard A, Tai YF, et al. Microglial activation correlates with severity in Huntington disease: A clinical and PET study. *Neurology.* 2006;66(11):1638–1643.

88. Politis M, Pavese N, Tai YF, et al. Microglial activation in regions related to cognitive function predicts disease onset in Huntington's disease: A multimodal imaging study. *Hum Brain Mapp.* 2011;32(2):258–270.

89. Kraft AD, Kaltenbach LS, Lo DC, Harry GJ. Activated microglia proliferate at neurites of mutant huntingtin-expressing neurons. *Neurobiol Aging.* 2012;33(3):621 e617–e633.

90. Kalonia H, Kumar P, Kumar A. Attenuation of proinflammatory cytokines and apoptotic process by verapamil and diltiazem against quinolinic acid induced Huntington like alterations in rats. *Brain Res.* 2011;1372:115–126.

91. Forrest CM, Mackay GM, Stoy N, et al. Blood levels of kynurenines, interleukin-23 and soluble human leucocyte antigen-G at different stages of Huntington's disease. *J Neurochem.* 2010;112(1):112–122.

92. Kalonia H, Kumar A. Suppressing inflammatory cascade by cyclo-oxygenase inhibitors attenuates quinolinic acid induced Huntington's disease-like alterations in rats. *Life Sci.* 2011;88(17–18):784–791.

93. Reiner A, Lafferty DC, Wang HB, Del Mar N, Deng YP. The group 2 metabotropic glutamate receptor agonist LY379268 rescues neuronal, neurochemical and motor abnormalities in R6/2 Huntington's disease mice. *Neurobiol Dis.* 2012;47(1):75–91.

94. Xifro X, Garcia-Martinez JM, Del Toro D, Alberch J, Perez-Navarro E. Calcineurin is involved in the early activation of NMDA-mediated cell death in mutant huntingtin knock-in striatal cells. *J Neurochem.* 2008;105(5):1596–1612.

95. Graham RK, Pouladi MA, Joshi P, et al. Differential susceptibility to excitotoxic stress in YAC128 mouse models of Huntington disease between initiation and progression of disease. *J Neurosci.* 2009;29(7):2193–2204.

96. Fan MM, Raymond LA. N-methyl-D-aspartate (NMDA) receptor function and excitotoxicity in Huntington's disease. *Progr Neurobiol.* 2007;81(5–6):272–293.

97. Andre VM, Cepeda C, Levine MS. Dopamine and glutamate in Huntington's disease: A balancing act. *CNS Neurosci Ther.* 2010;16(3):163–178.

98. Rebec GV, Conroy SK, Barton SJ. Hyperactive striatal neurons in symptomatic Huntington R6/2 mice: Variations with behavioral state and repeated ascorbate treatment. *Neuroscience.* 2006;137(1):327–336.

99. Kunig G, Leenders KL, Sanchez-Pernaute R, et al. Benzodiazepine receptor binding in Huntington's disease: [11C]flumazenil uptake measured using positron emission tomography. *Ann Neurol.* 2000;47(5):644–648.

100. Rekik L, Daguin-Nerriere V, Petit JY, Brachet P. gamma-Aminobutyric acid type B receptor changes in the rat striatum and substantia nigra following intrastriatal quinolinic acid lesions. *J Neurosci Res.* 2011;89(4):524–535.

101. Cepeda C, Starling AJ, Wu N, et al. Increased GABAergic function in mouse models of Huntington's disease: Reversal by BDNF. *J Neurosci Res.* 2004;78(6):855–867.

102. Yuen EY, Wei J, Zhong P, Yan Z. Disrupted GABAAR trafficking and synaptic inhibition in a mouse model of Huntington's disease. *Neurobiol Dis.* 2012;46(2):497–502.

103. Rebec GV, Barton SJ, Marseilles AM, Collins K. Ascorbate treatment attenuates the Huntington behavioral phenotype in mice. *Neuroreport.* 2003;14(9):1263–1265.

104. Sandhir R, Sood A, Mehrotra A, Kamboj SS. N-Acetylcysteine reverses mitochondrial dysfunctions and behavioral abnormalities in 3-nitropropionic acid-induced Huntington's disease. *Neurodegener Dis.* 2012;9(3):145–157.

105. Andreassen OA, Ferrante RJ, Dedeoglu A, Beal MF. Lipoic acid improves survival in transgenic mouse models of Huntington's disease. *Neuroreport.* 2001;12(15):3371–3373.

106. Hickey MA, Zhu C, Medvedeva V, Franich NR, Levine MS, Chesselet MF. Evidence for behavioral benefits of early dietary supplementation with coenzyme Q10 in a slowly progressing mouse model of Huntington's disease. *Mol Cell Neurosci.* 2012;49(2):149–157.

107. Smith KM, Matson S, Matson WR, et al. Dose ranging and efficacy study of high-dose coenzyme Q10 formulations in Huntington's disease mice. *Biochim Biophys Acta.* 2006;1762(6):616–626.

108. Yang L, Calingasan NY, Wille EJ, et al. Combination therapy with coenzyme Q10 and creatine produces additive neuroprotective effects in models of Parkinson's and Huntington's diseases. *J Neurochem.* 2009;109(5):1427–1439.

109. Silva-Adaya D, Perez-De La Cruz V, Herrera-Mundo MN, et al. Excitotoxic damage, disrupted energy metabolism, and oxidative stress in the rat brain: Antioxidant and neuroprotective effects of L-carnitine. *J Neurochem.* 2008;105(3):677–689.

110. Vamos E, Voros K, Vecsei L, Klivenyi P. Neuroprotective effects of L-carnitine in a transgenic animal model of Huntington's disease. *Biomed Pharmacother.* 2010;64(4):282–286.

111. Kumar P, Kumar A. Effect of lycopene and epigallocatechin-3-gallate against 3-nitropropionic acid induced cognitive dysfunction and glutathione depletion in rat: A novel nitric oxide mechanism. *Food Chem Toxicol.* 2009;47(10):2522–2530.

112. Wang X, Sirianni A, Pei Z, et al. The melatonin MT1 receptor axis modulates mutant huntingtin-mediated toxicity. *J Neurosci.* 2011;31(41):14496–14507.

113. Hickey MA, Zhu C, Medvedeva V, et al. Improvement of neuropathology and transcriptional deficits in CAG 140 knock-in mice supports a beneficial effect of dietary curcumin in Huntington's disease. *Mol Neurodegener.* 2012;7:12.

114. Kumar P, Padi SS, Naidu PS, Kumar A. Effect of resveratrol on 3-nitropropionic acid-induced biochemical and behavioural changes: Possible neuroprotective mechanisms. *Behav Pharmacol.* 2006;17(5–6):485–492.

115. Maher P, Dargusch R, Bodai L, Gerard PE, Purcell JM, Marsh JL. ERK activation by the polyphenols fisetin and resveratrol provides neuroprotection in multiple models of Huntington's disease. *Hum Mol Genet.* 2011;20(2):261–270.

116. Mahdy HM, Tadros MG, Mohamed MR, Karim AM, Khalifa AE. The effect of ginkgo biloba extract on 3-nitropropionic acid-induced neurotoxicity in rats. *Neurochem Int.* 2011;59(6):770–778.

117. Tasset I, Pontes AJ, Hinojosa AJ, de la Torre R, Tunez I. Olive oil reduces oxidative damage in a 3-nitropropionic acid-induced Huntington's disease-like rat model. *Nutr Neurosci.* 2011;14(3):106–111.

118. Colle D, Hartwig JM, Soares FA, Farina M. Probucol modulates oxidative stress and excitotoxicity in Huntington's disease models in vitro. *Brain Res Bull.* 2012;87(4–5):397–405.

119. Hathorn T, Snyder-Keller A, Messer A. Nicotinamide improves motor deficits and upregulates PGC-1alpha and BDNF gene expression in a mouse model of Huntington's disease. *Neurobiol Dis.* 2011;41(1):43–50.

120. Sorolla MA, Rodriguez-Colman MJ, Tamarit J, et al. Protein oxidation in Huntington disease affects energy production and vitamin B6 metabolism. *Free Radic Biol Med.* 2010;49(4):612–621.

121. Isaac MG, Quinn R, Tabet N. Vitamin E for Alzheimer's disease and mild cognitive impairment. *Cochrane Database Syst Rev.* 2008(3):CD002854.

122. Farina N, Isaac MG, Clark AR, Rusted J, Tabet N. Vitamin E for Alzheimer's dementia and mild cognitive impairment. *Cochrane Database Syst Rev.* 2012;11:CD002854.

123. Hamaguchi T, Ono K, Yamada M. REVIEW: Curcumin and Alzheimer's disease. *CNS Neurosci Ther.* 2010;16(5):285–297.

124. Hager K, Kenklies M, McAfoose J, Engel J, Munch G. Alpha-lipoic acid as a new treatment option for Alzheimer's disease—A 48-month follow-up analysis. *J Neural Transm Suppl.* 2007(72):189–193.

125. Dysken MW, Sano M, Asthana S, et al. Effect of vitamin E and memantine on functional decline in Alzheimer disease: The TEAM-AD VA cooperative randomized trial. *JAMA.* 2014;311(1):33–44.

126. Fiala M, Terrando N, Dalli J. Specialized pro-resolving mediators from omega-3 fatty acids improve amyloid-beta phagocytosis and regulate inflammation in patients with minor cognitive impairment. *J Alzheimers Dis.* 2015;48(2):293–301.

127. Chiu CC, Su KP, Cheng TC, et al. The effects of omega-3 fatty acids monotherapy in Alzheimer's disease and mild cognitive impairment: A preliminary randomized double-blind placebo-controlled study. *Prog Neuropsychopharmacol Biol Psychiatry.* 2008;32(6):1538–1544.

128. Shults CW, Oakes D, Kieburtz K, et al. Effects of coenzyme Q10 in early Parkinson disease: Evidence of slowing of the functional decline. *Arch Neurol.* 2002;59(10):1541–1550.

129. Vile GF, Winterbourn CC. Inhibition of adriamycin-promoted microsomal lipid peroxidation by beta-carotene, alpha-tocopherol and retinol at high and low oxygen partial pressures. *FEBS Lett.* 1988;238(2):353–356.

130. Niki E. Interaction of ascorbate and alpha-tocopherol. *Ann N Y Acad Sci.* 1987;498:186–199.

131. Prasad KN. Oxidative stress and proinflammatory cytokines may act as one of signals for regulating microRNAs expression in Alzheimer's disease. *Mech Ageing Dev.* 2017;162:63–71.

132. Wu H, Kong L, Tan Y, et al. C66 ameliorates diabetic nephropathy in mice by both upregulating NRF2 function via increase in miR-200a and inhibiting miR-21. *Diabetologia.* 2016;59:1558–1568.

133. Prasad KN. Simultaneous activation of Nrf2 and elevation of antioxidant compounds for reducing oxidative stress and chronic inflammation in human Alzheimer's disease. *Mech Ageing Dev.* 2016;153:41–47.

134. Itoh K, Chiba T, Takahashi S, et al. An Nrf2/small maf heterodimer mediates the induction of phase II detoxifying enzyme genes through antioxidant response elements. *Biochem Biophys Res Commun.* 1997;236(2):313–322.

135. Williamson TP, Johnson DA, Johnson JA. Activation of the Nrf2-ARE pathway by siRNA knockdown of Keap1 reduces oxidative stress and provides partial protection from MPTP-mediated neurotoxicity. *Neurotoxicology.* 2012;33(3):272–279.

136. Jaramillo MC, Zhang DD. The emerging role of the Nrf2-Keap1 signaling pathway in cancer. *Genes Dev.* 2013;27(20):2179–2191.

137. Li W, Khor TO, Xu C, et al. Activation of Nrf2-antioxidant signaling attenuates NFkappaB-inflammatory response and elicits apoptosis. *Biochem Pharmacol.* 2008;76(11):1485–1489.

138. Kim J, Cha YN, Surh YJ. A protective role of nuclear factor-erythroid 2-related factor-2 (Nrf2) in inflammatory disorders. *Mutat Res.* 2010;690(1–2):12–23.

139. Suh JH, Shenvi SV, Dixon BM, et al. Decline in transcriptional activity of Nrf2 causes age-related loss of glutathione synthesis, which is reversible with lipoic acid. *Proc Natl Acad Sci USA.* 2004;101(10):3381–3386.

140. Mostafavi-Pour Z, Ramezani F, Keshavarzi F, Samadi N. The role of quercetin and vitamin C in Nrf2-dependent oxidative stress production in breast cancer cells. *Oncol Lett.* 2017;13(3):1965–1973.

141. Katsuyama Y, Tsuboi T, Taira N, Yoshioka M, Masaki H. 3-O-Laurylglyceryl ascorbate activates the intracellular antioxidant system through the contribution of PPAR-gamma and Nrf2. *J Dermatol Sci.* 2016;82(3):189–196.

142. Xi YD, Yu HL, Ding J, et al. Flavonoids protect cerebrovascular endothelial cells through Nrf2 and PI3K from beta-amyloid peptide-induced oxidative damage. *Curr Neurovasc Res.* 2012;9(1):32–41.

143. Choi HK, Pokharel YR, Lim SC, et al. Inhibition of liver fibrosis by solubilized coenzyme Q10: Role of Nrf2 activation in inhibiting transforming growth factor-beta1 expression. *Toxicol Appl Pharmacol.* 2009;240(3):377–384.

144. Ji L, Liu R, Zhang XD, et al. N-acetylcysteine attenuates phosgene-induced acute lung injury via upregulation of Nrf2 expression. *Inhal Toxicol.* 2010;22(7):535–542.

145. Gao L, Wang J, Sekhar KR, et al. Novel n-3 fatty acid oxidation products activate Nrf2 by destabilizing the association between Keap1 and Cullin3. *J Biol Chem.* 2007;282(4):2529–2537.

146. Saw CL, Yang AY, Guo Y, Kong AN. Astaxanthin and omega-3 fatty acids individually and in combination protect against oxidative stress via the Nrf2-ARE pathway. *Food Chem Toxicol.* 2013;62:869–875.

147. Trujillo J, Chirino YI, Molina-Jijon E, Anderica-Romero AC, Tapia E, Pedraza-Chaverri J. Renoprotective effect of the antioxidant curcumin: Recent findings. *Redox Biol.* 2013;1(1):448–456.

148. Steele ML, Fuller S, Patel M, Kersaitis C, Ooi L, Munch G. Effect of Nrf2 activators on release of glutathione, cysteinylglycine and homocysteine by human U373 astroglial cells. *Redox Biol.* 2013;1(1):441–445.

149. Kode A, Rajendrasozhan S, Caito S, Yang SR, Megson IL, Rahman I. Resveratrol induces glutathione synthesis by activation of Nrf2 and protects against cigarette smoke-mediated oxidative stress in human lung epithelial cells. *Am J Physiol Lung Cell Mol Physiol.* 2008;294(3):L478–L488.

150. Zambrano S, Blanca AJ, Ruiz-Armenta MV, et al. The renoprotective effect of L-carnitine in hypertensive rats is mediated by modulation of oxidative stress-related gene expression. *Eur J Nutr.* 2013;52(6):1649–1659.

151. Eades G, Yang M, Yao Y, Zhang Y, Zhou Q. miR-200a regulates Nrf2 activation by targeting Keap1 mRNA in breast cancer cells. *J Biol Chem.* 25 2011;286(47):40725–40733.

152. Narasimhan M, Riar AK, Rathinam ML, Vedpathak D, Henderson G, Mahimainathan L. Hydrogen peroxide responsive miR153 targets Nrf2/ARE cytoprotection in paraquat induced dopaminergic neurotoxicity. *Toxicol Lett.* 2014;228(3):179–191.

153. Jin YN, Yu YV, Gundemir S, et al. Impaired mitochondrial dynamics and Nrf2 signaling contribute to compromised responses to oxidative stress in striatal cells expressing full-length mutant huntingtin. *PLoS One.* 2013;8(3):e57932.

154. Ellrichmann G, Petrasch-Parwez E, Lee DH, et al. Efficacy of fumaric acid esters in the R6/2 and YAC128 models of Huntington's disease. *PLoS One.* 2011;6(1):e16172.

155. Calkins MJ, Jakel RJ, Johnson DA, Chan K, Kan YW, Johnson JA. Protection from mitochondrial complex II inhibition in vitro and in vivo by Nrf2-mediated transcription. *Proc Natl Acad Sci USA.* 2005;102(1):244–249.

156. Bahramisharif A, van Gerven MA, Aarnoutse EJ, et al. Propagating neocortical gamma bursts are coordinated by traveling alpha waves. *J Neurosci.* 2013;33(48):18849–18854.

157. Abate A, Yang G, Dennery PA, Oberle S, Schroder H. Synergistic inhibition of cyclooxygenase-2 expression by vitamin E and aspirin. *Free Radic Biol Med.* 2000;29(11):1135–1142.

158. Fu Y, Zheng S, Lin J, Ryerse J, Chen A. Curcumin protects the rat liver from CCl4-caused injury and fibrogenesis by attenuating oxidative stress and suppressing inflammation. *Mol Pharmacol.* 2008;73(2):399–409.

159. Lee HS, Jung KK, Cho JY, et al. Neuroprotective effect of curcumin is mainly mediated by blockade of microglial cell activation. *Pharmazie.* 2007;62(12):937–942.

160. Rahman S, Bhatia K, Khan AQ, et al. Topically applied vitamin E prevents massive cutaneous inflammatory and oxidative stress responses induced by double application of 12-O-tetradecanoylphorbol-13-acetate (TPA) in mice. *Chem Biol Interact.* 2008;172(3):195–205.

161. Suzuki YJ, Aggarwal BB, Packer L. Alpha-lipoic acid is a potent inhibitor of NF-kappa B activation in human T cells. *Biochem Biophys Res Commun.* 1992;189(3):1709–1715.

162. Zhu J, Yong W, Wu X, et al. Anti-inflammatory effect of resveratrol on TNF-alpha-induced MCP-1 expression in adipocytes. *Biochem Biophys Res Commun.* 2008;369(2):471–477.

163. Barger SW, Goodwin ME, Porter MM, Beggs ML. Glutamate release from activated microglia requires the oxidative burst and lipid peroxidation. *J Neurochem.* 2007;101(5):1205–1213.

164. Dohare P, Hyzinski-Garcia MC, Vipani A, et al. The neuroprotective properties of the superoxide dismutase mimetic tempol correlate with its ability to reduce pathological glutamate release in a rodent model of stroke. *Free Radic Biol Med.* 2014;77:168–182.

165. Lu CW, Lin TY, Wang SJ. Quercetin inhibits depolarization-evoked glutamate release in nerve terminals from rat cerebral cortex. *Neurotoxicology.* 2013;39:1–9.

166. Hurtado O, De Cristobal J, Sanchez V, et al. Inhibition of glutamate release by delaying ATP fall accounts for neuroprotective effects of antioxidants in experimental stroke. *FASEB J.* 2003;17(14):2082–2084.

167. Santos PS, Campelo LM, Freitas RL, Feitosa CM, Saldanha GB, Freitas RM. Lipoic acid effects on glutamate and taurine concentrations in rat hippocampus after pilocarpine-induced seizures. *Arquivos de neuro-psiquiatria.* 2011;69(2B):360–364.

168. Chang Y, Huang SK, Wang SJ. Coenzyme Q10 inhibits the release of glutamate in rat cerebrocortical nerve terminals by suppression of voltage-dependent calcium influx and mitogen-activated protein kinase signaling pathway. *J Agric Food Chem.* 2012;60(48):11909–11918.

169. Yang TT, Wang SJ. Pyridoxine inhibits depolarization-evoked glutamate release in nerve terminals from rat cerebral cortex: A possible neuroprotective mechanism? *J Pharmacol Exp Ther.* 2009;331(1):244–254.

170. Hung KL, Wang CC, Huang CY, Wang SJ. Cyanocobalamin, vitamin B12, depresses glutamate release through inhibition of voltage-dependent Ca2+ influx in rat cerebrocortical nerve terminals (synaptosomes). *Eur J Pharmacol.* 2009;602(2–3):230–237.

171. Wang SJ, Wu WM, Yang FL, Hsu GS, Huang CY. Vitamin B2 inhibits glutamate release from rat cerebrocortical nerve terminals. *Neuroreport.* 2008;19(13):1335–1338.

172. Behl C, Davis J, Cole GM, Schubert D. Vitamin E protects nerve cells from amyloid beta protein toxicity. *Biochem Biophys Res Commun.* 1992;186(2):944–950.

173. Sandhu JK, Pandey S, Ribecco-Lutkiewicz M, et al. Molecular mechanisms of glutamate neurotoxicity in mixed cultures of NT2-derived neurons and astrocytes: Protective effects of coenzyme Q10. *J Neurosci Res.* 2003;72(6):691–703.

174. Brusa L, Orlacchio A, Moschella V, Iani C, Bernardi G, Mercuri NB. Treatment of the symptoms of Huntington's disease: Preliminary results comparing aripiprazole and tetrabenazine. *Mov Disord.* 2009;24(1):126–129.

175. de Yebenes JG, Landwehrmeyer B, Squitieri F, et al. Pridopidine for the treatment of motor function in patients with Huntington's disease (MermaiHD): A phase 3, randomised, double-blind, placebo-controlled trial. *Lancet Neurol.* 2011;10(12):1049–1057.

176. Huntington Study Group HART Investigators. A randomized, double-blind, placebo-controlled trial of pridopidine in Huntington disease. *Mov Disord.* 2013;28(10):1407–1415.

18 Micronutrients in Protecting Against Late Adverse Health-Effects of Diagnostic Radiation Doses

INTRODUCTION

Humans have been exposed to low doses of ionizing radiation from the background since their existence on planet Earth. In addition, humans are exposed to medical radiation exposures for the diagnostic and treatment of certain human diseases. Radiation workers are also exposed to radiation doses higher than non-radiation workers. These workers include those who are responsible for conducting diagnostic radiation procedures and those who are working with the nuclear industries. The crews of commercial flight also receive doses higher than those who do not fly. Frequent flyers are also exposed to radiation doses higher than those who fly infrequently.

It is established that ionizing radiation is a potent mutagen and carcinogen that can induce somatic and heritable mutations and neoplastic and certain nonneoplastic diseases; however, it is also used in the diagnosis and treatment of certain human diseases. Children are more sensitive to ionizing radiation on all criteria of damage, including cancer, than adults. Also, the time interval between radiation exposure and death in children is longer than in adults, which would allow increased risk of expression of deleterious effects in children more than in adults.[1,2]

Growing use of X-ray-based devices in the early diagnosis of human diseases has raised concerns about potential hazards of such procedures in increasing the risk of neoplastic and nonneoplastic diseases and somatic and heritable mutations in individuals receiving diagnostic doses of radiation. These risks also exist in radiation workers who are exposed to higher doses of ionizing radiation per year than non-radiation workers. The number of radiation workers has increased proportionally with increased diagnostic radiation procedures.

Efforts to develop protection against radiation damage began soon after the discovery of X-rays in 1895 by Dr. Roentgen, a German scientist. In 1927, Dr. Muller of Columbia University, USA, reported that X-ray caused gene mutations in *Drosophila melanogaster* (common fruit fly) and provided new impetus to develop effective physical and biological protection strategies against radiation damage. The initial physical concept of radiation protection involved three principles that can reduce dose levels: (1) lead shielding of unexposed areas, especially radiosensitive organs such as bone marrow, intestine, gonads, and thyroid, if possible; (2) increased distance between the radiation source and radiation workers or patients; and (3) reduction of radiation exposure time. Each of these physical principles has been very useful in reducing dose levels during diagnostic procedures, but they have limitations. For example, during fluoroscopy, it may not be possible to protect the gastrointestinal tract (one of the most radiosensitive organs) against radiation damage by lead shielding alone. Increasing the distance between the radiation source and individuals to be exposed may not be practical for many radiation workers, patients, civilian, or military personnel. Reducing radiation exposure time may also not be pertinent to all populations, except those that are involved in taking care of patients who have received gamma-emitting radioisotopes for medical purposes or who are responsible for radioactive decontamination as a result of nuclear accidents or attack.

To address the growing concerns of radiation-induced damage, the concept of ALARA (as low as reasonably achievable) with respect to dose was recommended by national and international radiation protection agencies for radiation workers and individuals receiving diagnostic doses of radiation.[3] At present, all radiologists and radiobiologists follow the principles of ALARA in order to reduce radiation doses to patients. Additional recommendations are being made to reduce the number of diagnostic procedures in patients, whenever possible in order to reduce the doses as much as possible.[4–6] These recommendations represent physical principles of radiation protection, and they have been very useful in reducing the diagnostic radiation doses to patients.

The search for nontoxic radioprotective agents, which can protect normal tissue against radiation damage began soon after World War II. In order to develop an effective biological radiation protection strategy, it is important to identify early cellular defects that initiate and promote damage following irradiation with diagnostic doses of radiation. It is now established that increased oxidative stress and chronic inflammation represent early events that are involved in the pathogenesis of low doses of radiation. Therefore, attenuation these two cellular defects may prevent radiation-induced late adverse effects of radiation. Extensive radiobiological studies identified numerous radioprotective agents. Unfortunately, most of them were toxic to humans; however, a few reviews have identified commonly used dietary and endogenous antioxidants that are nontoxic to humans and exhibit radioprotective properties.[7,8]

This chapter describes sources of low doses including background, diagnostic radiation procedures, radiation workers, and fight crews, and potential health risks of exposure to low doses of radiation. It discusses interaction of radiation with chemical, biological carcinogens, and tumor promoters, and describes radiation-induced neoplasm and nonneoplastic diseases. It presents current recommendations for radiation protection and proposes a novel concept of biological protection against low doses of radiation referred to as PAMARA (protection as much as reasonably achievable) that would complement the existing physical radiation protection concept of ALARA that refers to dose reduction.

SOURCES OF BACKGROUND RADIATION

The primary sources of background radiation are cosmic radiation, cosmogenic radionuclides, terrestrial radiation, and man made radiation (summarized from the fact of USNRC 1994). The level of cosmic radiation varies depending upon primarily on the altitude. For example, dose rate per year at sea level is 31 mrem (310 uSv); at 5,000 feet, it is 55 mrem (550 uSv); at 30,000 feet (normal jet liner), it is 1900 mrem; and at 80,000 (spy plane), it is 12,200 mrem.

Cosmic radionuclides arise primarily from the collision of highly energetic cosmic ray particles with atmospheric gases. The most important radionuclide produced is ^{14}C, but others, such as ^{3}H, ^{22}Na, and ^{7}Be are also produced. The ^{14}C in the atmosphere is rapidly oxidized to form $^{14}CO_2$, the majority of which is absorbed by the ocean. These radioactive isotopes are also released during nuclear testing. Nuclear reactors also generate ^{14}C that can leak out in case of an accident.

Several radioactive isotopes of varying physical half-lives are found on the earth. They include radioactive potassium (^{40}K, with a half-life of 1.28 billion years, emits both beta-and gamma-radiation) and radioactive rubidium (^{87}Rb with a half-life of 4.7 billion years, emits only beta-emitter), and alpha-radiation emitters naturally occurring isotopes ^{238}U with a half-life of 4.7 billion years, ^{235}U with a physical half-life of about 700 million years, and ^{232}Th with a half-life of 14.05 billion years.

Man made sources that contribute to the background radiation include weapon testing and use, nuclear reactors, and accidents in nuclear power plants. Many short-lived and long-lived radioisotopes are released into the atmosphere when nuclear testing is done or when a nuclear power plant accident occurs. They include primarily ^{131}I with a physical half-life of about 8 days, ^{137}Cs with a physical half-life of 30 years, and ^{90}Sr with a physical half-life of 28.1 years.

TABLE 18.1

Percentage Contribution of Radiation Dose to the Background Radiation from Various Sources

Radiation Sources	Percentage Contribution
Natural	
Radon and thorn	37
Cosmic (space)	5
Terrestrial (soil)	3
Internal	5
Total	50
Manmade	
Medical procedures	36
Consumer products	2
Nuclear medicine	12
Industrial and occupational	0.1
Total	50.1

Source: NCRP Report No. 160/2009, www.NCRPpublications.org.

The USNRC has estimated the total annual average background dose from natural sources is about 3.1 mSv. Radon and thoron gases contribute about 2.3rd of this exposure. Man made radiation sources that include medical, commercial, and industrial activities contribute about 3.1 mSv to annual exposure to the US population. Thus, total average annual whole-body dose to the US population may be 6.20 mSv. The percent contribution of radiation dose to the background radiation from the various sources is presented in Table 18.1.

The fact sheet of the Office of Radiation Protection of the Washington State Department of health suggests that the tobacco smoking can add additional about 2.8 mSv. The tobacco in cigarettes contains radioactive lead-210 (^{210}Pb), a beta-radiation producing isotope, which precipitates out of the atmosphere and deposits on the leaves of tobacco. This radioactive isotope decays to radioactive polonium-210 (^{210}PO), which is an alpha-emitter. The tobacco smokers receive radiation doses from ^{210}Pb that deposits on the surface of bones, and ^{210}PO that deposits in the liver, kidney, and spleen. The background radiation levels can vary depending upon the altitudes and soil rich in naturally occurring radioactive isotopes, such as 235U. About 140,000 people of the Indian states of Kerala and Chennai are exposed to background radiation of about 30 mSv per year, out of which 15 mSv is contributed by radon gas.

DOSE-ESTIMATE OF DIAGNOSTIC RADIATION PROCEDURES AND PER CAPITA DOSE

In 2006, approximately 395 million diagnostic procedures were performed with a per capita dose of 3.01 mSv (Table 18.2). The annual per capita dose from medical procedures has increased from 0.5 mSv in 1980 to 3.01 in 2006, a rise of 6-fold. Because of the potential health hazards of low doses of radiation, developing an effective radioprotective strategy that involves both physical and biological protection methods against potential damage from low doses of radiation has become an urgent issue for the present and future generations. Dose estimate from other diagnostic procedures are presented in Tables 18.3 and 18.4.

TABLE 18.2

Estimated Number of Diagnostic Radiation Procedures and per Capita Dose in 2006

Type of Procedures	Total Number of Procedures in Million	% of Total	Dose (mSv)
Diagnostic radiography and fluoroscopy	293	74	0.33
Interventional procedures	14	4	0.43
CT Scanning	67	17	1.47
Nuclear medicine studies	18	5	0.77
Total	395	100	3.01

Source: Mettler, F.A. Jr. et al., *Radiology*, 253, 520–531, 2009.

Note: Radiography includes X-ray-based procedures including mammograms.
        CT (computed tomography).

TABLE 18.3

Estimated Doses of Ionizing Radiation Delivered During Specific Diagnostic Procedures

Procedure Type	Effective Dose (mSv)
Chest or dental X-ray	0.01
Electron-beam CT (cardiac)	1.0–1.3
Electron-beam CT coronary angiography	1.5–2.0
Catheter coronary angiography	2.1–2.5
Electron-beam CT whole body	5.2
CT (head)	2.0
CT (abdomen)	10.0
Barium enema	7.0
Upper GI exam	3.0
IV Urogram	2.5
Lumbar spine	1.3
Mammogram	7.0
Passenger from Athens to New York	0.06
Occupational annual dose limit	50.0
General public annual dose limit	1.0
Background annual dose at sea level	1.0

Source: Prasad, K.N., *Br. J. Radiol.*, 78, 485–492, 2005.

Note: Occupational and general public dose limit does not include background radiation.

TABLE 18.4

Estimated Doses of Radiation from Selected Radioactive Nuclides Administered Once During Nuclear Medicine Procedures

Procedure Type	Effective Dose (mSv)
18F-Flurodeoxyglucose, 10 mCi	4.8
99mTc-MAA lung scan, 5 mCi	0.60
99mTc-HDP bone scan, 20 mCi	4.0
201Tl Thallium scan, 3 mCi	0.60

Source: Prasad, K.N., *Br. J. Radiol.*, 78, 485–492, 2005.

ESTIMATED DOSE RECEIVED BY RADIATION WORKERS

The effective dose and equivalent dose to radiation workers markedly differ from one procedure to another and from one country to another. In the USA, during a transcatheter aortic calve implantation, radiation workers received a significant higher effective dose (about 0.03 mSv) than other members who were not involved in this procedure.[9] In another study, the effective doses ranged from 0.02–38.0 uSV for diagnostic catheterizations, 0.17–31.2 uSv for percutaneous coronary interventions, 0.24–9.6 uSv for ablations, and 0.29–17.4 uSv for pacemaker or intracardiac defibrillator implantations.[10] In Netherlands, the effective dose for neurointerventional procedures was about 6.7 uSv.[11] In Poland, an effective dose for a cardiological angioplastic procedure was 2.5 mSv, whereas the effective dose to radiation workers from intravascular angioplastic procedures within the abdominal cavity and neuroradiological procedures was 4 mSv.[12] In Nigeria, the average annual dose to radiation workers increased from about 3.6 mSv in 1999 to about 7.7 mSv in 2001.[13]

ESTIMATED DOSE RECEIVED BY CREWS OF COMMERCIAL FLIGHT

The amount of radiation dose received by the commercial air crews differs depending upon the route of travel. The radiation dose rate during a fight from Paris to Buenos Aires is 0.3 mrem/h. Based on 700 hours flight time per year on a commercial airline, the air crews may receive a total annual effective dose of 210 mrem (2.10 mSv). This is below than 20 mSv recommended by the ICRP and FAA. Military and civilian pilots and flight attendants are exposed to increased levels of cosmic ionizing radiation of galactic and solar origin, and secondary radiation produced in the atmosphere, the aircraft structure and its contents, potential chemical carcinogens (fuel, jet engine exhausts, and cabin air pollutants), electromagnetic fields from cockpit instruments, and disrupted sleep pattern. In May 2000, the European Union (EU) adopted regulations that apply to the air carriers in all twenty seven nations requiring education on health risks of inflight radiation. In addition, assessment of radiation dose for all EU flight crewmembers required. International Commission on Radiation Protection (ICRP) has classified aircrews as radiation workers. Depending upon the flight patterns and altitudes, the annual dose range may vary from 0.2 to 5 mSv.[14] The average annual radiation dose equivalent of occupationally exposed adults in the USA is estimated to be about 1.1 mSv. Another study has reported that the average dose rate 4–5 microSv/h for long-haul pilots and 1–3 microSv/h for short-haul pilots, yielding an annual effective dose of 2–3 mSv for long-haul pilots and 1–2 mSv for short-haul pilots.[15] Another study reported that the average annual dose received varies from 3–6 mSv.[16]

HEALTH EFFECTS OF LOW DOSES OF RADIATION

EFFECTS OF BACKGROUND RADIATION ON HUMAN HEALTH

Doses from the background radiation have been presumed to be safe for human health, because humans have adapted to these doses and survived. Antioxidant defense system that can quench radiation-induced free radicals has helped them to adapt to background radiation successfully. Any dose of radiation can induce somatic and heritable mutations that can increases the risk of chronic diseases. Mutations that are caused by direct ionization may not be protected by antioxidant defense system; therefore, they can persist from one generation to another. It should be pointed out that radiation interacts with other mutagens present in the environment, diet, and lifestyle in a synergistic manner to enhance the risk of chronic diseases. Human suffer from varieties of chronic diseases. It is not possible to separate the contribution of background radiation alone to human diseases. Bases on the fact that radiation is a mutagenic and carcinogenic agent, background radiation must contribute to some extent to the risk of chronic diseases. Continuous exposure to background radiation of (3 rem or 0.03 Sv) per generation of 30 years would increase mutations by only about 1%–6% of the spontaneous mutation rate in humans. Because of interaction of radiation with other mutagenic substances present in the environment, diet and lifestyle; it is difficult to estimate with any accuracy the mutation rate induced by the background radiation alone. Although all mutations do not lead to cancer, but all cancer are preceded by mutations. The rate of spontaneous cancer in humans probably is the result of interaction between background radiation, and chemical and biological carcinogens, and tumor promoters present in the diet and environment.

INDUCTION OF MUTATIONS

Low doses of radiation can induce both somatic and heritable mutations. At present, the frequency of mutation in humans is based on mammalian genetics. It has been reported that the frequency of mutations in mice is dependent upon the dose rate and total dose.[17–19] The effect of dose rate on mutations in females is different from that observed in males. The mutation frequency in oocytes at a high dose rate is greater than that in spermatogonia; however, at a lower dose rate, it is much less than that in spermatogonia. The older mice are more sensitive to dose rate effect than the younger mice. The time interval between two fractionated doses is important for the production of mutations in the male mice.

INDUCTION OF RADIATION-INDUCED CANCER

Radiation-induced carcinogenesis is no different from that occur spontaneously or caused by chemical carcinogens/tumor promoters. It involves a gradual accumulation of multiple mutations over a long period of time. Radiation-induced human cancers have long latent periods; 10 years for leukemia and 30 years or more for solid tumors.[20] This implies that radiation-induced mutations (due to genetic mutations and/or chromosomal damage) that can be detected within 24 hours of radiation exposure are not directly responsible for the development of carcinogenesis in normal human cells, because such cells continue to divide and proliferate like unirradiated normal cells for a long time. However, radiation-induced mutations cause genetic instability in normal cells that can make these cells more sensitive to mutagenic changes caused by increased oxidative stress that continues to occur as a function of time. Such genetically unstable cells may continue to proliferate and differentiate like nonirradiated cells in spite of carrying genetic abnormalities for a long period of time until the expression of genes that regulate differentiation is altered. This defect in expression of differentiation genes prevents cells from going through normal pattern of differentiation and death; and thus, continues to divide. These cells are referred to as immortal cells, and they represent the first step in carcinogenesis. Immortalized cells can continue to proliferate and can form adenomas such as polyps in the colon or cysts in the breast. When some key cellular genes, oncogenes or antioncogenes, are altered by continued exposure to increased oxidative stress caused by mutagens, carcinogens, and/or tumor promoters, these cells then become fully transformed and can induce cancer when tested in the appropriate host.[21,22] The existence of a long-latent period for radiation-induced cancer provides an opportunity to intervene at any time after radiation exposure with appropriate radioprotective agents in order to reduce the risk of late adverse effects of radiation.

IMPACT OF CHEMICAL AND BIOLOGICAL CARCINOGENS, AND TUMOR PROMOTERS ON RADIATION-INDUCED CANCER

In addition to low doses of ionizing radiation from background radiation, diagnostic radiation procedures, frequent flying at the high altitudes, and working with radiation equipment, humans are also exposed to chemical and biological carcinogens and tumor promoters that can enhance the effect of low doses of radiation on neoplastic and non-plastic diseases. This has been demonstrated by the laboratory experiments primarily using high dose but nonlethal dose of radiation on the cell culture models. For example, X-radiation-induced transformation was enhanced by about 9-fold[23] by chemical carcinogens in normal mammalian cells. The incidence of transformation by X-irradiation was enhanced 12 fold by UV light.[24] X-irradiation also enhanced the level of ozone[25,26] and viral-induced[27] transformation in cell culture. Radiation doses that alone do not transform normal fibroblasts, but they do so when combined with a tumor promoter.[28] Ionizing radiation in combination with tobacco smoking increases the risk of lung cancer by about 50%. A low dose of radiation (20 mSv) does not produce detectable levels of mutations as measured by chromosomal damage; however, in the presence of caffeine (which inhibits repair of DNA damage), mutations become detectable.[28] The issue of interaction of radiation with other carcinogens and tumor promoters is often ignored when discussing the risk of radiation-induced cancer in children or adults.

Low doses of radiation (20 and 50 mSv) can act as a mitogen,[29] and lower doses (about 1 mSv) do not activate double-strand DNA break repair mechanisms.[30] This lack of repair after exposure to low doses of radiation can lead to accumulation of mutations that can increase the risk of cancer.

MODELS USED FOR RISK ESTIMATES OF RADIATION-INDUCED CANCER

Two models of risk estimate for radiation-induced cancer have been proposed. The first model proposes that cancer risk in humans following exposure to low doses of radiation (100 mSv or less) may be best estimated by a linear no-threshold relationship, since any dose has the potential to induce cancer. The most recent BEIR report supports this model.[31] This model of risk estimation for radiation-induced cancer can also be applied to children.[32] The second model suggests that there is a threshold-dose below which radiation may not induce cancer in humans.[33,34] The second model has relied primarily on mathematical modeling. Mathematical modeling may assume certain constant physical factors such as body weight[34] that may not reflect the inherent biological variations associated with radiation-induced carcinogenesis. These include differences in radiosensitivity with respect to age, organs, body mass, and differences in the efficacy of repair mechanisms.

CANCER RISKS IN POPULATIONS EXPOSED TO DIAGNOSTIC RADIATION PROCEDURES

ADULTS AND CHILDREN

The health risk of low doses of radiation include increased incidence of cancer, and certain non-neoplastic diseases, such as thyroid diseases, vision disorders, and micronuclei formation in the buccal mucosa following dental X-rays. Recently, a few excellent reviews have been published in support of the model of linear no-threshold model for radiation-induced cancer.[32,35] The typical radiation doses for an adult from a chest CT scan can range between 6 and 10 mSv.[36] The average annual dose from background radiation in the USA is approximately 3.1 mSv. Several radiation dose estimates for imaging studies in adults and children have been published.[36,37] A dose of from a CT scan may increase the risk of cancer in children by 1 in 1000 exposed individuals[4,38,39]; however, another study has reported that the lifetime cancer mortality risks for a 1-year-old child exposed to radiation dose from a CT scan are 0.18% (abdominal CT scan) and 0.07% (head CT scan). This risk estimate is an order of magnitude higher than for adults. It was further estimated that in 2001, approximately 600,000 abdominal and head CT scans were performed in children under the age of 15 years, and that 500 of the exposed children might die from cancer attributed to CT scan.[40] A Canadian study reported that an abdominal CT study in a 5-year-old child may increase lifetime risk of radiation-induced cancer by approximately 26.1 per 100,000 in female and 20.4 per 100,000 in male patients.[41] Another study performed in Israel estimated an increase of about 0.29% over the total number of patients who are eventually are expected to die from cancer.[6] If one considers the fact that patients receiving diagnostic doses of radiation and radiation workers may also be exposed to chemical and biological carcinogens, as well as tumor promoters that enhance radiation-induced cancer risk during their lifetime, the above estimates of cancer mortality risk could be higher.

TABLE 18.5

Estimated Increases in Cancer Risk from an Exposure to One Computed Tomography (CT) Scan

Source and Dose of Radiation	Increase in Cancer Risk in Exposed Individuals
One CT scan	1 per 1000[4,38,39]
	1 per 1200[40]
	2.9 per 1000[6]
	0.26 per 1000 female[41]
	0.2 per 1000 male[41]
15 mSv	1 per 750[17]
20 mSv	1 per 500[17]
25 mSv	1 per 400[17]

Note: The number in superscript refers to reference number.

The analysis of the risk of cancer on the basis of the annual number of diagnostic X-rays taken in UK and 14 other developing countries revealed the cumulative risk varied from 0.6% to 1.8%, whereas in Japan, which used the highest number of annual diagnostic X-rays, it was more than 3%.[42] BEIR report VII has estimated that a dose of 15 mSv may increase cancer risk by 1/750 cases. Others have estimated that coronary multislice CT (MSCT) scan that delivers patients about 20 mSv may increase the risk of cancer by 1/500; coronary stent by 1/400 for 25 mSv.[17] The estimates of cancer risk are presented in Table 18.5.

An epidemiologic study suggested that the increased risk of thyroid cancer was associated with exposure to multiple dental X-rays.[43] This association was independent of age, gender, nationality, and level of education.

If one considers the fact that children may be exposed to chemical and biological carcinogens, as well as tumor promoters that enhance radiation-induced cancer risk, these estimates of cancer mortality risk could be higher for children. It has been estimated that the risk of for hematopoietic tumors lasts for about 12 years and largely disappears within 30 years after irradiation. On the other hand, solid tumors seldom appear before 10 years after irradiation, and they may continue to appear for 30 years or more.[44]

CANCER RISK IN CHILDREN EXPOSED IN UTERO DURING ATOMIC BOMBING OF HIROSHIMA AND NAGASAKI

The incidence of cancer among children exposed in utero who were born between the days of the atomic bombing (August 6, 1945, in Hiroshima, and August 9, 1945, in Nagasaki) and May 1, 1946 was evaluated. The incidence of cancer during 1950–1984 increased by about 2- to 3-fold, depending upon the dose.[45] The incidence of breast cancer was higher among girls exposed to atomic bombing under the age of 10 years than those who were older at the time of bombing.[46] Among those girls who received 0.5 Gy or more, 10 cases of breast cancer were observed, in comparison to expected cases of 2 among nonirradiated girls.[47]

RISK OF CHILDHOOD CANCER AFTER IRRADIATION OF FETUSES

Most of the human data are based on the analysis of radiation exposed pregnant women of Hiroshima and Nagasaki or of pregnant women who received a radiation dose during diagnostic radiation procedure or radiation therapy of cancer. The effects of high doses of irradiation on the nonneoplastic diseases have been discussed in Chapter 19. It has been reported that an increase in crude cancer risk is directly proportional to the number of X-ray films or fetus dose.[48] The cancer risk was greater when fetuses received radiation doses during the first trimester. The authors estimated that 0.01 Gy (1 cGy) delivered to the fetus shortly before birth would cause an increase of 300–800 deaths per million before the age of 10 years due to cancer (572 ± 133). This corresponds to an annual absolute risk of 57 cancer deaths per million per rad during the period of observation of 10 years. Further analysis of radiation-induced cancer in children following radiation exposure to the fetuses confirmed the hypothesis of a linear relationship between fetal dose and the relative incidence of cancer[49–54]; however, the magnitude of the effect of fetal irradiation on the incidence of cancer has been questioned.[52] It has been estimated that exposure of fetuses to low levels of radiation increased the risk of leukemia in childhood by an excess relative coefficient of around 50 per Gy (equivalent to an excess absolute risk coefficient of about 3% per Gy).[55] It has been estimated that the proportion of childhood leukemia incidence in Great Britain attributable to natural background is about 15%–20%.[56] A significant increase in malignancy has been found even after 0.25 cGy to the human fetus.[51] Maternal smoking and irradiation with diagnostic doses during pregnancy increases the risk of childhood leukemia by more than 3-folds compared to irradiation alone.[57] The incidence of leukemia was higher among children irradiated with diagnostic doses of radiation *in utero*; the incidence was still higher if the mother had previously experienced miscarriage or stillbirth.[58] It has been reported that the incidence of childhood leukemia was 5 times more if the pregnant women received diagnostic doses of radiation during the first trimester; however, if the pregnant women received diagnostic doses of radiation during the second or third trimester, the incidence of cancer was only 1.47 fold higher than those who did not receive radiation during pregnancy.[48,49,59] A high incidence of tumors among children after the administration of radioactive iron (^{59}Fe) to pregnant women was reported.[60] The estimated fetus dose was 5–15 cGy. Among 634 children exposed, one leukemia and two sarcoma cases were found. No malignancies were observed in control group.

WOMEN RECEIVING GONADAL DOSES OF RADIATION BEFORE CONCEPTION

The studies on the effects of diagnostic doses of X-rays before conception are not sufficient to make any definitive conclusion. However, a few studies suggest a potential risk of nonneoplastic diseases. For example, it has been reported that young females who received diagnostic doses of radiation (0.5–7 cGy) before conception had 10 time more aneuploidy children out of which 8 were mongoloid than those who did not receive radiation.[61] A gonadal dose of about 5 cGy to the young women before conception produced an eye defect in subsequent children.[62] A gonadal dose of 5 R (about 5 cGy), which may be received by medical radiation exposure over 30 years, would increase the number of point mutations by about 1%.[63]

The estimated minimal spontaneous frequency of point mutations per generation due to naturally occurring mutagens is about 2%. This mutation rate contributes to less than half of the gross abnormalities, such as mental defects, hematological and endocrine defects, defects in vision and hearing, cutaneous and skeletal defects, and defects in the GI tract that occur after birth. It does not include those mutations whose effects are less drastic.

CANCER RISK AMONG RADIATION WORKERS

Assessment of cancer risk among radiation workers can be estimated only by epidemiologic studies. These studies thus far have produced conflicting results on the risk of neoplastic and nonneoplastic diseases. This may due to the fact that latent period after low doses of radiation is very high. In addition, radiation workers who worked during the 1940–1980s may have received higher accumulative doses than those who are working after because of advancement of technology of diagnostic radiation equipment that have reduce exposure to radiation workers. Recently employed radiation workers are difficult to evaluate for cancer risk because of insufficient time interval between irradiation and the risk of developing cancer. A review of published epidemiologic studies involving 400,000 radiation workers suggested that an accumulated dose of 100 mGy or 100 mSv was significantly associated with an increase in leukemia risk.[64] Another study analyzed the cancer risk among 67,562 radiation workers 23,580 males and 43,982 females employed during 1951–1987 in Canada. The results showed that the thyroid cancer incidence was significantly increased both among males and females, with a combined standardized incidence ration of 1.74.[65] At present, medical radiation workers in Canada are receiving much lower doses of radiation in comparison to those who were working during 1951–1987. The risk of cancer among these radiation workers remains unknown. In an epidemiologic study involving 56,436 US female radiologic technologists who were certified from 1925 to 1980, the incident of breast cancer was evaluated. The results showed that the increased incidence of cancer among those who were working before 1940 but not after that. Improvement in radiation technology and implementation in radiation protection standards have contribution to reduction of accumulative radiation doses.[66] Another study reported increased risk of leukemia among radiologists and technologists who were employed before 1950.[67] In a 15-counry collaborative cohort study involving 407,391 nuclear industry workers, the risk of radiation-induced cancer was evaluated.[68] The results showed that among 31 specific types of cancers, only for lung cancer a significant association was observed. However, for multiple myeloma and ill-defined and secondary cancers, a borderline significant association was observed. The same group of investigators found that among 600,000 nuclear industry workers who received an average cumulative dose of about 19.2 mSv, a strong association with improved health was found in most countries.[69] The incidence of thyroid cancer was evaluated among 73,080 radiologic technologists. The increased risk of thyroid cancer was observed among those who work for more than 5 years prior to 1950. The analysis of cancer risk among the South Korean radiation workers in nuclear power plants revealed no increase in cancer risk.[70] The risk of cataract formation among interventional cardiologists and associated nurses was evaluated in 116 radiation exposed individuals and 93 nonexposed individuals. The results showed that 38% of those who received cumulative lens dose of about 6.0 mSv developed cataract compared to 12% in unexposed individuals. Only 21% of the nurses and technicians who received cumulative lens dose of 1.5 mSv developed cataract.[71] The gene expression profiles are markedly altered in the peripheral lymphocytes of radiation workers.[72] Generally, radiation workers may receive whole-body irradiation that is like to induce heritable mutations that may appear in future generations.

The above epidemiologic studies provide no conclusive evidence for increased health risks among radiation workers. It should be emphasized that not all radiation workers receive same cumulative radiation doses. For example, radiation workers involved in interventional cardiology procedures may receive much higher accumulative doses per year than those responsible for chest or dental X-ray. In addition, environmental-, dietary-, and lifestyle-related factors may influence the radiation-induced carcinogenic processes. It is impossible to account for all external variables that could impact radiation-induced cancer risk in any epidemiologic studies. In my opinion, radiation workers should consider adopting a strategy that can provide biological protection against damage, no matter how small damage that might be.

CANCER RISK IN MILITARY AND CIVILIAN PILOTS AND FLIGHT ATTENDANTS

Several epidemiologic studies have evaluated the risk of cancer in these populations. Most studies suggest that the increase risk of prostate, melanoma, and other skin cancer, and acute myeloid leukemia in male pilots,[73–76] and breast cancer, melanoma,[75,77,78] and bone cancer[79,80] in female attendants. The incidence of acute myeloid leukemia and brain cancer did not change among flight crews from Denmark, Finland, Iceland, Norway, and Sweden.[76] Most epidemiologic studies have revealed that the risk of certain types of cancer increases among flight pilots and attendants. Since they receive whole-body irradiation, the risk of heritable mutations that may appear in future generations may also increase.

CANCER RISK AMONG FREQUENT FLYERS

Frequent flyers may receive extra radiation doses while going through X-ray scanners at the airport and while within the aircraft. They may receive accumulative radiation doses less than flight crews; but the risk of adverse health effects may exist in this population similar to that in flight crews. There are no epidemiologic studies to evaluate the risk of cancer or noncancerous diseases among frequent flyers. Since no radiation doses are considered safe, it is prudent to adopt a strategy to provide biological protection against the adverse health effects of radiation.

RISK OF LOW-DOSE RADIATION-INDUCED NONNEOPLASTIC DISEASES

Developing organisms constitute a highly dynamic system in which rapid cell proliferation, cell migration, and cell differentiation occur. Therefore, it is expected that radiation response of the human embryos as a whole or specific tissue, would markedly differ depending upon the stage of development. Several animal studies suggest that radiation-induced changes are similar in different species when they are irradiated at an equivalent stage of the development.[44,81] Many studies have shown that low radiation doses are harmful to the human fetus.[48,59,82] The central nervous system and optic tissues in developing fetuses are highly radiosensitive and small doses (0.05–0.1 Gy) may cause abnormalities in these organs. The extent of damage depends upon total dose, dose rate, LET (linear energy transfer), and mode of radiation delivery (single versus fractionated dose). The type and number of abnormalities may depend upon the age of the fetus and mode of radiation delivery.

The incidence of nonneoplastic diseases and intermediate health risks measured by certain specific biochemical markers were studied in children living in radiation-contaminated areas near the Chernobyl nuclear accident site. The incidence of thyroid gland enlargement and vision disorders, mostly dry-eye syndrome, was closely related to the levels of contamination.[20] Increased levels of oxidized conjugated dienes, products of lipid peroxidation, were found among these children. In another report, increased levels of spontaneous chemiluminescence, an indicator of enhanced oxygen radical activity, in leukocytes of children living in contaminated areas were observed.[83] The accuracy of these intermediate markers for predicting health risks after radiation exposure remains uncertain. Radiation exposure during interventional cardiovascular procedures can induce damage to DNA and can cause chromosomal aberrations.[84] Complex cytogenetic abnormalities among Japanese survivors of the atomic bomb were observed 20 years after radiation exposure. The micronucleus assay in exfoliated buccal cells is considered a useful and minimally invasive assay method for monitoring genetic damage in humans.[85] Dental X-ray can induce formation of micronuclei in buccal cells in both adults and children.[84,86] The significance of this observation in predicting cancer risk remains to be established following dental X-rays remain uncertain.

REDUCING OXIDATIVE STRESS AND INFLAMMATION BY SINGLE ANTIOXIDANTS IN HUMANS

It is now well established that irradiation cause damage by free radicals and inflammation; therefore attenuation of these cellular defects may reduce late adverse effects of diagnostic radiation. The questions remain how to simultaneously reduce oxidative stress and inflammation. Using high doses of radiation, several radioprotective agents have been identified in cell culture and animal models. Only limited studies have been conducted in humans with low doses of radiation. These studies are briefly described here.

An oral supplementation with alpha-lipoic acid for 28 days lowered the levels of lipid peroxidation among children chronically exposed to low doses of radiation in the area contaminated by the Chernobyl nuclear accident.[83] In another study, beta-carotene supplementation reduced cellular damage in the above population of children.[20] A combination of vitamin E and alpha-lipoic acid was more effective than the individual agents.[83] These studies in humans are very exciting, because they demonstrate that very low doses of radiation can increase oxidative stress and induce cellular damage that can be protected by antioxidants.

REDUCING DAMAGE BY MULTIPLE ANTIOXIDANTS IN HUMANS

A study has reported that irradiation of freshly isolated lymphocytes with a dose of 10 mGy of X-rays increased the number of cells with DNA double-strand breaks (DSBs) (Figure 18.1). Treatment of cells with a mixture of multiple antioxidants (Bioshield R1, a commercial preparation) before irradiation reduced the number of cells with DSBs. A similar result was obtained when the number of cells with DSBs was determined in the lymphocytes isolated from patients who received Bio-shield-R1 before a dose of 10 mGy[87] (Figure 18.2).

PROPOSED STRATEGY TO SIMULTANEOUSLY REDUCE OXIDATIVE STRESS AND INFLAMMATION

In order to simultaneously reduce oxidative stress and inflammation, it is essential to increase the levels of antioxidant enzymes and dietary and endogenous antioxidants at the same time. The levels of antioxidants can be increased by supplementation, but increasing the levels of antioxidant enzymes requires an activation of Nrf2 (Nuclear Factor-Erythroid-2-Related Factor 2).

ACTIVATION OF Nrf2 (NUCLEAR FACTOR-ERYTHROID-2-RELATED FACTOR 2)

Nrf2

The nuclear transcriptional factor, Nrf2 (nuclear factor-erythroid-2-related factor 2) belongs to the Cap "n" Collar (CNC) family that contains a conserved basic leucine zipper (bZIP) transcriptional factor.[88] Under physiological condition, Nrf2 is associated with Kelch-like ECH associated

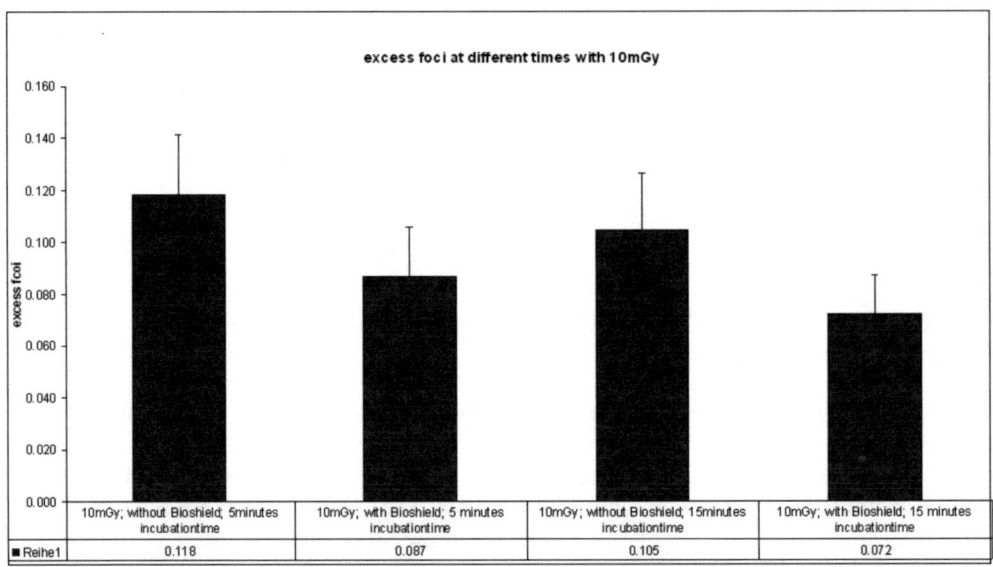

FIGURE 18.1 Freshly isolated human lymphocytes were irradiated with 10 mGy in the presence or absence of Bioshield-R1 and incubated for 5 min and 15 min. Bio-shield treatment reduced the number of cells with DNA double-strand breaks (DNA DSBs). (From Ehrlich, J.S. et al., Effect of proprietary combination of antioxidants/glutathione-elevating agents on X-ray induced DNA double-strand breaks, *Presented at the Annual Meeting of Society of Cardiovascular Computed Tomography*, 2011.)

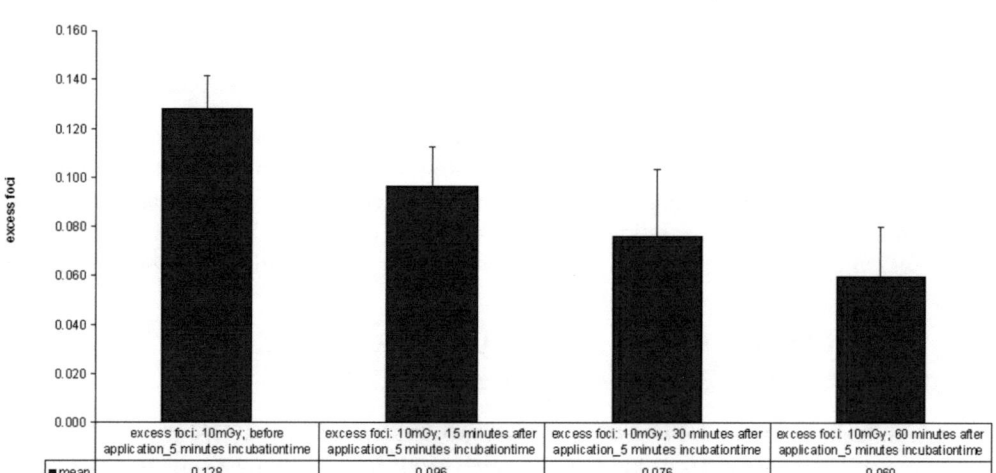

mean excess foci with different experimental setting at radiation of 10 mGy

	excess foci: 10mGy; before application_5 minutes incubationtime	excess foci: 10mGy; 15 minutes after application_5 minutes incubationtime	excess foci: 10mGy; 30 minutes after application_5 minutes incubationtime	excess foci: 10mGy; 60 minutes after application_5 minutes incubationtime
■ mean	0.128	0.096	0.076	0.060

FIGURE 18.2 Freshly isolated lymphocytes from patients who received Bio-shield-R1 before irradiation with a dose of 10 mGy. Bio-shield treatment reduced the number of cells with DNA double-stranded breaks (DNA DSBs). (From Ehrlich, J.S. et al., Effect of proprietary combination of antioxidants/glutathione-elevating agents on X-ray induced DNA double-strand breaks, *Presented at the Annual Meeting of Society of Cardiovascular Computed Tomography*, 2011.)

protein 1 (Keap1), which acts as an inhibitor of Nrf2.[89] Keap1 protein serves as an adaptor to link Nrf2 to the ubiquitin ligase CuI-Rbx1 complex for degradation by proteasomes and maintains the steady levels of Nrf2 in the cytoplasm. Nrf2-keap1 complex is primarily located in the cytoplasm; Keap1 acts as a sensor for ROS/electrophilic stress.

Activation of Nrf2 During Acute Oxidative Stress

During acute oxidative stress, ROS is needed to activate Nrf2 which then dissociates itself from Keap1-CuI-Rbx1 complex and translocates in the nucleus where it heterodimerizes with a small Maf protein, binds with ARE leading to increased expression of target genes coding for several cytoprotective enzymes including antioxidant enzymes.[90–92]

Failure to Activate Nrf2 During Chronic Oxidative Stress

During chronic oxidative stress, Nrf2 becomes resistant to ROS,[93–95] suggesting that activation of Nrf2 by a ROS-independent mechanism exists. This is evidenced by the fact that increased chronic oxidative stress occurs despite the presence of Nrf2 long after exposure to diagnostic radiation procedures. The question arises as to how to activate ROS-resistant Nrf2 in individuals who have received low doses of radiation.

Antioxidants Activate ROS-Resistant Nrf2

Some examples are vitamin E and genistein,[96] alpha-lipoic acid,[97] curcumin,[98] resveratrol,[99,100] omega-3-fatty acids,[101,102] glutathione,[103] NAC,[104] and coenzyme Q10.[105] Several plant-derived phytochemicals, such as epigallocatechin-3-gallate, carestol, kahweol, cinnamonyl-based compounds, zerumbone, lycopene and carnosol,[88,106,107] genistein,[96] allicin, a major organosulfur compound found in garlic,[108] sulforaphane, a organosulfur compound, found in cruciferous vegetables,[109] and kavalactones (methysticin, kavain, and yangonin).[110] The reasons for the activation of Nrf2 without ROS by antioxidant compounds are not known.

BINDING OF Nrf2 WITH ARE IN THE NUCLEUS

An activation of Nrf2 alone is not sufficient to increase the levels of antioxidant enzymes. Activated Nrf2 must bind with ARE in the nucleus for increasing the expression of target genes coding for antioxidant enzymes. This binding ability of Nrf2 with ARE was impaired in aged rats and this defect was restored by supplementation with alpha-lipoic acid.[97] It is unknown whether the binding ability of Nrf2 with ARE is impaired in individuals who have received diagnostic doses of radiation.

PROPOSED MICRONUTRIENTS FOR SIMULTANEOUSLY REDUCING OXIDATIVE STRESS AND INFLAMMATION

Activation of Nrf2 may not be sufficient to optimally reduce oxidative stress, because antioxidants compounds are also decreased during chronic oxidative stress[111–113]; therefore, their levels must also be simultaneously elevated. Activation of Nrf2[114,115] and some individual antioxidant compounds reduced chronic inflammation.[116–122]

A comprehensive micronutrient mixture containing multiple dietary antioxidant compounds (vitamin A, natural mixed carotenoids, vitamin C, vitamin E succinate, vitamin E acetate, mineral selenomethionine, curcumin, and resveratrol), endogenous antioxidants (alpha-lipoic acid, L-carnitine, and coenzyme Q10), a synthetic antioxidant N-acetylcysteine (NAC), omega-3-fatty acids, vitamin D3, and all B-vitamins for radiation protection is proposed. This mixture of micronutrients may optimally reduce oxidative stress and chronic inflammation by simultaneously enhancing the levels of antioxidant enzymes through activation of the Nrf2/ARE pathway, and elevating the levels of antioxidants. Daily consumption of this micronutrient mixture may reduce the risk of developing neoplastic and nonneoplastic diseases after irradiation with diagnostic doses of radiation.

Although the recommendation of ALARA can help to reduce the level of radiation dose to patients, this does not help to reduce the level of damage to those patients receiving diagnostic doses of radiation or to workers who are daily exposed to radiation doses higher than non-radiation workers. Daily consumption of proposed micronutrient mixture before and after diagnostic radiation procedures would help to extend the concept of ALARA from the dose to the biological protection.[123] This novel concept is referred to as PAMARA (protection as much as reasonably achievable), which was initially referred to as DALARA (damage as low reasonably achievable).[123,124]

CONCLUSIONS

Humans are exposed to low doses of ionizing radiation from the background, medical exposures, working in the radiation environment, and flying on commercial jets. The USNRC has estimated the total average annual whole-body dose to the US population is about 6.20 mSv (3.1 mSv from natural sources and 3.1 mSv from man made sources). The effects of these low doses on health risk are impossible to evaluate because of their interaction with other toxic agents in the environment. The rate of spontaneous cancer in humans probably is the result of these risk factors. The growing use of X-ray-based equipment in early diagnosis of human diseases has raised concerns about potential hazards of such procedures in increasing the risk of cancer, noncancerous diseases, and somatic and heritable mutations in patients and radiation workers. The developing fetuses are extremely sensitive to ionizing radiation; the types and severity of effect depend upon the dose, stage of development, and the mode of delivery of radiation (single dose, fractionation, or protraction). Exposure of fetuses at any stage of development to diagnostic doses of radiation increases the risk of childhood leukemia. The risk appears to be higher during the first trimester than during the second or third trimester. There appears to be no threshold dose for leukemia among children who received radiation in utero; however, for most organ defects, there appears to be a threshold dose. The physical radiation protection involves three principles: (a) lead shielding of the area not being exposed directly to radiation; (b) increasing distance between the radiation source and recipients; and (c) reducing the radiation exposure time. The adoption of concept of ALARA has reduced the dose levels to the patients and radiation workers. Since radiation induced damage by producing free radicals and inflammation, a mixture of micronutrients that may simultaneously decrease oxidative stress and inflammation by enhancing the levels of antioxidant enzymes through activation of the Nrf2/ARE pathway, as well as antioxidants, is proposed. This mixture of micronutrients would decrease the risk of late adverse effects of low doses of radiation. The implementation of this micronutrient strategy for biological protection PAMARA would extend the concept of ALARA from reduction in radiation doses to reduction in tissue damage.

REFERENCES

1. Prasad K. *Handbook of Radiobiology*, Second Edition. Boca Rotan, FL: CRC Press; 1995.
2. Kleinerman RA. Cancer risks following diagnostic and therapeutic radiation exposure in children. *Pediatr Radiol.* 2006;36(Suppl 2):121–125.
3. ICRP. 1990 Recommendations of the International Commission on Radaition Protection. *Ann ICRP.* 1991;21(1–3):1–201.
4. 1994–2004 TDoDs. *Lessoned Learned and New Challenges: Worshop.* Washington, DC: National Academic Press; 2008.
5. Brody AS, Frush DP, Huda W, Brent RL, American Academy of Pediatrics Section on Radiology. Radiation risk to children from computed tomography. *Pediatrics.* 2007;120(3):677–682.
6. Chodick G, Ronckers CM, Shalev V, Ron E. Excess lifetime cancer mortality risk attributable to radiation exposure from computed tomography examinations in children. *Isr Med Assoc J.* 2007;9(8):584–587.
7. Prasad KN. *Prevention and Mitigation of Damage after Low Radiation Doses.* Boca Raton, FL: CRC Press; 2012.
8. Weiss JF, Landauer MR. Protection against ionizing radiation by antioxidant nutrients and phytochemicals. *Toxicology.* 2003;189(1–2):1–20.
9. Sauren LD, van Garsse L, van Ommen V, Kemerink GJ. Occupational radiation dose during transcatheter aortic valve implantation. *Catheter Cardiovasc Interv.* 2011;78(5):770–776.
10. Kim KP, Miller DL, Balter S, et al. Occupational radiation doses to operators performing cardiac catheterization procedures. *Health Phys.* 2008;94(3):211–227.
11. Kemerink GJ, Frantzen MJ, Oei K, et al. Patient and occupational dose in neurointerventional procedures. *Neuroradiology.* 2002;44(6):522–528.
12. Staniszewska MA, Jankowski J. Personnel exposure during interventional radiologic procedures. *Med Pr.* 2000;51(6):563–571.
13. Ogundare FO, Balogun FA. Whole-body doses of occupationally exposed female workers in Nigeria (1999–2001). *J Radiol Prot.* 2003;23(2):201–208.
14. Waters M, Bloom TF, Grajewski B. The NIOSH/FAA Working Women's Health Study: Evaluation of the cosmic-radiation exposures of flight attendants. Federal Aviation Administration. *Health Phys.* 2000;79(5):553–559.
15. Bagshaw M. Cosmic radiation in commercial aviation. *Travel Med Infect Dis.* 2008;6(3):125–127.
16. Blettner M, Grosche B, Zeeb H. Occupational cancer risk in pilots and flight attendants: Current epidemiological knowledge. *Radiat Environ Biophys.* 1998;37(2):75–80.
17. Report BV. *Health Risks from Exposure to Low Levels of Ionizing Radiation.* Washington, DC: The National Academic Press; 2006.
18. Buring J, Hennekens, CH. Antioxidant vitamins in cancer: The Physicians' Health Study and Women's Health Study. In: Prasad K, Santamaria L, Williams RM, eds. *Nutrients in Cancer Prevention and Treatment.* Totowa, NJ: Humana Press; 1995:223.
19. Russell WL. The effect of radiation dose rate and fractionation onmutation in mice. In: Sagel FH, ed. *Repair from Genetic Radiation Damage and Differential Radiosensitivity in Germ Cells.* New york: Macmillan Press; 1963.

20. Ben-Amotz A, Yatziv S, Sela M, et al. Effect of natural beta-carotene supplementation in children exposed to radiation from the Chernobyl accident. *Radiat Environ Biophys.* 1998;37(3):187–193.

21. Hanson AJ, Prasad JE, Nahreini P, et al. Overexpression of amyloid precursor protein is associated with degeneration, decreased viability, and increased damage caused by neurotoxins (prostaglandins A1 and E2, hydrogen peroxide, and nitric oxide) in differentiated neuroblastoma cells. *J Neurosci Res.* 2003;74(1):148–159.

22. Hovland A, Nahreini P, Andreatta CP, Edwards-Prasad J, Prasad KN. Identifying genes involved in regulating differentiation of neuroblastoma cells. *J Neurosci Res.* 2001;64(3):302–310.

23. DiPaolo JA. In vitro morphologic transformation of syriam hamster cells by UV-irradiation is enhanced by X-irradiation and unaffected by chemicak carcinogen. *Int J Radiat Biol Relat Stud Phys Chem Med.* 1976;30(1):41–53.

24. Borek C, Ong A, Mason H, Donahue L, Biaglow JE. Selenium and vitamin E inhibit radiogenic and chemically induced transformation in vitro via different mechanisms. *Proc Natl Acad Sci USA.* 1986;83(5):1490–1494.

25. Pollock EJ, Todaro GJ. Radiation enhancement of SV40 transformation in 3T3 and human cells. *Nature.* 1968;219(5153):520–521.

26. Little JB. Influence of noncarcinogenic secondary factors on radiation carcinogenesis. *Radiat Res.* 1981;87(2):240–250.

27. Clark EP, Hahn GM, Little JB. Hyperthermic modulation of X-ray-induced oncogenic transformation in C3H 10T1/2 cells. *Radiat Res.* 1981;88(3):619–622.

28. Puck TT, Morse H, Johnson R, Waldren CA. Caffeine enhanced measurement of mutagenesis by low levels of gamma-irradiation in human lymphocytes. *Somat Cell Mol Genet.* 1993;19(5):423–429.

29. Suzuki K, Kodama S, Watanabe M. Extremely low-dose ionizing radiation causes activation of mitogen-activated protein kinase pathway and enhances proliferation of normal human diploid cells. *Cancer Res.* 2001;61(14):5396–5401.

30. Rothkamm K, Lobrich M. Evidence for a lack of DNA double-strand break repair in human cells exposed to very low X-ray doses. *Proc Natl Acad Sci USA.* 2003;100(9):5057–5062.

31. BEIR P. *National Council of the National Academies Committe to Assess Health Risks from Exposure to Low Levels of Ionizing Radiation.* Washington, DC: The National Academies Press; 2006.

32. Brenner DJ, Sachs RK. Estimating radiation-induced cancer risks at very low doses: Rationale for using a linear no-threshold approach. *Radiat Environ Biophys.* 2006;44(4):253–256.

33. Banauch GI, Alleyne D, Sanchez R, et al. Persistent hyperreactivity and reactive airway dysfunction in firefighters at the World Trade Center. *Am J Respir Crit Care Med.* 2003;168(1):54–62.

34. Bond VP, Benary V, Sondhaus CA. A different perception of the linear, nonthreshold hypothesis for low-dose irradiation. *Proc Natl Acad Sci USA.* 1991;88(19):8666–8670.

35. Altas E, Ertekin MV, Gundogdu C, Demirci E. L-carnitine reduces cochlear damage induced by gamma irradiation in guinea pigs. *Ann Clin Lab Sci.* 2006;36(3):312–318.

36. DeKosky ST, Williamson JD, Fitzpatrick AL, et al. Ginkgo biloba for prevention of dementia: A randomized controlled trial. *JAMA.* 2008;300(19):2253–2262.

37. Bayir H, Kochanek PM, Kagan VE. Oxidative stress in immature brain after traumatic brain injury. *Dev Neurosci.* 2006;28(4–5):420–431.

38. Dennis PA, Weinberg JB, Calhoun PS, et al. An investigation of vago-regulatory and health behavior accounts for increased inflammation in posttraumatic stress disorder. *J Psychosom Res.* 2016;83:33–39.

39. George JM. The synucleins. *Genome Biol.* 2002;3(1):REVIEWS3002.

40. Brenner D, Elliston C, Hall E, Berdon W. Estimated risks of radiation-induced fatal cancer from pediatric CT. *AJR Am J Roentgenol.* 2001;176(2):289–296.

41. Baum MK, Campa A, Lai S, et al. Effect of micronutrient supplementation on disease progression in asymptomatic, antiretroviral-naive, HIV-infected adults in Botswana: A randomized clinical trial. *JAMA.* 2013;310(20):2154–2163.

42. Berrington de Gonzalez A, Darby S. Risk of cancer from diagnostic X-rays: Estimates for the UK and 14 other countries. *Lancet.* 2004;363(9406):345–351.

43. Memon A, Godward S, Williams D, Siddique I, Al-Saleh K. Dental X-rays and the risk of thyroid cancer: A case-control study. *Acta Oncol.* 2010;49(4):447–453.

44. Radiations CotBEoI. *The Effects of Populations Exposure to Low Levels of Ionizing Radiation.* Washington, DC: National Academy Press; 1980.

45. Yoshimoto Y. Cancer risk among children of atomic bomb survivors. A review of RERF epidemiologic studies. Radiation effects research foundation. *JAMA.* 1990;264(5):596–600.

46. Yoshimoto Y, Kato H, Schull WJ. Risk of cancer among children exposed in utero to A-bomb radiations, 1950–1984. *Lancet.* 1988;2(8612):665–669.

47. Miller RW. Effects of prenatal exposure to ionizing radiation. *Health Phys.* 1990;59(1):57–61.

48. Stewart A, Kneale GW. Radiation dose effects in relation to obstetric X-rays and childhood cancers. *Lancet.* 1970;1(7658):1185–1188.

49. Stewart A, Webb J, Hewitt D. A survey of childhood malignancies. *Br Med J.* 1958;1(5086):1495–1508.

50. Doll R. Radiation hazards: 25 years of collaborative research. Sylvanus Thompson memorial lecture, 1980. *Br J Radiol.* 1981;54(639):179–186.

51. Newcombe HB, McGregor JF. Childhood cancer following obstetric radiography. *Lancet.* 1971;2(7734):1151–1152.

52. Shore FJ, Robertson JS, Bateman JL. Childhood cancer following obstetric radiography. *Health Phys.* 1973;24(2):258–260.

53. Mole RH. Childhood cancer after prenatal exposure to diagnostic X-ray examinations in Britain. *Br J Cancer.* 1990;62(1):152–168.

54. Williams PM, Fletcher S. Health effects of prenatal radiation exposure. *Am Fam Physician.* 2010;82(5):488–493.

55. Wakeford R. Childhood leukaemia following medical diagnostic exposure to ionizing radiation in utero or after birth. *Radiat Prot Dosimetry.* 2008;132(2):166–174.

56. Little MP, Wakeford R, Kendall GM. Updated estimates of the proportion of childhood leukaemia incidence in Great Britain that may be caused by natural background ionising radiation. *J Radiol Prot.* 2009;29(4):467–482.

57. Stjernfeldt M, Berglund K, Lindsten J, Ludvigsson J. Maternal smoking and irradiation during pregnancy as risk factors for child leukemia. *Cancer Detect Prev.* 1992;16(2):129–135.

58. Graham SL. Preconception, intrauterine and postnatal irradiation as related to leukemia. *Natl Cancer Inst Monogr.* 1966;19:342.

59. Macmahon B. Prenatal X-ray exposure and childhood cancer. *J Natl Cancer Inst.* 1962;28:1173–1191.

60. Hagstrom RM, Glasser SR, Brill AB, Heyssel RM. Long term effects of radioactive iron administered during human pregnancy. *Am J Epidemiol.* 1969;90(1):1–10.

61. Uchida IA, Holunga R, Lawler C. Maternal radiation and chromosomal aberrations. *Lancet.* 1968;2(7577):1045–1049.

62. Awa AA, Bloom AD, Yoshida MC, Meriishi S, Archer PG. Cytogenetic study of the offspring of atom bomb survivors. *Nature.* 1968;218(5139):367–368.

63. Herskowitz IH. Damage to offspring of irradiated women. *Prog Immunol Gynecol.* 1957;3:374.

64. Daniels RD, Schubauer-Berigan MK. A meta-analysis of leukaemia risk from protracted exposure to low-dose gamma radiation. *Occup Environ Med.* 2010;68(6):457–464.

65. Zielinski JM, Garner MJ, Band PR, et al. Health outcomes of low-dose ionizing radiation exposure among medical workers: A cohort study of the Canadian national dose registry of radiation workers. *Int J Occup Med Environ Health.* 2009;22(2):149–156.

66. Doody MM, Freedman DM, Alexander BH, et al. Breast cancer incidence in US radiologic technologists. *Cancer.* 2006;106(12):2707–2715.

67. Yoshinaga S, Mabuchi K, Sigurdson AJ, Doody MM, Ron E. Cancer risks among radiologists and radiologic technologists: Review of epidemiologic studies. *Radiology.* 2004;233(2):313–321.

68. Cardis E, Vrijheid M, Blettner M, et al. The 15-country collaborative study of cancer risk among radiation workers in the nuclear industry: Estimates of radiation-related cancer risks. *Radiat Res.* 2007;167(4):396–416.

69. Vrijheid M, Cardis E, Blettner M, et al. The 15-country collaborative study of cancer risk among radiation workers in the nuclear industry: Design, epidemiological methods, and descriptive results. *Radiat Res.* 2007;167(4):361–379.

70. Jeong M, Jin YW, Yang KH, Ahn YO, Cha CY. Radiation exposure and cancer incidence in a cohort of nuclear power industry workers in the Republic of Korea, 1992–2005. *Radiat Environ Biophys.* 2010;49(1):47–55.

71. Vano E, Kleiman NJ, Duran A, Rehani MM, Echeverri D, Cabrera M. Radiation cataract risk in interventional cardiology personnel. *Radiat Res.* 2010;174(4):490–495.

72. Fachin AL, Mello SS, Sandrin-Garcia P, et al. Gene expression profiles in radiation workers occupationally exposed to ionizing radiation. *J Radiat Res (Tokyo).* 2009;50(1):61–71.

73. Buja A, Lange JH, Perissinotto E, et al. Cancer incidence among male military and civil pilots and flight attendants: An analysis on published data. *Toxicol Ind Health.* 2005;21(10):273–282.

74. Band PR, Le ND, Fang R, et al. Cohort study of Air Canada pilots: Mortality, cancer incidence, and leukemia risk. *Am J Epidemiol.* 1996;143(2):137–143.

75. Hammer GP, Blettner M, Zeeb H. Epidemiological studies of cancer in aircrew. *Radiat Prot Dosimetry.* 2009;136(4):232–239.

76. Pukkala E, Aspholm R, Auvinen A, et al. Cancer incidence among 10,211 airline pilots: A Nordic study. *Aviat Space Environ Med.* 2003;74(7):699–706.

77. Sigurdson AJ, Ron E. Cosmic radiation exposure and cancer risk among flight crew. *Cancer Invest.* 2004;22(5):743–761.

78. Rafnsson V, Tulinius H, Jonasson JG, Hrafnkelsson J. Risk of breast cancer in female flight attendants: A population-based study (Iceland). *Cancer Causes Control.* 2001;12(2):95–101.

79. Pukkala E, Auvinen A, Wahlberg G. Incidence of cancer among finnish airline cabin attendants, 1967–1992. *BMJ.* 1995;311(7006):649–652.

80. Buja A, Mastrangelo G,. Perissinotto E, et al. Camcer incidence among female flight attendants: A meta-analysis of published data. *J Womens Health (Larchmt).* 2006;15:98–105.

81. Rugh R. X-irradiation effects on the human fetus. *J Pediatr.* 1958;52(5):531–538.

82. Schwarz GS. Radiation hazards to the human fetus in present-day society. Should a pregnant women be subjected to a diagnostic X-ray procedure? *Bull N Y Acad Med.* 1968;44(4):388–399.

83. Korkina LG, Afanas'ef IB, Diplock AT. Antioxidant therapy in children affected by irradiation from the Chernobyl nuclear accident. *Biochem Soc Trans.* 1993;21(Pt 3)(3):314S.

84. Angelieri F, de Oliveira GR, Sannomiya EK, Ribeiro DA. DNA damage and cellular death in oral mucosa cells of children who have undergone panoramic dental radiography. *Pediatr Radiol.* 2007;37(6):561–565.

85. Holland N, Bolognesi C, Kirsch-Volders M, et al. The micronucleus assay in human buccal cells as a tool for biomonitoring DNA damage: The HUMN project perspective on current status and knowledge gaps. *Mutat Res.* 2008;659(1–2):93–108.

86. Ribeiro DA, Angelieri F. Cytogenetic biomonitoring of oral mucosa cells from adults exposed to dental X-rays. *Radiat Med.* 2008;26(6):325–330.

87. Ehrlich JS, Brand R, Uder M, Kuefner M. Effect of proprietary combination of antioxidants/glutathione-elevating agents on X-ray induced DNA double-strand breaks. *Presented at the Annual Meeting of Society of Cardiovascular Computed Tomography,* 2011.

88. Jaramillo MC, Zhang DD. The emerging role of the Nrf2-Keap1 signaling pathway in cancer. *Genes Dev.* 2013;27(20):2179–2191.

89. Williamson TP, Johnson DA, Johnson JA. Activation of the Nrf2-ARE pathway by siRNA knockdown of Keap1 reduces oxidative stress and provides partial protection from MPTP-mediated neurotoxicity. *Neurotoxicology.* 2012;33(3):272–279.

90. Itoh K, Chiba T, Takahashi S, et al. An Nrf2/small Maf heterodimer mediates the induction of phase II detoxifying enzyme genes through antioxidant response elements. *Biochem Biophys Res Commun.* 1997;236(2):313–322.

91. Hayes JD, Chanas SA, Henderson CJ, et al. The Nrf2 transcription factor contributes both to the basal expression of glutathione S-transferases in mouse liver and to their induction by the chemopreventive synthetic antioxidants, butylated hydroxyanisole, and ethoxyquin. *Biochem Soc Trans.* 2000;28(2):33–41.

92. Chan K, Han XD, Kan YW. An important function of Nrf2 in combating oxidative stress: Detoxification of acetaminophen. *Proc Natl Acad Sci USA.* 2001;98(8):4611–4616.

93. Ramsey CP, Glass CA, Montgomery MB, et al. Expression of Nrf2 in neurodegenerative diseases. *J Neuropathol Exp Neurol.* 2007;66(1):75–85.

94. Chen PC, Vargas MR, Pani AK, et al. Nrf2-mediated neuroprotection in the MPTP mouse model of Parkinson's disease: Critical role for the astrocyte. *Proc Natl Acad Sci USA.* 2009;106(8):2933–2938.

95. Lastres-Becker I, Ulusoy A, Innamorato NG, et al. Alpha-synuclein expression and Nrf2 deficiency cooperate to aggravate protein aggregation, neuronal death, and inflammation in early-stage Parkinson's disease. *Hum Mol Genet.* 2012;21(14):3173–3192.

96. Xi YD, Yu HL, Ding J, et al. Flavonoids protect cerebrovascular endothelial cells through Nrf2 and PI3K from beta-amyloid peptide-induced oxidative damage. *Curr Neurovasc Res.* 2012;9(1):32–41.

97. Suh JH, Shenvi SV, Dixon BM, et al. Decline in transcriptional activity of Nrf2 causes age-related loss of glutathione synthesis, which is reversible with lipoic acid. *Proc Natl Acad Sci USA.* 2004;101(10):3381–3386.

98. Trujillo J, Chirino YI, Molina-Jijon E, Anderica-Romero AC, Tapia E, Pedraza-Chaverri J. Renoprotective effect of the antioxidant curcumin: Recent findings. *Redox Biol.* 2013;1(1):448–456.

99. Steele ML, Fuller S, Patel M, Kersaitis C, Ooi L, Munch G. Effect of Nrf2 activators on release of glutathione, cysteinylglycine and homocysteine by human U373 astroglial cells. *Redox Biol.* 2013;1(1):441–445.

100. Kode A, Rajendrasozhan S, Caito S, Yang SR, Megson IL, Rahman I. Resveratrol induces glutathione synthesis by activation of Nrf2 and protects against cigarette smoke-mediated oxidative stress in human lung epithelial cells. *Am j Physiol Lung Cell Mol Physiol.* 2008;294(3):L478–L488.

101. Gao L, Wang J, Sekhar KR, et al. Novel n-3 fatty acid oxidation products activate Nrf2 by destabilizing the association between Keap1 and Cullin3. *J Biol Chem.* 2007;282(4):2529–2537.

102. Saw CL, Yang AY, Guo Y, Kong AN. Astaxanthin and omega-3 fatty acids individually and in combination protect against oxidative stress via the Nrf2-ARE pathway. *Food Chem Toxicol.* 2013;62:869–875.

103. Song J, Kang SM, Lee WT, Park KA, Lee KM, Lee JE. Glutathione protects brain endothelial cells from hydrogen peroxide-induced oxidative stress by increasing nrf2 expression. *Exp Neurobiol.* 2014;23(1):93–103.

104. Ji L, Liu R, Zhang XD, et al. N-acetylcysteine attenuates phosgene-induced acute lung injury via upregulation of Nrf2 expression. *Inhal Toxicol.* 2010;22(7):535–542.

105. Choi HK, Pokharel YR, Lim SC, et al. Inhibition of liver fibrosis by solubilized coenzyme Q10: Role of Nrf2 activation in inhibiting transforming growth factor-beta1 expression. *Toxicol Appl Pharmacol.* 2009;240(3):377–384.

106. Bai H, Liu R, Chen HL, et al. Enhanced antioxidant effect of caffeic acid phenethyl ester and Trolox in combination against radiation induced-oxidative stress. *Chem Biol Interact.* 2014;207:7–15.

107. Cui L, Jeong H, Borovecki F, Parkhurst CN, Tanese N, Krainc D. Transcriptional repression of PGC-1alpha by mutant huntingtin leads to mitochondrial dysfunction and neurodegeneration. *Cell.* 2006;127(1):59–69.

108. Li XH, Li CY, Lu JM, Tian RB, Wei J. Allicin ameliorates cognitive deficits ageing-induced learning and memory deficits through enhancing of Nrf2 antioxidant signaling pathways. *Neurosci Lett.* 2012;514(1):46–50.

109. Bergstrom P, Andersson HC, Gao Y, et al. Repeated transient sulforaphane stimulation in astrocytes leads to prolonged Nrf2-mediated gene expression and protection from superoxide-induced damage. *Neuropharmacology.* 2011;60(2–3):343–353.

110. Wruck CJ, Gotz ME, Herdegen T, Varoga D, Brandenburg LO, Pufe T. Kavalactones protect neural cells against amyloid beta peptide-induced neurotoxicity via extracellular signal-regulated kinase 1/2-dependent nuclear factor erythroid 2-related factor 2 activation. *Mol Pharmacol.* 2008;73(6):1785–1795.

111. Song SM, Park YS, Lee A, et al. Concentrations of blood vitamin A, C, E, coenzyme Q10, and urine cotinine related to cigarette smoking exposure. *Korean J Lab Med.* 2009;29(1):10–16.

112. Galan P, Viteri FE, Bertrais S, et al. Serum concentrations of beta-carotene, vitamins C and E, zinc and selenium are influenced by sex, age, diet, smoking status, alcohol consumption, and corpulence in a general French adult population. *Eur J Clin Nutr.* 2005;59(10):1181–1190.

113. Adhikari D, Baxi J, Risal S, Singh PP. Oxidative stress and antioxidant status in cancer patients and healthy subjects, a case-control study. *Nepal Med Coll J.* 2005;7(2):112–115.

114. Li W, Khor TO, Xu C, et al. Activation of Nrf2-antioxidant signaling attenuates NFkappaB-inflammatory response and elicits apoptosis. *Biochem Pharmacol.* 2008;76(11):1485–1489.

115. Kim J, Cha YN, Surh YJ. A protective role of nuclear factor-erythroid 2-related factor-2 (Nrf2) in inflammatory disorders. *Mutat Res.* 2010;690(1–2):12–23.

116. Abate A, Yang G, Dennery PA, Oberle S, Schroder H. Synergistic inhibition of cyclooxygenase-2 expression by vitamin E and aspirin. *Free Radic Biol Med.* 2000;29(11):1135–1142.

117. Devaraj S, Tang R, Adams-Huet B, et al. Effect of high-dose alpha-tocopherol supplementation on biomarkers of oxidative stress and inflammation and carotid atherosclerosis in patients with coronary artery disease. *Am J Clin Nutr.* 2007;86(5):1392–1398.

118. Fu Y, Zheng S, Lin J, Ryerse J, Chen A. Curcumin protects the rat liver from CCl4-caused injury and fibrogenesis by attenuating oxidative stress and suppressing inflammation. *Mol Pharmacol.* 2008;73(2):399–409.

119. Lee HS, Jung KK, Cho JY, et al. Neuroprotective effect of curcumin is mainly mediated by blockade of microglial cell activation. *Pharmazie.* 2007;62(12):937–942.

120. Rahman S, Bhatia K, Khan AQ, et al. Topically applied vitamin E prevents massive cutaneous inflammatory and oxidative stress responses induced by double application of 12-O-tetradecanoylphorbol-13-acetate (TPA) in mice. *Chem Biol Interact.* 2008;172(3):195–205.

121. Suzuki YJ, Aggarwal BB, Packer L. Alpha-lipoic acid is a potent inhibitor of NF-kappa B activation in human T cells. *Biochem Biophys Res Commun.* 1992;189(3):1709–1715.

122. Zhu J, Yong W, Wu X, et al. Anti-inflammatory effect of resveratrol on TNF-alpha-induced MCP-1 expression in adipocytes. *Biochem Biophys Res Commun.* 2008;369(2):471–477.
123. Goel HC, Prasad J, Singh S, et al. Radioprotective potential of an herbal extract of Tinospora cordifolia. *J Radiat Res (Tokyo).* 2004;45(1):61–68.
124. Arora R, Gupta D, Chawla R, et al. Radioprotection by plant products: Present status and future prospects. *Phytother Res.* 2005;19(1):1–22.
125. Mettler FA Jr, Bhargavan M, Faulkner K, et al. Radiologic and nuclear medicine studies in the United States and worldwide: Frequency, radiation dose, and comparison with other radiation sources, 1950–2007. *Radiology.* 2009;253(2):520–531.
126. Prasad KN. Rationale for using multiple antioxidants in protecting humans against low doses of ionizing radiation. *Br J Radiol.* 2005;78(930):485–492.

19 Micronutrients in Protecting Against Lethal Doses of Ionizing Radiation

INTRODUCTION

Ionizing radiation refers to photon energy that can knock out a negatively charged electron from the orbit of an atom, leaving it positively charged and thus creating an ion pair after every such interaction. The process of creating an ion pair is referred to as ionization. Ionization radiation has been divided into two categories, low energy transfer (LET) radiation and high LET radiation. The low LET radiation includes X-rays, gamma-rays, and beta-rays that cause cellular damage primarily (about two-third of damage) by generating free radicals during radiation exposure. The high LET radiation includes proton radiation, neutron radiation, alpha-particle radiation, and other heavy particle radiation that cause initial cellular damage primarily by ionization, while free radicals also play role in the progression of damage. High LET radiation is generally 5–20 times more effective than the low LET radiation in causing damage, depending upon the type of radiation and criteria of radiation injury. If radiation damage is not repaired, chronic inflammation sets in motion that releases additional free radicals, pro-inflammatory cytokines, complement proteins, and adhesion molecules, all of which are toxic to cells. Thus, increased oxidative stress and chronic inflammation together participate in the progression of acute and late effects of irradiation.

Increased oxidative stress and pro-inflammatory cytokines regulate the expression of microRNAs causing death of neurons and glia cells in culture.[1] Since irradiation of mammalian cells produces ROS and pro-inflammatory cytokines, it may alter the expression of microRNAs that could affect radiosensitivity of cells.

Antioxidants regulate the expression of microRNAs.[1] Since antioxidants when administered before irradiation protect cells in vitro and in vivo against radiation injury by quenching free radicals and reducing inflammation,[2,3] it may protect against radiation injury by altering the expression of microRNAs. However, the direct effects of antioxidants on the levels of microRNAs in providing radiation protection before or after irradiation on normal cells have not been investigated.

Numerous protective agents against high doses of radiation using cell culture and primarily rodents have been identified. Among them antioxidants are the only agents that are considered nontoxic in humans for short-term and long-term consumption. Several studies showed that intraperitoneally administration of individual antioxidants shortly before irradiation protect against lethal doses of radiation in rodents.[4] These agents were ineffective when administered after irradiation. The observation of existence of long-lived free radicals[5,6] and elevated levels of pro-inflammatory cytokines[7–10] after irradiation suggests that these cellular defects should also be attenuated for optimal radiation protection. Only a few studies on the effect of administration of antioxidants before and after irradiation have been conducted.

This chapter briefly describes unit of radiation doses, high-dose-induced acute and chronic damage, and the role of microRNAs in mediating radiation injury. This chapter also discusses radiation protection studies primarily with antioxidants before and after irradiation, and treatment procedures for lethally irradiated individuals. In order to provide an optimal radiation protection in humans, it is essential to increase the levels of antioxidant enzymes by activating the Nrf2/ARE pathway as well as dietary and endogenous antioxidant compounds before and after irradiation. A mixture of micronutrients that would accomplish the above goal is proposed. This mixture of micronutrients in combination with radiation therapeutic approaches, for the treatment of individuals exposed to lethal doses of radiation is suggested. The role of this micronutrient mixture in reducing the risks of developing late-adverse effects of radiation among survivors of high doses of radiation is also suggested.

UNIT OF RADIATION DOSES

The current unit of low LET radiation dose is Gy (named after a famous radiobiologist, Dr. Gray), whereas the unit used for radiation protection recommendation is Sv (named after a famous health physicist, Dr. Sievert). The unit Sv accommodates any difference in relative biological effectiveness (RBE) between low and high LET radiation. RBE is a ratio of a dose to produce an effect by low LET radiation and a dose to produce the same effect by high LET radiation.

HIGH-DOSE RADIATION-INDUCED DAMAGE

The effects of high doses of radiation have been described in detail in several books including the one referred here.[4] The extent of damage depends upon the dose, dose-rate, mode of delivery (single versus fractionated dose), surface area irradiated (whole-body versus partial-body), and radiosensitivity of target organs. The most radiosensitive organs on the criterion of cell death include bone marrow, small intestine, hair follicles and gonads. The responses to high-dose radiation differ among mammals and are generally measured in terms of mortality rate and survival time after irradiation. The mortality rate can be measured as LD_{50} (dose that produces 50% lethality) or LD_{100} (dose that produces 100% lethality). The efficacy of radiation protection is generally expressed as dose reduction factor (DRF) that is the ratio of a dose that produces an effect in the presence of a radioprotective agent and a dose that produces the same effect in the absence of the same radioprotective agent. Other ways to express the efficacy of radioprotective agents can include increase in survival rate and survival time compared to irradiated control groups.

High doses of radiation up to 1.5 Gy do not cause lethality, but they can increase the risk of some late adverse effects, including cancer. They can induce chromosomal damage and gene mutations (somatic and heritable). High doses of radiation can cause lethality and produce organ specific syndrome. Radiation syndromes have been divided into three major categories: (1) bone marrow syndrome, (2) gastrointestinal (GI) syndrome, and (3) central nervous system (CNS) syndrome. Each radiation syndrome is characterized by specific doses, survival rate, survival time, and symptoms. High doses of radiation also cause acute or chronic damage to organ systems without causing lethality. *The Handbook of Radiobiology* has discussed radiation syndromes in great detail.[4]

BONE MARROW SYNDROME

The LD_{50} dose requirement to produce the bone marrow syndrome varies from one species to another (Table 19.1). The LD50 dose for rodents is about 3-fold higher than humans. The bone marrow syndrome is often expressed in terms of $^{30}LD_{50}$ (50% lethality within 30 days). The deaths occur within 30 days in most species; however, in humans, most death occurs after 30 days, and 50% will die within 60 days of exposure. Therefore, for humans, the dose of bone marrow syndrome is expressed as $^{60}LD_{50}$. The bone marrow syndrome is primarily caused by extensive damage to bone marrow and lymphatic system, and is characterized by nausea, vomiting, and fatigue. Infection and bleeding are prominent. The major cause of death is infection.

TABLE 19.1

Variations in Bone Marrow

Syndrome Doses in Different Species

Species	LD_{50} Value in Gy
Human	2.7–3.0
Monkey	3.98
Rodents (rat and mice)	8.5–9.0
Desert mice	11.0–12.0
Hamster	9.0
Rabbit	8.4
Dog	2.65
Sheep	1.55
Swine	1.95

Source: Data were summarized from Handbook of Radiobiology and other. Prasad, K., *Handbook of Radiobiology*, Second Edition, CRC Press, Boca Rotan, FL, 1995; Bond, V.P. ed., *Radiation Mortality in Different Species*, Igaku Shoin, Tokyo, Japan, Bond, V.P. and Sagahara, T. eds., *Comparative Cellular and Species Radiosensitivity*, Igaku Shoin, Tokyo, Japan, 1969.

GASTROINTESTINAL (GI) SYNDROME

The dose requirement for the GI syndrome varies between rodents and humans. In rodents, it is 12–40 Gy, and in humans, it is 5–40 Gy. The doses that produce GI syndrome cause 100% mortality in 3.5 days in rodents and 14 days in humans. The common signs and symptoms include loss of appetite, gastric complaint, nausea, vomiting, diarrheas (may be bloody in some cases), electrolyte imbalance, dehydration, hemoconcentration, and circulatory collapse, leading to death. The major cause of death is the denudation of villi of the small intestine; however, other factors such as infection, hemorrhage, and electrolyte imbalance contribute to the rate of progression of injury.

CENTRAL NERVOUS SYSTEM (CNS) SYNDROME

The doses of 50 Gy or more can produce CNS syndrome in both humans and rodents. This syndrome is characterized by period of agitation, marked apathy, followed by disorientation, balance problem, ataxia, diarrhea, vomiting, opisthotonus, convulsion, coma, and death within 24 hours. The major causes of death are increased inflammatory reactions damaging blood vessels, neurons, and enhanced intracranial pressure. The death occurs so soon that no treatment is possible.

HIGH-DOSE RADIATION-INDUCED DAMAGE TO ORGANS

The acute radiation responses to the skin are referred to as radiation dermatitis. The chronic responses to the skin may include development of necrosis that may occur following infection or high radiation doses that can damage blood vessels and connective tissues. Radiation-induced necrotic ulcer is difficult to heal because of damage to the blood vessels and connective tissues that interfere with the regeneration of epithelial cells. The hair follicles are very sensitive to radiation. During radiation therapy involving head region, loss of hair frequently occurs.

Radiation responses of the mucous membrane are referred to as radiation mucositis. The sequences of changes are similar to the skin, except that the changes are seen earlier than those observed in the skin. Radiation responses of nondividing organs such as lung (radiation pneumonitis), liver (radiation hepatitis), brain, bone, and muscle are characterized by acute inflammatory reactions that are followed by fibrosis (lung and liver) and necrosis (brain, muscle and bone). Radiation-induced necrosis is difficult to heal.

RISK OF DEVELOPING CANCER AMONG SURVIVORS OF HIGH DOSES OF RADIATION

Most data for the adverse effects of high doses of radiation come primarily from populations exposed to radiation following explosion of atom bomb in Hiroshima and Nagasaki and cancer survivors who received radiation therapy and/or chemotherapy. The late adverse health effects of high doses of radiation include both neoplastic and non-neoplastic diseases. High doses of radiation can induce cancer in all organs that have dividing cells or that have nondividing cells with a capacity to proliferate following an appropriate stimulus. The increase in leukemia incidence following radiation exposure can be seen within 10 years; however, the risk of solid tumor persists for 30 years or more after irradiation. Thyroid cancer, breast cancer and hematopoietic cancer are most frequent after irradiation. Thyroid cancer is generally found in children; however, a 10-fold increase in incidence of this cancer was observed in children living in Belarus, Russia, and Ukraine who were exposed to radioactive fallout following Chernobyl nuclear accident after 10 years of exposure.[11] Among children surviving the treatment of leukemia and brain tumor with standard therapy, the risk of developing secondary primary central nervous system tumors is high. Radiation exposure was associated with the increased risk of glioma and meningioma. Glioma occurred after a median of 9 years and meningioma after 17 years from initial cancer treatment.[12] The higher risk of secondary primary glioma in children survivors who were irradiated at an early age may suggest greater susceptibility of the developing brain to radiation. In addition of tumors of central nervous system, childhood survivors of cancer treatment appear to be associated with more than 9-fold increase in the risk of secondary sarcomas compared to general population.[13] An epidemiologic study reported that the survivors of childhood cancer treatment had increased risk for the second primary cancer, including non-melanoma skin cancer.[14] It has been reported that two patients who were treated for malignant disease by surgery and gamma-radiation (36–40 Gy fractionated doses) developed melanoma in tattoo sites used for marking a radiation field.[15] At present, there are no preventive strategies to reduce the risk of second primary tumors or recurrence of primary tumors in survivors of cancer treatment.

RISK OF DEVELOPING NON-NEOPLASTIC DISEASES AMONG SURVIVORS OF HIGH DOSES OF RADIATION

The ovarian and testicular failure has been reported among survivors of the treatment of childhood cancer with tumor therapeutic agents.[16,17] Patients who received radiation doses 10–40 Gy fractionated doses for the treatment of other malignant diseases developed hypothyroidism a few months to several years after radiation therapy.[18] Other non-neoplastic diseases include cataract and delayed necrosis in brain, muscle, auditory ossicles, and bone.[4] At present, there are no preventive strategies to reduce the risk of non-neoplastic diseases in survivors of childhood or adult cancer treatment.

MicroRNAs IN RADIATION DAMAGE

MicroRNAs

MicroRNAs (miRs) are evolutionarily conserved small noncoding single-stranded RNAs of approximately 22 nucleotides in length, and are present in all living organisms including humans.[19–22] The biogenesis of miRs is very complex and involves multiple biochemical steps. The majority of miRs are transcribed by RNA polymerase II (Pol II), while some are transcribed by RNA polymerase III (Pol III) from the noncoding region of the DNA to produce primary miRs (pri-miRs). Pri-miRs undergo a nuclear cleavage by ribonuclease III Drosa to generate precursor-miRs (pre-miRs) that migrate to the cytoplasm where they are further cleaved by ribonuclease III Dicer to ultimately form mature single-stranded miRs with the help of another protein argonaute (Ago).[21,23–25] Each miR binds to its complimentary sequences in the 3′-untranslated region (3′-UTR) of the mRNA, promotes degradation of the mRNA transcript, and prevents translation of the message of protein. In this manner, miRs regulate the translation of proapoptotic or antiapoptotic proteins from their respective mRNAs, depending upon whether they receive damaging or protective signal.

IRRADIATION ALTERS THE EXPRESSION OF MicroRNAs IN NORMAL CELLS

Although irradiation changes the expression of micoRNAs in both normal and cancer cells, this section describes these changes only in normal cells (Table 19.2). Alterations in the expression of microRNAs can lead to increase or decrease in radiosensitivity of normal cells.

TABLE 19.2

Relationship Between Radiation-Induced Alterations in the Expression of MicroRNAs and Radiosensitivity of Normal Cells

Cell Type	Upregulation	Downregulation	Radiosensitivity
IM9	33 microRNAs	0	Increase[26]
CD34+	miR-30	0	Increase[28]
CD34+	miR-30b, miR-30c, miR-30d	0	Increase[29]
Hfob		miR-30c	Decrease[29]
HLF	miR-140	0	Decrease[30]
RPE, HUVEC	miR-525-3p	0	Decrease[32]
HDMEC	miR-let-7g	miR-127	Increase[33]
HDMEC		miR-125a, miR-189	Decrease[33]
Skin (rat)	miR-214		Decrease[34]
WI-38		miR-155, miR-20a	Increase[35]
WI-38	miR-152, miR-410	miR-155, miR-20a[35]	
	miR-431, miR-493	miR-25, miR-15a	

Source: The number under radiosensitivity indicates reference number.

Note: IM9, human lymphoblastic cells; hFOB, human fetal osteoblasts; HLF, Human lung fibroblasts; RPE, retinyl pigment epithelial cells; HUVEC, human umbilical vein endothelial cells; HDMEC, human dermal microvascular endothelial cells; Wi-38, human lung fibroblasts.

Upregulation and down regulation of microRNAs after irradiation could be due to their increased transcription, processing by Drosa in the nucleus and Dicer in the cytoplasm or stability.

Irradiation of IM9 human lymphoblastic cells with 1 and 10 Gy increased the expression of 73 and 33 microRNAs by more than 2-fold, respectively,[26] suggesting that the number of overexpressed microRNAs is dose-dependent. Most of these microRNAs caused apoptosis, cell cycle arrest, and impaired DNA repair process; therefore, these microRNAs may play an important role in determining the radiosensitivity of these cells.[27]

Whole-body gamma-irradiation of CD2F1 mice with 7–12.5 Gy or irradiation of human hematopoietic CD34+ cells in culture with 0.2 or 4 Gy increased the expression of miR-30b and miR-30c in mouse tissue and serum, and in CD4+ cells.[28] In addition, increased levels of interleukin IL-1β were also found in mouse tissue, serum and CD34+ cells. Supplementation with delta-tocotrienol 24 hours before irradiation downregulated the expression of miR-30 and decreased the levels of IL-1β that protected against radiation-induced apoptosis in irradiated mice and CD34+ cells.[28] This study suggests that upregulation of the expression of miR-30 increased the radiosensitivity of these cells, whereas downregulation of the expression of miR-30 may provide protection against radiation damage.

Irradiation of human fetal osteoblast cell line (hFOB) and human hematopoietic progenitor CD34+ cells with gamma-radiation downregulated the expression of 14 microRNAs in hFOB and 16 microRNAs in CD34+ cell, whereas it also upregulated the expression of 18 microRNAs in hFOB cells and 15 microRNAs in CD34+ cells.[29] Additional studies showed that irradiation upregulated the expression of miR-30b, miR-30c, and miR-30d in CD34+ cells, but downregulated the expression of miR-30c in hFOB cells. Overexpression of miR-30c inhibited its target proteins REDD1 (regulated in development and DNA response-1) protein, which suppressed the levels of mTOR (mechanistic target of rapamycin) that promoted cell growth and cell proliferation.[29] These results suggest that miR-30c plays an important role in the progression of radiation injury by reducing the levels of REDD1.

Irradiation of human lung fibroblasts (HLFs) increased the expression of miR-140 that activates Nrf2 by inhibiting the levels Keap1.[30] Irradiation of these cells also increased the levels of BRCA1 (breast cancer 1) protein that interacts with Nrf2 and promotes its stability and activation.[31] Thus, increased expression of miR-140 and levels of BRCA1 protein) after irradiation represents a protective response.

Irradiation of retinal pigment epithelial cells (RPE cells) and human umbilical vein endothelial cells (HUVECs) increased the expression of miR-525-3p and deceased the levels of its target proteins ARRB1 (arrestin beta1) that inhibits NF-kB activity, and TNX1 (thioredoxin-1) and HSPA9 (heat shock protein family A member 9) that control cell proliferation.[32] Overexpression of miR-525-3p makes cells radioresistant.

Irradiation of primary human dermal microvascular endothelial cells (HDMEC) with 2 Gy increased the expression of miR-let7g, miR-16, miR-20a, miR-21, miR-29c, and decreased the expression of miR-18a, miR-125a, miR-127, miR-148b, miR-189, and miR-503. Decreased expression of miR-125a and miR-189 reduced radiosensitivity, while increased expression of miRlet-7g and decreased expression of miR-127 enhanced the radiosensitivity of these cells.[33]

Irradiation of rat skin increased the expression of miR-214 and decreased the levels of its target protein peroxiredoxin-6 (PRDX-6), and thereby, enhanced radiosensitivity. This is further supported by the fact that overexpression of PRDX-6 makes cell radioresistant.[34]

Irradiation human lung fibroblasts (WI 38) induced premature senescence by upregulating the expression of miR-152, miR-410, miR-431and, miR-493, and downregulating the expression of miR-155, miR-20a, miR-25, and miR-15a. These alterations in microRNAs expression were also found in replicative senescence.[35]

Irradiation of rat myocardium downregulated the expression of miR-1, miR-15b; however, it increased the expression of miR-21. Treatment of animals with Enbrel and Tadalafil restored the expression of these microRNAs to the levels of nonirradiated control. Therefore, it was suggested that these heart medications could be useful in mitigating radiation injury.[36]

Irradiation enhanced the expression of miR-34a more in young mice than in adult mice. Upregulated miR-34a reduced the levels of its target antiproapoptotic protein Bc2, and thereby, increased radiosensitivity of cells.[37] Serum level of miR-34a remained stable; therefore, it was suggested that it could be used as a marker of radiation injury. However, this microRNA could be upregulated by other stressors; therefore, it may not be specific to radiation injury,

MicroRNAs IN RADIATION-INDUCED BYSTANDARD EFFECT

Co-culture of unirradiated human fibroblasts (WSI) with alpha-radiation irradiated human keratinocytes (HaCat) revealed that the levels of ROS and DNA damage increased in unirradiated fibroblasts. The expression of miR-21 in bystandard fibroblasts was also enhanced. It was further demonstrated that downregulation of the expression of miR-21 abolished bystandard effects, while upregulation of miR-21 induced bystandard effects in fibroblasts.[38] Irradiation of human fetal lung fibroblasts (MRC-5) enhanced the expression of miR-21 that was detected in the medium that induced bystandard effect in unirradiated fibroblasts.[39] The expression of miR-663 was downregulated and the levels of its target protein TGF-beta1 (transforming growth factor-beta 1) increased in irradiated human fibroblasts, while in bystandard cells, the expression of miR-663 was upregulated and the levels of TGF-beta1 was decreased. The latter limits further transmission of bystandard signals.[40]

MicroRNAs AS BIOMARKERS OF RADIATION DAMAGE

The expression of five radiosensitive microRNAs miR-183-5p, miR-9-3p, miR-200-5p, miR-342-3p, and miR-574-5p showed dose-dependent changes in the serum of mice irradiated with high LET radiation such as carbon-ion, iron-ion, or low LET radiation X-rays. The alterations in the expression of these microRNAs were independent of LET.[41] Radiation therapeutic dose of 50 Gy delivered in fractionated dose of 2 Gy per day, 5 days per week increased the expression of miR-34a in the serum of patient with breast cancer.[42] Since oxidative stress generated by agents other than the ionizing radiation also alters the expression of microRNAs, it is not certain whether changes in the expression of microRNAs can be used as biomarkers specific to radiation doses. Additional studies are needed with appropriate controls to substantial the role of microRNAs as biomarkers of radiation exposure.

BRIEF HISTORY OF RADIATION PROTECTION STUDIES

Efforts to protect normal tissue were started soon after the discovery of X-rays by Dr. Roentgen in 1995. However, it was not until World War II when the search for radioprotective agents began in earnest. Extensive radiobiological research identified numerous agents which, when administered intraperitoneally (IP) shortly before irradiation, protected animals (primarily rodents) against radiation-induced mortality.[4,43,44] Some of these agents, when added prior to irradiation, were also effective in reducing chromosomal aberrations, gene mutations and DNA damage. Most of these agents were ineffective when administered IP after irradiation.

Agents, which reduce radiation damage, have been divided into two groups; radioprotective agents and radiation mitigating agents. Initially, agents, which provided radiation protection only when administered before irradiation, were called radioprotective agents. They were ineffective when administered after irradiation. Agents, which provided radiation protection only when administered after irradiation, were called mitigating agents. This strict differentiation between radioprotective and radiation mitigating agents may not be applicable now. This is due to the fact that long-lived free radicals and toxic products of inflammation contribute to the rate of progression of damage after irradiation. Therefore, in order to maximize the efficacy of any radioprotective agents, administration of these agents before and after irradiation may be necessary.

Most widely studied radioprotective agents include (SH) compounds like cysteamine, cysteamine and aminoethylisothiourea (AET), and a cysteamine analogue, amifostine. They were powerful radioprotective agents against radiation doses that produce bone marrow syndrome in rodents without producing any adverse effects; however, all were considered toxic in humans even at doses one-tenth or less.[4,43,45–48] The primary mechanisms of protection against radiation injury by these agents include scavenging of free radicals and production of hypoxia. The effects of radioprotective agents on inflammation were never investigated.

RADIATION PROTECTION STUDIES WITH ANTIOXIDANTS IN CELL CULTURE MODELS

Several studies revealed that dietary antioxidants such as vitamin A, vitamin E (alpha-tocopheryl acetate and alpha-tocopheryl succinate), vitamin C, selenium, and endogenous antioxidants such as alpha-lipoic acid, N-acetylcysteine, and L-carnitine, which are nontoxic to humans, produced varying degree of radiation protection. It has been shown that alpha-tocopheryl succinate (alpha-TS) and selenium, but not alpha-tocopheryl acetate reduced radiation-induced transformation in mammalian cells in culture; the combination of alpha-TS and selenium was more effective than the individual agents.[49,50] Natural beta-carotene was more effective than the synthetic one in reducing radiation-induced transformation in mammalian cells in culture.[51] Vitamin E (alpha tocopherol and alpha-tocopheryl succinate), vitamin C, and beta-carotene inhibited radiation-induced mutations, chromosomal damage, and lethality in mammalian cells in culture.[52–58] In addition, endogenous antioxidants such as N-acetylcysteine (NAC), a glutathione-elevating agent, attenuated radiation-induced toxicity in mammalian cells in culture.[59] Calcitriol, the hormonally active vitamin D metabolite, protected keratinocytes against radiation-induced caspase-dependent and -independent programmed cell death in mammalian cells in culture.[60]

It was thought earlier that any pharmacological agents couldn't modify the radiation damage produced by high LET radiation, because most of the damage is produced by direct ionization. However, recent studies with antioxidant and space radiation (proton radiation and HZE-particles radiation) revealed that antioxidants could protect against space radiation-induced injury. For example, space radiation induced cytotoxicity in human breast epithelial cells in culture and transformation in human thyroid cells in culture were protected by pre-treatment of these cells with a mixture of soy-derived Bowman-Birk inhibitor (BBI), ascorbic acid, coenzyme Q10, selenomethionine, and alpha-tocopheryl succinate.[61] It has been reported that the treatment of cultured of human thyroid epithelial cells with selenomethionine alone also protected against space radiation-induced increase in oxidative stress, cytotoxicity, and cell transformation, possibly by enhancing DNA repair machinery in irradiated cells.[62] These studies suggest that the early radiobiology concept that the effect of high LET radiation cannot be modified is not valid.

RADIATION PROTECTION STUDIES WITH ANTIOXIDANTS IN ANIMAL MODELS

Using animal models, several studies revealed that a single intraperitoneal (IP) or subcutaneous (SC) administrations of individual dietary or endogenous antioxidants shortly before whole-body gamma-irradiation with high doses enhanced the survival rate in varying degrees in rodents.[63–75] Intraperitoneal administration of vitamin E or L-carnitine before irradiation markedly reduced the risk of cataract in rats.[76,77] Pre-irradiation treatment of rats with vitamin E or L-carnitine alone significantly reduced severity of brain and retinal damage in rats; however, the combination of two did not provide an additive protective effect.[78] It has been reported that IP administration of L-carnitine reduced gamma-radiation-induced cochlear damage in guinea pigs.[79] Vitamin E administered IP before irradiation reduced radiation-induced damage to salivary glands.[80] Pre- or post-irradiation treatment of mice with NAC reduced radiation-induced liver injury.[81]

Melatonin, the chief secretory product of the pineal gland, exhibited strong radioprotective effects both in cell culture and in animal models.[82] Melatonin and vitamin E administered IP before irradiation reduced radiation-induced damage in brain.[83] Melatonin significantly reduced radiation-induced edema, necrosis, and neuronal degeneration, whereas vitamin E reduced only necrosis. The reasons for these differential effects of melatonin and vitamin E are unknown.

The radiation protection studies with antioxidants and high LET radiation performed in mammalian cells in culture were confirmed in animal models. For example, space radiation-induced increase in oxidative stress in mice was reduced by dietary supplementation with Bowman-Birk Inhibitor Concentrate (BBIC), L-selenomethionine, or a combination of N-acetylcysteine, sodium ascorbate, coenzyme Q10, alpha-lipoic acid, L-selenomethionine, and alpha-tocopheryl succinate.[84] Alpha-lipoic acid administered IP before whole-body irradiation significantly attenuated high LET radiation (^{56}Fe-beams)-induced impairment in the reference memory, apoptotic damage in cerebellum, and increased in DNA and markers of oxidative damage.[85]

In addition to standard dietary and endogenous antioxidants, herbal antioxidants when administered IP shortly before high doses of radiation also protected irradiated animals against radiation damage in animal models.[86–90]

A few studies have shown that a mixture of dietary antioxidants administered IP before and after radiation exposure reduced radiation-induced myelosuppression and oxidative stress in rodents.[84,91] They were ineffective when injected after irradiation. An oral administration of antioxidants before or after whole body X-irradiation was ineffective. It was thought that only free radicals generated during radiation exposure contribute to radiation injury; therefore, antioxidants were used only before irradiation.

Administration of manganese superoxide dismutase-plasmid liposome (MnSOD-PL) provided local radiation protection to the lung, esophagus, oral cavity, urinary bladder, and intestine when administered before gamma-irradiation.[92] It is not known whether MnSOD-PL can reduce the risk of late adverse effects of high doses of radiation. The relevance of this observation in humans remains uncertain.

RADIATION PROTECTION STUDY WITH A MIXTURE OF MULTIPLE ANTIOXIDANTS ADMINISTERED ORALLY BEFORE AND AFTER IRRADIATION IN SHEEP

The GI syndrome in sheep appears to be more sensitive than in rodents or humans. A pilot study was performed to evaluate the effects of a mixture of multiple dietary (vitamin A, vitamin C, vitamin E [d-alpha-tocopheryl succinate and d-alpha-tocopheryl acetate]) and selenomethionine, and endogenous antioxidants (NAC, R-alpha-lipoic acid, coenzyme Q10) in sheep, in collaboration with Dr. Jones of NASA, Houston, Dr. Maliev of Russian Academy of Sciences, and Dr. Popov of Canada.

The results showed that a dose of 4.41 Gy produced GI syndrome associated with a mild CNS syndrome in sheep, causing 100% lethality in 7 days, compared to a dose of 7–8 Gy in rodents, and about 6 Gy in humans. An oral administration of the antioxidant mixture daily for 7 days before and daily for 7 days after irradiation increased the survival time of irradiated sheep from 7 to 38 days. To our knowledge this is a first demonstration in which antioxidant treatment before and after irradiation increased the survival time of irradiated animals exhibiting GI syndrome by about 5-fold. It should be noted that these animals received no supportive care such as antibiotic, fluid replacement, or blood transfusion. The exact mechanisms of this high level of radiation protection in irradiated sheep exhibiting GI syndrome remain unknown. However, I suggest that in addition to scavenging free radicals during radiation exposure, the antioxidant mixture administered after irradiation also neutralized radiation-induced long-lived free radicals and reduced inflammation. It remains uncertain whether the continuation of antioxidant treatment after irradiation for a period longer than 7 days would have provided a better radiation protection. It also remains unknown whether the concentration of antioxidants used in this study represented an optimal dose. It is possible that the use of other treatment modalities such as restoration of electrolyte imbalance, blood transfusions, and antibiotic treatment in combination of multiple antioxidants may have increased the survival rate in irradiated sheep. At present, except for bone marrow transplant, no other strategy is available and approved for treating irradiated individuals exhibiting GI syndromes, but nearly all survivors of bone marrow transplants eventually die of host versus graft rejection.

RADIATION PROTECTION STUDY WITH A MIXTURE OF MULTIPLE ANTIOXIDANTS ADMINISTERED ORALLY BEFORE AND AFTER IRRADIATION IN RABBITS

A pilot study was performed to evaluate the effects of a mixture of multiple antioxidants (same as used in sheep) in collaboration with Dr. Jones of NASA, Houston, Dr. Maliev of Russian Academy of Sciences, and Dr. Popov of Canada.

The GI syndrome in rabbits appears to be more sensitive than in sheep. The results showed that a dose of 9.011 Gy produced GI syndrome associated with a CNS syndrome. About 25% of irradiated rabbits died of CNS syndrome within 4 hours; the remaining died within 7 days.

An oral administration of the mixture of antioxidants did not prolong the survival time of irradiated rabbits. This was expected because the dose used to produce GI syndrome was closer to a dose that produced CNS syndrome in a significant number of irradiated animals. However, the necropsy of those irradiated rabbits dying of CNS syndrome showed that damage to the lungs was markedly reduced in the antioxidant treated group in comparison to that observed in the placebo treated group (Figure 19.1).

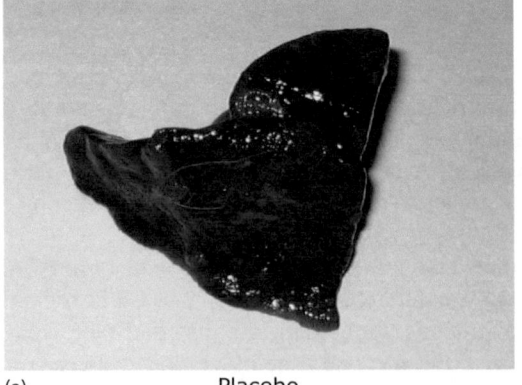
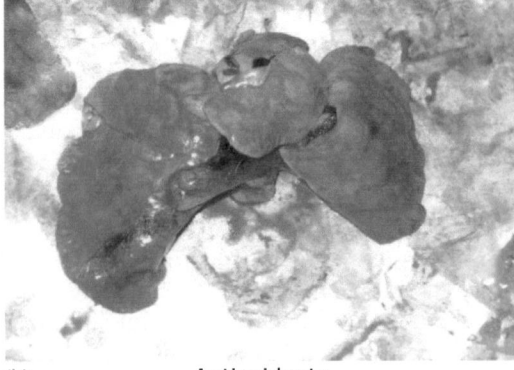

(a)   Placebo   (b)   Antioxidants

FIGURE 19.1 Protection of lung in rabbits exposed to CNS syndrome dose (9.011 Gy) by the mixture of dietary and endogenous antioxidants. The autopsy of irradiated rabbits receiving placebo (and died in 4 hours exhibiting central nervous system syndromes) revealed that lung was necrotic and without a lobular architecture (a), whereas antioxidant treated irradiated rabbits showed minimal pulmonary hemorrhage while maintaining the lobular architecture of the lung (b). This level of protection has never been achieved by any pharmacological or biological agents (unpublished observation, in collaboration with Drs. Jones of NASA, Houston, TX, and Maliev of Russian Academy of Sciences).

RADIATION PROTECTION STUDY WITH A MIXTURE OF MULTIPLE ANTIOXIDANTS ADMINISTERED ORALLY BEFORE IRRADIATION IN MICE

A pilot study was performed at the Armed Forces of Radiobiology Research Institute (AFRRI) to evaluate the effects of a mixture of multiple antioxidants (same as used in sheep) in mice. The results showed that a dose of 8.5 Gy produced bone marrow syndrome with a 100% lethality in 30 days. An oral administration of the antioxidant mixture daily for 7 days or 24 hours before whole-body gamma-irradiation increased the survival rate of irradiated animals from 0% to 40% (Table 19.3). Placebo treatment of irradiated mice was ineffective. To our knowledge, this level of protection has not been achieved by an oral administration of a single antioxidant or its derivatives before whole-body gamma-irradiation with a dose that produced bone marrow syndrome with a 100% mortality.

The results also revealed that placebo containing cellulose and dextrose administered orally exhibited radioprotective effect in mice at lower doses of radiation that is similar to that produced by the antioxidant mixture (data not shown). Thus, our initial assumption that the placebo used in this study was inert was found to be incorrect. It is interesting to point out that certain polysaccharides when administered IP shortly before whole-body irradiation have been reported to be of some radioprotective value in irradiated mice.[93–95] Therefore, it is not surprising that a mixture of cellulose and dextrose provided some degree of protection at lower doses; however, the protective effect of placebo was not observed at higher radiation doses in mice. In contrast to the observation made in mice, placebo treatment was totally ineffective in irradiated sheep and rabbits.

Additional approaches for radiation protection are being developed including vaccine,[96] anti-apoptotic peptides[97] and hormone derivative.[98] These approaches will require FDA approval before use in humans, because of their potential toxicity. Until then, the use of multiple dietary and endogenous antioxidants remains one of the best choices for protection against radiation injury in humans.

TABLE 19.3

Effect of an Antioxidant Mixture or Placebo Administered Orally at a Dose of 222.5 mg/kg of Body Weight 7 Days before Various Doses of Whole-Body Gamma-Irradiation on Survival in Mice

Agents	Dose (Gy)	% Survival
Placebo	7.5	90
Antioxidant mixture	7.5	80
Placebo	8	30
Antioxidant mixture	8	60
Placebo	8.5	0
Antioxidant mixture	8.5	40
Placebo	9.0	0
Antioxidant mixture	9.0	0
Placebo	9.25	0
Antioxidant mixture	9.25	0

Source: Antioxidant mixture contained neither microcrystalline cellulose nor dextrose, but it contained about 11% silica by weight. Doses administered orally to animals 7 days before irradiation were corrected for the presence of 11% silica. Each group contained 10 animals.

Based on the results of our present study and those published by others, and based on the fact that antioxidants neutralize free radicals and reduce inflammation that contribute to the progression of radiation damage, it is possible to develop formulations of micronutrients containing both dietary and endogenous antioxidants for reducing radiation damage produced by high doses of ionizing radiation in humans. Such formulations would be considered safe in humans.

RADIATION PROTECTION STUDY WITH A MIXTURE OF MULTIPLE ANTIOXIDANTS ADMINISTERED THROUGH THE DIET BEFORE AND AFTER IRRADIATION IN *DROSOPHILA MELANOGASTER*

A pilot study was performed to evaluate the effects of a mixture of multiple antioxidants (same as used in sheep) in collaboration with Dr. Sharmila Bhattacharya of NASA, Moffat Field, CA, on proton radiation-induced cancer in *Drosophila melanogaster* (fruit fly).

The female flies carrying mutant HOP (TUM-1) become very sensitive to develop leukemia-like cancer. Dietary supplementation with the antioxidant mixture 7 days daily before and for the entire observation period after irradiation prevented proton radiation-induced cancer in female fruit flies carrying mutant HOP (TUM-1). It is impossible to extrapolate data obtained from fruit flies to humans. However, the possibility exists that daily supplementation with a mixture of antioxidants may reduce the risk of cancer among survivors of high doses of radiation.

RADIATION PROTECTION STUDIES WITH ANTIOXIDANTS IN HUMANS

Direct radiation protection studies with antioxidants cannot be performed in humans for obvious reasons. The limited data on this issue primarily come from experiences of patients and radiation oncologists during radiation therapy of cancer or individuals exposed to high dose of radiation following an accident in nuclear plants. Administration of beta-carotene orally reduced the severity of radiation-induced mucositis during radiation therapy of the head and neck cancer.[99] A combination of dietary antioxidants was more effective in protecting normal tissue during radiation therapy than the individual agents.[100,101] Vitamin A and NAC may be effective against radiation-induced cancer.[102] Alpha-lipoic acid treatment alone for 28 days lowered lipid peroxidation among children chronically exposed to low doses of radiation daily in the area of contaminated by the Chernobyl nuclear accident.[103] In another study, supplementation with beta-carotene alone reduced cellular damage in the above population of children.[104] A combination of vitamin E and alpha-lipoic acid was more effective than the individual agents.[103] These studies strongly suggest that dietary and endogenous antioxidants can be of radioprotective value in humans.

RATIONALE FOR USING MULTIPLE ANTIOXIDANTS IN RADIATION PROTECTION

Some potentials rationales are described here:

1. Antioxidants show differential subcellular distribution and different mechanisms of action; therefore, a single antioxidant cannot protect all parts of the cell.
2. The body protects against oxidative damage by elevating antioxidant enzymes, and dietary and endogenous antioxidants; antioxidants neutralize free radicals by donating electrons to those molecules with unpaired electron, whereas antioxidant enzymes destroy free radicals by catalysis, converting them to harmless molecules such as water and oxygen. A single antioxidant cannot elevate both parts of antioxidant defense system.
3. The affinity of different antioxidants for free radicals differs, depending upon their solubility. For example, beta-carotene (BC) is more effective in quenching oxygen radicals than most other antioxidants.[105]

4. Both the aqueous and lipid compartments of the cell need to be protected together. Water-soluble antioxidants such as vitamin C and glutathione protect molecules in the aqueous environment of the cells, whereas lipid soluble antioxidants such as vitamin A and vitamin E protect molecules in the lipid compartment.

5. Vitamin E is more effective in quenching free radicals in a reduced oxygenated cellular environment, whereas vitamin A and beta-carotene (BC) are more effective in a higher oxygenated environment of the cells.[106]

6. BC can perform certain biological functions that cannot be produced by its metabolite vitamin A, and vice versa.[107,108] It has been reported that BC treatment enhances the expression of the connexin gene, which codes for a gap junction protein in mammalian fibroblasts in culture, whereas vitamin A treatment does not produce such an effect.[108] Vitamin A can induce differentiation in certain normal and cancer cells, whereas BC and other carotenoids do not.[109,110] Thus BC and vitamin A exhibit in part, different biological functions.

7. Vitamin C is important for recycling the oxidized form of alpha-tocopherol to the antioxidant form.[111]

8. Antioxidants produce cell protective proteins by altering the expression of different microRNAs.[1] For example, some antioxidants can activate Nrf2 by upregulating miR-200a that inhibits its target protein Keap1, whereas others activate Nrf2 by downregulating miR-21 that binds with 3′-UTR Nrf2 mRNA.[112]

9. D-alpha-tocopheryl succinate (alpha-TS) is the most effective form of vitamin E both in vitro and in vivo.[113,114] This form of vitamin E is more soluble than alpha-tocopherol and enters cells more easily than alpha-tocopherol. Alpha-TS is a powerful radioprotective agent in vitro and in vivo.[49,115]

10. Glutathione is effective in catabolizing H_2O_2 and anions. However, an oral supplementation with glutathione failed to significantly increase plasma levels of glutathione in human subjects,[116] suggesting that this tripeptide is completely hydrolyzed in the GI tract. Therefore, N-acetylcysteine and alpha-lipoic acid that increase the cellular levels of glutathione by different mechanisms should be added to a multiple micronutrient preparation.

    Other endogenous antioxidants, coenzyme Q_{10}, may also have some potential value in radiation protection.

11. Selenium is a cofactor of glutathione peroxidase, and Se-glutathione peroxidase increases the intracellular level of glutathione that is a powerful antioxidant and protects against radiation injury.

The use of a single antioxidant is not expected to produce optimal radiation protection against oxidative stress and inflammatory events, which contribute to radiation injury. For this reason, it is proposed that an elevation of the levels of antioxidant enzymes and dietary and endogenous antioxidants may be essential for simultaneously reducing oxidative stress and inflammation. Oral supplementation can increase the levels of dietary and endogenous antioxidants; however, elevation of the levels of antioxidant enzymes requires an activation of Nrf2. Therefore it is essential to understand the regulation of activation of Nrf2.

ACTIVATION OF Nrf2 (NUCLEAR FACTOR-ERYTHROID-2-RELATED FACTOR 2)

Nrf2

The nuclear transcriptional factor, Nrf2 (nuclear factor-erythroid-2-related factor 2) belongs to the Cap "n" Collar (CNC) family that contains a conserved basic leucine zipper (bZIP) transcriptional factor.[117] Under physiological condition, Nrf2 is associated with Kelch-like ECH associated protein 1 (Keap1), which acts as an inhibitor of Nrf2.[118] Keap1 protein serves as an adaptor to link Nrf2 to the ubiquitin ligase CuI-Rbx1 complex for degradation by proteasomes and maintains the steady levels of Nrf2 in the cytoplasm. Nrf2-keap1 complex is primarily located in the cytoplasm; Keap1 acts as a sensor for ROS/electrophilic stress.

ACTIVATION OF Nrf2 DURING ACUTE OXIDATIVE STRESS

During acute oxidative stress, ROS is needed to activate Nrf2 which then dissociates itself from Keap1-CuI-Rbx1 complex and translocates in the nucleus where it heterodimerizes with a small Maf protein, binds with ARE leading to increased expression of target genes coding for several cytoprotective enzymes including antioxidant enzymes.[119–121]

ACTIVATION OF Nrf2 DURING ACUTE PHASE OF IRRADIATION

Exposure to high doses of radiation generates excessive amounts of ROS during and soon after irradiation; therefore, activation of Nrf2 as a protective response is expected. Indeed, irradiation of mammalian cells activates Nrf2.[122] If the dose is high, it can overtake protective response of Nrf2 that can lead to lethality. However treatment of cells with the activators of Nf2 before irradiation would protect against radiation damage. This was demonstrated by an experiment in which treatment of human skin fibroblasts with an activator of Nrf2 (sulforaphane) before irradiation reduced radiation damage.[123]

FAILURE TO ACTIVATE Nrf2 DURING RADIATION-INDUCED CHRONIC PHASE OF IRRADIATION

During chronic oxidative stress, Nrf2 becomes resistant to ROS,[124–126] suggesting that activation of Nrf2 by a ROS-independent mechanism exists. This is evidenced by the fact that increased chronic oxidative stress occurs despite the presence of Nrf2 in chemical-induced cancer (see Chapter 7) in other chronic diseases.[127] No studies have been performed on the levels of Nrf2 during expression of late effects in survivors of high doses of radiation. However, increased oxidative stress occurs during chronic phase of irradiation.[128,129] This implies that Nrf2 became resistant to ROS during expression of late effects of radiation. The question arises as to how to activate ROS-resistant Nrf2 during progression of radiation injury.

ANTIOXIDANTS ACTIVATE ROS-RESISTANT Nrf2

Some examples are vitamin E and genistein,[130] alpha-lipoic acid,[131] curcumin,[132] resveratrol,[133,134] omega-3-fatty acids,[135,136] glutathione,[137] NAC,[138] and coenzyme Q10.[139] Several plant-derived phytochemicals, such as epigallocatechin-3-gallate, carestol, kahweol, cinnamonyl-based compounds, zerumbone, lycopene and carnosol,[117,140,141] genistein,[130] allicin, a major organosulfur compound found in garlic,[142] sulforaphane, a organosulfur compound, found in cruciferous vegetables,[143] and kavalactones (methysticin, kavain, and yangonin).[144] The reasons for the activation of Nrf2 without ROS by antioxidant compounds are not known.

BINDING OF Nrf2 WITH ARE IN THE NUCLEUS

An activation of Nrf2 alone is not sufficient to increase the levels of antioxidant enzymes. Activated Nrf2 must bind with ARE in the nucleus for increasing the expression of target genes coding for antioxidant enzymes. This binding ability of Nrf2 with ARE was impaired in aged rats and this defect was restored by supplementation with alpha-lipoic acid.[131] It is unknown whether the binding ability of Nrf2 with ARE is impaired during progression of radiation injury.

REDUCING OXIDATIVE STRESS LEVEL FOR RADIATION PROTECTION

Activation of Nrf2 may not be sufficient to optimally reduce oxidative stress, because antioxidant compounds are also decreased during chronic oxidative stress[145–147]; therefore, their levels must also be simultaneously elevated.

REDUCING INFLAMMATION LEVEL FOR RADIATION PROTECTION

Activation of Nrf2[148,149] and some individual antioxidant compounds reduced chronic inflammation.[7,150–155]

PROPOSED MICRONUTRIENTS FOR RADIATION PROTECTION

A comprehensive micronutrient mixture containing multiple dietary antioxidant compounds (vitamin A, natural mixed carotenoids, vitamin C, vitamin E succinate, vitamin E acetate, curcumin, resveratrol, and mineral selenomethionine), endogenous antioxidants (alpha-lipoic acid, L-carnitine, and coenzyme Q10), a synthetic antioxidant N-acetylcysteine (NAC), omega-3-fatty acids, vitamin D3, zinc, and all B-vitamins is proposed. This mixture of micronutrients may optimally reduce oxidative stress and chronic inflammation by simultaneously enhancing the levels of antioxidant enzymes through activation of the Nrf2/ARE pathway, and elevating the levels of antioxidants. This mixture when administered before and after irradiation may provide optimal radiation protection against lethal doses of radiation. No iron, copper, or manganese would be included because these trace minerals are known to interact with vitamin C to produce free radicals. These trace minerals are absorbed from the intestinal tract more in the presence of antioxidants than in their absence that could results in increased body stores of these minerals. Increased iron stores have been linked to increased risk of several chronic diseases. The micronutrient for reducing acute effects of high doses of radiation should be administered twice a day (morning and evening with meal, if possible) as soon as possible after radiation exposure, and continued throughout the observation period of at least 60 days, and then switch to micronutrient formulation for reducing the late adverse effects for the entire lifespan.

GUIDELINES FOR THE MANAGEMENT OF LARGE NUMBER OF PEOPLE IRRADIATED WITH LETHAL DOSES OF RADIATION

In the events of terrorist attack by nuclear devices, unintended nuclear conflicts, or accidents in a nuclear plant, physicians, radiation physicists, radiation biologists, nurses, and other health-care professionals and their private or public hospitals will assume responsibility of treating individuals exposed to high doses of radiation. Under the above scenarios, radiation exposures may result in a few to mass casualties. In order to provide a guideline for the management of large number radiation exposed individuals, the Strategic National Stockpile Radiation Working Group developed a consensus document.[156,157] This document recommends that individual radiation dose is estimated by determining the time of onset and severity of nausea, vomiting, decline in peripheral lymphocyte counts over several hours or days after irradiation, and appearance of chromosomal aberrations (including dicentrics and ring forms) in peripheral blood lymphocytes. In addition, documentation of clinical signs and symptoms characteristics of bone marrow syndrome, GI syndrome, and CNS syndrome or skin responses over time is essential in order to provide a rational basis for the selection therapeutic agents and expected prognosis of the exposed individuals. The potential therapeutic agents may include replacement therapy (antibiotics, and transfusion of blood and electrolytes when indicated), which is most suitable for treating individuals exposed to doses that produce bone marrow syndrome. However, for those individuals who are exposed to doses that produce GI syndrome, additional agents such as certain cytokines, bone marrow or stem cells transplant should be administered. The explosion of nuclear devices containing radioactive iodine, immediate supplementation with potassium iodide may be necessary. The administration of potassium iodide will not be effective if taken several hours after exposure to radioactive Iodine. It is also not affective against other radioactive isotopes.

RADIATION MITIGATING AGENTS

The radiation mitigating agents can be grouped into two broad categories: (1) chemical agents and (2) biological agents.

CHEMICAL AGENTS FOR MITIGATING RADIATION INJURY

ANTIBIOTICS, BLOOD, AND ELECTROLYTES

The effectiveness of antibiotics in protecting against high doses of radiation that produce bone marrow syndrome is observed only when infection is present after irradiation. This is due to the fact that infection is the major cause of death in irradiated animals dying of bone marrow syndrome. In addition, loss of electrolytes and depletion of platelets and leukocytes occur after irradiation; therefore, transfusion with electrolytes and blood when indicated becomes necessary to prevent the irradiated individuals from dying of bone marrow syndrome. They are ineffective in reducing mortality in irradiated animals or humans exposed to doses that cause GI syndrome.

ERYTHROPOIETIN

The survival of mice irradiated whole-body with a dose of 10 Gy increased from 0% to 40% when erythropoietin administered after irradiation.[158] The DRF value of erythropoietin dose (10 units) injected 1 hour after whole-body irradiation with a dose of 6.51 Gy is 1.12.[159] The efficacy of erythropoietin in irradiated individual has not been evaluated, but it is an FDA-approved drug that is used in certain human diseases to boost hemoglobin levels; therefore, it can be used as a radiation therapeutic agent in humans.

STATINS

Statins are commonly used to lower cholesterol levels in humans. They exhibit both antioxidant and anti-inflammatory activities; therefore, it is expected that they will be of some radioprotective value. Indeed, pravastatin administered through drinking water daily 3 days before and 14 days after irradiation of surgically exteriorized small intestine with a dose of 19 Gy protected intestinal injury, but it did not protect tumor cells in culture against radiation injury.[160] Pravastatin also reduced radiation-induce skin lesions in mice when administered daily for 28 days.[161] The efficacy of statins in treating radiation exposed individuals remains uncertain. It is very interesting to note that they mimic the effects of antioxidants in reducing radiation injury. These statins are FDA approved drugs; and therefore, can be used in the short-term management of radiation injury in humans.

CYTOKINES AND GROWTH FACTORS

Interleukin-4 (IL-4) injected once or for 5 consecutive days 2 hours after whole-body irradiation of mice with doses of 7–10 Gy increased the survival of irradiated animals in the presence of poor recovery of hematopoietic system.[162] The cytokines IL-4 and IL-13 appear to have pleiotropic effects affecting both pathological changes and tissue remodeling. Comparing the effects of IL-13 Ralpha2

(IL-13 receptor alpha2) in irradiated wild-type mice and IL-4 receptor alpha gene deficient mice revealed that IL-13Ralpha2 plays a major role in regeneration of epithelial cells after irradiation.[163]

Pre- or post-irradiation of mice treated with recombinant murine (rM) colony-stimulating factor-granulocyte-macrophage (CSF-gm) or recombinant human (rh) CSF-granulocyte reduced radiation damage. These growth factors were injected 20 hours before irradiation or soon after irradiation.[164] The efficacy of recombinant human interleukin-3 (rhIL-3) and granulocyte-macrophage colony-stimulating factor (GM-CSF) on the peripheral lymphocytes of rhesus monkey after whole-body irradiation with a dose of 3 Gy gamma-radiation was evaluated. The results showed that GM-CSF alone or GM-CSF + rhIL-3 reduced radiation-induced apoptosis in peripheral lymphocytes. The combination was more effective than the individual agents.[165] Acidic or basic fibroblast factor (FGF-1 or FGF-2) injected intravenously 24 hours before or 1 hour after whole-body irradiation with a dose of 7–18 Gy reduced radiation-induced apoptosis in crypt stem cells of intestine of mice.[166] These growth factors can be used in the management of radiation injury associated with GI syndrome in humans.

BIOLOGICAL AGENTS FOR MITIGATING RADIATION INJURY

BONE MARROW AND NEWBORN LIVER CELLS TRANSPLANT

Bone marrow transplant is often administered intravenously to irradiated individuals exposed to doses of radiation that produce GI syndrome, because replacement therapy is not effective in increasing the survival of irradiated individuals. On the other hand, bone marrow transplantation can save many irradiated individuals dying from GI syndrome; however, these individuals die within a few years because of host versus graft rejection events.

A recent study has revealed that transplantation of newborn liver cells (as a source of hematopoietic stem cells) plus new born thymus markedly improved the survival rate of mice irradiated with a dose that produced GI syndrome.[167] The relevance of this observation in the treatment of irradiated individuals remains uncertain.

THE CHERNOBYL EXPERIENCE IN TREATING IRRADIATED INDIVIDUALS

On April 26, 1986, the world's most serious nuclear accident occurred at the Chernobyl nuclear power station in the former Soviet Union, releasing excessive amounts of radioactive substances into the atmosphere.[168] The care and treatment of individuals receiving high doses of radiation has been discussed in a book.[169] The medical response to this emergency involved 5 phases: assessment/containment, reduction of radiation exposure, estimation of dose to individuals, and treatment of irradiated individuals.

Assessments were made on important parameters such as amount and type of radioactive released. Measures to contain the spread of radioactivity were carried out. To limit the radiation exposure to individuals located near the reactor, massive evacuations were conducted. Within 36 hours of the accident, 45,000 persons were evacuated, and 2 weeks later, 90,000 additional individuals were evacuated.

In order to reduce the dose to exposed individual, exposed persons are thoroughly washed. In the event of exposure to radioactive ^{131}Iodine, a dose of potassium iodide is recommended as soon as possible in order to block the uptake of ^{131}Iodine by the thyroid gland. An oral administration of potassium iodide 2 hours after exposure to ^{131}I will reduce the uptake by the gland by 80%, and 6 hours after, by about 30%.[170]

After ingestion of $^{3}H_2O$ (radioactive water), most of the radioactivity can be removed from the body in a few days by excessive drinking of cold water; however, if ^{3}H were present as ^{3}H-thymidine that incorporated into DNA, the above treatment would be useless. Chelating agents can remove certain radioactive metals by binding with them, but they could be toxic in humans if not properly monitored.

Physical dosimeter, such as the use of individual radiation meters or film badges, was of limited value at Chernobyl, because the monitoring devices were either unrecoverable or destroyed by the high radiation doses. Biological dosimeter proved more effective at providing information on exposure levels, but demanded enormous amounts of medical and technical expertise and resources. Furthermore, there were limitations to the accuracy of the doses because of thermal and chemical injuries that have an impact on biological damage.[171]

About 200 people were exposed to large doses of whole-body radiation. One hundred and five received about 1–2 Gy or more; 33 received less than 6 Gy; and 10 received 6 Gy or more. Thirteen persons received dose of 5.6–13.4 Gy that produced GI syndrome received bone marrow transplant.[171] Two transplanted patients who received an estimated dose of 5.6 and 8.7 Gy were surviving 3 years after the accident. Six irradiated patients received fetal liver transplant. Most died in about 3 months, and two patients who survived 3 years also died primarily due to host versus graft rejection.

The studies discussed above suggest that the current treatment of irradiated patients exposed to doses that produce GI syndrome is not effective; therefore, additional approaches should be developed.

PROPOSED MICRONUTRIENT MIXTURE FOR THE TREATMENT OF BONE MARROW SYNDROME

The persons exposed to doses that produce bone marrow syndrome should be treated like any other hematologic disorders. Although treatment with replacement therapy (blood transfusion and antibiotics when indicated) can save all 50% of exposed individual who otherwise will die,[172,173] this treatment may not protect survivors from late adverse-health effects. In addition, the requirements of antibiotic and blood transfusion per individual are so great that only a few individuals can be treated in any one medical institution. Supplementation with the proposed micronutrient mixture may reduce mortality, and in combination with replacement therapy, may improve survival rates more than produced by replacement therapy alone. Micronutrient mixture can be administered orally before and after irradiation for 30 days in rodents and 60 days for humans, while continued supplement with micronutrients may reduce the late adverse effects of high dose radiation. No studies have been conducted to investigate these possibilities.

PROPOSED MICRONUTRIENT MIXTURE FOR THE TREATMENT OF GI SYNDROME

The replacement therapy that includes administration of antibiotics, transfusion blood, and electrolyte when indicated can increase the survival time of irradiated individuals by about 2-fold, from 14 to 28 days in humans. Only bone marrow transplant can save the irradiated individuals dying from the GI syndrome, but all die later because of host versus graft reactions. Supplementation with the proposed micronutrient mixture may reduce mortality, and in combination with replacement therapy, may improve survival rates. Micronutrient mixture can be administers orally before and after irradiation for 30 days, if rodents survive 3.5 days, and in case of humans for 60 days if they survive 14 days. No studies have been performed to test this possibility.

CONCLUSIONS

High doses of ionizing radiation cause extensive damage to organ systems including lethality, depending upon the total dose, dose-rate, modes of delivery (single dose versus fractionated dose), and surface area irradiated (whole-body versus partial body). High LET (linear energy transfer) radiation (proton, neutron, alpha-particles and other heavy particles radiation) is 5–20 times more effective than the low LET radiation (X-rays and gamma-rays). In humans, the $^{60}LD_{50}$

(dose producing 50% mortality in 60 days) for bone marrow syndrome is about 3 Gy. The $^{7}LD_{100}$ (dose producing 100% mortality in 7 days) for gastrointestinal (GI) syndrome is 6 Gy. The CNS syndrome is produced by doses 50 Gy or more and 100% mortality occur within 24 hours. Irradiation of mammalian cells alters the expression of microRNAs that allow the translation of proapoptotic proteins from their respective mRNAs. Irradiation also activates Nrf2 by ROS generated during irradiation, which is a protective response. Nrf2 becomes resistant to ROS during chronic oxidative stress that occurs as a late effect of radiation. Several antioxidants and phytochemicals activate ROS-resistant Nrf2. Numerous radioprotective agents have been identified utilizing cell culture, animal, and human models, but except for antioxidants, all are found to be toxic in humans. The previous radiation protection studies with individual antioxidants in animal models have utilized primarily intraperitoneal (IP) route of administration, and occasionally, subcutaneous (SC) route. These routes of administration are not relevance to humans. In most previous radiation protection studies, individual antioxidant was administered only before irradiation. In view of the fact that irradiation of cells produces long-lived free radicals, treatment with antioxidants before and after irradiation becomes necessary in order to produce an optimal protection. Using a mixture of micronutrient formulation containing dietary and endogenous antioxidants, we have demonstrated that oral administration of antioxidants before irradiation increased the survival time of gamma-irradiated sheep exposed to GI syndrome dose form 7 to 38 days without any other therapeutic intervention. The same mixture of antioxidants administered orally 7 days before irradiation protected lung of irradiated rabbits, which died of CNS syndrome within 4 hours. The same mixture of antioxidants administered orally 7 days before irradiation increased the survival of irradiated rats exposed to doses that produce bone marrow syndrome from 0%–40% without any other therapeutic intervention. Except for replacement therapy (antibiotics, transfusion of blood, and electrolyte, when indicated), most other approaches are not effective in increasing the survival rate of animals irradiated with high doses of radiation that can produce GI syndrome. Transplantations with bone marrow or hematopoietic stem cells are effective in improving the survival rate of individuals exposed to doses of radiation that produce GI syndrome, but all later die because of host versus graft rejection events. I have proposed a mixture of micronutrients when administered orally before and after irradiation may protect against high doses of irradiation. This micronutrient mixture in combination with the replacement therapy may increase the survival rates of lethally irradiated animals or humans more than that produced by replacement therapy alone. This micronutrient mixture also may reduce the risk of developing neoplastic and non-neoplastic diseases when consumed daily for the entire lifetime.

REFERENCES

1. Prasad KN. Oxidative stress and pro-inflammatory cytokines may act as one of signals for regulating microRNAs expression in Alzheimer'sdisease. *Mech Ageing Dev*. 2017;162:63–71.
2. Weiss JF, Landauer MR. Radioprotection by antioxidants. *Ann N Y Acad Sci*. 2000;899:44–60.
3. Prasad KN. *Prevention and Mitigation of Acute Radiation Sickness (ARS)*. Boca Raton, FL: CRC Press; 2012.
4. Prasad K. *Handbook of Radiobiology, Second Edition*. Boca Rotan, FL: CRC Press; 1995.
5. Kumagai J, Masui K, Itagaki Y, et al. Long-lived mutagenic radicals induced in mammalian cells by ionizing radiation are mainly localized to proteins. *Radiat Res*. 2003;160(1):95–102.
6. Waldren CA, Vannais DB, Ueno AM. A role for long-lived radicals (LLR) in radiation-induced mutation and persistent chromosomal instability: counteraction by ascorbate and RibCys but not DMSO. *Mutat Res*. 2004;551(1–2):255–265.
7. Abate A, Yang G, Dennery PA, Oberle S, Schroder H. Synergistic inhibition of cyclooxygenase-2 expression by vitamin E and aspirin. *Free Radic Biol Med*. 2000;29(11):1135–1142.
8. Fedorocko P, Egyed A, Vacek A. Irradiation induces increased production of haemopoietic and proinflammatory cytokines in the mouse lung. *Int J Radiat Biol*. 2002;78(4):305–313.
9. Mizutani N, Fujikura Y, Wang YH, et al. Inflammatory and anti-inflammatory cytokines regulate the recovery from sublethal X-irradiation in rat thymus. *Radiat Res*. 2002;157(3):281–289.

10. Popp W, Plappert U, Muller WU, et al. Biomarkers of genetic damage and inflammation in blood and bronchoalveolar lavage fluid among former German uranium miners: A pilot study. *Radiat Environ Biophys*. 2000;39(4):275–282.

11. Demidchik YE, Saenko VA, Yamashita S. Childhood thyroid cancer in Belarus, Russia, and Ukraine after Chernobyl and at present. *Arq Bras Endocrinol Metabol*. 2007;51(5):748–762.

12. Neglia JP, Robison LL, Stovall M, et al. New primary neoplasms of the central nervous system in survivors of childhood cancer: A report from the Childhood Cancer Survivor Study. *J Natl Cancer Inst*. 2006;98(21):1528–1537.

13. Henderson TO, Whitton J, Stovall M, et al. Secondary sarcomas in childhood cancer survivors: A report from the Childhood Cancer Survivor Study. *J Natl Cancer Inst*. 2007;99(4):300–308.

14. Meadows AT, Friedman DL, Neglia JP, et al. Second neoplasms in survivors of childhood cancer: Findings from the Childhood Cancer Survivor Study cohort. *J Clin Oncol*. 2009;27(14):2356–2362.

15. Bartal AH, Cohen Y, Robinson E. Malignant melanoma arising at tattoo sites used for radiotherapy field marking. *Br J Radiol*. 1980;53(633):913–914.

16. Stillman RJ, Schinfeld JS, Schiff I, et al. Ovarian failure in long-term survivors of childhood malignancy. *Am J Obstet Gynecol*. 1981;139(1):62–66.

17. Sherins RJ, Olweny CL, Ziegler JL. Gynecomastia and gonadal dysfunction in adolescent boys treated with combination chemotherapy for Hodgkin's disease. *N Engl J Med*. 1978;299(1):12–16.

18. Rubin P, Casarett GW. *Clinical Radiation Pathology*. Philadelphia, PA: W.B. Saunder; 1968.

19. Lee RC, Feinbaum RL, Ambros V. The C. elegans heterochronic gene lin-4 encodes small RNAs with antisense complementarity to lin-14. *Cell*. 1993;75(5):843–854.

20. Wightman B, Ha I, Ruvkun G. Posttranscriptional regulation of the heterochronic gene lin-14 by lin-4 mediates temporal pattern formation in C. elegans. *Cell*. 1993;75(5):855–862.

21. Macfarlane LA, Murphy PR. MicroRNA: Biogenesis, function and role in cancer. *Curr Genomics*. 2010;11(7):537–561.

22. Londin E, Loher P, Telonis AG, et al. Analysis of 13 cell types reveals evidence for the expression of numerous novel primate- and tissue-specific microRNAs. *Proc Natl Acad Sci U S A*. 2015;112(10):E1106–E1115.

23. Denli AM, Tops BB, Plasterk RH, Ketting RF, Hannon GJ. Processing of primary microRNAs by the Microprocessor complex. *Nature*. 2004;432(7014):231–235.

24. Lee Y, Ahn C, Han J, et al. The nuclear RNase III Drosha initiates microRNA processing. *Nature*. 2003;425(6956):415–419.

25. Hutvagner G, McLachlan J, Pasquinelli AE, Balint E, Tuschl T, Zamore PD. A cellular function for the RNA-interference enzyme Dicer in the maturation of the let-7 small temporal RNA. *Science*. 2001;293(5531):834–838.

26. Cha HJ, Shin S, Yoo H, et al. Identification of ionizing radiation-responsive microRNAs in the IM9 human B lymphoblastic cell line. *Int J Oncol*. 2009;34(6):1661–1668.

27. Mao A, Liu Y, Zhang H, Di C, Sun C. MicroRNA expression and biogenesis in cellular response to ionizing radiation. *DNA Cell Biol*. 2014;33(10):667–679.

28. Li XH, Ha CT, Fu D, Landauer MR, Ghosh SP, Xiao M. Delta-tocotrienol suppresses radiation-induced microRNA-30 and protects mice and human CD34+ cells from radiation injury. *PLoS One*. 2015;10(3):e0122258.

29. Li XH, Ha CT, Fu D, Xiao M. Micro-RNA30c negatively regulates REDD1 expression in human hematopoietic and osteoblast cells after gamma-irradiation. *PLoS One*. 2012;7(11):e48700.

30. Duru N, Gernapudi R, Zhang Y, et al. NRF2/miR-140 signaling confers radioprotection to human lung fibroblasts. *Cancer Lett*. 2015;369(1):184–191.

31. Gorrini C, Baniasadi PS, Harris IS, et al. BRCA1 interacts with Nrf2 to regulate antioxidant signaling and cell survival. *J Exp Med*. 2013;210(8):1529–1544.

32. Kraemer A, Barjaktarovic Z, Sarioglu H, et al. Cell survival following radiation exposure requires miR-525-3p mediated suppression of ARRB1 and TXN1. *PLoS One*. 2013;8(10):e77484.

33. Wagner-Ecker M, Schwager C, Wirkner U, Abdollahi A, Huber PE. MicroRNA expression after ionizing radiation in human endothelial cells. *Radiat Oncol*. 2010;5:25.

34. Zhang S, Wang W, Gu Q, et al. Protein and miRNA profiling of radiation-induced skin injury in rats: The protective role of peroxiredoxin-6 against ionizing radiation. *Free Radic Biol Med*. 2014;69:96–107.

35. Wang Y, Scheiber MN, Neumann C, Calin GA, Zhou D. MicroRNA regulation of ionizing radiation-induced premature senescence. *Int J Radiat Oncol Biol Phys*. 2011;81(3):839–848.

36. Kura B, Yin C, Frimmel K, et al. Changes of microRNA-1, -15b and -21 levels in irradiated rat hearts after treatment with potentially radioprotective drugs. *Physiol Res.* 2016;65 Suppl 1:S129–S137.

37. Liu C, Zhou C, Gao F, et al. MiR-34a in age and tissue related radio-sensitivity and serum miR-34a as a novel indicator of radiation injury. *Int J Biol Sci.* 2011;7(2):221–233.

38. Tian W, Yin X, Wang L, et al. The key role of miR-21-regulated SOD2 in the medium-mediated bystander responses in human fibroblasts induced by alpha-irradiated keratinocytes. *Mutat Res.* 2015;780:77–85.

39. Xu S, Ding N, Pei H, et al. MiR-21 is involved in radiation-induced bystander effects. *RNA Biol.* 2014;11(9):1161–1170.

40. Hu W, Xu S, Yao B, et al. MiR-663 inhibits radiation-induced bystander effects by targeting TGFB1 in a feedback mode. *RNA Biol.* 2014;11(9):1189–1198.

41. Wei W, He J, Wang J, et al. Serum microRNAs as early indicators for estimation of exposure degree in response to ionizing irradiation. *Radiat Res.* 2017;188(3):342–354.

42. Halimi M, Shahabi A, Moslemi D, et al. Human serum miR-34a as an indicator of exposure to ionizing radiation. *Radiat Environ Biophys.* 2016;55(4):423–429.

43. Thomson J. *Radiation Protection in Mammals.* New York: Reinhold; 1962.

44. Weiss JF, Landauer MR. History and development of radiation-protective agents. *Int J Radiat Biol.* 2009;85(7):539–573.

45. Capizzi RL, Oster W. Chemoprotective and radioprotective effects of amifostine: An update of clinical trials. *Int J Hematol.* 2000;72(4):425–435.

46. Allalunis-Turner MJ, Walden TL, Jr., Sawich C. Induction of marrow hypoxia by radioprotective agents. *Radiat Res.* 1989;118(3):581–586.

47. Anne PR. Phase II trial of subcutaneous amifostine in patients undergoing radiation therapy for head and neck cancer. *Semin Oncol.* 2002;29(6 Suppl 19):80–83.

48. Weiss JF, Landauer MR. Protection against ionizing radiation by antioxidant nutrients and phytochemicals. *Toxicology.* 2003;189(1–2):1–20.

49. Borek C, Ong A, Mason H, Donahue L, Biaglow JE. Selenium and vitamin E inhibit radiogenic and chemically induced transformation in vitro via different mechanisms. *Proc Natl Acad Sci U S A.* 1986;83(5):1490–1494.

50. Radner BS, Kennedy AR. Suppression of X-ray induced transformation by vitamin E in mouse C3H/10T1/2 cells. *Cancer Lett.* 1986;32(1):25–32.

51. Kennedy AR, Krinsky NI. Effects of retinoids, beta-carotene, and canthaxanthin on UV- and X-ray-induced transformation of C3H10T1/2 cells *in vitro.* *Nutr Cancer.* 1994;22(3):219–232.

52. Ushakova T, Melkonyan H, Nikonova L, et al. Modification of gene expression by dietary antioxidants in radiation-induced apoptosis of mice splenocytes. *Free Radic Biol Med.* 1999;26(7–8):887–891.

53. Konopacka M, Widel M, Rzeszowska-Wolny J. Modifying effect of vitamins C, E, and beta-carotene against gamma-ray-induced DNA damage in mouse cells. *Mutat Res.* 1998;417(2–3):85–94.

54. Gaziev AI, Podlutsky A, Panfilov BM, Bradbury R. Dietary supplements of antioxidants reduce hprt mutant frequency in splenocytes of aging mice. *Mutat Res.* 1995;338(1–6):77–86.

55. Chandrashekara S, Anilkumar T, Jamuna S. Complementary and alternative drug therapy in arthritis. *J Assoc Physicians India.* 2002;50:225–227.

56. O'Connor MK, Malone JF, Moriarty M, Mulgrew S. A radioprotective effect of vitamin C observed in Chinese hamster ovary cells. *Br J Radiol.* 1977;50(596):587–591.

57. Gottlober P, Steinert M, Weiss M, et al. The outcome of local radiation injuries: 14 years of follow-up after the Chernobyl accident. *Radiat Res.* 2001;155(3):409–416.

58. Konopacka M, Rzeszowska-Wolny J. Antioxidant vitamins C, E, and beta-carotene reduce DNA damage before as well as after gamma-ray irradiation of human lymphocytes in vitro. *Mutat Res.* 2001;491(1–2):1–7.

59. Wu W, Abraham L, Ogony J, Matthews R, Goldstein G, Ercal N. Effects of N-acetylcysteine amide (NACA), a thiol antioxidant on radiation-induced cytotoxicity in Chinese hamster ovary cells. *Life Sci.* 2008;82(21–22):1122–1130.

60. Langberg M, Rotem C, Fenig E, Koren R, Ravid A. Vitamin D protects keratinocytes from deleterious effects of ionizing radiation. *Br J Dermatol.* 2009;160(1):151–161.

61. Kennedy AR, Zhou Z, Donahue JJ, Ware JH. Protection against adverse biological effects induced by space radiation by the Bowman-Birk inhibitor and antioxidants. *Radiat Res.* 2006;166(2):327–332.

62. Kennedy AR, Ware JH, Guan J, et al. Selenomethionine protects against adverse biological effects induced by space radiation. *Free Radic Biol Med.* 2004;36(2):259–266.

63. de Moraes Ramos FM, Schonlau F, Novaes PD, Manzi FR, Boscolo FN, de Almeida SM. Pycnogenol protects against Ionizing radiation as shown in the intestinal mucosa of rats exposed to X-rays. *Phytother Res.* 2006;20(8):676–679.

64. Kumar B, Jha MN, Cole WC, Bedford JS, Prasad KN. D-alpha-tocopheryl succinate (vitamin E) enhances radiation-induced chromosomal damage levels in human cancer cells, but reduces it in normal cells. *J Am Coll Nutr.* 2002;21(4):339–343.

65. Kumar KS, Srinivasan V, Toles R, Jobe L, Seed TM. Nutritional approaches to radioprotection: Vitamin E. *Mil Med.* 2002;167(2 Suppl):57–59.

66. Manda K, Ueno M, Moritake T, Anzai K. Alpha-lipoic acid attenuates X-irradiation-induced oxidative stress in mice. *Cell Biol Toxicol.* 2007;23(2):129–137.

67. Mansour HH, Hafez HF, Fahmy NM, Hanafi N. Protective effect of N-acetylcysteine against radiation induced DNA damage and hepatic toxicity in rats. *Biochem Pharmacol.* 2008;75(3):773–780.

68. Mutlu-Turkoglu U, Erbil Y, Oztezcan S, Olgac V, Toker G, Uysal M. The effect of selenium and/or vitamin E treatments on radiation-induced intestinal injury in rats. *Life Sci.* 2000;66(20):1905–1913.

69. Satyamitra M, Devi PU, Murase H, Kagiya VT. In vivo radioprotection by alpha-TMG: Preliminary studies. *Mutat Res.* 2001;479(1–2):53–61.

70. Shirazi A, Ghobadi G, Ghazi-Khansari M. A radiobiological review on melatonin: A novel radioprotector. *J Radiat Res (Tokyo).* 2007;48(4):263–272.

71. Sridharan S, Shyamaladevi CS. Protective effect of N-acetylcysteine against gamma ray induced damages in rats—Biochemical evaluations. *Indian J Exp Biol.* 2002;40(2):181–186.

72. Srinivasan M, Sudheer AR, Pillai KR, Kumar PR, Sudhakaran PR, Menon VP. Lycopene as a natural protector against gamma-radiation induced DNA damage, lipid peroxidation, and antioxidant status in primary culture of isolated rat hepatocytes in vitro. *Biochim Biophys Acta.* 2007;1770(4):659–665.

73. Harapanhalli RS, Yaghmai V, Giuliani D, Howell RW, Rao DV. Antioxidant effects of vitamin C in mice following X-irradiation. *Res Commun Mol Pathol Pharmacol.* 1996;94(3):271–287.

74. Narra VR, Harapanhalli RS, Howell RW, Sastry KS, Rao DV. Vitamins as radioprotectors *in vivo.* I. Protection by vitamin C against internal radionuclides in mouse testes: Implications to the mechanism of damage caused by the Auger effect. *Radiat Res.* 1994;137(3):394–399.

75. Ramakrishnan N, Wolfe WW, Catravas GN. Radioprotection of hematopoietic tissues in mice by lipoic acid. *Radiat Res.* 1992;130(3):360–365.

76. Karslioglu I, Ertekin MV, Kocer I, et al. Protective role of intramuscularly administered vitamin E on the levels of lipid peroxidation and the activities of antioxidant enzymes in the lens of rats made cataractous with gamma-irradiation. *Eur J Ophthalmol.* 2004;14(6):478–485.

77. Kocer I, Taysi S, Ertekin MV, et al. The effect of L-carnitine in the prevention of ionizing radiation-induced cataracts: A rat model. *Graefes Arch Clin Exp Ophthalmol.* 2007;245(4):588–594.

78. Sezen O, Ertekin MV, Demircan B, et al. Vitamin E and L-carnitine, separately or in combination, in the prevention of radiation-induced brain and retinal damages. *Neurosurg Rev.* 2008;31(2):205–213; discussion 213.

79. Altas E, Ertekin MV, Gundogdu C, Demirci E. L-carnitine reduces cochlear damage induced by gamma irradiation in Guinea pigs. *Ann Clin Lab Sci.* Summer 2006;36(3):312–318.

80. Ramos FM, Pontual ML, de Almeida SM, Boscolo FN, Tabchoury CP, Novaes PD. Evaluation of radioprotective effect of vitamin E in salivary dysfunction in irradiated rats. *Arch Oral Biol.* 2006;51(2):96–101.

81. Liu Y, Zhang H, Zhang L, et al. Antioxidant N-acetylcysteine attenuates the acute liver injury caused by X-ray in mice. *Eur J Pharmacol.* 2007;575(1–3):142–148.

82. Vijayalaxmi, Reiter RJ, Tan DX, Herman TS, Thomas CR, Jr. Melatonin as a radioprotective agent: A review. *Int J Radiat Oncol Biol Phys.* 2004;59(3):639–653.

83. Erol FS, Topsakal C, Ozveren MF, et al. Protective effects of melatonin and vitamin E in brain damage due to gamma radiation: An experimental study. *Neurosurg Rev.* 2004;27(1):65–69.

84. Guan J, Stewart J, Ware JH, Zhou Z, Donahue JJ, Kennedy AR. Effects of dietary supplements on the space radiation-induced reduction in total antioxidant status in CBA mice. *Radiat Res.* 2006;165(4):373–378.

85. Manda K, Ueno M, Anzai K. Memory impairment, oxidative damage, and apoptosis induced by space radiation: Ameliorative potential of alpha-lipoic acid. *Behav Brain Res.* 2008;187(2):387–395.

86. Goel HC, Prasad J, Singh S, Sagar RK, Kumar IP, Sinha AK. Radioprotection by an herbal preparation of Hippophae rhamnoides, RH-3, against whole body lethal irradiation in mice. *Phytomedicine.* 2002;9(1):15–25.

87. Gupta ML, Tyagi S, Flora SJ, et al. Protective efficacy of semi purified fraction of high altitude podophyllum hexandrum rhizomes in lethally irradiated Swiss albino mice. *Cell Mol Biol (Noisy-le-grand)*. 2007;53(5):29–41.

88. Lee TK, Johnke RM, Allison RR, O'Brien KF, Dobbs LJ, Jr. Radioprotective potential of ginseng. *Mutagenesis*. 2005;20(4):237–243.

89. Shimoi K, Masuda S, Shen B, Furugori M, Kinae N. Radioprotective effects of antioxidative plant flavonoids in mice. *Mutat Res*. 1996;350(1):153–161.

90. Goyal PK, Gehlot P. Radioprotective effects of Aloe vera leaf extract on Swiss albino mice against whole-body gamma irradiation. *J Environ Pathol Toxicol Oncol*. 2009;28(1):53–61.

91. Blumenthal RD, Lew W, Reising A, et al. Anti-oxidant vitamins reduce normal tissue toxicity induced by radio-immunotherapy. *Int J Cancer*. 2000;86(2):276–280.

92. Greenberger JS, Epperly MW. Review. Antioxidant gene therapeutic approaches to normal tissue radioprotection and tumor radiosensitization. *In Vivo*. 2007;21(2):141–146.

93. Guenechea G, Albella B, Bueren JA, et al. AM218, a new polyanionic polysaccharide, induces radioprotection in mice when administered shortly before irradiation. *Int J Radiat Biol*. 1997;71(1):101–108.

94. Patchen ML, MacVittie TJ, Solberg BD, D'Alesandro MM, Brook I. Radioprotection by polysaccharides alone and in combination with aminothiols. *Adv Space Res*. 1992;12(2–3):233–248.

95. Ross WM, Peeke J. Radioprotection conferred by dextran sulfate given before irradiation in mice. *Exp Hematol*. 1986;14(2):147–155.

96. Maliev VP, D; Jones, JA; Casey, RC. Mechanisms of action of anti-radiation vaccine in reducing the biological impact of high-dose gamma-irradiation. *J Adv Space Res*. 2007;40:586–590.

97. McConnell KW, Muenzer JT, Chang KC, et al. Anti-apoptotic peptides protect against radiation-induced cell death. *Biochem Biophys Res Commun*. 2007;355(2):501–507.

98. Stickney DR, Dowding C, Garsd A, et al. 5-Androstenediol stimulates multilineage hematopoiesis in rhesus monkeys with radiation-induced myelosuppression. *Int Immunopharmacol*. 2006;6(11):1706–1713.

99. Mills EE. The modifying effect of beta-carotene on radiation and chemotherapy induced oral mucositis. *Br J Cancer*. 1988;57(4):416–417.

100. Jaakkola K, Lahteenmaki P, Laakso J, Harju E, Tykka H, Mahlberg K. Treatment with antioxidant and other nutrients in combination with chemotherapy and irradiation in patients with small-cell lung cancer. *Anticancer Res*. 1992;12(3):599–606.

101. Lamson DW, Brignall MS. Antioxidants in cancer therapy; their actions and interactions with oncologic therapies. *Altern Med Rev*. 1999;4(5):304–329.

102. Sminia P, van der Kracht AH, Frederiks WM, Jansen W. Hyperthermia, radiation carcinogenesis, and the protective potential of vitamin A and N-acetylcysteine. *J Cancer Res Clin Oncol*. 1996;122(6):343–350.

103. Korkina LG, Afanas'ef IB, Diplock AT. Antioxidant therapy in children affected by irradiation from the Chernobyl nuclear accident. *Biochem Soc Trans*. 1993;21(Pt 3)(3):314S.

104. Ben-Amotz A, Yatziv S, Sela M, et al. Effect of natural beta-carotene supplementation in children exposed to radiation from the Chernobyl accident. *Radiat Environ Biophys*. 1998;37(3):187–193.

105. Krinsky NI. Antioxidant functions of carotenoids. *Free Radic Biol Med*. 1989;7(6):617–635.

106. Vile GF, Winterbourn CC. Inhibition of adriamycin-promoted microsomal lipid peroxidation by beta-carotene, alpha-tocopherol, and retinol at high and low oxygen partial pressures. *FEBS Lett*. 1988;238(2):353–356.

107. Hazuka MB, Edwards-Prasad J, Newman F, Kinzie JJ, Prasad KN. Beta-carotene induces morphological differentiation and decreases adenylate cyclase activity in melanoma cells in culture. *J Am Coll Nutr*. 1990;9(2):143–149.

108. Zhang LX, Cooney RV, Bertram JS. Carotenoids up-regulate connexin43 gene expression independent of their provitamin A or antioxidant properties. *Cancer Res*. 1992;52(20):5707–5712.

109. Carter CA, Pogribny M, Davidson A, Jackson CD, McGarrity LJ, Morris SM. Effects of retinoic acid on cell differentiation and reversion toward normal in human endometrial adenocarcinoma (RL95-2) cells. *Anticancer Res*. 1996;16(1):17–24.

110. Meyskens Jr FL. Role of Vitamin A and its derivatives in the treatment of human cancer. In: Prasad KN, Santamaria L, Williams RM, eds. *Nutrients in Cancer Prevention and Treatment*. Totowa, NJ: Humana Press; 1995:349–362.

111. Niki E. Interaction of ascorbate and alpha-tocopherol. *Ann N Y Acad Sci*. 1987;498:186–199.

112. Wu H, Kong L, Tan Y, et al. C66 ameliorates diabetic nephropathy in mice by both upregulating NRF2 function via increase in miR-200a and inhibiting miR-21. *Diabetologia*. 2016;59:1558–1568.

113. Prasad KN, Kumar B, Yan XD, Hanson AJ, Cole WC. Alpha-tocopheryl succinate, the most effective form of vitamin E for adjuvant cancer treatment: A review. *J Am Coll Nutr*. 2003;22(2):108–117.

114. Schwartz JL. Molecular and biochemical control of tumor growth following treatment with carotenoids or tocopherols. In: Prasad KN, Santamaria L, Williams RM, eds. *Nutrients in Cancer Prevention and Treatment.* Totowa, NJ: Humana Press; 1995:287–316.

115. Singh VK, Brown DS, Kao TC. Alpha-tocopherol succinate protects mice from gamma-radiation by induction of granulocyte-colony stimulating factor. *Int J Radiat Biol.* 2010;86(1):12–21.

116. Witschi A, Reddy S, Stofer B, Lauterburg BH. The systemic availability of oral glutathione. *Eur J Clin Pharmacol.* 1992;43(6):667–669.

117. Jaramillo MC, Zhang DD. The emerging role of the Nrf2-Keap1 signaling pathway in cancer. *Genes Dev.* 2013;27(20):2179–2191.

118. Williamson TP, Johnson DA, Johnson JA. Activation of the Nrf2-ARE pathway by siRNA knockdown of Keap1 reduces oxidative stress and provides partial protection from MPTP-mediated neurotoxicity. *Neurotoxicology.* 2012;33(3):272–279.

119. Itoh K, Chiba T, Takahashi S, et al. An Nrf2/small Maf heterodimer mediates the induction of phase II detoxifying enzyme genes through antioxidant response elements. *Biochem Biophys Res Commun.* 1997;236(2):313–322.

120. Hayes JD, Chanas SA, Henderson CJ, et al. The Nrf2 transcription factor contributes both to the basal expression of glutathione S-transferases in mouse liver and to their induction by the chemopreventive synthetic antioxidants, butylated hydroxyanisole, and ethoxyquin. *Biochem Soc Trans.* 2000;28(2):33–41.

121. Chan K, Han XD, Kan YW. An important function of Nrf2 in combating oxidative stress: Detoxification of acetaminophen. *Proc Natl Acad Sci USA.* 2001;98(8):4611–4616.

122. Sekhar KR, Freeman ML. Nrf2 promotes survival following exposure to ionizing radiation. *Free Radic Biol Med.* 2015;88(Pt B):268–274.

123. Mathew ST, Bergstrom P, Hammarsten O. Repeated Nrf2 stimulation using sulforaphane protects fibroblasts from ionizing radiation. *Toxicol Appl Pharmacol.* 2014;276(3):188–194.

124. Ramsey CP, Glass CA, Montgomery MB, et al. Expression of Nrf2 in neurodegenerative diseases. *J Neuropathol Exp Neurol.* 2007;66(1):75–85.

125. Chen PC, Vargas MR, Pani AK, et al. Nrf2-mediated neuroprotection in the MPTP mouse model of Parkinson's disease: Critical role for the astrocyte. *Proc Natl Acad Sci USA.* 2009;106(8):2933–2938.

126. Lastres-Becker I, Ulusoy A, Innamorato NG, et al. Alpha-synuclein expression and Nrf2 deficiency cooperate to aggravate protein aggregation, neuronal death, and inflammation in early-stage Parkinson's disease. *Hum Mol Genet.* 2012;21(14):3173–3192.

127. Prasad KN. Simultaneous activation of Nrf2 and elevation of antioxidant compounds for reducing oxidative stress and chronic inflammation in human Alzheimer's disease. *Mech Ageing Dev.* 2016;153:41–47.

128. Datta K, Suman S, Kallakury BV, Fornace AJ, Jr. Exposure to heavy ion radiation induces persistent oxidative stress in mouse intestine. *PLoS One.* 2012;7(8):e42224.

129. Szumiel I. Ionizing radiation-induced oxidative stress, epigenetic changes and genomic instability: The pivotal role of mitochondria. *Int J Radiat Biol.* 2015;91(1):1–12.

130. Xi YD, Yu HL, Ding J, et al. Flavonoids protect cerebrovascular endothelial cells through Nrf2 and PI3K from beta-amyloid peptide-induced oxidative damage. *Curr Neurovasc Res.* 2012;9(1):32–41.

131. Suh JH, Shenvi SV, Dixon BM, et al. Decline in transcriptional activity of Nrf2 causes age-related loss of glutathione synthesis, which is reversible with lipoic acid. *Proc Natl Acad Sci USA.* 2004;101(10):3381–3386.

132. Trujillo J, Chirino YI, Molina-Jijon E, Anderica-Romero AC, Tapia E, Pedraza-Chaverri J. Renoprotective effect of the antioxidant curcumin: Recent findings. *Redox Biol.* 2013;1(1):448–456.

133. Steele ML, Fuller S, Patel M, Kersaitis C, Ooi L, Munch G. Effect of Nrf2 activators on release of glutathione, cysteinylglycine, and homocysteine by human U373 astroglial cells. *Redox Biol.* 2013;1(1):441–445.

134. Kode A, Rajendrasozhan S, Caito S, Yang SR, Megson IL, Rahman I. Resveratrol induces glutathione synthesis by activation of Nrf2 and protects against cigarette smoke-mediated oxidative stress in human lung epithelial cells. *Am J Physiol Lung Cell Mol Physiol.* 2008;294(3):L478–L488.

135. Gao L, Wang J, Sekhar KR, et al. Novel n-3 fatty acid oxidation products activate Nrf2 by destabilizing the association between Keap1 and Cullin3. *J Biol Chem.* 26 2007;282(4):2529–2537.

136. Saw CL, Yang AY, Guo Y, Kong AN. Astaxanthin and omega-3 fatty acids individually and in combination protect against oxidative stress via the Nrf2-ARE pathway. *Food Chem Toxicicol.* 2013;62:869–875.

137. Song J, Kang SM, Lee WT, Park KA, Lee KM, Lee JE. Glutathione protects brain endothelial cells from hydrogen peroxide-induced oxidative stress by increasing nrf2 expression. *Exp Neurobiol.* 2014;23(1):93–103.

138. Ji L, Liu R, Zhang XD, et al. N-acetylcysteine attenuates phosgene-induced acute lung injury via up-regulation of Nrf2 expression. *Inhal Toxicol.* 2010;22(7):535–542.

139. Choi HK, Pokharel YR, Lim SC, et al. Inhibition of liver fibrosis by solubilized coenzyme Q10: Role of Nrf2 activation in inhibiting transforming growth factor-beta1 expression. *Toxicol Appl Pharmacol.* 2009;240(3):377–384.

140. Bai H, Liu R, Chen HL, et al. Enhanced antioxidant effect of caffeic acid phenethyl ester and Trolox in combination against radiation induced-oxidative stress. *Chem Biol Interact.* 2014;207:7–15.

141. Cui L, Jeong H, Borovecki F, Parkhurst CN, Tanese N, Krainc D. Transcriptional repression of PGC-1alpha by mutant huntingtin leads to mitochondrial dysfunction and neurodegeneration. *Cell.* 2006;127(1):59–69.

142. Li XH, Li CY, Lu JM, Tian RB, Wei J. Allicin ameliorates cognitive deficits ageing-induced learning and memory deficits through enhancing of Nrf2 antioxidant signaling pathways. *Neurosci Lett.* 2012;514(1):46–50.

143. Bergstrom P, Andersson HC, Gao Y, et al. Repeated transient sulforaphane stimulation in astrocytes leads to prolonged Nrf2-mediated gene expression and protection from superoxide-induced damage. *Neuropharmacology.* 2011;60(2–3):343–353.

144. Wruck CJ, Gotz ME, Herdegen T, Varoga D, Brandenburg LO, Pufe T. Kavalactones protect neural cells against amyloid beta peptide-induced neurotoxicity via extracellular signal-regulated kinase 1/2-dependent nuclear factor erythroid 2-related factor 2 activation. *Mol Pharmacol.* 2008;73(6):1785–1795.

145. Song SM, Park YS, Lee A, et al. Concentrations of blood vitamin A, C, E, coenzyme Q10 and urine cotinine related to cigarette smoking exposure. *Korean J Lab Med.* 2009;29(1):10–16.

146. Galan P, Viteri FE, Bertrais S, et al. Serum concentrations of beta-carotene, vitamins C and E, zinc, and selenium are influenced by sex, age, diet, smoking status, alcohol consumption, and corpulence in a general French adult population. *Eur J Clin Nutr.* 2005;59(10):1181–1190.

147. Adhikari D, Baxi J, Risal S, Singh PP. Oxidative stress and antioxidant status in cancer patients and healthy subjects, a case-control study. *Nepal Med Coll J.* 2005;7(2):112–115.

148. Li W, Khor TO, Xu C, et al. Activation of Nrf2-antioxidant signaling attenuates NFkappaB-inflammatory response and elicits apoptosis. *Biochem Pharmacol.* 2008;76(11):1485–1489.

149. Kim J, Cha YN, Surh YJ. A protective role of nuclear factor-erythroid 2-related factor-2 (Nrf2) in inflammatory disorders. *Mutat Res.* 2010;690(1–2):12–23.

150. Devaraj S, Tang R, Adams-Huet B, et al. Effect of high-dose alpha-tocopherol supplementation on biomarkers of oxidative stress and inflammation and carotid atherosclerosis in patients with coronary artery disease. *Am J Clin Nutr.* 2007;86(5):1392–1398.

151. Fu Y, Zheng S, Lin J, Ryerse J, Chen A. Curcumin protects the rat liver from CCl4-caused injury and fibrogenesis by attenuating oxidative stress and suppressing inflammation. *Mol Pharmacol.* 2008;73(2):399–409.

152. Lee HS, Jung KK, Cho JY, et al. Neuroprotective effect of curcumin is mainly mediated by blockade of microglial cell activation. *Pharmazie.* 2007;62(12):937–942.

153. Rahman S, Bhatia K, Khan AQ, et al. Topically applied vitamin E prevents massive cutaneous inflammatory and oxidative stress responses induced by double application of 12-O-tetradecanoylphorbol-13-acetate (TPA) in mice. *Chem Biol Interact.* 2008;172(3):195–205.

154. Suzuki YJ, Aggarwal BB, Packer L. Alpha-lipoic acid is a potent inhibitor of NF-kappa B activation in human T cells. *Biochem Biophys Res Commun.* 1992;189(3):1709–1715.

155. Zhu J, Yong W, Wu X, et al. Anti-inflammatory effect of resveratrol on TNF-alpha-induced MCP-1 expression in adipocytes. *Biochem Biophys Res Commun.* 2008;369(2):471–477.

156. Waselenko JK, MacVittie TJ, Blakely WF, et al. Medical management of the acute radiation syndrome: Recommendations of the Strategic National Stockpile Radiation Working Group. *Ann Intern Med.* 2004;140(12):1037–1051.

157. Coleman CN, Hrdina C, Bader JL, et al. Medical response to a radiologic/nuclear event: Integrated plan from the Office of the Assistant Secretary for Preparedness and Response, Department of Health and Human Services. *Ann Emerg Med.* 2009;53(2):213–222.

158. Naidu NV, Reddi OS. Effect of post-treatment with erythropoietin(s) on survival and erythropoietic recovery in irradiated mice. *Nature.* 1967;214(5094):1223–1224.

159. Vittorio PV, Whitfield JF, Rixon RH. The radioprotective and therapeutic effects of imidazole and erythropoietin on the erythropoiesis and survival of irradiated mice. *Radiat Res.* 1971;47(1):191–198.

160. Haydont V, Gilliot O, Rivera S, et al. Successful mitigation of delayed intestinal radiation injury using pravastatin is not associated with acute injury improvement or tumor protection. *Int J Radiat Oncol Biol Phys.* 2007;68(5):1471–1482.

161. Holler V, Buard V, Gaugler MH, et al. Pravastatin limits radiation-induced vascular dysfunction in the skin. *J Invest Dermatol.* 2009;129(5):1280–1291.

162. Van der Meeren A, Gaugler MH, Mouthon MA, Squiban C, Gourmelon P. Interleukin 4 promotes survival of lethally irradiated mice in the absence of hematopoietic efficacy. *Radiat Res.* 1999;152(6):629–636.

163. Kawashima R, Kawamura YI, Kato R, Mizutani N, Toyama-Sorimachi N, Dohi T. IL-13 receptor alpha2 promotes epithelial cell regeneration from radiation-induced small intestinal injury in mice. *Gastroenterology.* 2006;131(1):130–141.

164. Talmadge JE, Tribble H, Pennington R, et al. Protective, restorative, and therapeutic properties of recombinant colony-stimulating factors. *Blood.* 1989;73(8):2093–2103.

165. Cui YF, Yang H, Luo QL, et al. Radioprotection of recombinant human interleukin-3 and granulocyte-macrophage colony-stimulating factor on peripheral lymphocytes of rhesus monkey irradiated by 3.0 Gy gamma-rays. *Zhongguo Wei Zhong Bing Ji Jiu Yi Xue.* 2004;16(1):22–25.

166. Okunieff P, Mester M, Wang J, et al. *In vivo* radioprotective effects of angiogenic growth factors on the small bowel of C3H mice. *Radiat Res.* 1998;150(2):204–211.

167. Ryu T, Hosaka N, Miyake T, et al. Transplantation of newborn thymus plus hematopoietic stem cells can rescue supralethally irradiated mice. *Bone Marrow Transplant.* 2008;41(7):659–666.

168. Perry AR, Iglar AF. The accident at Chernobyl: Radiation doses and effects. *Radiol Technol.* 1990;61(4):290–294.

169. Carder TA. *Handling of Radiation Accident Patients by Paramedical and Hospital Personnel*, 2nd Edition. Boca Raton, FL: CRC Press; 1993.

170. Blakely J. *The Care of Radiation Casualties.* Springfield, IL: Charlec C Thomas; 1968.

171. Baranov A, Gale RP, Guskova A, et al. Bone marrow transplantation after the Chernobyl nuclear accident. *N Engl J Med.* 1989;321(4):205–212.

172. Bond VP, ed. *Radiation Mortality in Different Species.* Tokyo, Japan: Igaku Shoin; 1969; Bond VP, Sagahara T, eds. *Comarative Cellular and Species Radiosensitivity.* Tokyo, Japan: Igaku Shoin.

173. Bond VP, Fliedner TM, Aychambeau JO. *Mammalian Radiation Lethality.* New York: Academic Press; 1965.

20 Micronutrients in Prevention and Improvement of the Standard Therapy in Arthritis

INTRODUCTION

The term arthritis is derived from the Greek word *arthro*, meaning joint, and it refers to inflammation, and thus called joint inflammation. This is one of major health concerns throughout the world including the United States. There are several forms of arthritis. The major forms include rheumatoid arthritis (RA), osteoarthritis (OA), and juvenile rheumatoid arthritis (JRA). RA and OA are the commonest form of arthritis in adults. The analysis of the published results suggests that increased oxidative stress and inflammation play a central role in the initiation and progression of arthritis, although in most cases, inflammation precedes oxidative stress. Data on the role of oxidative stress and inflammation were presented in Chapter 17 of the first edition of this book. Since then, new studies supporting the role of these cellular defects in the pathogenesis of arthritis have been published. Therefore attenuation of these cellular abnormalities may reduce the risk of developing arthritis. Previous studies on the effects of individual antioxidants in human arthritis have produced inconsistent results varying from no effect to minimal improvement in clinical outcomes. The potential reasons for the in consistent results are discussed later in this chapter. The questions remain how to simultaneously reduce oxidative stress and inflammation in patients with arthritis.

The treatment with methotrexate or anti-cytokine therapy alone or in combination has produced significant relief in arthritis symptoms for certain period of time. These agents do not significantly reduce oxidative stress and are toxic. Therefore, additional approaches should be developed to improve the management of arthritis by standard therapy.

This chapter describes briefly the prevalence, cost, and major types of arthritis and their symptoms, and presents additional evidence for the role of oxidative stress and inflammation in the initiation and progression of arthritis. Previous studies with the effect of individual antioxidants on the symptoms of arthritis are described. A novel hypothesis that increasing the levels of oxidative stress and inflammation at the same time requires an increase in the levels of antioxidant enzymes as well as dietary and endogenous antioxidants is proposed. A mixture of micronutrients that may accomplish the above goal is suggested. In addition, this chapter proposes that this micronutrient mixture in combination with standard therapy may improve the clinical outcomes in arthritis.

PREVALENCE AND COST OF ARTHRITIS

Projected increase in prevalence of arthritis as the population grows and becomes older.

Year	Prevalence in Million
2005	46
2015	54
2020	63
2030	72

Source: The Centers for Disease Control and Prevention (CDC), 2018.

Prevalence of arthritis by age between 2013 and 2015.

Age (Years)	Percent of Population
18–44	7.1
45–64	29.3
65 and over	49.6

Source: The Centers for Disease Control and Prevention (CDC), 2018.

Prevalence of arthritis by gender.

Gender	Percent of Population
Men	18.1
Women	23.5

Source: The Centers for Disease Control and Prevention (CDC), 2018.

Prevalence of arthritis by ethnicity.

Ethnicity	Prevalence in Million
Hispanic adults	4.4
Non-Hispanic white adults	41.3
Non-Hispanic black adults	6.1
Non-Hispanic Asian adults	1.5

Source: The Centers for Disease Control and Prevention (CDC), 2018.

Prevalence of arthritis by body weight.

Body Weight	Percent of Population
Normal/Underweight	16
Overweight	23
Obesity	31

Source: The Centers for Disease Control and Prevention (CDC), 2018.

Although arthritis remains a major health concern of all racial/ethnic groups, the disabling effects of arthritis (arthritis-attributable activity limitations, work limitations, and severe pain) affect racial/ethnic minority more severely. A 2007 CDC study estimated that about 294,000 children under the age of 18 years in the USA suffer from JRA. It is now estimated that 300,000 American children have chronic arthritis (Arthritis Foundation, 2018).

Cost: The CDC has reported that the total cost of arthritis and other rheumatic conditions in the USA increased from $128.00 billion ($88.8 billion in direct medical cost and $47.0 billion in lost wages) in 2003 to $304 billion ($140 billion on direct medical cost and $164 billion in lost wages) in 2013.

TYPES OF ARTHRITIS

There are 100 different forms of arthritis that affect joints, the tissue surrounding the joint, and other connective tissues. Arthritis, in general, involves the breakdown of the cartilage that protects the joint. Cartilage allows smooth movements of the joints and absorbs shock when pressure is placed on the joints such as experience during walking, running or playing sports. The major causes of arthritis include autoimmune disease, injury to the bones, and general wear and tear on joints during aging, and bacterial or viral infection. The most common ones are RA, OA, and JRA. Some characteristics features of each of them are briefly described below.

RHEUMATOID ARTHRITIS (RA)

RA is considered an inflammatory disease of the joints and typically occurs in joints on both sides of the body such as hands, wrists, or knees. This symmetry generally helps distinguish rheumatoid arthritis from other types of arthritis. The primary symptoms include joint pain and swelling, reduced ability to move the joint, stiffness, especially in the morning or after sitting for long periods, warmth around a joint, redness of the skin around a joint, and fatigue. RA affects people differently. In most individuals, the joint symptoms develop gradually over several years; however, in some cases it may progress rapidly, while in others it may persist for a limited period and then enter a period of remission. This disease is more common in women than in men, but men are affected more severely than women. It generally appears in middle age or old age and also can be inherited from parents.

RA is characterized by the presence of inflammatory immune cells into the joints and joint-lining tissue (synovium). These inflammatory cells release reactive oxygen species (ROS), pro-inflammatory cytokines, prostaglandins, adhesion molecules, and complement proteins, all of which are toxic to cells. They can cause joint irritation, wearing down of cartilage, swelling, and production of excessive amounts of joint fluid within the joint. The progression of damage to the cartilage can cause narrowing of the space between the bones, and eventually may rub against each other leading to severe pain. In addition, the excessive proliferation and migration of synoviocytes play an important role in the pathophysiology of RA.

OSTEOARTHRITIS (OA)

OA is a degenerative joint disease and is the most common form of arthritis. It is characterized by focal and progressive loss of hyaline cartilage of joints. The pathological changes include narrowing of the space between the bones, osteophytes and bone sclerosis. The major symptoms include pain, swelling, and stiffness. The incidence of OA in women is higher than in men. It generally occurs after the age of 50 years. The most common sites are knee, hip, and hand.

Chondrocytes are the only cell type present in mature cartilage, and their death may contribute to the metabolic and structural changes in cartilage of patients with OA. Increased apoptotic cell death was found in the lesion areas compared to that in non-lesioned areas of the cartilage from same patients with osteoarthritis, while apoptotic cells are rarely seen in normal cartilage.[1] Chondrocyte apoptosis appears to be correlated with the age and severity of the disease.[2] In addition to apoptotic cells, cartilage also contained necrotic materials formed from dead cells. Since cartilage does not have phagocytes because of its avascular nature, dead cells are not removed, and thus form membrane-enclosed structure resembling matrix vesicles.[3] These structures may contribute to matrix mineralization or degradation in OA.

The risk factors include excess body mass, joint injury (sports, work, or trauma), excessive mechanical stress, heavy lifting, knee bending and repetitive motions, structural abnormal alignment, and muscle weakness. In addition, advancing age and genetics are important risk factor for developing OA.

JUVENILE RHEUMATOID ARTHRITIS (JRA)

JRA is the most common childhood arthritis. This is considered an autoimmune disease in which immune cells attack healthy cells of the joint causing inflammatory reactions that release toxic chemical species, which cause progressive damage to the joints and their surrounding tissues causing redness, swelling, pain, and stiffness. Some children with JRA outgrow the illness. As a matter of fact, the symptoms of JRA disappear in over about 50% of affected children. JRA may cause chronic fever and anemia and can affect the heart, lungs, eyes, and nervous system. These arthritic episodes may last for several weeks and then may recur with less severe symptoms. This disease can impair bone development and weaken fine motor skills. The incidence of JRA in girls is higher than in boys. Transient JRA may follow certain infections.

EVIDENCE FOR THE ROLE OF OXIDATIVE STRESS

There are numerous articles that have been published supporting the role of increased oxidative stress in the initiation and progression of arthritis in humans.[4–8] Animal studies also confirmed the role of oxidative stress in the etiology of arthritis.[9–11] Only arbitrarily selected references have been used in this section.

The blood levels of RA patients revealed a marked increase in ROS, lipid peroxidation, protein oxidation, DNA damage, and a decrease in the activities of antioxidant enzymes, and the levels of vitamin C and glutathione compared to healthy controls.[12] In a clinical study, the levels of DNA damage in the peripheral lymphocytes and plasma total oxidative damage markers were elevated in patients with RA compared to healthy controls. The levels of thiobarbituric acid-reactive substances (TBARS), lipid hydroperoxide, conjugated diene, protein oxidation (carbonyl), and DNA adduct (8-hydroxyguanosine) were significantly higher, whereas the levels of glutathione, and the activities of glutathione peroxidase and CuZn SOD in the blood were lowered compared to healthy controls. In addition, the levels of above markers of oxidative damage were significantly higher, and catalase activity lowered in the synovial fluid of RA patients compared to healthy subjects.[13]

In a clinical study, a 2- to 8-fold increase in the production of superoxide by the phagocytes from RA patients was observed, when compared to healthy subjects or patients with non-rheumatic disease.[5] The enhanced NADPH oxidase-dependent superoxide generation correlated well with the elevated plasma levels of TNF-α. Removal of circulating TNF-α by the dialysis of patient blood or inhibition of NADPH oxidase activity by prednisolone treatment normalized the elevated levels of ROS production to the levels of control subjects and correlated with the clinical improvements.[5] The leukocyte but not neutrophil mitochondria from the patients with RA produced 5-fold more ROS than those obtained from control subjects, and this correlated well with the increased plasma levels of TNFα.[14] This study suggests that mitochondrial defects are also associated with RA.

A clinical study involving 30 patients with RA, 15 patients with OA, and 15 patients with systemic lupus erythematosus (SLE) showed that the levels of 3-nitrotyrosine in synovial fluid and sera of patients with RA and OA were elevated compared to SLE.[15] The levels of 3-nitrotyrosine also correlated with the disease activity. High levels of nitrated type III collagen was found in synovial tissues of the patients with RA and knee OA compared to healthy controls. In addition, the serum levels of nitrated type III collagen was elevated in patients with OA 1.5-fold more than in healthy control subjects.[16] In patients with OA, the erythrocyte levels of MDA and activities of SOD, glutathione peroxidase, and plasma glutathione-s-transferase increased, whereas the erythrocyte levels of glutathione and ascorbic acid and plasma vitamin E decreased compared to those in healthy control subjects.[17] Macrophages and T-cells from RA patients produced more NO than that produced by these cells obtained from healthy subjects. TNF-α also increased production of NO in T cells obtained from RA patients. Overproduction NO may contribute to the T-cell dysfunction that is commonly found in the inflamed joint.[18] The synovial fluid neutrophils from RA patients are activated to produce increased amounts of ROS within the cells.[19] It has been reported that aldehydic products, primarily the 4-hydroxy-2-alkenals, form adducts with proteins that make them highly immunogenic, which can induce pathogenic antibodies in RA.[20]

Although oxidative damage was higher in patients with active RA and inactive RA, the levels of antioxidant enzymes and glutathione levels in these patients were higher than in control healthy subjects.[21] This suggests that elevated levels of selected antioxidant defense system were not sufficient to overcome oxidative damage and that enhanced oxidative stress participated in the progression of RA. In another study, high levels of oxidative stress and nitrosylative stress occurred in the presence of elevated levels of SOD in patients with RA.[22] The serum levels of reactive oxygen metabolites (ROM) was associated with CRP and Disease Activity score 28-erythrocyte sedimentation rate (DAS28-ESR), and MMP3 (matrix metalloproteinase 3) in RA patients.[23] The activity of SOD and the levels of glutathione and –SH groups were lower and lipid peroxidation level were higher in RA patients than in healthy control subjects, while the activities of CAT and GSG-Px did not differ between two groups.[24]

A case-control study revealed that smoking increased the risk of oxidative stress-induced RA,[25] and the effectiveness of anti-TNF-α therapy was reduced in smokers with RA.[26]

A review has shown that increased oxidative stress play a central role in pathophysiology of OA.[27] Among reactive aldehydes, 4-hydroxynonenal (HNE) is considered the most reactive species, and like ROS, HNE can induce various biological effects including apoptosis. Antioxidants such as N-acetylcysteine (NAC), and overexpression of glutathione-s-transferase A4-4 reduced HNE production and inhibited apoptosis in several cells. The levels of HNE were higher in synovial fluid of patients with OA than those found in healthy subjects.[28] It has been demonstrated that HNE can induce transcriptional and posttranscriptional modifications of type II collagen and matrix metalloproteinase-13 (MMP-13), resulting in extracellular matrix in cartilage from patients with OA.[28]

The number of CD4+ lymphocytes was lower in RA patients compared to control subjects. In addition, these cells from RA patients had increased levels of markers of oxidative stress and inflammation.[29] Treatment with anti-TNF-α reduces oxidative stress and improved symptoms in patients with RA.[30] This suggests that the source of free radicals was inflammatory reactions. Anti-TNF-α treatment enhanced the serum levels of soluble Fas (sFas) in RA patients compare to control or those RA patients receiving no anti-TNF-α, and improved clinical outcomes.[31]

EVIDENCE FOR THE ROLE OF INFLAMMATION

Rheumatoid arthritis (RA) is considered a chronic inflammatory disease. During the active phase of the disease, the plasma levels of pro-inflammatory cytokines, interleukin-6 (IL-6), interleukin-1β (IL-1β), tumor necrosis factor-alpha (TNF-α), and active-phase proteins are elevated.[32,33] Arachidonic acid metabolites, such as leukotrienes B4 (LTB4), play an important role in the pathogenesis of RA. The levels of LTB4 were low in the cultured media of rheumatoid arthritis synovial fibroblast (RASF), but the major LTB4 receptor (BLT2) was expressed in RASF. The addition of LTB4 markedly increased expression of TNF-α and IL-1β at the mRNA and protein levels, suggesting that LTB4 contributes to the damage associated with RA via increasing the levels of pro-inflammatory cytokines.[34] In addition to leukocytes, RASF produced a number of inflammatory mediators that recruit, retain, and activate immune cells and resident parenchymal cells in the joints in order to promote tissue destruction.

Several studies have reported the presence of increased number of mast cells in the synovial tissues and fluids of patients with RA, and at the sites of cartilage damage.[35] Activated mast cells were found in a significant number of specimens obtained from patients with RA. Activated mast cells release potent mediators, including histamine, heparin, proteinases, leukotrienes, and multi-functional cytokines, such as TNF-α, IL-6, and IL-1β, that contribute to tissue destruction in the joints. It has been reported that the serum levels of TNF-α, soluble TNF-α receptors (sTNF-Rp55 and sTNF-R p75), but not TNF-β, are good markers of RA.[36] The increased expression of IL-23 gene was found in all samples of synovial membranes, whereas the expression of IL-17A was found only in subset of synovial membranes. Both IL-23 and IL-17A co-localized in the synovial membranes. These results were interpreted to suggest that IL-17 by itself may not be important in the pathogenesis of RA, but it may amplify the inflammatory responses.[37] Activation of mast cells in RA synovial explants released increased amounts of PGE2 that contributes to the pathogenesis of RA.[38] RA is also associated with increased arterial stiffness. It has been reported that elevated plasma levels of osteopontin, a cytokine, contribute to the arterial stiffness in RA patients.[39] Both cathepsin K and S proteins were present in synovium from patients with RA and OA. Cathepsin-K protein was present in synovium fibroblasts, and stromal multinucleated giant cells, and, to a lesser degree, in CD68+macrophage-like-synoviocytes. In contrast to cathepsin-K, cathepsin-S expression was primarily located in CD68+macrophage-like synoviocytes, endothelial cells of blood vessels.[40] Both IL-1β and TNF-α increased cathepsin-K expression in RA- and OA-derived synovial fibroblasts. It appears that both cathepsin-K and $-$S participate in the degradation of cartilage in RA and OA.

In an animal model of RA, it was demonstrated that TNF-α plays an important role in joint swelling, whereas IL-1β plays a significant role in degeneration of cartilage.[41] Overexpression of IL-18 increased both joint inflammation and cartilage destruction in mice. Overexpression of IL-18 gene in IL-1 deficient mice induced joint inflammation without any cartilage damage; however, in vitro study suggested that IL-18-induced cartilage damage was dependent upon the presence of IL-1β. On the other hand, overexpression of IL-18 in TNF-α deficient mice showed that TNF-α was partly responsible for IL-18-induced joint swelling and influx of inflammatory cells, but that it had no role in IL-18-induced cartilage damage.[42] Toll-like receptors (TLRs) may contribute to the pathogenesis of RA. The presence of endogenous ligand for TLR has been found in the joints of RA patients. It has been reported that IL-1β-induced local joint inflammation, cartilage proteoglycan depletion, and bone degeneration are dependent on TLR4 activation. On the other hand, TNF-α-induced RA pathology was less dependent upon TLR4 or TLR-2. Furthermore, IL1-1beta-induced expression of cathepsin-K, a marker of osteoclast activity, was dependent on TLR4 activation.[43] A review of several studies indicates that autoantigen recognition by specific T-cell is important to the development of rheumatoid sinovitis.[44] The involvement of T-cells in the pathogenesis of RA is supported by the fact the numerous T-cell carrying activation markers were found in RA synovium. These T-cells appear to participate in the complex network of cell- and mediator-driven biochemical events that cause joint destruction. The transgenic k/BxN mice develop an inflammatory joint disease with many features characteristic of RA. This model is based on a T-cell receptor transgene, KRN that recognizes the foreign antigen, bovine RNase, and the ubiquitously expressed self-antigen, glucose-6-phosphate isomerase (GPI). Using this model it has been demonstrated that autoimmune response is initiated at the levels of both adaptive and innate immune systems.[45]

Pro-inflammatory cytokines such as IL-1β appears to be involved in the pathogenesis of OA through the production of catabolic enzymes and inflammatory mediators. Induction of heme oxygenase (HO-1) appears to exert anti-inflammatory effects. Induction of HO-1 by cobalt protoporphyrin IX increased the viability of primary culture of chondrocytes by inhibiting apoptosis, oxidative stress and reducing the production of prostaglandin E2.[46] In addition to pro-inflammatory cytokines, matrix metalloproteinases (MMPs), and other catabolic factors contribute to the pathogenesis of cartilage damage in OA. Pro-inflammatory cytokines such as Il-1β down-regulated H0-1, whereas IL-10 up-regulated HO-1 in OA chondrocytes.[47] Activation of HO-1 significantly reduced IL-1β-induced damage to cartilage. It also inhibited MMP activity and expression of collagenases MMP-1, and MMP-13 at protein and mRNA levels.[47]

Elevated levels of PGE2 play a significant role in the pathogenesis of arthritis. The levels of protein and mRNA of an inducible microsomal prostaglandin synthase-1 (mPGES-1) were higher in OA cartilage compared to normal cartilage.[48]

Increased levels of CRP were associated with severity of depression and pain in RA patients,[49] suggesting that depression and pain are associated with RA. RA enhances the risk of cardiovascular disease, independent of traditional risk factors. Angiotensin II (Ang II), a pro-inflammatory agent, plays a role in the pathogenesis of RA and other autoimmune diseases.[50] Inhibitors of Ang II reduced inflammation, the risk of cardiovascular disease, and autoimmune disease.

Interleukin-10 (IL-10) acts an anti-inflammatory cytokine in RA. Other members of IL-10 include IL-19, IL-20, IL-22, IL-24, and IL-26, and distant related cytokines are IL-28A, IL-28B, and IL-29. The mRNA levels of IL-10 and IL-19 were increased in synovial fluid mononuclear cells (SFMCs) from RA patients compared to peripheral blood MCs from RA patients or healthy control volunteers IL-20 and IL-22 mRNAs levels were also elevated in RA SFMCs, but their expression was lower than that of IL-10 and IL-19.[51] Further study showed that IL-1beta increased the levels of IL-19 in peripheral blood MCs, suggesting that elevated levels of IL-1β in RA joints contribute to the increased levels of IL-19 mRNA. Differential distributions of IL-10 family among different forms of arthritis are described here.[52]

Cytokines	Increased	Compared to
Serum IL-20	RA, PsA	OA, HC, SF
Serum IL-24	RA, PsA, OA	HC, SFPsA
Serum IL-19	OA, HC	RA, PsA
SF IL-19	PsA, RA	OA

Note: PsA, Psoriatic arthritis; HC, healthy control; SF, synovial fluid; SFPsA, synovial fluid from PsA patients.

It was further demonstrated that IL-19 appears to be involved in the joint inflammation, whereas IL-20 and IL-24 may contribute to the systemic inflammation.[52] Circulating IL-33 land its soluble receptor ST2 levels were higher in RA than those in OA, but they were undetectable in serum or SF of patients with psoriatic arthritis.[53] Pro-inflammatory cytokines IL-7 and thymic stromal lymphopoietin (TSLP) had an additive effect on the production of TH17 cytokines in human RA dendritic cell and T-cell co-cultures, and increased arthritis associated with inflammation in mice.[54] Since IL-7 and TSLP mediated their action via a common receptor IL-7R, inhibitors of IL-7R may be useful in preventing the effects of both cytokines in RA patients.

ROLE OF ANTIOXIDANTS IN ARTHRITIS

STUDIES ON ANIMAL MODELS OF ARTHRITIS

In collagen-induced arthritis in rats, it was observed that intradermal administration of a low molecular weight mimetic of SOD improved clinical symptoms and degenerative changes in the joint and paw, and reduced the levels of nitrotyrosine (a marker of protein oxidation) and DNA damage.[55] Similar results were obtained with Cu, ZN-SOD mimetic in collagen-induced arthritis in rats.[56] In collagen-induced arthritis in mice, it was found that depletion of vitamin from the diet induced increased expressions of joint tissue TNF-α and IL-1β, and increased levels of circulating macrophages chemoattractant protein-1, nitric oxide, and PGE2. However, supplementation with vitamin E or quercetin restored these markers to control levels.[57] Supplementation with quercetin reduced inflammatory markers and increased plasma antioxidant capacity in rat adjuvant arthritis.[58]

In an experimental rabbit inflammatory arthritis model (intra-articular injection of lipopolysaccharide), intra-articular injection of resveratrol protected cartilage against the development of chemical-induced inflammatory arthritis.[59] In a rat model of adjuvant arthritis, administration of L-carnitine and alpha-lipoic acid reduced markers of oxidative damage and inflammation.[60] In collagen-induced arthritis in mice, supplementation with alpha-lipoic acid reduced the incidence of arthritis and prevented bone erosion.[61] It also decreased the levels of ROS in lymphocytes obtained from inguinal lymph nodes, and the levels of TNF-α, IL-1β, and IL-6 in the paws.

In a mice model of arthritis, supplementation with epigallocatechin-3-gallate (EGCG) improved clinical symptoms and reduced histological scores of arthritis.[62] Administration of EGCG reduced inflammation, cardiovascular, and RA risks.[63] Catechins EGCG, epicatechin-3-gallate (ECG), and epicatechin (EC) differently affect the levels of inflammatory markers. EGCG and ECG inhibited IL-6 and IL-8 and MMP-2 levels and COX-2 activity in primary human RA synovial fibroblasts, while EC did not.[64]

Tamarind (*Tamarinds indica*) seed extract reduced adjuvant-induced arthritis in animals by reducing the markers of inflammatory events and oxidative damage. It also attenuated arthritis-mediated degradation of cartilage/bone.[65] Administration of Boswellia serrata gum resign extract reduced collagen-induced arthritis in rats by reducing the markers of chronic inflammation and oxidative stress and enhancing the levels of antioxidant enzymes.[66]

Treatment of synoviocytes cells (obtained from patients with RA) in culture with resveratrol inhibited proliferation of synoviocytes and induced apoptosis by activation of caspase-3.[67] In a rat model of RA (induced by streptococcal cell wall), administration of turmeric inhibited joint inflammation and periarticular joint destruction and prevented activation of NF-kappaB and decreased the levels of markers of inflammation.[68]

Treatment of bovine disc cells in culture with beta-fibroblastic growth factor (bFGF) or IL-1 increased the production of MMP-13 that was attenuated by the treatment with resveratrol; therefore, it was concluded that resveratrol treatment may slow the progression of intervertebral disc degeneration.[69] Resveratrol treatment of RA fibroblast-like synoviocytes induced apoptosis by activating caspase-8 that releases mitochondrial cytochrome.[70]

HUMAN CELL CULTURE MODELS OF ARTHRITIS

Pretreatment with alpha-lipoic acid inhibited TNF-alpha-induced activation of NF-kappaB pathway in cultures of fibroblast-like synovial cells from patients with RA.[71]

Treatment of RA synovial fibroblasts in culture with epigallocatechin-3-gallate suppressed TNF-alpha-induced production of matrix metalloproteinase-1 (MMP-1) and MMP-3 that play a significant role in destruction of cartilage and bone in RA joint.[72]

Animal studies have shown that 1alpha, 25-dihydroxyvitamin D3 (vitamin D3) upregulated matrix metalloproteinases (MMPs) that playa a major role in the degeneration of cartilage in the joints. It has been found that vitamin D3 is produced in the synovial fluid of arthritic joints, and vitamin D3 receptors are located in RA synovial tissues and at the site sites of cartilage damage.[73] Vitamin D3 treatment of monolayer cultures of RA synovial fibroblasts did not affect the basal production of MPP or PGE2; however, it suppressed the production of MPP and PGE2 in IL-1β-stimulated RA synovial fibroblasts.

STUDIES ON HUMAN RA AND OA

A review of 20 randomized clinical trials in which the effects of individual antioxidants such as vitamins A, C, and E or selenium or their combination in the treatment of inflammatory arthritis and OA revealed inconsistent results.[74,75] Most of these studies were of poor quality with respect to selection of number, types, and doses of antioxidants, and treatment periods. Therefore, no conclusion with respect to efficacy of antioxidant supplements to improve the symptoms in patients with RA or OA can be drawn from these studies. A double-blind, randomized, placebo-controlled trial supplementation with coenzyme Q10 reduced markers of oxidative stress and inflammation in RA patients.[76] Vitamin D deficiency was observed in RA patients with moderate disease activity.[77]

In the Women's Health Study involving 39,144 subjects without RA, supplementation with 600 IU of vitamin E alone taken every other day was not associated with a significant reduction in the risk of developing RA.[78] An open pilot study involving 8 non-smoking female patients with RA who received non-steroidal anti-inflammatory drug and/or second line of medication showed that antioxidant supplementation decreased the number of swollen and painful joints and improved general health and decreased Disease Activity Score from 28 to 1.6.[79] A randomized, double-blind, placebo-controlled trials involving 20 patients with RA showed that supplementation with quercetin plus vitamin C or alpha-lipoic acid for a period of 4 weeks did not change the levels of inflammation markers or disease severity.[80] Supplementation with fish oil and evening primrose oil reduced RA severity, and attenuated the markers of inflammation and oxidative stress and enhanced the activities of antioxidant enzymes.[81] Despite of contradictory results with individual antioxidants some studies continue to suggest that diet rich in antioxidants and omega-3 fatty acids with or without standard medications may improve the efficacy of therapy.[32,82,83]

The nocturnal plasma concentration of melatonin in patients with RA was higher than in healthy control subjects. In addition, melatonin was found in the synovial fluid of RA patients and synovial macrophages express specific binding sites. These studies suggested that melatonin may promote progression of RA.[84] In a clinical study involving 20 patients with JRA and 20 health age- and sex-matched controls, the serum levels of melatonin were elevated compared to controls, suggesting that melatonin may play a promoting role in JRA.[85]

PREVENTION STRATEGIES

In most chronic diseases such as Alzheimer's disease and Parkinson's disease, increased oxidative stress precedes other cellular defects including chronic inflammation in the initiation and progression of these diseases.[86,87] In contrast, in many cases, inflammation precedes oxidative stress in the development and progression of RA and OA. Since antioxidants and phytochemicals reduce inflammation and oxidative stress, they should be useful in prevention, and in combination with standard therapy, in improved management of RA and OA.

POTENTIAL REASONS FOR INCONSISTENT RESULTS

Limited human studies on antioxidants presented above produced inconsistent results varying from no effect to minimal improvement in the clinical outcomes in patients with arthritis. The reasons for individual antioxidants producing inconsistent results in humans RA or OA are not known; however, some potentials causes are described here: (a) antioxidants show differential subcellular distribution and different mechanisms of action; therefore, a single antioxidant cannot protect all parts of the cell; (b) a single antioxidant in a high internal oxidative environment in high-risk patients is oxidized and can then itself act as a prooxidant rather than as an antioxidant; (c) the body protects against oxidative damage by elevating antioxidant enzymes, and dietary and endogenous antioxidants; (d) antioxidants neutralize free radicals by donating electrons to those molecules with unpaired electron, whereas antioxidant enzymes destroy free radicals by catalysis, converting them to harmless molecules such as water and oxygen. Therefore, both of these agents should be enhanced to achieve substantial protection against oxidative damage and inflammation; (e) the affinity of different antioxidants for free radicals differs, depending upon their solubility; (f) both the aqueous and lipid compartments of the cell need to be protected together. Water-soluble antioxidants such as vitamin C and glutathione protect molecules in the aqueous environment of the cells, whereas lipid soluble antioxidants such as vitamin A and vitamin E protect molecules in the lipid compartment; (g) vitamin E is more effective in quenching free radicals in a reduced oxygenated cellular environment, whereas vitamin C and alpha-tocopherol are more effective in a higher oxygenated environment of the cells[88]; (h) vitamin C is important for recycling the oxidized form of alpha-tocopherol to the antioxidant form[89]; (i) antioxidants produce cell protective proteins by altering the expression of different microRNAs.[90] For example, some antioxidants can activate Nrf2 by upregulating miR-200a that inhibits its target protein Keap1, whereas others activate Nrf2 by downregulating miR-21 that binds with 3'-UTR Nrf2 mRNA.[91]

The use of a single micronutrient is not expected to produce optimal protection against oxidative stress and inflammatory events, which contribute to the initiation and progression of RA. For this reason, it is proposed that an elevation of the levels of antioxidant enzymes and dietary and endogenous antioxidants may be essential for simultaneously reducing these cellular defects in arthritis. Oral supplementation can increase the levels of dietary and endogenous antioxidants; however, an elevation of the levels of antioxidant enzymes requires an activation of Nrf2. Therefore, it is essential to understand the regulation of activation of Nrf2.

ACTIVATION OF Nrf2 (NUCLEAR FACTOR-ERYTHROID-2-RELATED FACTOR 2)

Nrf2

The nuclear transcriptional factor, Nrf2 (nuclear factor-erythroid-2-related factor 2) belongs to the Cap "n" Collar (CNC) family that contains a conserved basic leucine zipper (bZIP) transcriptional factor.[92] Under physiological condition, Nrf2 is associated with Kelch-like ECH associated protein 1 (Keap1), which acts as an inhibitor of Nrf2.[93] Keap1 protein serves as an adaptor to link Nrf2 to the ubiquitin ligase CuI-Rbx1 complex for degradation by proteasomes and maintains the steady levels of Nrf2 in the cytoplasm. Nrf2-keap1 complex is primarily located in the cytoplasm; Keap1 acts as a sensor for ROS/electrophilic stress.

ACTIVATION OF Nrf2 DURING ACUTE OXIDATIVE STRESS

During acute oxidative stress, ROS is needed to activate Nrf2 which then dissociates itself from Keap1-CuI-Rbx1 complex and translocates in the nucleus where it heterodimerizes with a small Maf protein, binds with ARE leading to increased expression of target genes coding for several cytoprotective enzymes including antioxidant enzymes.[94–96]

FAILURE TO ACTIVATE Nrf2 DURING CHRONIC OXIDATIVE STRESS

During chronic oxidative stress, Nrf2 becomes resistant to ROS,[97–99] suggesting that activation of Nrf2 by a ROS-independent mechanism exists. This is evidenced by the fact that increased chronic oxidative stress occurs despite the presence of Nrf2 in arthritis. The question arises as to how to activate ROS-resistant Nrf2 in arthritis.

ANTIOXIDANTS ACTIVATE ROS-RESISTANT Nrf2

Some examples are vitamin E and genistein,[100] alpha-lipoic acid,[101] curcumin,[102] resveratrol,[103,104] omega-3-fatty acids,[105,106] glutathione,[107] NAC,[108] and coenzyme Q10.[109] Several plant-derived phytochemicals, such as epigallocatechin-3-gallate, carestol, kahweol, cinnamonyl-based compounds, zerumbone, lycopene and carnosol,[92,110,111] genistein,[100] allicin, a major organosulfur compound found in garlic,[112] sulforaphane, a organosulfur compound, found in cruciferous vegetables,[113] and kavalactones (methysticin, kavain, and yangonin).[114] The reasons for the activation of Nrf2 without ROS by antioxidant compounds are not known.

Binding of Nrf2 with ARE in the Nucleus

An activation of Nrf2 alone is not sufficient to increase the levels of antioxidant enzymes. Activated Nrf2 must bind with ARE in the nucleus for increasing the expression of target genes coding for antioxidant enzymes. This binding ability of Nrf2 with ARE was impaired in aged rats and this defect was restored by supplementation with alpha-lipoic acid.[101] It is unknown whether the binding ability of Nrf2 with ARE is impaired in arthritis.

Importance of Activation of Nrf2 in Arthritis

Antibody-induced arthritis was more severe in Nrf2-knockout mice than in wild-type mice. In addition, increased number of spontaneously fractured bones was observed in Nrf2-knockout mice.[115,116] These data suggest that the functional Nrf2 is essential for reducing oxidative stress and inflammation in arthritis.

REDUCING OXIDATIVE STRESS LEVEL

Activation of Nrf2 may not be sufficient to optimally reduce oxidative stress, because antioxidants compounds are also decreased during chronic oxidative stress[117–119]; therefore, their levels must also be simultaneously elevated.

REDUCING INFLAMMATION LEVEL

Activation of Nrf2[120,121] and some individual antioxidant compounds reduced markers of inflammation.[122–128]

PROPOSED MICRONUTRIENTS FOR SIMULTANEOUSLY REDUCING OXIDATIVE STRESS AND INFLAMMATION IN ARTHRITIS

Because of the failure to produce optimal benefits in improving the symptoms of arthritis with single antioxidants, a comprehensive micronutrient mixture is proposed. This mixture contains multiple dietary antioxidant compounds (vitamin A, natural mixed carotenoids, vitamin C, vitamin E succinate, vitamin E acetate, curcumin, and resveratrol), endogenous antioxidants (alpha-lipoic acid, L-carnitine, and coenzyme Q10), a synthetic antioxidant N-acetylcysteine (NAC), vitamin D3, omega-3-fatty acids, zinc, and all B-vitamins. This mixture of micronutrients may optimally reduce oxidative stress and chronic inflammation by simultaneously enhancing the levels of antioxidant enzymes through activation of the Nrf2/ARE pathway, and elevating the levels of antioxidants.

PRIMARY PREVENTION OF ARTHRITIS

The purpose of primary prevention is to protect healthy individuals from developing arthritis. Older individuals and individuals who are carrying mutated gene for RA are suitable subjects for the primary prevention studies. At present, there are no strategies to prevent or delay the onset of RA in individuals with mutated genes. The proposed mixture of micronutrients may be effective in preventing or delaying the onset of symptoms of arthritis in these individuals. This possibility is indirectly supported by the experiments on the fruit flies described here.

The gene HOP (TUM-1) is essential for the development of *Drosophila melanogaster* (fruit fly). A mutation in this gene markedly increases the risk of developing a leukemia-like tumor in female flies. In collaboration with Dr. Bhattacharya of NASA Moffat Field, CA, we observed that whole-body irradiation of these flies with proton radiation dramatically increased the incidence of cancer compared to that observed in unirradiated female flies. Treatment with a mixture of multiple anti-oxidants before and after irradiation blocked the development of proton radiation-induced cancer in female fruit flies.[129] This is the first evidence that genetic basis of a disease can be prevented by multiple antioxidants, at least in fruit flies.

TREATMENT STRATEGIES OF ARTHRITIS

The current treatment strategies involve multiple agents including low-dose methotrexate, anti-cytokines, non-steroidal, anti-inflammatory drugs (NSAIDs) individually or in combination. Supplementation with individual antioxidants has produced inconsistent results. Some patients with arthritis used complementary medical approaches with for reducing the pain.

LOW-DOSE METHOTREXATE (MTX)

Methotrexate, a folate inhibitor, initially was used for the treatment of cancer. Low-dose MTX is considered a gold standard for the treatment of RA and has been for decades.[130–134] MTX is an immunosuppressive drug, which causes apoptosis via increased oxidative damage to proliferating cells in the joints of the patients with active RA. MTX has one of the best efficacy and toxicity ratios. It improves signs and symptoms of RA and physical function, and inhibits radiographic progression of cartilage damage, but to a smaller degree, compared to anti-TNF therapy. The proposed mechanisms of action include inhibition of T-cell proliferation, inhibition of transmethylation reactions required for the prevention of T-cell toxicity, interference with glutathione metabolism leading to alterations in recruitment of monocytes and other cells to the inflamed joints, and promotion of the release of the endogenous anti-inflammatory mediator adenosine. One case of an acute erythro-leukemia was detected during low-dose MTX therapy. In spite of this rare case of cancer, low-dose MTX remains the first choice for the initial treatment of RA.

ANTI-CYTOKINES THERAPY

The discovery anti-cytokine inhibitors, primarily TNF-alpha inhibitors, have revolutionized the treatment RA. However, severe side effects that include allergy, tuberculosis, opportunistic infections, demyelization, and cancer occur in some individuals. In a clinical study involving 29 patients with active RA and 25 healthy control, it was observed that anti-TNF-alpha therapy rapidly decreased the influx of leukocytes into inflamed joints, but did not impair neutrophil chemotaxis and production of ROS.[135] In a clinical study on 55 RA patients who were unresponsive to convention doses (3 mg/kg of body weight) of anti-TNF-alpha (infliximab), the effects of doses and frequency of infliximab infusions were evaluated. The results showed that changing the frequency of infliximab infusions in active RA group was more effective than increasing the dose of infliximab for improving the clinical outcomes.[136] The antioxidant capacity of HDL-cholesterol decreased in patients with RA. Anti-TNF therapy with infliximab improved antioxidant capacity after 6 months of therapy that may explain the protective effect of anti-TNF-therapy on cardiovascular morbidity in RA.[137] Angiogenesis is an important factor in remodeling of bone components in both normal and pathological condition. Angiopoietin (ANG) family of growth factors regulates angiogenesis. Ang-1 appears to stabilize new blood vessels by recruiting mesenchymal cells and promoting their differentiation into vascular smooth muscle. The osteoblasts obtained from patients with RA, OA, and healthy subjects spontaneously secreted significant amounts of ANG-1. Stimulation with TNF-alpha or interferon-gamma (IFN-gamma) had no significant effect on AGN-1 secretion; however, the combination of TNF-alpha and IFN-gamma caused dose- and time-dependent decreased in ANG-1 secretion.[138] Thus, over-production of these cytokines may interfere with the remodeling of bone components in patients with RA or OA by decreasing the secretion of ANG-1. Treatment with anti-TNF-alpha therapy with infliximab reduces the levels of some adhesion molecules that are elevated in patients with active RA.[139]

Extensive clinical studies have been performed on disease-modifying anti-rheumatic drugs (DMARDs), also called biologics, which include abatacept, adalimumab, anakinra, etanercept, infliximab, and rituximab, in patients with RA. Among these adalimumab, etanercept, and infliximab are TNF-alpha inhibitors, whereas anakinra is an IL-1 receptor antagonist. A detailed review on the relative efficacy and toxicity of these biologics reported that anakinra was less effective than others, and that etanercept caused fewer withdrawals due to toxicity than infliximab, anakinra, and adalimumab.[140] Certolizumab pegol is a PEGylated humanized Fab monoclonal antibody that neutralizes both membrane-bound and soluble TNF-α. In a randomized, double-blind, placebo-controlled trial involving 982 RA patients with an inadequate response to methotrexate alone, the efficacy certolizumab pegol in combination with methotrexate was determined. The results showed that treatment with certolizumab pegol in combination with methotrexate improved signs and symptoms of RA, inhibited the progression of structural joint damage, and improved physical function compared to control patients receiving placebo in combination with methotrexate.[141,142] This TNF-α inhibitor alone or in combination with methotrexate was generally well tolerated. The most common reported adverse event was infection.[142,143] The combination of adalimumab and methotrexate was superior to either adalimumab alone or methotrexate alone in improving signs and symptoms of RA, inhibiting radiographic progression of disease and enhancing disease remission period.[144] The beneficial effects of TNF-α inhibitors in combination with methotrexate were similar in older and younger patients with RA.[145]

In a randomized and placebo-controlled clinical investigation involving 359 patients with active RA in whom the response to methotrexate was inadequate, the efficacy of tocilizumab, a humanized anti-IL-6 receptor antibody, alone or in combination with methotrexate in patients with RA was evaluated. The results showed that a 20% improvement on the criterion of American College of Rheumatology score (ACR20 response) was observed in 61%–63% of patients receiving tocilizumab alone, and in 63%–74% patients receiving both tocilizumab and methotrexate. Tocilizumab was mostly well tolerated, and the safety profiles were similar to those of other biologics.[146] In a clinical study involving 499 RA patients with inadequate response to one or more TNF-α inhibitors, the efficacy of tocilizumab in combination with methotrexate was evaluated. The results showed that a 20% improvement in ACR score was observed in about 30%–50% of patients receiving tocilizumab in combination with methotrexate, depending upon the dose of tocilizumab; however, only 10% of control subjects receiving placebo showed such an improvement.[147] Similar beneficial effects of tocilizumab in combination with methotrexate were observed in another clinical study in which RA patients showed an inadequate response to methotrexate.[148] Treatment with an IL-6 blocking drug reduced the levels oxidative stress that was associated with reduction in joint damage and vascular degeneration in RA patients.[149]

The patients with JRA, who failed standard dose of methotrexate, showed increased disease severity associated with enhanced levels of IL-6 and TNF-α. Increased methotrexate dose was associated with reduction in the levels of IL-1α, IL-1β, IL-Ra, and IL-6; however, drug-induced decrease in the 71-joint Juvenile Arthritis Disease Activity Score (JADAS) was associated with reduction in IL-6 and TNFα. Treatment with Evanescent (ETN) decreased JADAS and increased TNF-α by 7-fold.[150] Another study on JRA revealed that treatment with ETN decreased the levels of IL-6 during inactive phase of the disease. Serum concentrations of TNF-α was higher in JRA patients during inactive phase of the disease compared to those in the active phase of the disease. The average value of serum TNFα enhanced several times irrespective clinical improvement following treatment with ETN.[151] JRA patients treated with ETN not only showed reduction in JADAS scores and CRP, but they also revealed attenuation of the levels of total cholesterol, low-density lipoprotein cholesterol, and triglycerides without any change in the levels of high-density lipoprotein cholesterol.[152]

TOXICITY OF MTX AND ANTI-CYTOKINE THERAPY

The common adverse effects of combined therapy with MTX and anti-cytokine therapy included increased incidence of infection, gastrointestinal symptoms, rash, and headache. Several cases of cancer have been reported in patients receiving etanercept, a TNF-alpha inhibitor.[153] The rate of tuberculosis in non-white patients with RA receiving anti-TNF-alpha was 6-fold higher than white patients with RA, and that the patients receiving infliximab or adalimumab 3–4-fold higher rate of tuberculosis than those receiving etanercept.[154] In addition, non-tuberculosis mycobacterial infections were observed in patients receiving anti-TNF-alpha inhibitors with or without methotrexate or prednisone.[155]

TREATMENT WITH GLUCOSAMINE AND CHONDROITIN

In a clinical study involving 46 patients with OA and 22 patients with RA, supplementation with glucosamine sulfate, chondroitin sulfate, and quercetin together for a period of 3 months showed a significant improvement in pain symptoms, daily physical activities (walking and climbing up and down stairs), and visual analogue scale. It also altered the synovial fluid properties. These effects of supplementation were not observed in patients with RA.[156] In a randomized, double-blind, placebo-controlled trial, the Glucosamine/Chondroitin Arthritis Intervention Trial (GAIT), 1583 OA patients received daily 1500 mg of glucosamine, 1200 mg of chondroitin sulfate individually or in combination, 200 mg of celecoxib or placebo for a period of 24 weeks. Up to 4000 mg of acetaminophen was allowed as rescue analgesia. The patients were stratified according to the intensity of knee pain yielding 1229 patients with mild pain and 354 patients with moderate to severe pain. The primary end point was a 20% decrease in knee pain from baseline data. The results showed that overall, the treatment with glucosamine and chondroitin sulfate was not significantly better compared to placebo in reducing knee pain by 20%. However, in patients with moderate to severe knee pain, the above treatment decreased the knee pain by about 25%.[157] The response rate in the celecoxib group was 10% higher than in placebo group, whereas in group receiving both glucosamine and chondroitin sulfate, it was about 6.5% higher than in placebo group. The above clinical study was extended to evaluate the effect of glucosamine and chondroitin sulfate, alone or in combination, celecoxib, and placebo on progressive loss of joint space and width (JSW) in 572 patients with knee OA who satisfied radiographic criteria (Kellgren/Lawrence grade 2 (K/L grade 2) or KL grade 3. At the end of observation period of 24 months, there was no significant difference in all treated groups compared to the placebo group. However, in KL-grade 2 group, a trend toward improvement of JSW was observed relative to the placebo group.[158] It has been reported that glucosamine sulfate is more effective than glucosamine chloride.[159] In a randomized, double-blind, placebo-controlled trial involving 622 patients with knee OA, the effect of glucosamine sulfate on changes in JSW was evaluated in 309 patients receiving daily once a day 400 mg of glucosamine sulfate and 313 patients receiving placebo for 2 years. The results showed that a significant reduction in minimum JSW loss occurred in the supplemented group compared to placebo group. The percentage of patients with radiographic progression of JSW was significantly reduced in the supplemented group compared to the placebo group. In addition, the knee pain was significantly improved in the supplemented group compared to the placebo group.[160] In a clinical study involving 89 patients with knee OA, supplementation with glucosamine chloride and chondroitin sulfate with or without exercise did not improve physical function, pain, or mobility after 1 month of treatment.[161]

TREATMENT WITH NON-STEROIDAL ANTI-INFLAMMATORY DRUGS (NSAIDs)

Chronic pain from arthritis remains one of the major problems that can cause disability and poor quality of life. Despite increased concerns of long-term toxicity of NSAIDs, especially cyclooxygenase-2 inhibitors, these drugs remain one of the viable options for managing the pain associated with RA.[162]

TREATMENT WITH COMPLEMENTARY MEDICINE

The patients with RA also utilize complementary and alternative medicine approaches to improve the symptoms of the disease. These include nutritional supplements, touch therapy, mind-body therapy, Reiki, acupuncture, herbal medicine, pulsed electromagnetic field, homeopathy, Ayurveda, and yoga.[163–165] A well-designed clinical study on any of the above complementary and alternative approaches has not been performed. The varying degrees of reduction in the joint pain in RA patients were reported in these studies.

In a clinical study involving 89 patients (90% female), supplementation with rose-hip powder (5 g/day) for a period of 6 months did not improve the pain intensity compared to the placebo group; it improved the Physician Global Evaluation of Disease activity.[166] Although L-carnitine and alpha-lipoic acid reduced MTX-induced oxidative damage in animal models,[167,168] it remains uncertain whether these antioxidants will have similar effects without interfering with the efficacy of MTX treatment in patients with RA or OA.

In rat model of RA, supplementation with MTX and probiotic bacteria Colinfant (COL) significantly inhibited inflammation and destructive arthritis-associated changes.[169]

PROPOSED MICRONUTRIENT MIXTURE IN COMBINATION WITH STANDARD THERAPY IN PATIENTS WITH ARTHRITIS

The treatment with MTX alone in combination with and anti-cytokine medications produced beneficial effects in patients with RA; however, significant adverse side effects of these treatments include infections such as non-tuberculosis and tuberculosis bacteria, gastrointestinal symptoms, rash, headache, and cancer. Therefore, additional approaches should be developed in order to enhance the efficacy of current therapy in RA and OA patients. The utilization of proposed micronutrient mixture in combination with standard therapy may improve the management of RA and OA by reducing oxidative stress and inflammation. Clinical studies should be initiated to test the above possibility. It is expected that the proposed micronutrient mixture would enhance the efficacy of standard therapy by increasing its response rates and decreasing its toxicity.

DIET AND LIFESTYLE RECOMMENDATIONS FOR HIGH RISK POPULATIONS AND PATIENTS WITH ARTHRITIS

A balanced diet containing low fat and high fiber with plenty of fruits and vegetables is suggested. Reducing consumption of inflammatory food items, such as refined sugar, fatty red meats, milk and milk products, cured meats, and alcohol is suggested. Lifestyle recommendations include daily moderate exercise, reduced stress, no tobacco smoking, and maintaining normal weight.

CONCLUSIONS

Arthritis is considered an inflammatory disease and primarily occurs in the form of rheumatoid arthritis (RA), osteoarthritis (OA), and juvenile rheumatoid arthritis (JRA). This disease is characterized by swelling, pain, and degenerative changes in the joints. OA is the most common form of arthritis in adults. Arthritis affects a large number of people throughout the world including the USA, and mostly occurs in older individuals. Extensive studies in human and animal models show that increased oxidative stress and inflammation are the early cellular events that initiate and promote arthritis. In most cases, inflammation precedes oxidative stress. Thus, attenuation of these two cellular defects may reduce the risk of developing arthritis among high- risk populations such as older individuals and those carrying mutated gene for arthritis. Previous studies on human arthritis with single antioxidants produced inconsistent results. The potential reasons for this are discussed. In order to reduce oxidative stress and inflammation, it is essential to increase the levels of antioxidant enzymes through activating the Nrf2/ARE pathway, as well as the levels of dietary and endogenous antioxidants by supplementa-tion. A mixture of micronutrients to achieve the above goal is proposed. At present, there are no effec-tive preventive strategies to reduce the risk of RA. The proposed micronutrient mixture may reduce the risk of developing arthritis. Low-dose methotrexate (MTX) therapy is considered a gold standard for the initial treatment of arthritis. High doses of methotrexate and anti-cytokine therapy alone or in combination have been useful in improving the symptoms of arthritis. The combination of MTX and anti-cytokine therapy has produced better results than either agent alone. Nevertheless, the current treatments are not considered an optimal, and they produce severe side effects in some individuals. The proposed micronutrients in combination with standard therapy may help in improved management of arthritis. The effectiveness proposed micronutrient mixture in prevention and improved management of arthritis should be tested by well-designed clinical trials.

REFERENCES

1. Kim HA, Lee YJ, Seong SC, Choe KW, Song YW. Apoptotic chondrocyte death in human osteoarthri-tis. *J Rheumatol*. 2000;27(2):455–462.
2. Mistry D, Oue Y, Chambers MG, Kayser MV, Mason RM. Chondrocyte death during murine osteoar-thritis. *Osteoarthr Cartil*. 2004;12(2):131–141.
3. Hashimoto S, Ochs RL, Komiya S, Lotz M. Linkage of chondrocyte apoptosis and cartilage degradation in human osteoarthritis. *Arthritis Rheum*. 1998;41(9):1632–1638.
4. Altindag O, Karakoc M, Kocyigit A, Celik H, Soran N. Increased DNA damage and oxidative stress in patients with rheumatoid arthritis. *Clin Biochem*. 2007;40(3–4):167–171.
5. Miesel R, Hartung R, Kroeger H. Priming of NADPH oxidase by tumor necrosis factor alpha in patients with inflammatory and autoimmune rheumatic diseases. *Inflammation*. 1996;20(4):427–438.
6. Mirshafiey A, Mohsenzadegan M. The role of reactive oxygen species in immunopathogenesis of rheu-matoid arthritis. *Iran J Allergy Asthma Immunol*. 2008;7(4):195–202.
7. Bauerova K, Bezek A. Role of reactive oxygen and nitrogen species in etiopathogenesis of rheumatoid arthritis. *Gen Physiol Biophys*. 1999;18:15–20.
8. Hitchon CA, El-Gabalawy HS. Oxidation in rheumatoid arthritis. *Arthritis Res Ther*. 2004;6(6):265–278.
9. Nemirovskiy OV, Radabaugh MR, Aggarwal P, et al. Plasma 3-nitrotyrosine is a biomarker in animal mod-els of arthritis: Pharmacological dissection of iNOS' role in disease. *Nitric Oxide*. 2009;20(3):150–156.
10. Strosova M, Tomaskova I, Ponist S, et al. Oxidative impairment of plasma and skeletal muscle sarcoplas-mic reticulum in rats with adjuvant arthritis—Effects of pyridoindole antioxidants. *Neuro Endocrinol Lett*. 2008;29(5):706–711.
11. Strosova M, Karlovska J, Spickett CM, et al. Modulation of SERCA in the chronic phase of adjuvant arthritis as a possible adaptation mechanism of redox imbalance. *Free Radic Res*. 2009;43(9):852–864.
12. Mateen S, Moin S, Khan AQ, Zafar A, Fatima N. Increased reactive oxygen species formation and oxi-dative stress in rheumatoid arthritis. *PLoS One*. 2016;11(4):e0152925.
13. Seven A, Guzel S, Aslan M, Hamuryudan V. Lipid, protein, DNA oxidation and antioxidant status in rheumatoid arthritis. *Clin Biochem*. 2008;41(7–8):538–543.
14. Miesel R, Murphy MP, Kroger H. Enhanced mitochondrial radical production in patients which rheu-matoid arthritis correlates with elevated levels of tumor necrosis factor alpha in plasma. *Free Radic Res*. 1996;25(2):161–169.
15. Khan F, Siddiqui AA. Prevalence of anti-3-nitrotyrosine antibodies in the joint synovial fluid of patients with rheumatoid arthritis, osteoarthritis, and systemic lupus erythematosus. *Clin Chim Acta*. 2006;370(1–2):100–107.

16. Richardot P, Charni-Ben Tabassi N, Toh L, et al. Nitrated type III collagen as a biological marker of nitric oxide-mediated synovial tissue metabolism in osteoarthritis. *Osteoarthr Cartil.* 2009;17(10):1362–1367.

17. Surapaneni KM, Venkataramana G. Status of lipid peroxidation, glutathione, ascorbic acid, vitamin E, and antioxidant enzymes in patients with osteoarthritis. *Indian J Med Sci.* 2007;61(1):9–14.

18. Nagy G, Clark JM, Buzas E, et al. Nitric oxide production of T lymphocytes is increased in rheumatoid arthritis. *Immunol Lett.* 2008;118(1):55–58.

19. Cedergren J, Forslund T, Sundqvist T, Skogh T. Intracellular oxidative activation in synovial fluid neutrophils from patients with rheumatoid arthritis but not from other arthritis patients. *J Rheumatol.* 2007;34(11):2162–2170.

20. Kurien BT, Scofield RH. Autoimmunity and oxidatively modified autoantigens. *Autoimmun Rev.* 2008;7(7):567–573.

21. Garcia-Gonzalez A, Gaxiola-Robles R, Zenteno-Savin T. Oxidative stress in patients with rheumatoid arthritis. *Rev Invest Clin.* 2015;67(1):46–53.

22. Veselinovic M, Barudzic N, Vuletic M, et al. Oxidative stress in rheumatoid arthritis patients: Relationship to diseases activity. *Mol Cell Biochem.* 2014;391(1–2):225–232.

23. Nakajima A, Aoki Y, Shibata Y, et al. Identification of clinical parameters associated with serum oxidative stress in patients with rheumatoid arthritis. *Mod Rheumatol.* 2014;24(6):926–930.

24. Staron A, Makosa G, Koter-Michalak M. Oxidative stress in erythrocytes from patients with rheumatoid arthritis. *Rheumatol Int.* 2012;32(2):331–334.

25. Navarro-Compan V, Melguizo-Madrid E, Hernandez-Cruz B, et al. Interaction between oxidative stress and smoking is associated with an increased risk of rheumatoid arthritis: A case-control study. *Rheumatology (Oxford).* 2013;52(3):487–493.

26. Chang K, Yang SM, Kim SH, Han KH, Park SJ, Shin JI. Smoking and rheumatoid arthritis. *Int J Mol Sci.* 2014;15(12):22279–22295.

27. Vaillancourt F, Fahmi H, Shi Q, et al. 4-hydroxynonenal induces apoptosis in human osteoarthritic chondrocytes: The protective role of glutathione-S-transferase. *Arthritis Res Ther.* 2008;10(5):R107.

28. Morquette B, Shi Q, Lavigne P, Ranger P, Fernandes JC, Benderdour M. Production of lipid peroxidation products in osteoarthritic tissues: New evidence linking 4-hydroxynonenal to cartilage degradation. *Arthritis Rheum.* 2006;54(1):271–281.

29. Lo Gullo A, Mandraffino G, Sardo MA, et al. Circulating progenitor cells in rheumatoid arthritis: Association with inflammation and oxidative stress. *Scand J Rheumatol.* 2014;43(3):184–193.

30. Cacciapaglia F, Anelli MG, Rizzo D, et al. Influence of TNF-alpha inhibition on oxidative stress of rheumatoid arthritis patients. *Reumatismo.* 2015;67(3):97–102.

31. Romano E, Terenzi R, Manetti M, et al. Disease activity improvement in rheumatoid arthritis treated with tumor necrosis factor-alpha inhibitors correlates with increased soluble Fas levels. *J Rheumatol.* 2014;41(10):1961–1965.

32. Miggiano GA, Gagliardi L. Diet, nutrition, and rheumatoid arthritis. *Clin Ter.* 2005;156(3):115–123.

33. Taylor PC, Feldmann M. Anti-TNF biologic agents: Still the therapy of choice for rheumatoid arthritis. *Nat Rev Rheumatol.* 2009;5(10):578–582.

34. Xu S, Lu H, Lin J, Chen Z, Jiang D. Regulation of TNFalpha and IL1beta in rheumatoid arthritis synovial fibroblasts by leukotriene B4. *Rheumatol Int.* 2009;30(9):1183–1189.

35. Woolley DE, Tetlow LC. Mast cell activation and its relation to proinflammatory cytokine production in the rheumatoid lesion. *Arthritis Res.* 2000;2(1):65–74.

36. Robak T, Gladalska A, Stepien H. The tumor necrosis factor family of receptors/ligands in the serum of patients with rheumatoid arthritis. *Eur Cytokine Netw.* 1998;9(2):145–154.

37. Stamp LK, Easson A, Pettersson L, Highton J, Hessian PA. Monocyte derived interleukin (IL)-23 is an important determinant of synovial Il-17A expression in rheumatoid arthritis. *J Rheumatol.* 2009;36(11):2403–2408.

38. Tetlow LC, Harper N, Dunningham T, Morris MA, Bertfield H, Woolley DE. Effects of induced mast cell activation on prostaglandin E and metalloproteinase production by rheumatoid synovial tissue in vitro. *Ann Rheum Dis.* 1998;57(1):25–32.

39. Bazzichi L, Ghiadoni L, Rossi A, et al. Osteopontin is associated with increased arterial stiffness in rheumatoid arthritis. *Mol Med.* 2009;15(11–12):402.

40. Hou WS, Li W, Keyszer G, et al. Comparison of cathepsins K and S expression within the rheumatoid and osteoarthritic synovium. *Arthritis Rheum.* 2002;46(3):663–674.

41. van den Berg WB, Joosten LA, van de Loo FA. TNF alpha and IL-1 beta are separate targets in chronic arthritis. *Clin Exp Rheumatol.* 1999;17(6 Suppl 18):S105–S114.

42. Joosten LA, Smeets RL, Koenders MI, et al. Interleukin-18 promotes joint inflammation and induces interleukin-1-driven cartilage destruction. *Am J Pathol.* 2004;165(3):959–967.

43. Abdollahi-Roodsaz S, Joosten LA, Koenders MI, van den Brand BT, van de Loo FA, van den Berg WB. Local interleukin-1-driven joint pathology is dependent on toll-like receptor 4 activation. *Am J Pathol.* 2009;175(5):2004–2013.

44. Fournier C. Where do T cells stand in rheumatoid arthritis? *Joint Bone Spine.* 2005;72(6):527–532.

45. Mandik-Nayak L, Allen PM. Initiation of an autoimmune response: Insights from a transgenic model of rheumatoid arthritis. *Immunol Res.* 2005;32(1–3):5–13.

46. Megias J, Guillen MI, Clerigues V, et al. Heme oxygenase-1 induction modulates microsomal prostaglandin E synthase-1 expression and prostaglandin E(2) production in osteoarthritic chondrocytes. *Biochem Pharmacol.* 2009;77(12):1806–1813.

47. Guillen M, Megias J, Gomar F, Alcaraz M. Haem oxygenase-1 regulates catabolic and anabolic processes in osteoarthritic chondrocytes. *J Pathol.* 2008;214(4):515–522.

48. Li X, Afif H, Cheng S, et al. Expression and regulation of microsomal prostaglandin E synthase-1 in human osteoarthritic cartilage and chondrocytes. *J Rheumatol.* 2005;32(5):887–895.

49. Kojima M, Kojima T, Suzuki S, et al. Depression, inflammation, and pain in patients with rheumatoid arthritis. *Arthritis Rheum.* 2009;61(8):1018–1024.

50. Chang Y, Wei W. Angiotensin II in inflammation, immunity and rheumatoid arthritis. *Clin Exp Immunol.* 2015;179(2):137–145.

51. Alanara T, Karstila K, Moilanen T, Silvennoinen O, Isomaki P. Expression of IL-10 family cytokines in rheumatoid arthritis: Elevated levels of IL-19 in the joints. *Scand J Rheumatol.* 2010;39(2):118–126.

52. Scrivo R, Conigliaro P, Riccieri V, et al. Distribution of interleukin-10 family cytokines in serum and synovial fluid of patients with inflammatory arthritis reveals different contribution to systemic and joint inflammation. *Clin Exp Immunol.* 2015;179(2):300–308.

53. Talabot-Ayer D, McKee T, Gindre P, et al. Distinct serum and synovial fluid interleukin (IL)-33 levels in rheumatoid arthritis, psoriatic arthritis, and osteoarthritis. *Joint Bone Spine.* 2012;79(1):32–37.

54. Hillen MR, Hartgring SA, Willis CR, et al. The additive inflammatory in vivo and in vitro effects of IL-7 and TSLP in arthritis underscore the therapeutic rationale for dual blockade. *PLoS One.* 2015;10(6):e0130830.

55. Salvemini D, Mazzon E, Dugo L, et al. Amelioration of joint disease in a rat model of collagen-induced arthritis by M40403, a superoxide dismutase mimetic. *Arthritis Rheum.* 2001;44(12):2909–2921.

56. Garcia-Gonzalez A, Lotz M, Ochoa JL. Anti-inflammatory activity of superoxide dismutase obtained from Debaryomyces hansenii on type II collagen induced arthritis in rats. *Rev Invest Clin.* 2009;61(3):212–220.

57. Choi EJ, Bae SC, Yu R, Youn J, Sung MK. Dietary vitamin E and quercetin modulate inflammatory responses of collagen-induced arthritis in mice. *J Med Food.* 2009;12(4):770–775.

58. Gardi C, Bauerova K, Stringa B, et al. Quercetin reduced inflammation and increased antioxidant defense in rat adjuvant arthritis. *Arch Biochem Biophys.* 2015;583:150–157.

59. Elmali N, Baysal O, Harma A, Esenkaya I, Mizrak B. Effects of resveratrol in inflammatory arthritis. *Inflammation.* 2007;30(1–2):1–6.

60. Tastekin N, Aydogdu N, Dokmeci D, et al. Protective effects of L-carnitine and alpha-lipoic acid in rats with adjuvant arthritis. *Pharmacol Res.* 2007;56(4):303–310.

61. Lee EY, Lee CK, Lee KU, et al. Alpha-lipoic acid suppresses the development of collagen-induced arthritis and protects against bone destruction in mice. *Rheumatol Int.* 2007;27(3):225–233.

62. Morinobu A, Biao W, Tanaka S, et al. (-)-Epigallocatechin-3-gallate suppresses osteoclast differentiation and ameliorates experimental arthritis in mice. *Arthritis Rheum.* 2008;58(7):2012–2018.

63. Riegsecker S, Wiczynski D, Kaplan MJ, Ahmed S. Potential benefits of green tea polyphenol EGCG in the prevention and treatment of vascular inflammation in rheumatoid arthritis. *Life Sci.* 2013;93(8):307–312.

64. Fechtner S, Singh A, Chourasia M, Ahmed S. Molecular insights into the differences in anti-inflammatory activities of green tea catechins on IL-1beta signaling in rheumatoid arthritis synovial fibroblasts. *Toxicol Appl Pharmacol.* 2017;329:112–120.

65. Sundaram MS, Hemshekhar M, Santhosh MS, et al. Tamarind seed (tamarindus indica) extract ameliorates adjuvant-induced arthritis via regulating the mediators of cartilage/bone degeneration, inflammation and oxidative stress. *Sci Rep.* 2015;5:11117.

66. Umar S, Umar K, Sarwar AH, et al. Boswellia serrata extract attenuates inflammatory mediators and oxidative stress in collagen induced arthritis. *Phytomedicine.* 2014;21(6):847–856.

67. Tang LL, Gao JS, Chen XR, Xie X. Inhibitory effect of resveratrol on the proliferation of synovio-cytes in rheumatoid arthritis and its mechanism in vitro. *Zhong Nan Da Xue Xue Bao Yi Xue Ban*. 2006;31(4):528–533.

68. Funk JL, Frye JB, Oyarzo JN, et al. Efficacy and mechanism of action of turmeric supplements in the treatment of experimental arthritis. *Arthritis Rheum*. 2006;54(11):3452–3464.

69. Li X, Phillips FM, An HS, et al. The action of resveratrol, a phytoestrogen found in grapes, on the inter-vertebral disc. *Spine (Phila Pa 1976)*. 2008;33(24):2586–2595.

70. Byun HS, Song JK, Kim YR, et al. Caspase-8 has an essential role in resveratrol-induced apoptosis of rheumatoid fibroblast-like synoviocytes. *Rheumatology (Oxford)*. 2008;47(3):301–308.

71. Lee CK, Lee EY, Kim YG, Mun SH, Moon HB, Yoo B. Alpha-lipoic acid inhibits TNF-alpha induced NF-kappa B activation through blocking of MEKK1-MKK4-IKK signaling cascades. *Int Immunopharmacol*. 2008;8(2):362–370.

72. Yun HJ, Yoo WH, Han MK, Lee YR, Kim JS, Lee SI. Epigallocatechin-3-gallate suppresses TNF-alpha-induced production of MMP-1 and -3 in rheumatoid arthritis synovial fibroblasts. *Rheumatol Int*. 2008;29(1):23–29.

73. Tetlow LC, Woolley DE. The effects of 1 alpha,25-dihydroxyvitamin D(3) on matrix metalloproteinase and prostaglandin E(2) production by cells of the rheumatoid lesion. *Arthritis Res*. 1999;1(1):63–70.

74. Canter PH, Wider B, Ernst E. The antioxidant vitamins A, C, E and selenium in the treatment of arthri-tis: A systematic review of randomized clinical trials. *Rheumatology (Oxford)*. 2007;46(8):1223–1233.

75. Pattison DJ, Winyard PG. Dietary antioxidants in inflammatory arthritis: Do they have any role in etiol-ogy or therapy? *Nat Clin Pract Rheumatol*. 2008;4(11):590–596.

76. Abdollahzad H, Aghdashi MA, Asghari Jafarabadi M, Alipour B. Effects of coenzyme Q10 supple-mentation on inflammatory cytokines (TNF-alpha, IL-6) and oxidative stress in rheumatoid arthritis patients: A randomized controlled trial. *Arch Med Res*. 2015;46(7):527–533.

77. Lo Gullo A, Mandraffino G, Bagnato G, et al. Vitamin D status in rheumatoid arthritis: Inflammation, arterial stiffness and circulating progenitor cell number. *PLoS One*. 2015;10(8):e0134602.

78. Karlson EW, Shadick NA, Cook NR, Buring JE, Lee IM. Vitamin E in the primary prevention of rheu-matoid arthritis: The Women's Health Study. *Arthritis Rheum*. 2008;59(11):1589–1595.

79. van Vugt RM, Rijken PJ, Rietveld AG, van Vugt AC, Dijkmans BA. Antioxidant intervention in rheu-matoid arthritis: Results of an open pilot study. *Clin Rheumatol*. 2008;27(6):771–775.

80. Bae SC, Jung WJ, Lee EJ, Yu R, Sung MK. Effects of antioxidant supplements intervention on the level of plasma inflammatory molecules and disease severity of rheumatoid arthritis patients. *J Am Coll Nutr*. 2009;28(1):56–62.

81. Vasiljevic D, Veselinovic M, Jovanovic M, et al. Evaluation of the effects of different supplementation on oxidative status in patients with rheumatoid arthritis. *Clin Rheumatol*. 2016;35(8):1909–1915.

82. Darlington LG, Stone TW. Antioxidants and fatty acids in the amelioration of rheumatoid arthritis and related disorders. *Br J Nutr*. 2001;85(3):251–269.

83. Rennie KL, Hughes J, Lang R, Jebb SA. Nutritional management of rheumatoid arthritis: A review of the evidence. *J Hum Nutr Diet*. 2003;16(2):97–109.

84. Maestroni GJ, Sulli A, Pizzorni C, Villaggio B, Cutolo M. Melatonin in rheumatoid arthritis: Synovial macrophages show melatonin receptors. *Ann N Y Acad Sci*. 2002;966:271–275.

85. El-Awady HM, El-Wakkad AS, Saleh MT, Muhammad SI, Ghaniema EM. Serum melatonin in juvenile rheumatoid arthritis: Correlation with disease activity. *Pak J Biol Sci*. 2007;10(9):1471–1476.

86. Prasad KN, Bondy SC. Inhibition of early upstream events in prodromal Alzheimer's disease by use of targeted antioxidants. *Curr Aging Sci*. 2014;7(2):77–90.

87. Prasad KN. Simultaneous activation of Nrf2 and elevation of dietary and endogenous antioxidants for prevention and improved managment of Parkinson's disease. In: Bondy SCC, ed. *Inflammation, Aging and Oxidative Stress*. New York: Springer; 2016:277–301.

88. Vile GF, Winterbourn CC. Inhibition of adriamycin-promoted microsomal lipid peroxidation by beta-carotene, alpha-tocopherol, and retinol at high and low oxygen partial pressures. *FEBS Lett*. 1988;238(2):353–356.

89. Niki E. Interaction of ascorbate and alpha-tocopherol. *Ann N Y Acad Sci*. 1987;498:186–199.

90. Prasad KN. Oxidative stress and pro-inflammatory cytokines may act as one of signals for regulating microRNAs expression in Alzheimer's disease. *Mech Ageing Dev*. 2017;162:63–71.

91. Wu H, Kong L, Tan Y, et al. C66 ameliorates diabetic nephropathy in mice by both upregulating NRF2 function via increase in miR-200a and inhibiting miR-21. *Diabetologia*. 2016;59:1558–1568.

92. Jaramillo MC, Zhang DD. The emerging role of the Nrf2-Keap1 signaling pathway in cancer. *Genes Dev*. 2013;27(20):2179–2191.

93. Williamson TP, Johnson DA, Johnson JA. Activation of the Nrf2-ARE pathway by siRNA knockdown of Keap1 reduces oxidative stress and provides partial protection from MPTP-mediated neurotoxicity. *Neurotoxicology.* 2012;33(3):272–279.

94. Itoh K, Chiba T, Takahashi S, et al. An Nrf2/small Maf heterodimer mediates the induction of phase II detoxifying enzyme genes through antioxidant response elements. *Biochem Biophys Res Commun.* 1997;236(2):313–322.

95. Hayes JD, Chanas SA, Henderson CJ, et al. The Nrf2 transcription factor contributes both to the basal expression of glutathione S-transferases in mouse liver and to their induction by the chemopreventive synthetic antioxidants, butylated hydroxyanisole, and ethoxyquin. *Biochem Soc Trans.* 2000;28(2):33–41.

96. Chan K, Han XD, Kan YW. An important function of Nrf2 in combating oxidative stress: Detoxification of acetaminophen. *Proc Natl Acad Sci USA.* 2001;98(8):4611–4616.

97. Ramsey CP, Glass CA, Montgomery MB, et al. Expression of Nrf2 in neurodegenerative diseases. *J Neuropathol Exp Neurol.* 2007;66(1):75–85.

98. Chen PC, Vargas MR, Pani AK, et al. Nrf2-mediated neuroprotection in the MPTP mouse model of Parkinson's disease: Critical role for the astrocyte. *Proc Natl Acad Sci USA.* 2009;106(8):2933–2938.

99. Lastres-Becker I, Ulusoy A, Innamorato NG, et al. Alpha-synuclein expression and Nrf2 deficiency cooperate to aggravate protein aggregation, neuronal death, and inflammation in early-stage Parkinson's disease. *Hum Mol Genet.* 2012;21(14):3173–3192.

100. Xi YD, Yu HL, Ding J, et al. Flavonoids protect cerebrovascular endothelial cells through Nrf2 and PI3K from beta-amyloid peptide-induced oxidative damage. *Curr Neurovasc Res.* 2012;9(1):32–41.

101. Suh JH, Shenvi SV, Dixon BM, et al. Decline in transcriptional activity of Nrf2 causes age-related loss of glutathione synthesis, which is reversible with lipoic acid. *Proc Natl Acad Sci USA.* 2004;101(10):3381–3386.

102. Trujillo J, Chirino YI, Molina-Jijon E, Anderica-Romero AC, Tapia E, Pedraza-Chaverri J. Renoprotective effect of the antioxidant curcumin: Recent findings. *Redox Biol.* 2013;1(1):448–456.

103. Steele ML, Fuller S, Patel M, Kersaitis C, Ooi L, Munch G. Effect of Nrf2 activators on release of glutathione, cysteinylglycine, and homocysteine by human U373 astroglial cells. *Redox Biol.* 2013;1(1):441–445.

104. Kode A, Rajendrasozhan S, Caito S, Yang SR, Megson IL, Rahman I. Resveratrol induces glutathione synthesis by activation of Nrf2 and protects against cigarette smoke-mediated oxidative stress in human lung epithelial cells. *Am J Physiol Lung Cell Mol Physiol.* 2008;294(3):L478–L488.

105. Gao L, Wang J, Sekhar KR, et al. Novel n-3 fatty acid oxidation products activate Nrf2 by destabilizing the association between Keap1 and Cullin3 *J Biol Chem.* 2007;282(4):2529–2537.

106. Saw CL, Yang AY, Guo Y, Kong AN. Astaxanthin and omega-3 fatty acids individually and in combination protect against oxidative stress via the Nrf2-ARE pathway. *Food Chem Toxicol.* 2013;62:869–875.

107. Song J, Kang SM, Lee WT, Park KA, Lee KM, Lee JE. Glutathione protects brain endothelial cells from hydrogen peroxide-induced oxidative stress by increasing nrf2 expression. *Exp Neurobiol.* 2014;23(1):93–103.

108. Ji L, Liu R, Zhang XD, et al. N-acetylcysteine attenuates phosgene-induced acute lung injury via upregulation of Nrf2 expression. *Inhal Toxicol.* 2010;22(7):535–542.

109. Choi HK, Pokharel YR, Lim SC, et al. Inhibition of liver fibrosis by solubilized coenzyme Q10: Role of Nrf2 activation in inhibiting transforming growth factor-beta1 expression. *Toxicol Appl Pharmacol.* 2009;240(3):377–384.

110. Bai H, Liu R, Chen HL, et al. Enhanced antioxidant effect of caffeic acid phenethyl ester and Trolox in combination against radiation induced-oxidative stress. *Chem Biol Interact.* 2014;207:7–15.

111. Cui L, Jeong H, Borovecki F, Parkhurst CN, Tanese N, Krainc D. Transcriptional repression of PGC-1alpha by mutant huntingtin leads to mitochondrial dysfunction and neurodegeneration. *Cell.* 2006;127(1):59–69.

112. Li XH, Li CY, Lu JM, Tian RB, Wei J. Allicin ameliorates cognitive deficits ageing-induced learning and memory deficits through enhancing of Nrf2 antioxidant signaling pathways. *Neurosci Lett.* 2012;514(1):46–50.

113. Bergstrom P, Andersson HC, Gao Y, et al. Repeated transient sulforaphane stimulation in astrocytes leads to prolonged Nrf2-mediated gene expression and protection from superoxide-induced damage. *Neuropharmacology.* 2011;60(2–3):343–353.

114. Wruck CJ, Gotz ME, Herdegen T, Varoga D, Brandenburg LO, Pufe T. Kavalactones protect neural cells against amyloid beta peptide-induced neurotoxicity via extracellular signal-regulated kinase 1/2-dependent nuclear factor erythroid 2-related factor 2 activation. *Mol Pharmacol.* 2008;73(6):1785–1795.

115. Wruck CJ, Fragoulis A, Gurzynski A, et al. Role of oxidative stress in rheumatoid arthritis: Insights from the Nrf2-knockout mice. *Ann Rheum Dis.* 2011;70(5):844–850.

116. Maicas N, Ferrandiz ML, Brines R, et al. Deficiency of Nrf2 accelerates the effector phase of arthritis and aggravates joint disease. *Antioxid Redox Signal.* 2011;15(4):889–901.

117. Song SM, Park YS, Lee A, et al. Concentrations of blood vitamin A, C, E, coenzyme Q10, and urine cotinine related to cigarette smoking exposure. *Korean J Lab Med.* 2009;29(1):10–16.

118. Galan P, Viteri FE, Bertrais S, et al. Serum concentrations of beta-carotene, vitamins C and E, zinc, and selenium are influenced by sex, age, diet, smoking status, alcohol consumption, and corpulence in a general French adult population. *Eur J Clin Nutr.* 2005;59(10):1181–1190.

119. Adhikari D, Baxi J, Risal S, Singh PP. Oxidative stress and antioxidant status in cancer patients and healthy subjects, a case-control study. *Nepal Med Coll J.* 2005;7(2):112–115.

120. Li W, Khor TO, Xu C, et al. Activation of Nrf2-antioxidant signaling attenuates NFkappaB-inflammatory response and elicits apoptosis. *Biochem Pharmacol.* 2008;76(11):1485–1489.

121. Kim J, Cha YN, Surh YJ. A protective role of nuclear factor-erythroid 2-related factor-2 (Nrf2) in inflammatory disorders. *Mutat Res.* 2010;690(1–2):12–23.

122. Abate A, Yang G, Dennery PA, Oberle S, Schroder H. Synergistic inhibition of cyclooxygenase-2 expression by vitamin E and aspirin. *Free Radic Biol Med.* 2000;29(11):1135–1142.

123. Devaraj S, Tang R, Adams-Huet B, et al. Effect of high-dose alpha-tocopherol supplementation on biomarkers of oxidative stress and inflammation and carotid atherosclerosis in patients with coronary artery disease. *Am J Clin Nutr.* 2007;86(5):1392–1398.

124. Fu Y, Zheng S, Lin J, Ryerse J, Chen A. Curcumin protects the rat liver from CCl4-caused injury and fibrogenesis by attenuating oxidative stress and suppressing inflammation. *Mol Pharmacol.* 2008;73(2):399–409.

125. Lee HS, Jung KK, Cho JY, et al. Neuroprotective effect of curcumin is mainly mediated by blockade of microglial cell activation. *Pharmazie.* 2007;62(12):937–942.

126. Rahman S, Bhatia K, Khan AQ, et al. Topically applied vitamin E prevents massive cutaneous inflammatory and oxidative stress responses induced by double application of 12-O-tetradecanoylphorbol-13-acetate (TPA) in mice. *Chem Biol Interact.* 2008;172(3):195–205.

127. Suzuki YJ, Aggarwal BB, Packer L. Alpha-lipoic acid is a potent inhibitor of NF-kappa B activation in human T cells. *Biochem Biophys Res Commun.* 1992;189(3):1709–1715.

128. Zhu J, Yong W, Wu X, et al. Anti-inflammatory effect of resveratrol on TNF-alpha-induced MCP-1 expression in adipocytes. *Biochem Biophys Res Commun.* 2008;369(2):471–477.

129. Prasad KN. *Etiology of Alzheimer's Disease Prevention and Improved Management by Micronutrients.* Boca Raton, FL: CRC Press; 2015.

130. Herman S, Zurgil N, Langevitz P, Ehrenfeld M, Deutsch M. Methotrexate selectively modulates TH1/TH2 balance in active rheumatoid arthritis patients. *Clin Exp Rheumatol.* 2008;26(2):317–323.

131. Cronstein BN. Low-dose methotrexate: A mainstay in the treatment of rheumatoid arthritis. *Pharmacol Rev.* 2005;57(2):163–172.

132. Fiehn C. Methotrexate in rheumatology. *Z Rheumatol.* 2009;60(1):1–4.

133. Swierkot J, Szechinski J. Methotrexate in rheumatoid arthritis. *Pharmacol Rep.* 2006;58(4):473–492.

134. Braun J, Rau R. An update on methotrexate. *Curr Opin Rheumatol.* 2009;21(3):216–223.

135. den Broeder AA, Wanten GJ, Oyen WJ, Naber T, van Riel PL, Barrera P. Neutrophil migration and production of reactive oxygen species during treatment with a fully human anti-tumor necrosis factor-alpha monoclonal antibody in patients with rheumatoid arthritis. *J Rheumatol.* 2003;30(2):232–237.

136. Edrees AF, Misra SN, Abdou NI. Anti-tumor necrosis factor (TNF) therapy in rheumatoid arthritis: Correlation of TNF-alpha serum level with clinical response and benefit from changing dose or frequency of infliximab infusions. *Clin Exp Rheumatol.* 2005;23(4):469–474.

137. Popa C, van Tits LJ, Barrera P, et al. Anti-inflammatory therapy with tumour necrosis factor alpha inhibitors improves high-density lipoprotein cholesterol antioxidative capacity in rheumatoid arthritis patients. *Ann Rheum Dis.* 2009;68(6):868–872.

138. Kasama T, Isozaki T, Odai T, et al. Expression of angiopoietin-1 in osteoblasts and its inhibition by tumor necrosis factor-alpha and interferon-gamma. *Transl Res.* 2007;149(5):265–273.

139. Gonzalez-Gay MA, Garcia-Unzueta MT, De Matias JM, et al. Influence of anti-TNF-alpha infliximab therapy on adhesion molecules associated with atherogenesis in patients with rheumatoid arthritis. *Clin Exp Rheumatol.* 2006;24(4):373–379.

140. Singh JA, Christensen R, Wells GA, et al. Biologics for rheumatoid arthritis: An overview of cochrane reviews. *Cochrane Database Syst Rev.* 2009;4:CD007848.

141. Keystone E, Heijde D, Mason D Jr, et al. Certolizumab pegol plus methotrexate is significantly more effective than placebo plus methotrexate in active rheumatoid arthritis: Findings of a 52-week, phase III, multicenter, randomized, double-blind, placebo-controlled, parallel-group study. *Arthritis Rheum.* 2008;58(11):3319–3329.

142. Smolen J, Landewe RB, Mease P, et al. Efficacy and safety of certolizumab pegol plus methotrexate in active rheumatoid arthritis: The RAPID 2 study. A randomised controlled trial. *Ann Rheum Dis.* 2009;68(6):797–804.

143. Duggan ST, Keam SJ. Certolizumab pegol: In rheumatoid arthritis. *BioDrugs.* 2009;23(6):407–417.

144. Breedveld FC, Weisman MH, Kavanaugh AF, et al. The PREMIER study: A multicenter, randomized, double-blind clinical trial of combination therapy with adalimumab plus methotrexate versus methotrexate alone or adalimumab alone in patients with early, aggressive rheumatoid arthritis who had not had previous methotrexate treatment. *Arthritis Rheum.* 2006;54(1):26–37.

145. Koller MD, Aletaha D, Funovits J, Pangan A, Baker D, Smolen JS. Response of elderly patients with rheumatoid arthritis to methotrexate or TNF inhibitors compared with younger patients. *Rheumatology (Oxford).* 2009;48(12):1575–1580.

146. Maini RN, Taylor PC, Szechinski J, et al. Double-blind randomized controlled clinical trial of the interleukin-6 receptor antagonist, tocilizumab, in European patients with rheumatoid arthritis who had an incomplete response to methotrexate. *Arthritis Rheum.* 2006;54(9):2817–2829.

147. Emery P, Keystone E, Tony HP, et al. IL-6 receptor inhibition with tocilizumab improves treatment outcomes in patients with rheumatoid arthritis refractory to anti-tumor necrosis factor biologicals: Results from a 24-week multicentre randomised placebo-controlled trial. *Ann Rheum Dis.* 2008;67(11):1516–1523.

148. Nishimoto N, Miyasaka N, Yamamoto K, et al. Study of active controlled tocilizumab monotherapy for rheumatoid arthritis patients with an inadequate response to methotrexate (SATORI): Significant reduction in disease activity and serum vascular endothelial growth factor by IL-6 receptor inhibition therapy. *Mod Rheumatol.* 2009;19(1):12–19.

149. Hirao M, Yamasaki N, Oze H, et al. Serum level of oxidative stress marker is dramatically low in patients with rheumatoid arthritis treated with tocilizumab. *Rheumatol Int.* 2012;32(12):4041–4045.

150. Funk RS, Chan MA, Becker ML. Cytokine biomarkers of disease activity and therapeutic response after initiating methotrexate therapy in patients with juvenile idiopathic arthritis. *Pharmacotherapy.* 2017;37(6):700–711.

151. Kaminiarczyk-Pyzalka D, Adamczak K, Mikos H, Klimecka I, Moczko J, Niedziela M. Proinflammatory cytokines in monitoring the course of disease and effectiveness of treatment with etanercept (ETN) of children with oligo- and polyarticular juvenile idiopathic arthritis (JIA). *Clin Lab.* 2014;60(9):1481–1490.

152. De Sanctis S, Marcovecchio ML, Gaspari S, et al. Etanercept improves lipid profile and oxidative stress measures in patients with juvenile idiopathic arthritis. *J Rheumatol.* 2013;40(6):943–948.

153. Rousseau A, Taberne R, Siberchicot F, Fricain JC, Zwetyenga N. TNF-alpha inhibitor etanercept and oral cavity carcinoma. *Rev Stomatol Chir Maxillofac.* 2009;110(5):306–308.

154. Dixon WG, Hyrich KL, Watson KD, et al. Drug-specific risk of tuberculosis in patients with rheumatoid arthritis treated with anti-TNF therapy: Results from the British Society for Rheumatology Biologics Register (BSRBR). *Ann Rheum Dis.* 2009;69(3):522–528.

155. Winthrop KL, Chang E, Yamashita S, Iademarco MF, LoBue PA. Nontuberculous mycobacteria infections and anti-tumor necrosis factor-alpha therapy. *Emerg Infect Dis.* 2009;15(10):1556–1561.

156. Matsuno H, Nakamura H, Katayama K, et al. Effects of an oral administration of glucosamine-chondroitin-quercetin glucoside on the synovial fluid properties in patients with osteoarthritis and rheumatoid arthritis. *Biosci Biotechnol Biochem.* 2009;73(2):288–292.

157. Clegg DO, Reda DJ, Harris CL, et al. Glucosamine, chondroitin sulfate, and the two in combination for painful knee osteoarthritis. *N Engl J Med.* 2006;354(8):795–808.

158. Sawitzke AD, Shi H, Finco MF, et al. The effect of glucosamine and/or chondroitin sulfate on the progression of knee osteoarthritis: A report from the glucosamine/chondroitin arthritis intervention trial. *Arthritis Rheum.* 2008;58(10):3183–3191.

159. Bruyere O, Reginster JY. Glucosamine and chondroitin sulfate as therapeutic agents for knee and hip osteoarthritis. *Drugs Aging.* 2007;24(7):573–580.

160. Kahan A, Uebelhart D, De Vathaire F, Delmas PD, Reginster JY. Long-term effects of chondroitins 4 and 6 sulfate on knee osteoarthritis: The study on osteoarthritis progression prevention, a two-year, randomized, double-blind, placebo-controlled trial. *Arthritis Rheum.* 2009;60(2):524–533.

161. Messier SP, Mihalko S, Loeser RF, et al. Glucosamine/chondroitin combined with exercise for the treatment of knee osteoarthritis: A preliminary study. *Osteoarthr Cartil.* 2007;15(11):1256–1266.

162. Ross E. Update on the management of pain in arthritis and the use of cyclooxygenase-2 inhibitors. *Curr Pain Headache Rep.* 2009;13(6):455–459.

163. Efthimiou P, Kukar M. Complementary and alternative medicine use in rheumatoid arthritis: Proposed mechanism of action and efficacy of commonly used modalities. *Rheumatol Int.* 2009;30(5):571–586.

164. Chandrashekara S, Anilkumar T, Jamuna S. Complementary and alternative drug therapy in arthritis. *J Assoc Physicians India.* 2002;50:225–227.

165. Zaman T, Agarwal S, Handa R. Complementary and alternative medicine use in rheumatoid arthritis: An audit of patients visiting a tertiary care centre. *Natl Med J India.* 2007;20(5):236–239.

166. Willich SN, Rossnagel K, Roll S, et al. Rose hip herbal remedy in patients with rheumatoid arthritis—A randomized controlled trial. *Phytomedicine.* 2009;17(2):87–93.

167. Sener G, Eksioglu-Demiralp E, Cetiner M, et al. L-Carnitine ameliorates methotrexate-induced oxidative organ injury and inhibits leukocyte death. *Cell Biol Toxicol.* 2006;22(1):47–60.

168. Dadhania VP, Tripathi DN, Vikram A, Ramarao P, Jena GB. Intervention of alpha-lipoic acid ameliorates methotrexate-induced oxidative stress and genotoxicity: A study in rat intestine. *Chem Biol Interact.* 2009;183(1):85–97.

169. Rovensky J, Stančíková M, Uteseny J, Bauerova K, Jurcovicova J. Treatment of adjuvant-induced arthritis with the combination of methotrexate and probiotic bacteria Escherichia coli O83 (Colinfant). *Folia Microbiol.* 2009;54:359–363.

21 Misconceptions about the Functions and Value of Antioxidants in Health and Disease

INTRODUCTION

In recent years, many popular magazines, prestigious newspapers, internationally respected scientific journals, and books have described new advances in research into the function of antioxidants and their potential role in optimal health, disease prevention, and treatment of chronic diseases. Unfortunately, many of these scientific articles have produced contradictory results regarding the usefulness of antioxidants in human health, disease prevention, or treatment. As a result, a number of misconceptions, concerning the value of antioxidant exist among most physicians and other health professionals. This has created confusion in the minds of consumers, although most continue to take supplemental nutrition with or without the knowledge of their doctors. This chapter attempts to clarify some of the misconceptions regarding the value of antioxidants in health and disease that exist at this time.

MISCONCEPTION 1

Misconception: Antioxidants have only one function—reduce oxidative stress by neutralizing free radicals by donating an electron to the molecule with an unpaired electron.

Fact: This belief is only partly correct. Antioxidants have additional functions that do not involve neutralizing free radicals. Normally, under acute oxidative stress, ROS is needed to activate Nrf2 (nuclear factor erythroid-2-related factor-2), which migrates from the cytoplasm to the nucleus where it binds with ARE (antioxidant response element) that allows transcription cytoprotective enzymes including antioxidant enzymes. However, under chronic oxidative stress, activation of Nrf2 becomes resistant to ROS. Certain antioxidant activate ROS-resistant Nrf2. Antioxidants also alter expression of microRNAs, which are single stranded small of RNAs of 22–25 nucleotide transcribed from the non-coding region of DNA. These microRNAs allow translation of anti-apoptotic proteins or pro-apoptotic proteins depending upon whether they have received protective signals from antioxidants or damaging signals from ROS and pro-inflammatory cytokines.

MISCONCEPTION 2

Misconception: A single antioxidant is sufficient to simultaneously reduce oxidative stress and chronic inflammation that are found in human chronic diseases.

Fact: This idea is totally incorrect. The human body has an antioxidant defense system against oxidative damage represented by antioxidant enzymes, as well as antioxidants that we consume from diet and antioxidants that are made in the body. Therefore, it is essential to enhance the levels of antioxidant enzymes through the activation of Nrf2 pathway and antioxidants in order to simultaneously reduce oxidative stress and chronic inflammation. A single antioxidant commonly used in clinical study to evaluate its effectiveness in reducing the risk or progression of chronic diseases cannot achieve the above goal. Additionally, a single antioxidant in the high oxidative environment found in chronic diseases is oxidized and then acts as a prooxidant rather than as an antioxidant. For these reasons, continued use of a single antioxidant in the prevention of human diseases has no scientific merit.

MISCONCEPTION 3

Misconception: Beta-carotene has only one function. It acts as a precursor of vitamin A (retinol).

Fact: This belief is partly correct. Beta-carotene acts as a precursor of vitamin A, but it performs other biological function in the cells that cannot be produced by vitamin A. For example, beta-carotene enhances the transcription of connexin gene, but vitamin A cannot. Vitamin A induces cell differentiation in normal and cancer cells, but beta-carotene cannot.

MISCONCEPTION 4

Misconception: Activation of Nrf2 is sufficient to reduce oxidative stress.

Fact: This notion is not true. Activated Nrf2 must bind with ARE in the nucleus in order to increase the transcription genes coded for antioxidant enzymes. This binding of Nrf2 with ARE is impaired in older age. Supplementation with alpha-lipoic acid restores the ability of Nrf2 to bind with ARE.

MISCONCEPTION 5

Misconception: It is essential to add iron, copper, and manganese to a multivitamin preparation in order to enhance the health benefits.

Fact: This notion is dangerous. Although trace amounts of iron, copper, and manganese are essential for your health, slight excess of the free form of these trace minerals in the body can increase the risk of most chronic diseases. Additionally, these trace minerals are absorbed from the intestinal tract faster than in their absence that would saturate their respective binding proteins leading to increased levels of free form of iron, copper, and manganese.

MISCONCEPTION 6

Misconception: All forms of vitamin E have same function.

Fact: This belief is incorrect. D-alpha-tocopheryl succinate is the most effective form of vitamin E as anticancer agents, while *d*-alpha-tocopheryl acetate or *d*-alpha-tocopherol has no effect on cancer cells.

MISCONCEPTION 7

Misconception: Taking a multivitamin once a day is sufficient for your optimal health.

Fact: This may be incorrect. Biological half-lives of ingredients in a multivitamin preparation markedly vary depending upon their solubility. Variation in the levels of vitamin E succinate produces marked alterations in the expression of genes. Taking multivitamin once a day may create large fluctuations in the levels of antioxidants that could alter genetic activity. Prolonged hypergenetic activity can cause an error leading to mutations some of which could be harmful. Therefore, taking a multivitamin twice a day (half in the morning and half in the evening with meals) may reduce the levels of variations in the amounts of antioxidants in the plasma.

MISCONCEPTION 8

Misconception: Supplemented vitamins should be consumed for your optimal health only when you have a deficiency for that vitamin.

Fact: This belief in not valid. In order to defend increased levels of oxidative stress and chronic inflammation, which occur during aging, in individual with a family history of a disease, and in persons with an early or established phase of chronic diseases, it is essential to increase the levels of antioxidant enzymes and dietary and endogenous antioxidants. The correction of deficiency must be done. However, this approach may not provide optimal protection against oxidative damage.

MISCONCEPTION 9

Misconception: A balanced diet is sufficient for maintaining optimal health and disease prevention.

Fact: The concept of a balanced diet is very general. A balanced diet alone may not be adequate for optimal health and disease prevention. Trying to obtain the optimal levels of dietary and endogenous (made in the body) antioxidants at the appropriate times through a balanced diet only may not be possible or practical. In addition, all the food we consume on a daily basis contains both protective and toxic substances. In order to maximize the intake of protective substances, supplementary micronutrients, including antioxidants, are important.

MISCONCEPTION 10

Misconception: The more supplementary micronutrients, including antioxidants, you take, the better you will feel.

Fact: This belief can be dangerous. Consuming excessive quantities of certain micronutrients may cause severe damage. For instance, taking large amounts of vitamin A (10,000 IU or more per day over a long period of time) may lead to liver and skin toxicity and can increase the risk of birth defects in pregnant women. Excessive intakes of selenium at doses 500 mcg or more per day over a long period of time can cause cataracts, an eye disease in which the lens becomes opaque. Taking excessive quantities of vitamin B6—50 mg or more per day over an extended period of time—can induce peripheral neuropathy, or numbness in the extremities, a condition that is reversible upon discontinuation.

MISCONCEPTION 11

Misconception: Most supplementary micronutrients, including antioxidants, pass out of the body in the urine and feces, so why take them?

Fact: This misconception has no scientific justification. Approximately 10 percent of most orally ingested antioxidants are absorbed from the intestinal tract. Consuming higher doses of antioxidants, therefore, can lead to increased levels of these nutrients and their products in the urine and feces. The presence of excessive amounts of antioxidants in the intestinal tract may be beneficial, however, even if they are not totally absorbed into the blood stream. For example, increased amounts of vitamin C or vitamin E (alpha-tocopherol) are needed in the stomach to lower the levels of nitrosamine, a potent cancer-causing agent, which is formed from nitrite-containing foods such as bacon, sausage, hot dogs, or cured meats. Additionally, enhanced levels of toxic substances such as mutagens and carcinogens are formed during digestion of food, and absorption of these toxic chemicals from the intestinal tract could have adverse health effects over a long period of time. Supplementation with vitamin C and vitamin E reduced the levels of these toxic substances during digestion. The combination of two antioxidants was more effective than the individual agent. For these reasons, higher than normal amounts of antioxidants in the feces or urine should not be considered wasteful, since they have beneficial effects in the body even without being completely absorbed.

MISCONCEPTION 12

Misconception: Antioxidants affect both normal and cancer cells in the same manner.

Fact: Normal cells and cancer cells respond to antioxidants in a different manner. High doses of antioxidants kill the cancer cells and reduce their growth by bypassing Nrf2-induced resistant to apoptosis. Antioxidants have no significant effect on the growth of normal cells.

MISCONCEPTION 13

Misconception: All fat-soluble antioxidants are toxic to humans.

Fact: Only vitamin A when taken at high doses over a long period of time or during pregnancy can produce some toxic effects. It can produce bone fracture in older individuals. The safety window for vitamin A is very narrow.

MISCONCEPTION 14

Misconception: Natural and synthetic antioxidants have similar effects.

Fact: This belief is not true. Natural beta-carotene can reduce the formation of radiation-induced cancer, whereas synthetic beta-carotene cannot. Also, cells prefer to use natural vitamin E rather than the synthetic version.

MISCONCEPTION 15

Misconception: Supplementary vitamin C causes kidney stones.

Fact: This has not been observed in normal adults. If the urine becomes acidic, some of the waste products in the kidneys may solidify and form stones, but this biological phenomenon usually occurs if there is an imbalance in body chemistry, such as if acidic pH cannot be neutralized in the blood. The body normally neutralizes any acidic solution it takes in. In certain specific disease conditions in which one's body has lost this capacity, one should not take vitamin C in large amounts.

The link between vitamin C intake and kidney stones is derived from two observations: (1) a person taking vitamin C at high doses sometimes shows increased excretion of oxalic acid in the urine, and (2) many people who have kidney stones also have higher than normal levels of oxalic acid in the urine. These two separate observations have been interpreted to mean that high doses of vitamin C can heighten the risk of kidney stones. These observations may be unrelated. There are no published data to support the conclusion that high doses of vitamin C produce kidney stones in healthy people. Millions of people around the world consume high doses of vitamin C, but no increase in the risk of kidney stones has been reported in any region of the world.

MISCONCEPTION 16

Misconception: Frozen fruit and vegetable juices or antioxidant-supplemented water or fruit and vegetable juices maintain when stored in the refrigerator.

Fact: Frozen fruit or vegetable juices may provide some antioxidants to your body, provided you drink them within a few hours of preparation. When they are stored in a cold place and exposed to light and/or air, however, antioxidants—particularly vitamin C—in solution rapidly deteriorate. After about 24 hours, more than 50% of vitamin C is lost. Antioxidant-rich fruit or vegetable juices in cartons or opaque glass may have more antioxidants than those in clear plastic or glass containers. Repeated opening and closing of the bottles diminishes antioxidant levels as well.

MISCONCEPTION 17

Misconception: If you take supplementary micronutrients that include antioxidants, you do not have to worry about a balanced diet or a modification in lifestyle.

Fact: Supplementary micronutrients, a healthy diet (one that is low fat and high fiber), and lifestyle modification (meaning no tobacco smoking or consumption, regular exercise, increased consumption of fruits and vegetables, meditation, and so on) are equally important for optimal health and disease prevention.

At this time, many misconceptions exist regarding the value of antioxidant micronutrients in health and in disease prevention and treatment. A few have been discussed in this chapter. Putting these misconceptions to rest is a challenge for researchers, physicians, other health professionals, and educators. Improving the health of the general population depends upon the success of educating health professionals and others about these misconceptions. Removing these misconceptions is equally important in order to promote the correct utilization of antioxidant micronutrient supplements for an optimal health and disease prevention.

CONCLUSIONS

I hope the misconceptions discussed in this chapter may further clarify the potential useful role of micronutrients, especially antioxidants in optimal health and prevention and improved management of chronic diseases. The recommendations of micronutrients for achieving the above goal are described in previous chapters that may provide valuable guidelines as to why, when, and how to use micronutrients for optimal health.

22 Dietary Reference Intakes of Selected Micronutrients

INTRODUCTION

The changes in the nutritional guidelines have evolved significantly since World War II due to a rapid expansion of knowledge in nutrition and health. The nutritional guidelines referred to as Recommended Dietary Allowances (RDAs) were first established in 1941. The Food and Nutrition Board of the USA subsequently revised them every 5–10 years.

RDA (DRI)

RDA refers to the value of the daily dietary intake level of a nutrient considered sufficient to meet the requirements of 97%–98% of healthy individuals of different ages and gender. Because of rapid growth of research on the role of nutrients in human health, the Food and Nutrition Board of the Institute of Medicine (IOM) of the USA in collaboration with Health Canada, updated the values of RDAs and renamed them as Dietary Reference Intakes (DRIs) in 1998. Since then, the DRIs values are used by both the USA and Canada. The DRA values of selected nutrients are listed in Tables 22.1 through 22.21. The DRI values are not currently used in nutrition labeling, but the RDA values of nutrients continue to be used for this purpose. The DRI values for carotenoids, alpha-lipoic acid, N-acetylcysteine, coenzyme Q10, and L-carnitine have not been determined.

TABLE 22.1
Dietary Reference Intakes (DRIs) of Antioxidants

Antioxidant Type	Age	RDA/AI* (µg/d)	UL (µg/d)
Vitamin A	Infants		
	0–6 mo	400*	600
	7–12 mo	500*	600
	Children		
	1–3 y	300	600
	4–8 y	400	900
	Males		
	9–13 y	600	1,700
	14–18 y	900	2,800
	19 y and over	900	3,000
	Females		
	9–13 y	600	1,700
	14–18 y	700	2,800
	19 y and over	700	3,000
	Pregnancy		
	≤18 y	750	2,800
	19–50 y	770	3,000
	Lactation		
	≤18 y	1,200	2,800
	19–50 y	1,300	3,000

Note: The values are adapted and summarized from the table of the Dietary Reference Intakes (DRI) published by www.nap.edu. RDA refers to Recommended Dietary Allowance; AI* to Adequate Intakes, and UL to Tolerable Upper Intake Value. 1 µg of retinol equals 1 µg of RAE (retinol activity equivalent); 1 IU (international unit) of retinol equals 0.3 µg of retinol; and 2 µg of beta-carotene equals 1 µg of retinol.

TABLE 22.2
Dietary Reference Intakes (DRIs) of Antioxidants

Antioxidant Type	Age	RDA/AI* (mg/d)	UL (mg/d)
Vitamin C	Infants		
	0–6 mo	40*	ND
	7–12 mo	50*	ND
	Children		
	1–3 y	15	400
	4–8 y	25	650
	Males		
	9–13 y	45	1,200
	14–18 y	75	1,800
	19 y and over	90	2,000
	Females		
	9–13 y	45	1,200
	14–18 y	65	1,800
	19 y and over	75	2,000

Note: The values are adapted and summarized from the table of the Dietary Reference Intakes (DRI) published by www.nap.edu. RDA refers to Recommended Dietary Allowance; AI* to Adequate Intakes, and UL to Tolerable Upper Intake Value. ND (not determined).

TABLE 22.3
Dietary Reference Intakes (DRIs) of Antioxidants

Antioxidant Type	Age	RDA/AI* (mg/d)	UL (mg/d)
Vitamin E	Infants		
	0–6 mo	4*	ND
	7–12 mo	5*	ND
	Children		
	1–3 y	6	200
	4–8 y	7	300
	Males		
	9–13 y	11	600
	14–18 y	15	800
	19 y and over	15	1,000
	Females		
	9–13 y	11	600
	14–18 y	15	800
	19 y and over	15	1,000
	Pregnancy		
	≤18 y	15	800
	19–50 y	15	1,000
	Lactation		
	≤18 y	19	800
	19–50 y	19	1,000

Note: The values are adapted and summarized from the table of the Dietary Reference Intakes (DRI) published by www.nap.edu. RDA refers to Recommended Dietary Allowance; AI* to Adequate Intakes, and UL to Tolerable Upper Intake Value. ND (not determined). 1 IU of vitamin E equals 0.66 mg of d- and 0.45 mg of *dl*-alpha-tocopherol.

TABLE 22.4
Dietary Reference Intakes (DRIs) of Vitamins

Vitamin Type	Age	RDA/AI* (µg/d)	UL (µg/d)
Vitamin D	Infants		
	0–12 mo	5*	25
	Children		
	1–8 y	5*	50
	Males		
	9–50 y	5*	50
	50–70 y	10*	50
	>70 y	15*	50
	Females		
	9–50 y	5*	50
	50–70 y	10*	50
	>70 y	15*	50
	Pregnancy		
	≤18–50 y	5*	50
	Lactation		
	≤18–50 y	5*	50

Note: The values are adapted and summarized from the tables of the Dietary Reference Intakes (DRI) published by www.nap.edu. RDA refers to Recommended Dietary Allowance; AI* to Adequate Intakes, and UL to Tolerable Upper Intake Value. 1 µg of cholecalciferol equals 40 IU (international unit) of Vitamin D.

TABLE 22.5
Dietary Reference Intakes (DRIs) of Vitamins

Vitamin Type	Age	RDA/AI* (mg/d)	UL (mg/d)
Vitamin B1 (Thiamin)	Infants		
	0–6 mo	0.2*	ND
	7–12 mo	0.3*	ND
	Children		
	1–3 y	0.5	ND
	4–8 y	0.6	ND
	Males		
	9–13 y	0.9	ND
	14 y and over	1.2	ND
	Females		
	9–13 y	0.9	ND
	14–18 y	1.0	ND
	19 y and over	1.1	ND
	Pregnancy		
	≤18–50 y	1.4	ND
	Lactation		
	≤18–50 y	1.4	ND

Note: The values are adapted and summarized from the tables of the Dietary Reference Intakes (DRI) published by www.nap.edu. RDA refers to Recommended Dietary Allowance; AI* to Adequate Intakes, and UL to Tolerable Upper Intake Value... ND (not determined).

TABLE 22.6
Dietary Reference Intakes (DRIs) of Vitamins

Vitamin Type	Age	RDA/AI* (mg/d)	UL (mg/d)
Vitamin B2 (Riboflavin)	Infants		
	0–6 mo	0.3*	ND
	7–12 mo	0.4*	ND
	Children		
	1–3 y	0.5	ND
	4–8 y	0.6	ND
	Males		
	9–13 y	0.9	ND
	14 y and over	1.3	ND
	Females		
	9–13 y	0.9	ND
	14–18 y	1.0	ND
	19 y and over	1.1	ND
	Pregnancy		
	≤18–50 y	1.4	ND
	Lactation		
	≤18–50 y	1.6	ND

Note: The values are adapted and summarized from the table of the Dietary Reference Intakes (DRI) published by www.nap.edu. RDA refers to Recommended Dietary Allowance; AI* to Adequate Intakes, and UL to Tolerable Upper Intake Value. ND (not determined).

TABLE 22.7
Dietary Reference Intakes (DRIs) of Vitamins

Vitamin Type	Age	RDA/AI* (mg/d)	UL (mg/d)
Vitamin B6	Infants		
	0–6 mo	0.1*	ND
	7–12 mo	0.3*	ND
	Children		
	1–3 y	0.5	30
	4–8 y	0.6	40
	Males		
	9–13 y	1.0	60
	14–50 y	1.3	80
	50–70 y and over	1.7	100
	Females		
	9–13 y	1.0	60
	14–18 y	1.2	80
	19–30 y	1.3	100
	50 y and over	1.5	100
	Pregnancy		
	≤18 y	1.9	80
	19–50 y	1.9	100
	Lactation		
	≤18 y	2.0	80
	19–50 y	2.0	100

Note: The values are adapted and summarized from the table of the Dietary Reference Intakes (DRI) published by www.nap.edu. RDA refers to Recommended Dietary Allowance; AI* to Adequate Intakes, and UL to Tolerable Upper Intake Value. ND (not determined).

TABLE 22.8

Dietary Reference Intakes (DRIs) of Vitamins

Vitamin Type	Age	DA/AI* (µg/d)	UL (µg/d)
Vitamin B12 (Cobalamin)	Infants		
	0–6 mo	0.4*	ND
	7–12 mo	0.5*	ND
	Children		
	1–3 y	0.9	ND
	4–8 y	1.2	ND
	Males		
	9–13 y	1.08	ND
	14 y and over	2.4	ND
	Females		
	9–13 y	1.8	ND
	14 y and over	2.4	ND
	Pregnancy		
	≤18–50 y	2.6	ND
	Lactation		
	≤18–50 y	2.8	ND

Note: The values are adapted and summarized from the table of the Dietary Reference Intakes (DRI) published by www.nap.edu. RDA refers to Recommended Dietary Allowance; AI* to Adequate Intakes, and UL to Tolerable Upper Intake Value. ND (not determined).

TABLE 22.9

Dietary Reference Intakes (DRIs) of Vitamins

Vitamin Type	Age	RDA/AI* (mg/d)	UL (mg/d)
Pantothenic acid	Infants		
	0–6 mo	1.7*	ND
	7–12 mo	1.8*	ND
	Children		
	1–3 y	2*	ND
	4–8 y	2*	ND
	Males		
	9–13 y	4*	ND
	14 y and over	5*	ND
	Females		
	9–13 y	4*	ND
	14 y and over	5*	ND
	Pregnancy		
	≤18–50 y	6*	ND
	Lactation		
	≤18–50 y	7*	ND

Note: The values are adapted and summarized from the table of the Dietary Reference Intakes (DRI) published by www.nap.edu. RDA refers to Recommended Dietary Allowance; AI* to Adequate Intakes, and UL to Tolerable Upper Intake Value. ND (not determined).

TABLE 22.10

Dietary Reference Intakes (DRIs) of Vitamins

Vitamin Type	Age	RDA/AI* (mg/d)	UL (mg/d)
Niacin	Infants		
	0–6 mo	2*	ND
	7–12 mo	0.4*	ND
	Children		
	1–3 y	6.0	10
	4–8 y	8.0	15
	Males		
	9–13 y	12	20
	14–50 y	16	30
	50–70 y and over	16	35
	Females		
	9–13 y	12	20
	14–18 y	14	30
	19 y and over	14	35
	Pregnancy		
	≤18 y	18	30
	19–50 y	18	35
	Lactation		
	≤18 y	17	30
	19–50 y	17	35

Note: The values are adapted and summarized from the table of the Dietary Reference Intakes (DRI) published by www.nap.edu. RDA refers to Recommended Dietary Allowance; AI* to Adequate Intakes, and UL to Tolerable Upper Intake Value. ND (not determined).

TABLE 22.11
Dietary Reference Intakes (DRIs) of Vitamins

Vitamin Type	Age	RDA/AI* (µg/d)	UL (µg/d)
Folate	Infants		
	0–6 mo	65*	ND
	7–12 mo	80*	ND
	Children		
	1–3 y	150	300
	4–8 y	200	400
	Males		
	9–13 y	300	600
	14–18 y	400	800
	19 y and over	400	1,000
	Females		
	9–13 y	300	600
	14–18 y	400	800
	19 y and over	400	1,000
	Pregnancy		
	≤18 y	600	800
	19–50 y	600	1,000
	Lactation		
	≤18 y	500	800
	19–50 y	500	1,000

Note: The values are adapted and summarized from the table of the Dietary Reference Intakes (DRI) published by www.nap.edu. RDA refers to Recommended Dietary Allowance; AI* to Adequate Intakes, and UL to Tolerable Upper Intake Value. ND (not determined).

TABLE 22.12
Dietary Reference Intakes (DRIs) of Micronutrients

Micronutrient Type	Age	RDA/AI* (μg/d)	UL (μg/d)
Biotin	Infants		
	0–6 mo	0.5*	ND
	7–12 mo	0.6*	ND
	Children		
	1–3 y	8*	ND
	4–8 y	12*	ND
	Males		
	9–13 y	20	ND
	14–18 y	25	ND
	19 y and over	30	ND
	Females		
	9–13 y	20	ND
	14–18 y	25	ND
	19 y and over	30	ND
	Pregnancy		
	≤18 y	30*	ND
	19–50 y	30*	ND
	Lactation		
	≤18 y	35*	ND
	19–50 y	35*	ND

Note: The values are adapted and summarized from the table of the Dietary Reference Intakes (DRI) published by www.nap.edu. RDA refers to Recommended Dietary Allowance; AI* to Adequate Intakes, and UL to Tolerable Upper Intake Value. ND (not determined).

TABLE 22.13
Dietary Reference Intakes (DRIs) of Minerals

Mineral Type	Age	RDA/AI* (mg/d)	UL (mg/d)
Calcium	Infants		
	0–6 mo	210*	ND
	7–12 mo	270*	ND
	Children		
	1–3 y	500*	2,500
	4–8 y	800*	2,500
	Males		
	9–18 y	1,300*	2,500
	19–50 y	1,000*	2,500
	51 y and over	1,200*	2,500
	Females		
	9–18 y	1,300*	2,500
	19–50 y	1,000*	2,500
	51 y and over	1,200*	2,500
	Pregnancy		
	≤18 y	1,300*	2,500
	19–50 y	1,000*	2,500
	Lactation		
	≤18 y	1,300*	2,500
	19–50 y	1,000*	2,500

Note: The values are adapted and summarized from the table of the Dietary Reference Intakes (DRI) published by www.nap.edu. RDA refers to Recommended Dietary Allowance; AI* to Adequate Intakes, and UL to Tolerable Upper Intake Value. ND (not determined).

TABLE 22.14
Dietary Reference Intakes (DRIs) of Minerals

Mineral Type	Age	RDA/AI* (mg/d)	UL (mg/d)
Magnesium	Infants		
	0–6 mo	30*	ND
	7–12 mo	75*	ND
	Children		
	1–3 y	80	65
	4–8 y	130	110
	Males		
	9–13 y	240	350
	14–18 y	410	350
	19–30 y	400	350
	31 y and over	420	350
	Females		
	9–13 y	240	350
	14–18 y	360	350
	31 y and over	320	350
	Pregnancy		
	≤18 y	400	350
	19–30 y	350	350
	31–50 y	360	350
	Lactation		
	≤18 y	360	350
	31–50 y	320	350

Note: The values are adapted and summarized from the table of the Dietary Reference Intakes (DRI) published by www.nap.edu. RDA refers to Recommended Dietary Allowance; AI* to Adequate Intakes, and UL to Tolerable Upper Intake Value. ND (not determined).

TABLE 22.15
Dietary Reference Intakes (DRIs) of Minerals

Mineral Type	Age	RDA/AI* (mg/d)	UL (mg/d)
Manganese	Infants		
	0–6 mo	0.003*	ND
	7–12 mo	0.6*	ND
	Children		
	1–3 y	1.2*	2
	4–8 y	1.5*	3
	Males		
	9–13 y	1.9*	6
	14–18 y	2.2*	9
	19 y and over	2.3*	11
	Females		
	9–13 y	1.6*	6
	14–18 y	1.6*	9
	19 y and over	1.8*	11
	Pregnancy		
	≤18 y	2.0*	9
	19–50 y	2.0*	11
	Lactation		
	≤18 y	2.6*	9
	19–50 y	2.6*	11

Note: The values are adapted and summarized from the table of the Dietary Reference Intakes (DRI) published by www.nap. edu. RDA refers to Recommended Dietary Allowance; AI* to Adequate Intakes, and UL to Tolerable Upper Intake Value. ND (not determined).

TABLE 22.16
Dietary Reference Intakes (DRIs) of Minerals

Mineral Type	Age	RDA/AI* (µg/d)	UL (µg/d)
Chromium	Infants		
	0–6 mo	0.2*	ND
	7–12 mo	5.5*	ND
	Children		
	1–3 y	11*	ND
	4–8 y	15*	ND
	Males		
	9–13 y	25*	ND
	14–50 y	35*	ND
	51 y and over	30*	ND
	Females		
	9–13 y	21*	ND
	14–18 y	24*	ND
	19–50 y	25*	ND
	Pregnancy		
	≤18 y	29*	ND
	19–50 y	30*	ND
	Lactation		
	≤18 y	44*	ND
	19–50 y	45*	ND

Note: The values are adapted and summarized from the table of the Dietary Reference Intakes (DRI) published by www.nap.edu. RDA refers to Recommended Dietary Allowance; AI* to Adequate Intakes, and UL to Tolerable Upper Intake Value. ND (not determined).

TABLE 22.17
Dietary Reference Intakes (DRIs) of Minerals

Mineral Type	Age	RDA/AI* (μg/d)	UL (μg/d)
Copper	Infants		
	0–6 mo	200*	ND
	7–12 mo	220*	ND
	Children		
	1–3 y	340	1,000
	4–8 y	440	3,000
	Males		
	9–13 y	700	5,000
	14–18 y	890	8,000
	19 y and over	900	10,000
	Females		
	9–13 y	700	5,000
	14–18 y	890	8,000
	19 y and over	900	10,000
	Pregnancy		
	≤18 y	1,000	8,000
	19–50 y	1,000	10,000
	Lactation		
	≤18 y	1,300	8,000
	19–50 y	1,300	10,000

Note: The values are adapted and summarized from the table of the Dietary Reference Intakes (DRI) published by www.nap.edu. RDA refers to Recommended Dietary Allowance; AI* to Adequate Intakes, and UL to Tolerable Upper Intake Value. ND (not determined).

TABLE 22.18
Dietary Reference Intakes (DRIs) of Minerals

Mineral Type	Age	RDA/AI* (mg/d)	UL (mg/d)
Iron	Infants		
	0–6 mo	0.27*	40
	7–12 mo	11	40
	Children		
	1–3 y	7	40
	4–8 y	10	40
	Males		
	9–13 y	8	40
	14–18 y	11	45
	19 y and over	8	45
	Females		
	9–13 y	8	40
	14–18 y	15	45
	19–50 y	18	45
	50 y and over	8	45
	Pregnancy		
	≤18–50 y	27	45
	Lactation		
	≤18 y	10	45
	19–50 y	9	45

Note: The values are adapted and summarized from the table of the Dietary Reference Intakes (DRI) published by www.nap.edu. RDA refers to Recommended Dietary Allowance; AI* to Adequate Intakes, and UL to Tolerable Upper Intake Value. ND (not determined).

TABLE 22.19
Dietary Reference Intakes (DRIs) of Minerals

Mineral Type	Age	RDA/AI* (µg/d)	UL (µg/d)
Selenium	Infants		
	0–6 mo	15*	45
	7–12 mo	20*	60
	Children		
	1–3 y	20	90
	4–8 y	30	150
	Males		
	9–13 y	40	280
	14 y and over	55	400
	Females		
	9–13 y	40	280
	14 y and over	55	400
	Pregnancy		
	≤18–50 y	60	400
	Lactation		
	≤18–50 y	70	400

Note: The values are adapted and summarized from the table of the Dietary Reference Intakes (DRI) published by www.nap.edu. RDA refers to Recommended Dietary Allowance; AI* to Adequate Intakes, and UL to Tolerable Upper Intake Value. ND (not determined).

TABLE 22.20
Dietary Reference Intakes (DRIs) of Minerals

Mineral Type	Age	RDA/AI* (mg/d)	UL (mg/d)
Phosphorus	Infants		
	0–6 mo	100*	ND
	7–12 mo	275*	ND
	Children		
	1–3 y	460	3,000
	4–8 y	500	3,000
	Males		
	9–18 y	1,250	4,000
	19–70 y	700	4,000
	>70 y	700	3,000
	Females		
	9–18 y	1,250	4,000
	19–70 y	700	4,000
	>70 y	700	3,000
	Pregnancy		
	≤18 y	1,250	3,500
	19–50 y	700	3,500
	Lactation		
	≤18 y	1,250	4,000
	19–50 y	700	4,000

Note: The values are adapted and summarized from the table of the Dietary Reference Intakes (DRI) published by www. nap.edu. RDA refers to Recommended Dietary Allowance; AI* to Adequate Intakes, and UL to Tolerable Upper Intake Value. ND (not determined).

TABLE 22.21
Dietary Reference Intakes (DRIs) of Minerals

Mineral Type	Age	RDA/AI* (mg/d)	UL (mg/d)
Zinc	Infants		
	0–6 mo	2*	4
	7–12 mo	3	5
	Children		
	1–3 y	3	7
	4–8 y	5	12
	Males		
	9–13 y	8	23
	14–18 y	11	34
	19 y and over	11	40
	Females		
	9–13 y	8	23
	14–18 y	9	34
	19 y and over	8	40
	Pregnancy		
	≤18 y	12	34
	19–50 y	11	40
	Lactation		
	≤18 y	13	34
	19–50 y	12	40

Note: The values are adapted and summarized from the table of the Dietary Reference Intakes (DRI) published by www.nap.edu. RDA refers to Recommended Dietary Allowance; AI* to Adequate Intakes, and UL to Tolerable Upper Intake Value. ND (not determined).

ADEQUATE INTAKE (AI)

AI refers to the value of a nutrient for which no RDA has been established, but the value established may be sufficient for everyone in the demographic group.

TOLERABLE UPPER INTAKE LEVEL (UL)

This is the maximum level of daily nutrient intake that is likely to pose no risk of adverse health effects. The UL value represents total intake of a nutrient from food, water, and supplements.

RDA, AI, or UL values of nutrients are expected to be adequate for individuals for normal growth and survival; however, the values of micronutrients needed for prevention or improved management of human diseases are not known at this time. The data on doses obtained from the use of a single micronutrient in prevention or treatment of human diseases should not be extrapolated to the doses of the same micronutrient present in a multiple micronutrient preparation. Generally, whenever a single micronutrient is used in the laboratory or clinical studies, high doses of a micronutrient are needed to observe any biological effects. Low doses of the same micronutrient may be needed when used in combination with multiple micronutrients for the same effects.

CONCLUSIONS

The initial nutritional guidelines, Recommended Dietary Allowances (RDAs), have been replaced by Dietary Reference Intakes (DRIs), and are currently used by the USA and Canada. The DRI values of nutrients are sufficient for the growth and development of the 97%–98% of the healthy individuals. The DRI values for carotenoids, alpha-lipoic acid, N-acetylcysteine, coenzyme Q10, and L-carnitine have not been determined. The optimal value needed for prevention or improved management of human diseases is not known. Studies are in progress to establish these values.

Index

Note: Page numbers in italic and bold refer to figures and tables, respectively.